Practical Avian Medicine

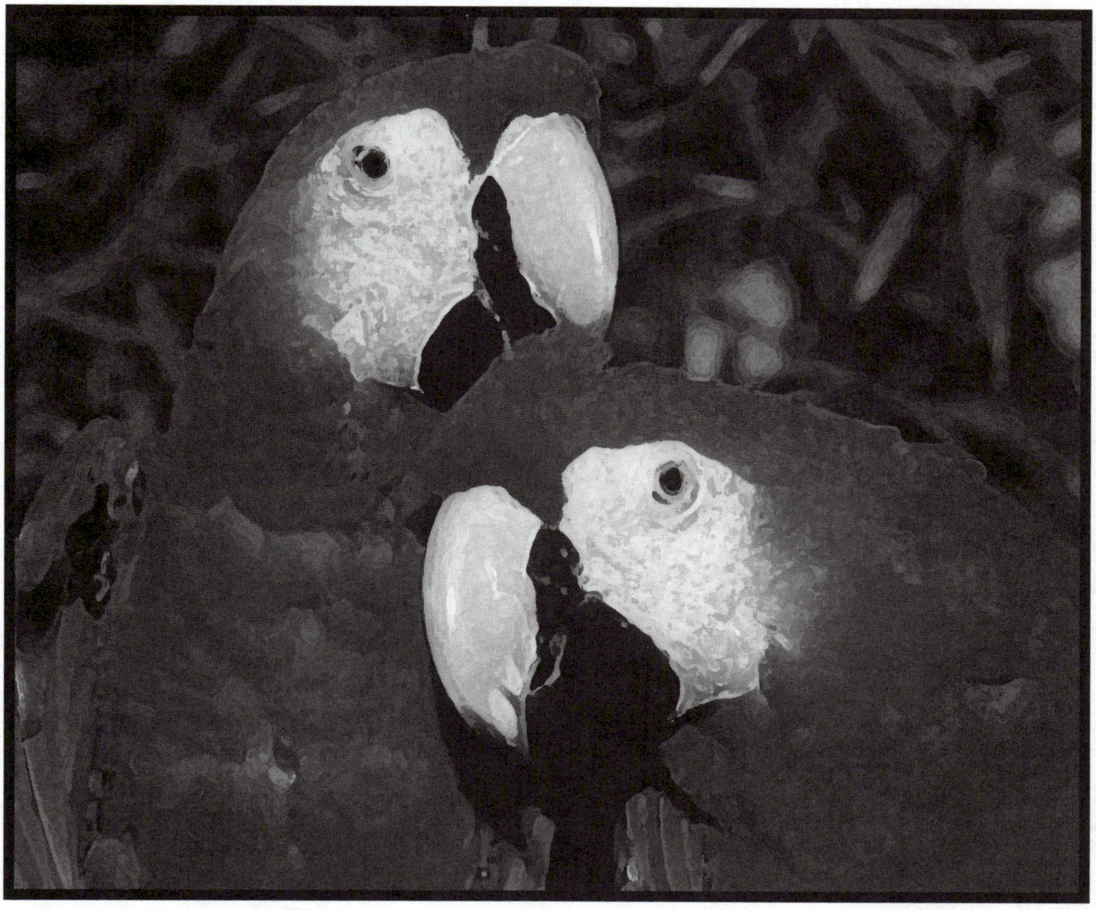

Heidi L. Hoefer, DVM, Editor and Reviewer

The
COMPENDIUM
COLLECTION

FOREWORD

The Compendium Collections gather together the best, most practical information from the pages of the *Compendium on Continuing Education for the Practicing Veterinarian.* As the knowledge base within veterinary medicine has expanded, so too have the sources from which to cull information. In order to provide our readers with the latest, most applicable answers, we have drawn from other pertinent veterinary material for this collection. Included are four articles from *Perspectives—A Resource for Women in Veterinary Medicine* and one article from the out-of-print VLS book, *Dermatology for the Small Animal Practitioner* (Nesbitt GH, Ackerman LJ (eds), 1991). In addition, several articles were written specifically for this publication.

Although not from the pages of *Compendium*, these additional articles were found by our editors to be in keeping with the editorial and educational standards that have been established by previous Collections. The information provided herein, therefore, provides a well-rounded reference for the practitioner involved with or interested in practical avian medicine.

Published by Veterinary Learning Systems
Trenton, New Jersey

Printed in U.S.A.

ISBN 1-884254-34-9

PREFACE

The pet bird industry has grown exponentially during the past decade and may represent the fastest growing field in veterinary medicine today. In 1994, the Pet Industry Joint Advisory Council estimated that there are 31 million pet birds (not including breeding stock). The 17.7% of U.S. households that own birds has an average of 4.2 birds each, a statistic that provides further testament that birds have a well-established place as household pets. The veterinary industry also reflects this growth. Since its inception in 1980, the Association of Avian Veterinarians has grown to more than 3,300 members worldwide. In 1993, the American Board of Veterinary Practitioners (ABVP) began certifying veterinarians in the avian practice specialty. The rapidly changing and advancing field of avian medicine brings with it the need for up-to-date, easily accessible information. This Compendium Collection was assembled in response to that need.

The collection covers a variety of clinical issues and has been organized into convenient sections that expedite retrieval of information. Within the broad areas of anatomy, cytology, dermatology, diseases, emergency care, radiography, surgery, and orthopedics are several articles that address specific topics of practical interest to clinicians. While most of the articles come from previous *Compendium* issues, three new papers have been written specifically for this collection. In addition, many of the previously published articles have been updated to reflect new information. The articles cover issues as they relate to pet or caged birds, although two articles feature raptors and one concerns the ostrich. Overall, the collection is designed to offer readers a succinct approach to pertinent issues in avian medicine and surgery.

With the recognition of birds as beloved companions and pets comes a higher expectation for appropriate and sophisticated veterinary care. As the body of veterinary knowledge increases, we are compelled to learn all that we can about the various species that we treat. I hope this collection provides a framework on which to build a higher standard of avian care. We owe it to our clients, to ourselves as health care professionals, and to those delightful little creatures that enchant and enrich our lives.

I want to thank all the authors for their time, effort, and knowledge. Collectively, their contributions reflect many years of experience in avian practice. I hope you enjoy reading this collection as much as I have.

Heidi L. Hoefer, DVM
Diplomate, ABVP–Avian Practice
Staff Veterinarian
Avian and Exotic Animal Service
The Animal Medical Center
New York, New York

CONTENTS

AVIAN SURGERY AND ORTHOPEDICS

AVIAN DERMATOLOGY

MISCELLANEOUS

The Avian Cardiovascular System

Karen Rosenthal, DVM, MS, ABVP

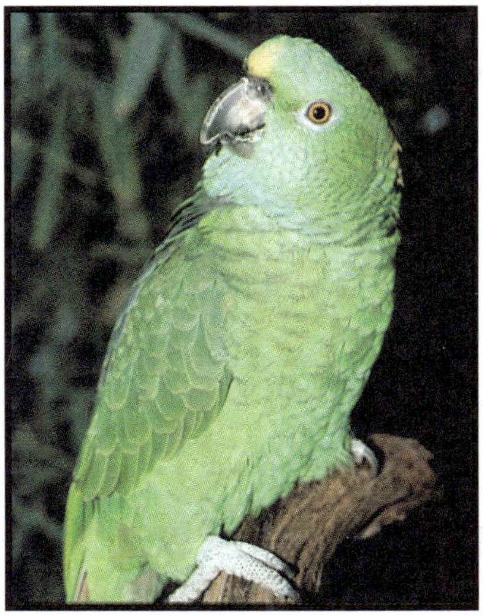

Photography by Joan Balzarini

The avian circulatory system is quite similar to that of mammals. A major difference in anatomy and function of the avian circulatory system is apparent in the renal blood supply where two afferent pathways are present. Other differences include the relatively large-sized avian heart and its fast rate of beating, which leads to a greater cardiac output than is found in mammals.

Anatomically, the avian and mammalian hearts are quite similar. The avian heart also has four chambers, two atria and two ventricles, but the tricuspid valve found in the mammalian heart is just a muscular flap in birds. A major difference noted in the structure of the avian circulatory system is the ascending aorta which curves to the right in birds. That is because the avian aorta, in contrast to mammals, is derived from the right fourth arterial arch and the right dorsal aorta.

Originally published in January/February 1995 *Perspectives*

Avian Cardiovascular System

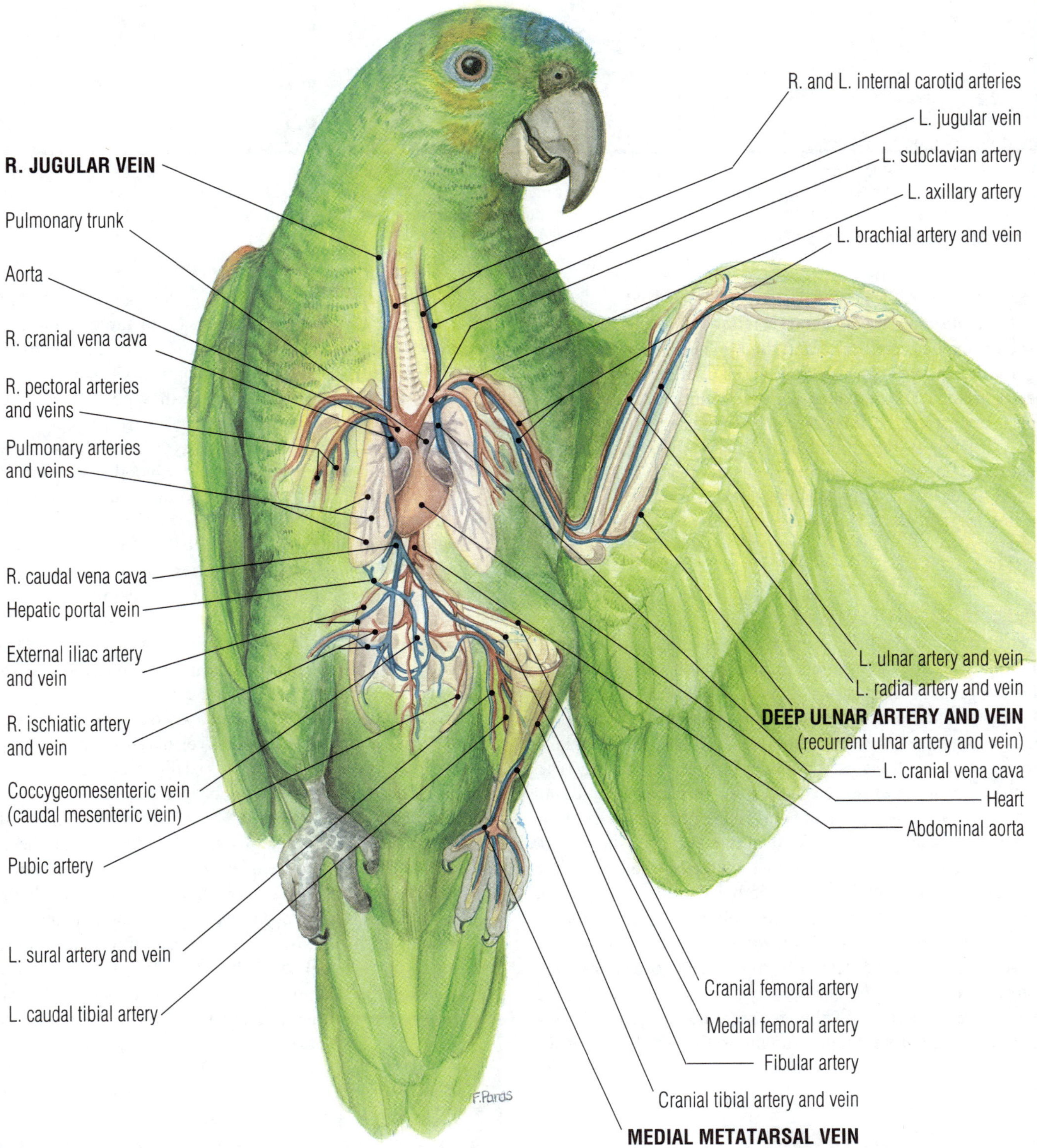

Cardiovascular system of the Amazon parrot. *Turn to page 9 for a schematic of the avian renal portal system.*

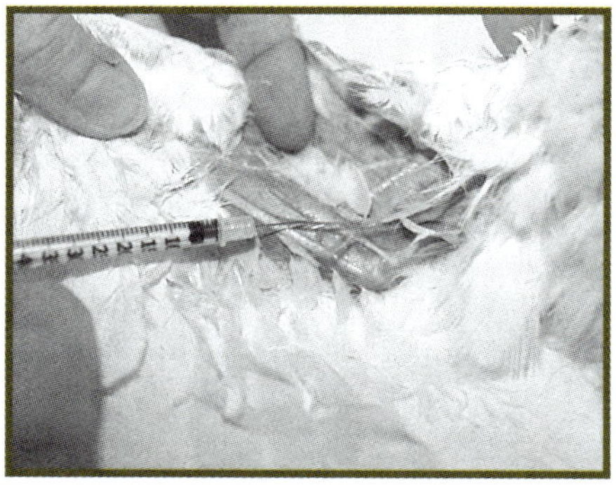

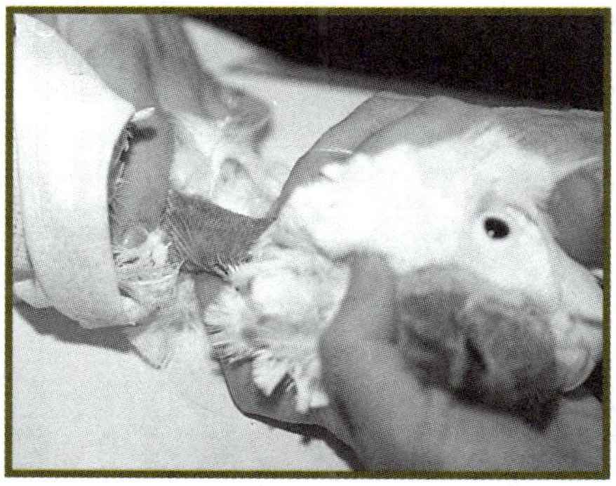

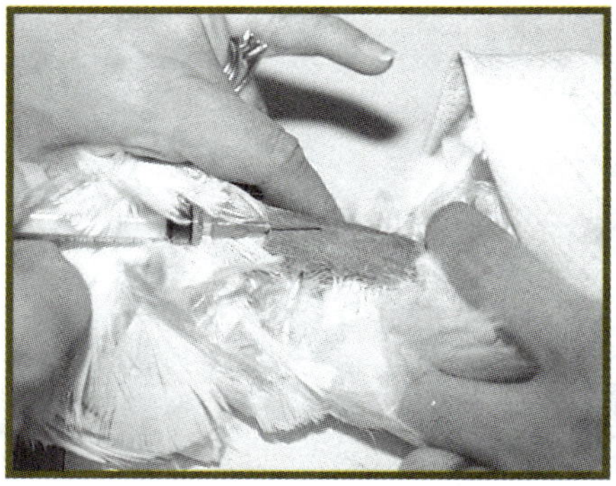

From Left: 1) Site for venipuncture of the avian ulnar vein in a cockatoo; 2) Proper holding technique for venipuncture of the right jugular vein in a cockatoo. The body is wrapped in a towel and the holder places a finger in the thoracic inlet. The venipuncturist holds the head with one hand and uses the other hand to draw blood. The jugular vein is apparent in the center of the neck; 3) Site for venipuncture of the avian right jugular vein in a cockatoo. Photographs courtesy of Dr. Karen Rosenthal.

CROSSCURRENT EXCHANGE SYSTEM

The avian lung has a unique anatomical arrangement between the blood capillaries and the air capillaries. The blood capillaries intersect the air capillaries at right angles in the parabronchus. This is called a crosscurrent exchange system and it appears to be inherently more efficient than the uniform pooling system found in the mammalian lung. In the avian system, more oxygen rich air can reach oxygen poor blood. Therefore, this arrangement is more efficient in pulling oxygen from the respired air than is the mammalian system.

THERMOREGULATION

The avian circulatory system is used as a means of heat regulation. It is not uncommon to have owners describe their bird's legs and feet as "hot." This is an accurate observation. During heat stress, blood flow to the legs is greatly increased and the unfeathered areas of the legs are used as heat radiators. Conversely, the avian circulatory system is also used as a means to prevent excessive heat loss. In some aquatic and wading birds, the arteries and veins in the proximal part of the leg form a countercurrent tibiotarsal rete system. This rete, or network of vessels, functions by transferring heat from the warmer arteries emanating from the body's core to the colder veins bringing blood from the extremities. This prevents excessive heat loss at the extremities and heat is conserved by returning it to the core. The veins must be in close approximation with the arteries for this to occur and this is why the rete exists. The advantage of this countercurrent system is that blood flow, therefore oxygen supply, to the distal parts of the extremities is maintained without incurring a high level of heat loss.

RENAL PORTAL SYSTEM

One of the most important differences between mammals and birds is the existence in birds of the renal portal system (see Schematic on facing page). Clinicians who treat birds should be aware of this anatomical difference as it has great practical implications. Basically, any substance injected into the lower half of the bird's body may go through the renal system before it is routed throughout the rest of the body, including the liver. Drugs that are nephrotoxic pose an even greater risk in this type of system as they go directly to the kidneys before they can be metabolized by other organs. The avian kidney is supplied with two types of afferent blood pathways—the normal arteriole afferent blood system and the afferent venous blood via the renal portal system. A common efferent venous system drains both the renal portal system and the arterial blood supply. The renal portal veins carry blood to the kidney tubules and act like arteries rather than like veins. The renal portal veins do not go to the glomerulus but rather bathe the tubules. This means that substances injected into the legs, agents absorbed by the intestines, or metabolic wastes from the lower part of the body will be excreted first by the tubules before they enter the general circulation.

Blood from the lower half of the body does not always flow into the renal portal system. The liver may receive the blood directly as it bypasses the kidneys. This is accomplished by venous valves and also by the coccygeomesenteric vein. The valves are located at the juncture of the renal vein and the iliac vein. Under the influence of substances such as cholinergic and adrenergic agents, the valves are either opened or closed. If the valve is closed, blood flows into the kidney and bathes the renal tubules. If it is open, it flows into the hepatic portal system and the liver. There is conflicting information available regarding whether the valves are always opened or always closed; it is still not clear which agents open and which

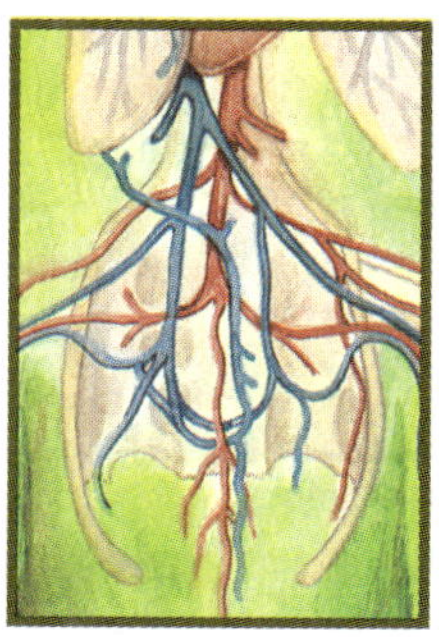

agents close the valves. For the practitioner's purposes, it is probably safest to assume that the valves are always closed. From a physiological standpoint, this scenario would appear to be the most logical, because otherwise wastes would not be removed from the kidneys. On the other hand, there are many factors yet to be studied in connection with this characteristic that is so unique to birds.

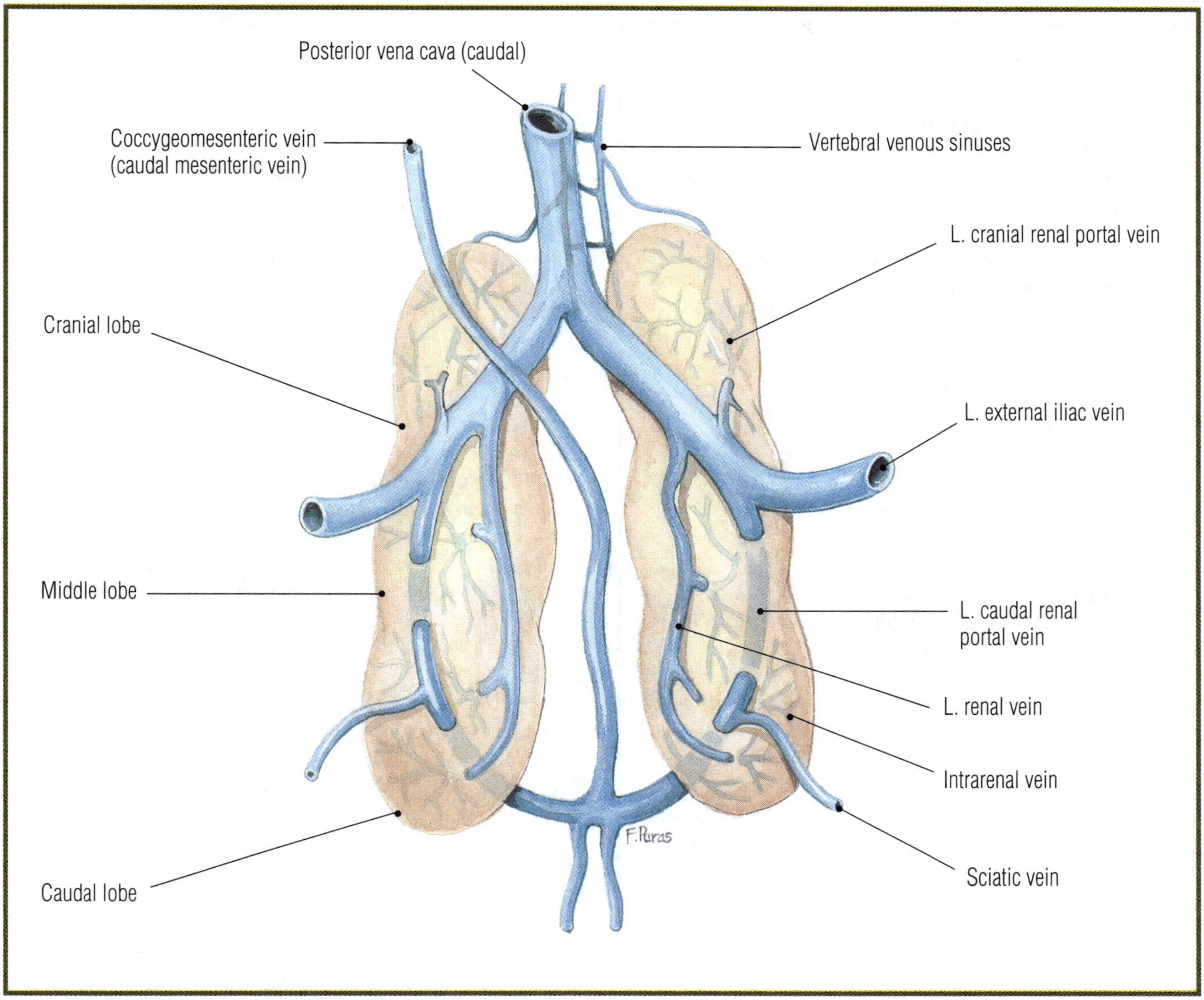

Illustration by Felecia J. Paras

Schematic of the avian renal portal system.

COCCYGEOMESENTERIC VEIN

A unique avian vessel is the coccygeomesenteric vein. This is also known as the caudal mesenteric vein and it drains the lower half of the body including the large intestine, cloaca, and rectum. This vein has the unique property of emptying both into the hepatic portal system and the renal portal system but not into both at the same time. It is the link between the two systems. Blood in this vessel normally flows toward the kidneys. The flow also can be reversed, which causes the blood to be directed toward the hepatic portal system where it effectively bypasses the renal tubules.

LYMPHATIC SYSTEM

Like mammals, birds have a lymphatic system that accompanies the blood vessels. There are typically two lymphatic vessels for each blood vessel. Avian lymphatics have relatively fewer valves than mammalian lymphatic vessels and therefore have a less "beaded" appearance.

VENIPUNCTURE SITES

Favorite venipuncture sites in birds are few due to their unique anatomy; there are fewer accessible peripheral vessels in birds than there are in mammals. Those vessels that are accessible, even on the largest of psittacine species, are not very big.

Commonly used vessels in birds include the wing vein (the deep ulnar vein becomes accessible for blood collection at the elbow where it becomes subcutaneous), the medial metatarsal vein, and the jugular vein.

- **Wing vein.** The wing vein (deep ulnar vein) is found near the ventral aspect of the elbow. Although venipuncture at

BLOOD COMPONENTS

Avian blood components differ in substantial ways from mammalian blood components. When looking at an avian blood smear, the nucleated red blood cells are the first indication of these differences.

The granulocytic leukocytes of birds are the heterophils, eosinophils, and basophils:

- The heterophils are the equivalent of the mammalian neutrophil. The nucleus is lobed and the clear cytoplasm contains eosinophilic granules.
- The eosinophils are distinct in that they have intensely red granules in a blue staining cytoplasm. The nucleus is also lobed.
- The basophils have a nonlobed nucleus with clear cytoplasm containing purple granules.

Lymphocytes and monocytes are also found in avian blood:

- Lymphocytes have a nonlobed nucleus with a high nucleus-to-cytoplasm ratio. They vary in size from small to large.
- Monocytes are the largest leukocyte in avian blood. They have a finely granular cytoplasm with a blue gray appearance and the nucleus can be round to bilobed.

Thrombocytes are the avian equivalent of mammalian platelets. They differ from platelets in that they are nucleated. They have a pyknotic, dark purple nucleus with a colorless cytoplasm.

KEY DIFFERENCES

AVIAN VS. MAMMALIAN CARDIOVASCULAR SYSTEM

- Renal portal system and the coccygeomesenteric vein
- Larger heart and fast rate of beating
- Countercurrent tibiotarsal rete system and its unique role in thermoregulation in some avians
- Crosscurrent exchange system in the lungs
- Hematology

this site is relatively easy to accomplish, it is a less than ideal place for venipuncture. Firm pressure must be applied for a number of minutes after venipuncture in order to avoid a large hematoma; there are some patients in which this is not acceptable. For example, anemic patients may lose a significant and devastating amount of blood through a wing vein hematoma. Also, if the patient has already deteriorated, the added stress of handling to avoid a hematoma may further compromise the patient.

- **Medial metatarsal vein.** Located along the medial side of the tarsometatarsus, the medial metatarsal vein can be accessed for venipuncture in many birds. The small size of this vessel limits its usefulness when larger samples are required.

- **Jugular vein.** In almost all birds, the right jugular vein is larger than the left and many consider it the vein of choice for venipuncture. The jugular veins are found in the apteria along the sides of the neck. To obtain a blood sample from a jugular vein, the vein is held off at the thoracic inlet and the feathers are parted along the neck revealing the featherless tract area.

Toenail clipping is often advocated as a method of blood collection, but in birds, it is probably the least acceptable route. The practice is painful for the bird and blood collected from the toenail generally is contaminated with tissue fluid. Poor circulation to this area also may result in hematologic values that are not an accurate representation of whole body values.

About the Author

Dr. Rosenthal, who is board certified in avian practice, is a Staff Veterinarian for the avian and exotic pet service of The Animal Medical Center in New York City.

RESOURCES

King, AS and McLelland, J. *Birds: Their Structure and Function.* Bailliere Tindall, Philadelphia, 1984

Ritchie, BW, Harrison, GJ, and Harrison, LR, eds. *Avian Medicine: Principles and Applications.* Wingers, Inc. Lake Worth, FL. 1994.

Sturkie, PD, ed. *Avian Physiology.* Springer-Verlag, New York, 1986.

The Avian Gastrointestinal System

PART ONE OF A TWO PART SERIES

R. Avery Bennett, DVM, MS, Diplomate ACVS
Sharon L. Deem, DVM, PhD

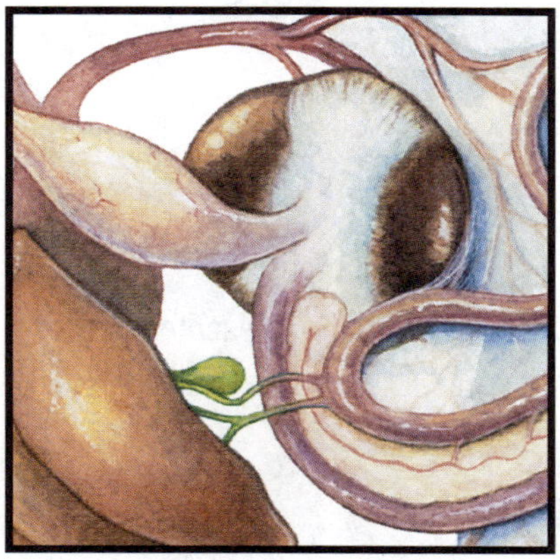

Illustration by Felecia J. Paras

ALTHOUGH THE GASTROINTESTINAL tracts (GITs) of different avian species are, in general, much closer in design than those of different mammalian species, there are idiosyncrasies worth noting. Most of these adaptations are dictated by the particular bird's diet (i.e., carnivorous raptors, granivorous poultry, or omnivorous psittacines), and are designed to provide the optimum in food digestion and absorption. Additionally, the anatomy and physiology of the avian GIT has been influenced by the need to fly; hence its shorter length, optimal efficiency, and reduced volume, which, in turn, results in reduced weight.

While much of the research on avian gastroenterology (especially in physiology) has been carried out on poultry, this article emphasizes the GIT of the most commonly treated avian patients in private practice: psittacines (namely, true parrots). The lack of research on these types of birds, however, means that many of the unique features of the psittacine GIT are not fully understood.

Originally published in September/October 1995 *Perspectives*

The Gastrointestinal Tract

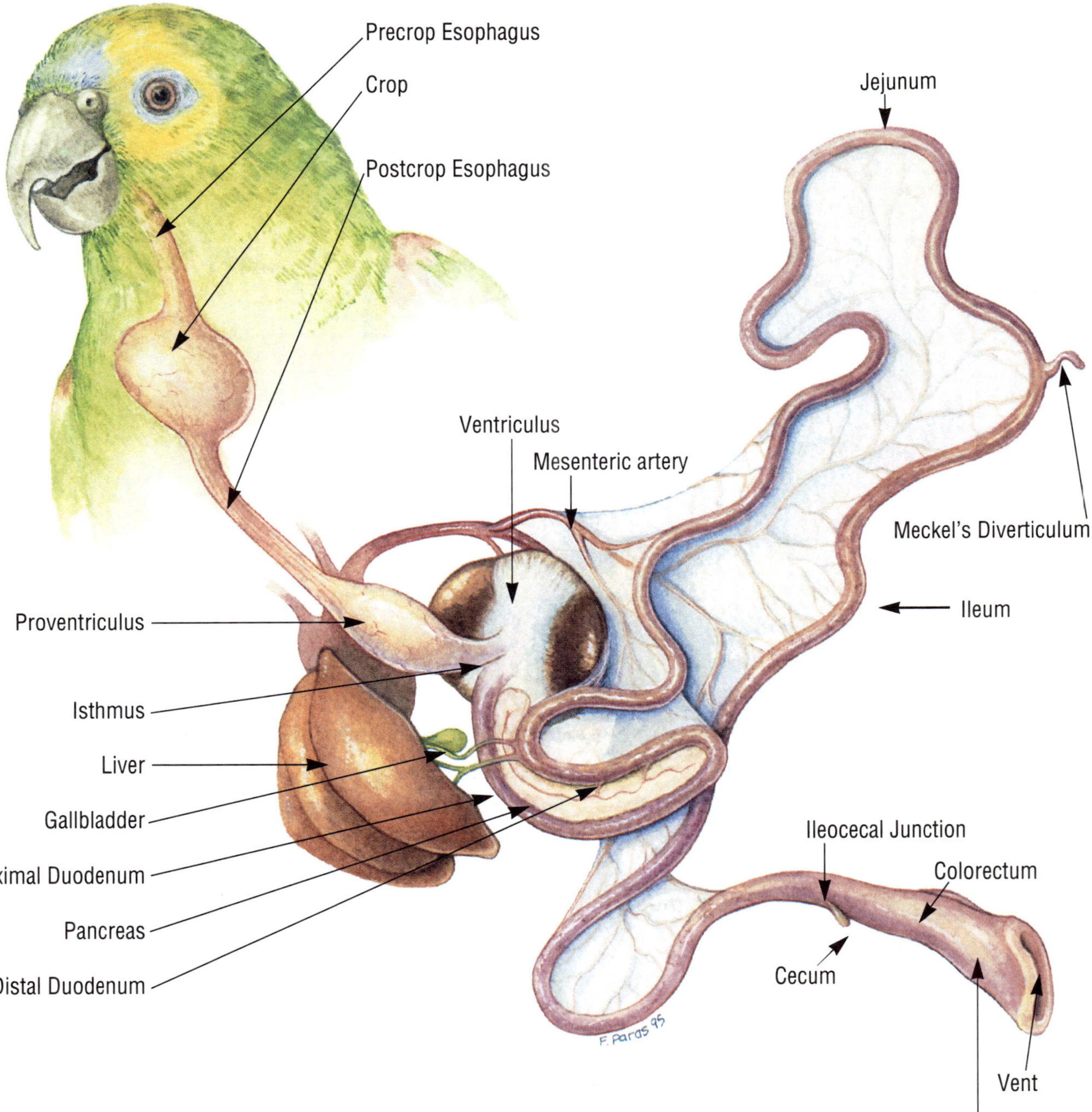

Illustration by Felecia J. Paras

The psittacine upper gastrointestinal system showing the crop, proventriculus, and ventriculus. The system is not placed as it would appear anatomically, but extended in this illustration to enhance visibility of all its parts.

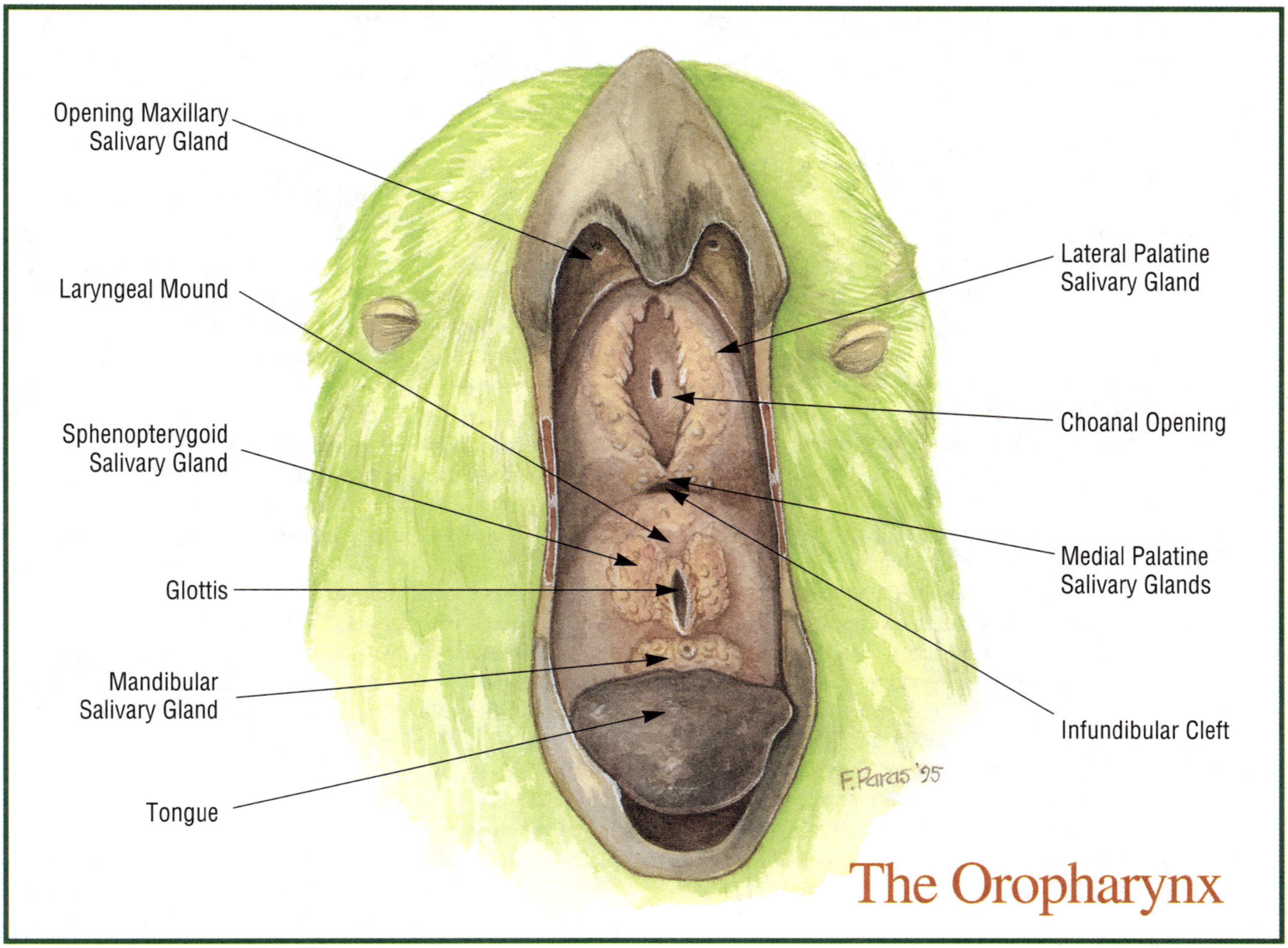

Illustration by Felecia J. Paras

THE BEAK

Adaptations to the avian diet start with this specialized structure. The beak is composed of bone, a vascular layer, a germinal layer, and a keratinized surface (see "Unique Features of the Avian Integumentary System," *Perspectives*, May/June 1995, pp. 17–23). In psittacine birds, both the upper and lower jaw are connected to the skull by moving joints, allowing these birds to move both the upper and lower beak. The keratin layer covering the beak is the **rhamphotheca**. This is further divided into the **rhinotheca** covering the upper beak and the **gnathotheca** covering the lower beak. The **culmen** is the dorsal midline ridge of the rhinotheca and the **gonys** is the ventral midline ridge of the gnathotheca. **Tomia** are the cutting edges of the rhamphotheca which are used to remove the hulls of seeds. Birds use their beaks for prehension of food, preparation and delivery of food to the esophagus, and, in psittacines, for locomotion. The beak grows continuously but the growth rate varies with species and function.

CLINICAL ADVISORY

Bacterial, mycotic (candidiasis), parasitic (knemidokoptiasis), and viral (psittacine beak and feather disease) infections may result in damage to and necrosis of the beak. Trauma to the beak and its germinal layer also occurs with some degree of frequency. Any conditions which affect the germinal layer of the beak can affect beak growth and conformation. Liver disease has been linked to beak overgrowth, especially in budgerigars.

THE OROPHARYNX

Birds do not have glossopalatine arches which, in mammals, divide the oral cavity and pharynx, or a soft palate, which separates the nasal and oral pharynx. Instead, birds have a single cavity called the **oropharynx**. This cavity is lined by stratified squamous epithelium and contains numerous papillae. These papillae are directed aborad and help move food into the esophagus. Papillae are arranged either randomly or in transverse rows on the roof of the oropharynx; along the margins of the choana and infundibular cleft; on the tongue; and on the laryngeal mound.

The **choana** is an opening in the hard palate along the midline connecting the nasal cavity and the oropharynx. The choana closes reflexively during swallowing to prevent food from entering the nasal cavity. In birds with hypovitaminosis A, the choanal papillae are frequently short and blunted as a result of squamous metaplasia (see Clinical Advisory below for more information).

The **infundibular cleft** is located just caudal to the choana. It contains the slit-like openings of the bilateral pharyngotympanic tubes (equivalent to eustachian tubes). The openings of these tubes are not covered as they are in mammals. This prevents pressure from building up in the middle ear when the bird changes altitude during flight. The wall of the infundibular cleft contains lymphatic tissue called **pharyngeal tonsils**.

KEY DIFFERENCES

Avian Versus Mammalian Gastrointestinal System

- Birds have two stomachs and, in some species, a crop
- Birds have oxynticopeptic cells in the proventriculus that have two functions
- Birds lack glossopalatine arches and a soft palate, creating a single structure called the oropharynx
- Birds have uncovered pharyngotympanic tubes
- The esophagus is located on the right side of neck. Length and diameter are greater than in mammals, allowing for passage of proportionately larger food items

The Tongue

Psittacines are the only group of avian species with intrinsic muscles in the tongue. In most birds, tongue movement is a result of the attachment of the hyobranchial apparatus to the caudal aspect of the tongue. The **entoglossal bone** is located within the tongue and is a part of the hyoid apparatus. This structure is paired in psittacines. In budgerigars, the two bones are bifurcated at the rostral tip. The structure of the tongue varies with species and dietary adaptations. The tongue's few taste buds are located at its base. Other taste buds are located on the palate, the floor of the oropharynx, and the laryngeal mound, a structure that is formed by the prominent muscles and cartilages of the glottis at the base of the tongue.

Salivary Glands

Salivary glands are abundant in the avian oropharynx. The maxillary salivary glands are located in the roof of the oropharynx, while the palatine glands are at the angle of the mouth and on the lateral walls of the oropharynx. Sphenopterygoid salivary glands are within the floor of the oropharynx. These glands are most developed in birds that eat dry food items and are least developed in water birds. They are totally absent in great cormorants. In some species, amylase is also a component of saliva, aiding in digestion. Eating and parasympathetic stimulation initiate salivary secretion.

CLINICAL ADVISORY

In birds with hypovitaminosis A, a condition that is reversible with proper diet, squamous metaplasia results in occlusion of the salivary gland ducts. This predisposes them to the development of secondary bacterial infections and abscessation. Abscesses are commonly located around the choana, the laryngeal mound, and under the tongue.

Candidiasis and trichomoniasis cause the formation of diphtheritic plaques in the oropharynx. Pox virus causes the formation of proliferative masses in the mouth and esophagus. Pigeon herpesvirus infection results in the formation of a diphtheritic membrane over the surface of the oropharynx and esophagus.

SWALLOWING

Food is prehended by the beak, held by sticky mucus secreted by the salivary glands, and moved by the tongue. The choana, infundibular cleft, and laryngeal mound close reflexively as food passes over. Papillae on the tongue, roof of the mouth, and the laryngeal mound help move food in an aborad direction. Repeated, rapid, rostral to caudal movements of the tongue roll the food into the caudal oropharynx. Once the food reaches the laryngeal mound, similar movements allow papillae to "rake" the food into the proximal esophagus where esophageal peristalsis moves the food in an aborad direction.

Drinking is accomplished in a similar manner but is aided by gravity: most birds hold their heads up while moving the tongue and laryngeal mound, thereby allowing water to move into the caudal oropharynx. Psittacines, however, are able to lap water because of their intrinsic tongue muscles while hummingbirds are able to suck nectar through their tubular tongues. Columbiformes (pigeon type birds) can also generate suction and usually immerse the beak during drinking.

ESOPHAGUS

The esophagus in birds lies immediately under the skin on the right side of the neck (opposite the left-sided location in mammals). Its location makes it easily accessible for placement of an esophagostomy tube. As the esophagus is longer and of a larger diameter than that of mammals, birds are able to swallow very large whole food items. There also are longitudinal folds which help increase distensibility. This feature allows for the passage of large tubes for enteral feeding and diagnostic sample collection, as well as for passage of large endoscopes and instruments for diagnostic purposes and foreign body removal. (Note: Using a large tube helps prevent accidental tracheal intubation if the tube is too large to pass through the glottis.)

Keratinized stratified squamous epithelium lines the esophagus. There are many subepithelial mucous glands, particularly within the thoracic esophagus, to help lubricate the food for passage into the proventriculus. As in mammals, the smooth muscle layers of the esophagus are circular on the inside and longitudinal on the outside. They are innervated by the vagus nerve and motility is influenced by excitement and fear.

The **ingluvies** or crop is a dilated portion of the esophagus just cranial to the thoracic inlet. Its structure and function vary with species and diet. It is absent in owls, gulls, and penguins where food passes directly into the proventriculus or is stored in the tubular esophagus. The ingluvies is located immediately below and firmly attached to the skin of the thoracic inlet making it easily palpable. Both the esophagus and ingluvies are the site of food storage and softening.

In psittacines, the crop is relatively large and oriented transversely across the thoracic inlet. Ingluviotomy incisions are generally made in the left pouch to avoid the jugular vein, carotid artery, and the entrance and exit openings of the ingluvies. The ultrastructure of the ingluvies is similar to the remainder of the esophagus except that mucous glands are absent. Gram-positive bacteria and a small number of *Candida* sp are normally found in the crop. Its pH is acidic (4 to 6) in most species. The external carotid arteries supply the esophagus and ingluvies with blood; the jugular veins receive their venous drainage.

Crop Idiosyncrasies

Male birds of some species (pigeons, sage grouse, ostriches, and great bustards) have esophageal diverticula that inflate with air, creating a chamber for resonating sound during sexual displays. In columbiformes, crop milk is produced by both males and females to feed hatchlings; its production is stimulated by prolactin. The milk has the gross appearance of mammalian milk but has no calcium or carbohydrates. Composed of desquamated epithelial cells that are high in fat and protein, crop milk initially is the sole source of food for squabs. As the squabs matures, the parents gradually mix in other food items. Psittacines, finches, greater flamingos, and emperor penguins also produce crop secretions for feeding neonates.

CLINICAL ADVISORY

Diagnostic samples can be obtained from the ingluvies by passing a tube into the crop and instilling sterile, physiologic saline, then aspirating a sample back. The sample should be examined by direct wet mount for trichomonads and centrifuged for cytologic evaluation. Yeast and bacterial infections are diagnosed on cytology. The sample may also be submitted for culture and sensitivity testing.

FOOD TRANSPORT

The esophageal mucous glands produce mucus to lubricate food carried by peristalsis to the proventriculus. Motility is affected by the presence of food within the ventriculus. When the ingluvies contracts, eliminating the pouches, the food moves past the ingluvies and into the proventriculus. If the ventriculus is full, food either stays in the crop or within the esophagus (in species that do not have a crop).

CLINICAL ADVISORY

Esophageal paresis or paralysis may occur with heavy metal intoxication resulting in stasis and impaction. Retroperistalsis is responsible for regurgitation, a normal function in some species. In many birds, neonates are fed regurgitated food which has been moistened and partially digested. Regurgitation is also a part of courtship display for many species, including psittacines. Many companion psittacines, for example, will court their owners and regurgitate to them. This should not be confused with regurgitation associated with pathologic conditions.

ASSESSING GI DYSFUNCTION

Gastrointestinal (GI) disease is common in companion birds, but patients often have nonspecific clinical signs. Anorexia, dysphagia, regurgitation, vomiting, constipation, diarrhea, and/or tenesmus in a patient should alert the clinician to a possible gastrointestinal problem. Weight loss and weakness may be better indicators of gastrointestinal involvement in a chronic disease. Because birds eliminate both urine and feces when they void, it is important for the practitioner to distinguish between diarrhea and polyuria when patients are presented for diarrhea: the distinction may be difficult for clients to determine. (Note: In diarrhea, the stool is simply soft. In polyuria, there is a marked increase in urine.)

The diagnostic approach for birds suspected of having GI disease should include a thorough history and physical exam; ingluvies (crop) and fecal samples for evaluation by Gram stain, acid-fast stain, Wright's stain and parasite examination by direct wet mount and flotation techniques; CBC and chemistry panel; radiology and endoscopy; and/or laparoscopy.

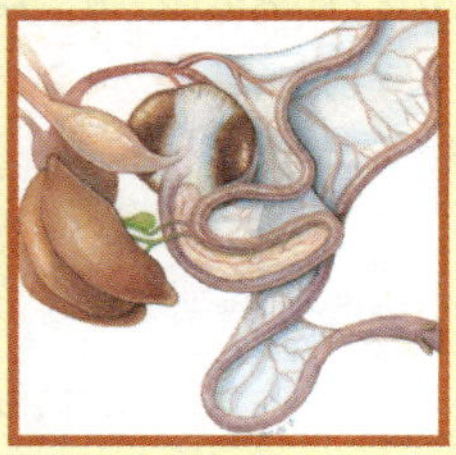

THE STOMACH

The avian stomach consists of two parts: the orad glandular portion, called the **proventriculus**, and the aborad muscular portion, called the **ventriculus**. These are separated by a narrow region called the **isthmus** or intermediate zone. The stomach lies to the left of midline and is dorsal to the liver. It is covered by the fat-filled posthepatic septum (the avian equivalent of the omentum). There is no distinct lower esophageal sphincter and the loss of longitudinal esophageal folds is the only grossly discernible distinction between the esophagus and proventriculus.

The avian stomach has one of two basic conformations depending on the species. In carnivorous and piscivorous birds that swallow large, whole prey, there is little distinction between the ventriculus and the proventriculus. These structures form one large, relatively thin-walled stomach that is easily distensible to accommodate food items. This type of stomach is much easier to close following proventriculotomy as it can be easily inverted. More commonly, as in companion birds, the proventriculus is thick walled and glandular, and the ventriculus is very thick and muscular with a defined isthmus separating the two components. Because the proventriculus is thick and relatively nondistensible with this type of stomach, closure of a proventriculotomy is much more difficult and prone to leakage.

THE PROVENTRICULUS

The glandular stomach produces and releases gastric fluid containing pepsinogen, hydrochloric acid, and mucus. There are only two cell populations: epithelial cells, which produce mucus, and **oxynticopeptic cells**, which produce both pepsino-

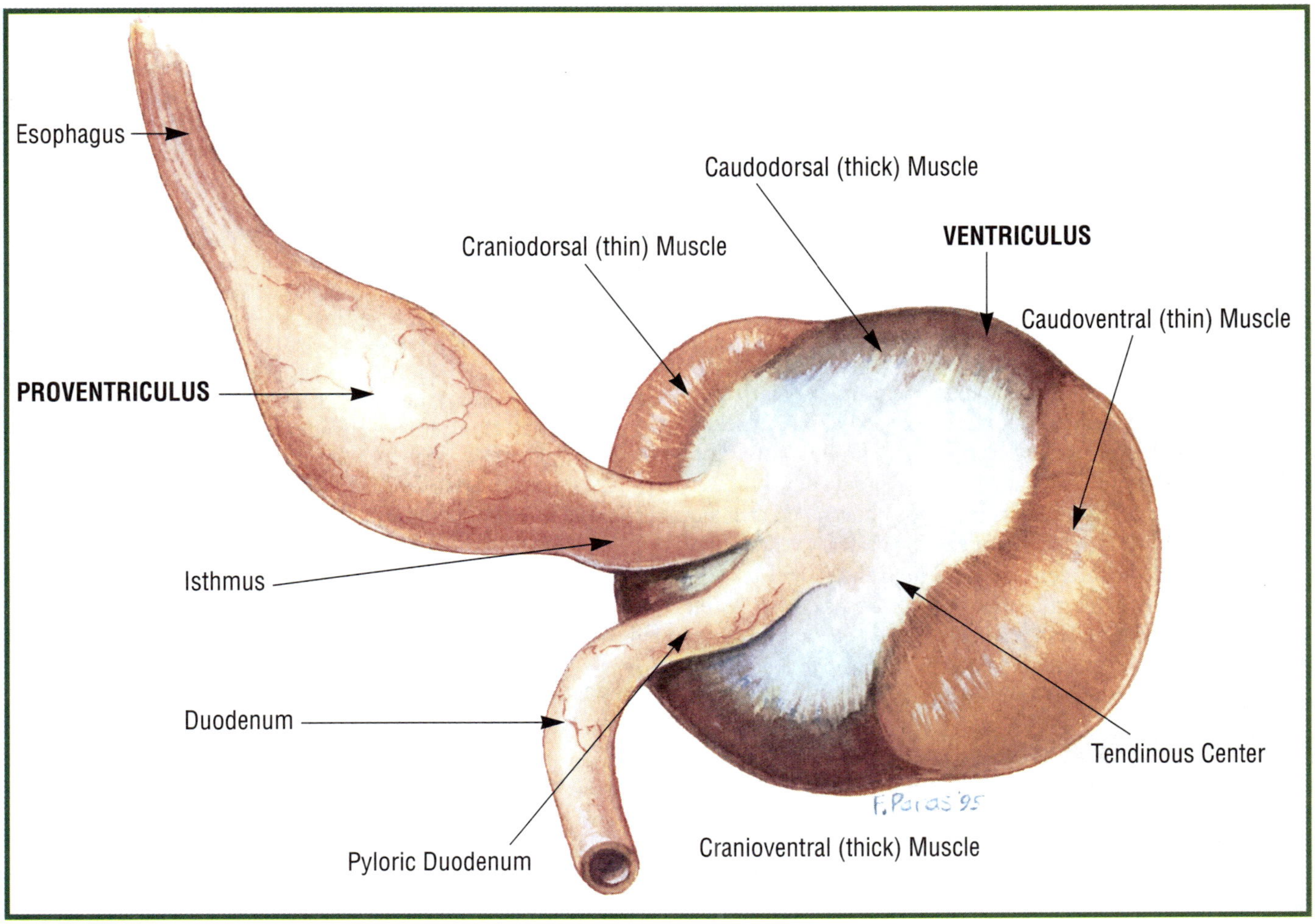

Illustration by Felecia J. Paras

The stomach is not placed as it would appear anatomically but extended in this illustration to enhance visibility of all its parts.

gen and hydrochloric acid. This is in contrast to the mammalian stomach where the chief cells produce pepsinogen and the parietal cells produce hydrochloric acid, but is parallel to the oxynticopeptic cells of other nonmammalian vertebrate stomachs. The distribution of these glands is throughout the proventriculus in most birds. In owls they occur in longitudinal tracts and in ostriches they are localized in a circular patch on the greater curvature.

CLINICAL ADVISORY

Radiographically, the proventriculus can be visualized dorsal to the liver on the lateral projection. Enlargement of the proventriculus can be associated with neuropathic gastric dilation, impaction, proventricular stasis, or even a recent meal, and is not necessarily diagnostic of a specific condition. Plumbism can cause gastric stasis. Foreign bodies may lodge in either the ventriculus or the proventriculus. Regurgitation of proventricular contents into the crop can lead to sour crop, with decreased GIT motility, associated distension of the crop, and foul smelling proventricular contents. Proventricular dilatation syndrome (neuropathic gastric dilation and encephalomyelitis) is believed to be caused by a virus. This disease is characterized by lymphocytic and monocytic infiltration of the splanchnic nerves of the tunica muscularis in the entire GIT. Clinical signs are the result of decreased motility, malabsorption, and maldigestion.

The isthmus or intermediate zone varies with species but is generally characterized as a transition from the glandular to the muscular stomach and thus has histologic characteristics of each. There is a gradual transition from the columnar mucus-producing epithelium of the proventriculus to the characteristic ventricular glands. The compound glands of the proventriculus are lost, but the surface is smooth without the papillae characteristic of the ventriculus. Most gastric neoplasms occur here. In birds with a large diameter isthmus, the ventriculus can be approached through a proventriculotomy and the contents of the ventriculus explored by passing instruments through the isthmus into the ventriculus.

THE VENTRICULUS

This is the site of protein digestion and mechanical breakdown of food. It is very muscular with the muscles being best developed in species such as granivorous birds and psittacines that eat relatively indigestible food . The ventriculus lies to the left of midline and can be palpated just caudal to the sternum on the left side as a firm mass. This is a normal structure and should not be confused with a coelomic mass.

The outer longitudinal muscle of the proventriculus is absent and the four muscle masses of the ventriculus are derived from the inner, circular, smooth muscle layer. In species of birds with a large, distensible ventriculus, both the inner circular and outer longitudinal muscles are retained. The two pair of opposing muscles include the thick caudodorsal and cranioventral muscles and the thin caudoventral and craniodorsal muscles (see stomach detail on page 17). These circular muscles attach to a central tendinous aponeurosis on both the right and left sides of the ventriculus. The high myoglobin content of these smooth muscles accounts for the dark color of the ventriculus. The thin muscles are lighter in color and form the cranial and caudal blind sacs. Because the thinner muscles are easier to close and heal better than the thick proventricular muscles, this is the location of choice for ventriculotomy incisions. These muscles contract in an asynchronous manner to create rotary crushing action in the lumen for mechanical digestion of food. Intraluminal pressures up to 200 mg/Hg have been recorded in chickens.

The tough, rough lining of the ventriculus is called the **cuticle** or **koilin**. It is formed by the secretions of two populations of cells within the ventriculus, creating vertical rods and horizontal matrix. It is composed of a complex of proteins and carbohydrates devoid of keratin. The vertical rods and horizontal matrix are indistinct and the cuticle is poorly developed in carnivorous and piscivorous birds.

Within the surface of the ventriculus are crypts into which groups of 5 to 8 tubular glands empty. Their secretions form firm vertical rods which extend above the surface of the cuticle as projections called **dentate processes**. The cells on the surface of the crypts and the mucosa of the ventriculus also produce secretions that flow over the surface and entrap desquamated cells and debris. This material remains soft until exposed to hydrochloric acid whereupon it hardens. This allows it to spread over the surface of the ventriculus to create the horizontal layers of the cuticle. The cuticle is constantly turning over as it is worn by the grinding action of the ventriculus. It is thickest in the area of the thick muscle and thinnest in the areas of the thin muscle. The cuticle has longitudinal folds and its characteristic yellow, green, or brown color is a result of bile reflux stains on its surface.

The pyloric region of the ventriculus is on the right side and marks the junction of the duodenum to the ventriculus. Its structure varies but, histologically, it shares features of both the ventriculus and the duodenum. In some species, the pylorus is a subtle narrowing (chickens), while in others it is a large pouch-like dilation (heron and cormorant). Food moves back and forth between the ventriculus and proventriculus by sequential contraction of the thin muscles, the duodenum, the thick muscles, and the proventriculus.

Egestion or casting occurs in raptors as a mechanism to eliminate indigestible components from the ventriculus. The pellets generally contain skin, feathers, fur, and bones. Owls generally cast after each meal and their pellets usually contain bone. Hawks cast or attempt to cast (when no pellet is present) daily at dawn. Because the material is in their stomach longer, bones are usually digested and not part of the pellet. The frequency of egestion is also a function of the amount of indigestible material eaten, the amount of fat and protein in the food, and the quantity of food. The pellet is formed in the ventriculus and vomited out.

CLINICAL ADVISORY

Foreign bodies, heavy metal intoxication, and hyperacidity may cause the development of erosions or ulcers in the ventriculus. Neurotrophic gastric dilation also affects the ventriculus. Impaction may be caused by foreign bodies or muscular stasis. Hypovitaminosis E can cause muscle degeneration and ventricular stasis.

NEXT ISSUE:

About the Authors

Dr. Bennett and Dr. Deem are on the staff of the Wildlife and Zoological Medicine Service, Department of Small Animal Clinical Sciences, University of Florida, Gainesville, Florida.

References

Duke GE: Alimentary canal: Anatomy, regulation of feeding, and motility, in Sturkie PD (ed): *Avian Physiology*, ed 4. New York, Springer-Verlag, 1986, pp 269–288.

Duke GE: Alimentary canal: Secretion and digestion, special digestive functions, and absorption, in Sturkie PD (ed): *Avian Physiology*, ed 4. New York, Springer-Verlag, 1986, pp 289–302.

King AS, McLelland J: Coelomic cavities, in *Birds—Their Structure and Function*. Philadelphia, Bailliere Tindall, 1984, pp 79–83.

King AS, McLelland J: Digestive system, in *Birds—Their Structure and Function*. Philadelphia, Bailliere Tindall, 1984, pp 84–109.

Lumeij JT: Gastoenterology, in Ritchie BW, Harrison GJ, Harrison LR (eds): *Avian Medicine: Principles and Application*. Lake Worth, Florida, Wingers Publishing, 1994, pp 482–521.

McKibben JS, Harrison, GJ: Clinical anatomy (with emphasis on the Amazon parrot), in Harrison GJ, Harrison LR (eds): *Clinical Avian Medicine and Surgery*. Philadelphia, WB Saunders Co, 1986, pp 31–66.

McLelland J: Digestive system, in *A Color Atlas of Avian Anatomy*. Philadelphia, WB Saunders Co, 1991, pp 47–65.

McLelland J: Peritoneum and peritoneal cavities, in *A Color Atlas of Avian Anatomy*. Philadelphia, WB Saunders Co, 1991, pp 65–88.

Rosenthal K: Unique features of the avian integumentary system. *Perspectives* May/June 1995, pp 17–23.

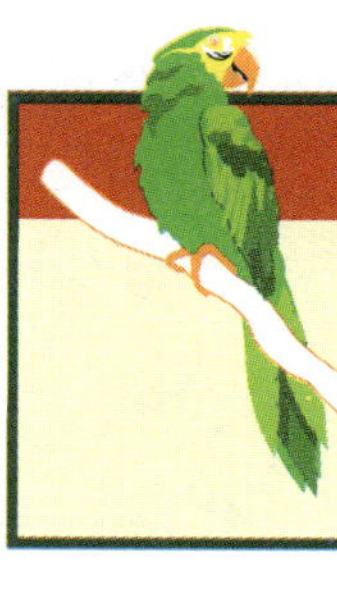

RESOURCES

Association of Avian Veterinarians
P.O. Box 811720
Boca Raton, Florida 33481
Phone: (407)393-8901

The Avian Gastrointestinal System

PART TWO OF A TWO PART SERIES

Sharon L. Deem, DVM, PhD
R. Avery Bennett, DVM, MS, Diplomate ACVS

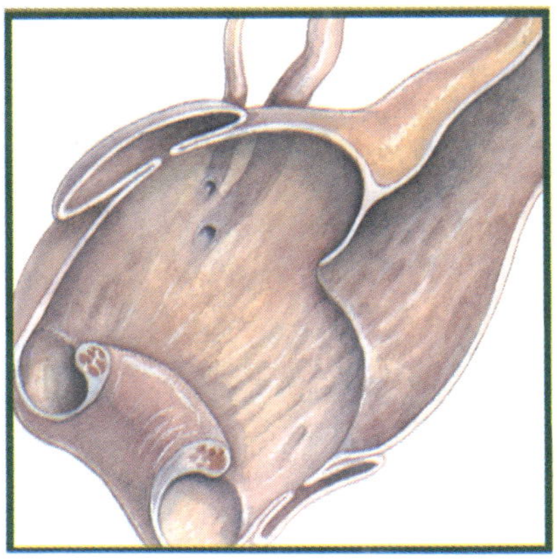

Illustration by Felecia J. Paras

THE GASTROINTESTINAL TRACTS (GITs) of different avian species have several key differences that are dictated by diet and influenced by the need to fly. Part I of this two part series covered food transport from the esophagus through the ventriculus. This article focuses on the liver, pancreas, and lower GIT of psittacines, the most commonly treated avian patients in private practice.

Updated from original publication in November/December 1995 *Perspectives*

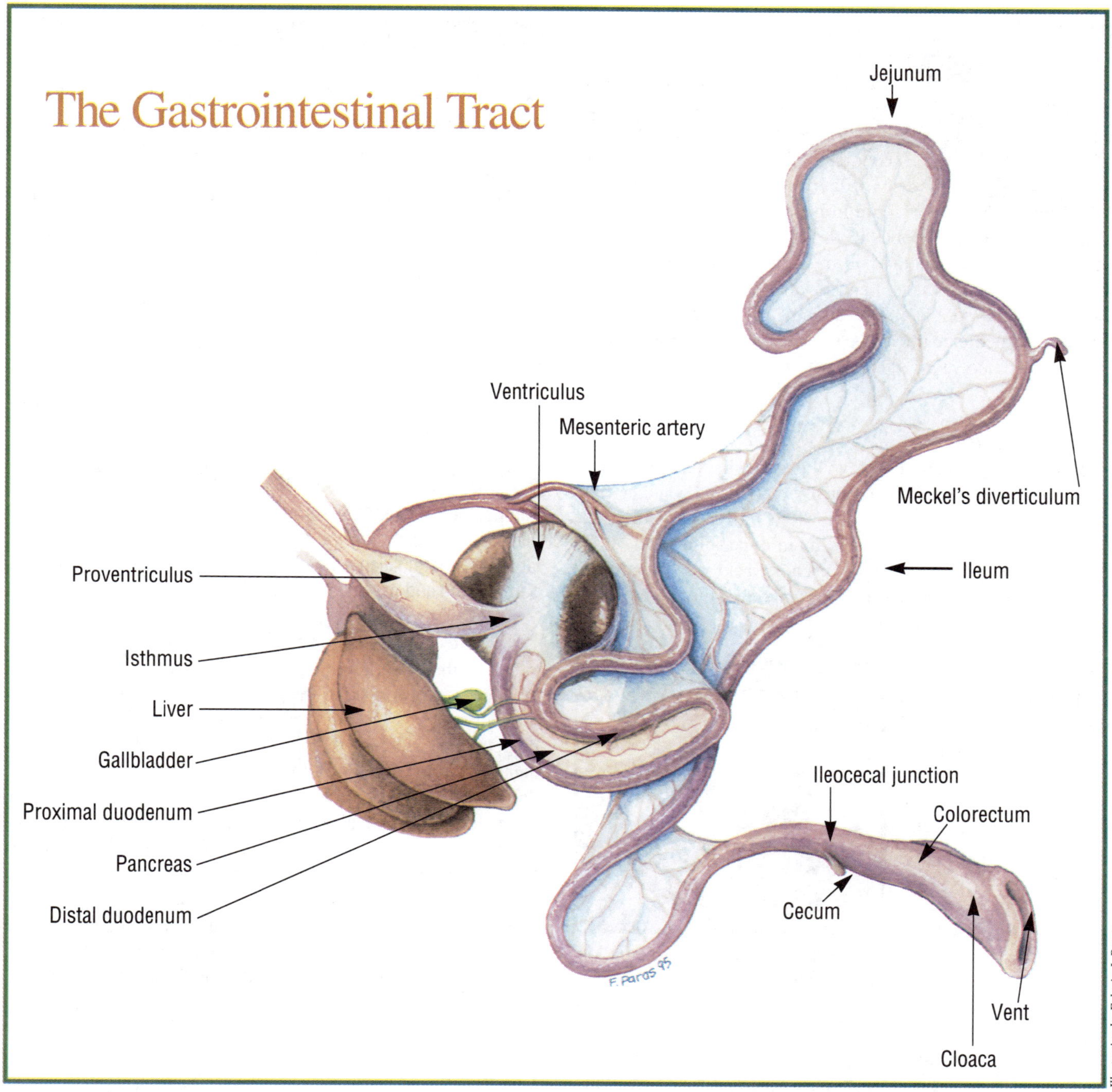

Illustration by Felecia J. Paras

The psittacine liver, pancreas, and lower gastrointestinal system. Anatomy and function of the proventriculus and ventriculus were covered in Part I. Note: *The system is not placed as it would appear anatomically, but extended in this illustration to enhance visibility of all its parts.*

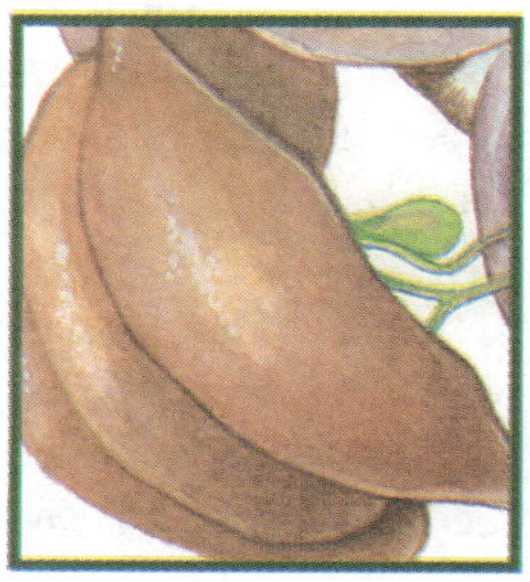

THE LIVER

In birds, there are two main liver lobes (right and left) which surround the apex of the heart and join cranially at the midline. In most species, the right lobe is larger than the left and one or the other lobe is frequently subdivided. The lobe which is subdivided varies with the species. The liver itself is covered by a fat-filled posthepatic septum. Portal circulation is well developed but there are no well defined hepatic triads or lobules. The caudal vena cava enters the dorsal portion of the right lobe. In newly hatched chicks, the liver is a yellow color because of the high fat content resulting from absorption of the yolk.

The Gallbladder

A gallbladder is present in many species of birds but is ab-

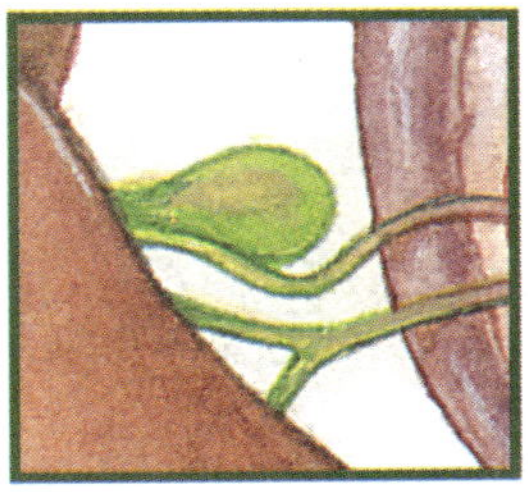

sent in psittaciformes, columbiformes, and ostriches. In species with a gallbladder, the **hepatocystic duct** carries bile from the right lobe of the liver to the gallbladder and the **cysticoenteric duct** carries bile from the gallbladder to the duodenum. The **common hepatoenteric duct** transports bile from both lobes to the duodenum. These last two ducts open into the aborad portion of the ascending duodenum. In birds that do not have a gall bladder (e.g., psittacines), bile flows from the right liver lobe directly to the duodenum via the **right hepatoenteric duct**. The common hepatoenteric duct and the right hepatoenteric duct empty into the ascending duodenum.

The Role of Bile

Bile plays an important role in digestion. Its main function is to aid in the emulsification of dietary fats. It also contains amylase and activates pancreatic lipase. Cholic, allocholic, and chenodeoxycholic acids are the main avian bile acids. In 10 species of wild birds, chenodeoxycholic acid was found to be the main bile acid produced. In carnivorous birds, cholic and allocholic acids predominate.

THE PANCREAS

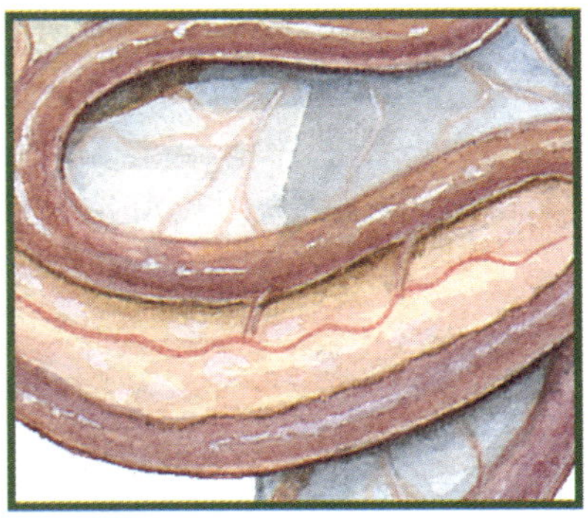

The pancreas lies within the duodenal loop. It is pale-pink to yellow in color and has a distinctly lobulated appearance. It is comprised of three lobes with one to three ducts. In most species (except pigeons and mallard ducks) the dorsal and ventral lobes are fused. The splenic lobe originates from either the dorsal or the ventral lobe and extends craniad. The ducts open in the ascending duodenum near the bile ducts.

The exocrine function of the pancreas is derived from the secretions of the tubuloacinar glands, which are lined by zymogen columnar cells. These cells produce the proenzyme precursors of amylase, lipase, trypsin, and chymotrypsin which must be activated by enterokinase. This process prevents the pancreas from being digested by its own secretions. Water and bicarbonate are also produced by the pancreas and secreted into the duodenum. The pancreatic enzymes function best in a high pH environment which is created by the bicarbonate. Pancreatic secretion is mediated by the vagus nerve and can be blocked by atropine. Humoral factors (secretin and vasoactive intestinal peptide: VIP) have also been identified in the intestines of birds and stimulate the release of pancreatic secretions. Force feeding results in a decrease in the release of digestive enzymes from the pancreas as compared with self feeding.

CLINICAL ADVISORY

With pancreatic insufficiency and maldigestion, the feces contain excess amounts of fat and amylum and have a pale tan, greasy, voluminous appearance.

COELOMIC CAVITIES

The avian coelomic cavities are a group of 16 separate cavities; eight air sacs and eight cavities of the coelom proper. It is imperative to know the anatomy of the various cavities when performing surgical approaches. Two of the coelomic cavities are pleural and one is the pericardial cavity. The remaining five cavities (left and right ventral hepatic, left and right dorsal hepatic, and intestinal) comprise the peritoneal cavities and are formed by five double layered sheets of peritoneum. Birds lack a true omentum, as is found in mammals; however, the **posthepatic septum** resembles the mammalian omentum.

CLINICAL ADVISORY

The posthepatic septum is important in restricting the spread of diseases by separating the peritoneum into distinct parts. Similar to the mammalian omentum, the peritoneum helps to close perforations and provides a supply of blood.

LOWER GASTROINTESTINAL TRACT

Unlike the avian upper GIT in which there are many adaptations necessary for flight, the lower GIT is very similar to that of mammals. A few general anatomical and physiological points will be addressed prior to examining individual components of the lower GIT. Both the small and large intestines are thin walled with a small diameter making surgical procedures difficult. The epithelial layers (from the lumen outward) consist of mucosa, submucosa, inner circular muscle, outer longitudinal muscle, and the serosa. Villi are present on the mucosa in both the small and large intestines of all species; however, there is great variation in their structure among species. The villi of carnivorous birds, for example, are well developed whereas those of herbivorous birds are flattened and leaflike. These variations provide the most efficient means of digestion for the bird's diet.

Circulatory Aspects

The arterial supply to the gastrointestinal tract is primarily from three major arteries; the coeliac artery (supplying the glandular and muscular stomachs, duodenum, and spleen), the anterior mesenteric artery (supplying the rest of the small intestines), and the caudal mesenteric artery (supplying the rectum and cloaca). Birds have a well developed capillary network to supply the GIT. Lacteals, present in mammals, are absent in all species of birds.

The three major venous drainage vessels are the gastroduodenal vein (draining the glandular and muscular stomachs), the anterior mesenteric vein (draining the small intestines), and the coccygeomesenteric vein (draining the rectum and cloaca). The first two of these vessels anastomose with the hepatic portal vein, whereas the coccygeomesenteric vein anastomoses with either the hepatic portal and/or the renal portal veins. Therefore, blood from the rectum and cloaca can flow to either the liver or the kidney.

Lymphatic Aspects

Lymph follicles (Peyer's patches) are diffusely distributed throughout the lamina propria and provide lymph drainage for the lower GIT. Birds lack true mesenteric lymph nodes. However, there are some indications that extrabursal sites of B-cell differentiation occur in gut-associated lymphoid tissue. An additional form of immunologic defense is provided by the migration of mediator-secreting cells from the bursa into the germinal centers of the cecal tonsils where they monitor the microenvironment of the ceca.

KEY DIFFERENCES

Avian Versus Mammalian Gastrointestinal System

- Birds lack a true omentum, lacteal vessels, and mesenteric lymph nodules
- Structures that are unique to the avian lower GIT include paired ceca, Meckel's diverticulum (the yolk sac and duct remnant), coelomic cavities, the bursa of Fabricius (vestigial in adult birds), and the cloaca
- Birds have a unique, continuous antiperistalsis which originates in the cloaca and allows water and electrolyte reabsorption to occur in the colon and ceca

Neurologic Aspects

Neurologic control of the avian GIT consists of three anatomically separate components. A submucosal nerve plexus innervates blood vessels and glands. The myenteric nerve plexus, located between the two muscle layers, is involved in coordinating gastric and duodenal motility. Extrinsic innervation, including both pre- and postganglionic cholinergic fibers, is controlled by either vagal or sympathetic pathways.

Small Intestines

The avian small intestines consist of the duodenum, jejunum, and ileum, although the histologic demarcation among the three is unclear. The duodenum is a U-shaped loop originating on the right side of the ventriculus and separated from the latter by the pylorus, a structure which prevents solid food from exiting the ventriculus. The duodenum is the most ventral of the intestines and is easily identified at postmortem against the ventral body wall.

CLINICAL ADVISORY

Care must be taken during celiotomy to avoid iatrogenic laceration of the duodenum and pancreas.

A hepatoduodenal ligament attaches the duodenum to the liver cranially. The pancreas is located on the antimesenteric surface of the ascending portion of the duodenum. The pancreatic and bile ducts open into the ascending duodenum.

The jejunum and ileum consist of many narrow U-shaped loops located in the right side of the abdomen at the end of the long dorsal mesentery which suspends them in the coelomic cavity. The jejunum and ileum are separated arbitrarily by **Meckel's (vitelline) diverticulum**, the remnant of the yolk sac and the remnant of the yolk duct into the intestine. The diverticulum is located on the antimesenteric surface, opposite the distal branches of the cranial mesenteric artery. In healthy chicks the yolk sac should be absorbed at approximately 10 days after hatching, leaving a scar tissue remnant (Meckel's diverticulum). The rate of yolk sac absorption is variable. Altricial birds absorb the yolk sac rapidly while precocial birds absorb theirs more slowly. Since altricial birds are fed by the parents soon after hatching they do not need to rely on the yolk for early nutrition. Precocial birds, on the other hand, must learn to eat on their own which can take several days. During this time, they are nourished by the yolk sac.

Chemical Digestion and Nutrient Absorption

The small intestines are the primary site of chemical digestion and nutrient absorption, processes which involve both intestinal and pancreatic enzymes. Passive diffusion along a concentration gradient and active transport via Na^+ carrier-mediated transport occur. Minerals such as calcium and phosphorus are also absorbed in the small intestine with the greatest absorption in the duodenum and jejunum and the least absorption in the ileum. Calcium absorption is highest in females when the mineral is needed for egg shell production.

Enzymes important in digestion are produced in both the intestines and the pancreas. The duodenum secretes amylase, lipase, dipeptidases, and saccharidases, but not lactase. Hormones involved in the regulation of gastric and intestinal actions (secretin and VIP) are also secreted in the duodenum.

CLINICAL ADVISORY

Both primary intestinal and secondary systemic disease can lead to disorders of the small intestines. Enteritis is frequently diagnosed and often is associated with diarrhea. Etiologies of primary enteritis include bacterial, viral, and parasitic. Psittacines have a predominantly gram positive microflora. A large percentage of gram negative bacteria should alert the clinician to the possibility of a bacterial enteritis.

Problems associated with a retained yolk sac also occur and are often noted in the first few days to weeks after hatching.

Septic omphalitis and failure of retraction prior to hatching are two potentially fatal conditions.

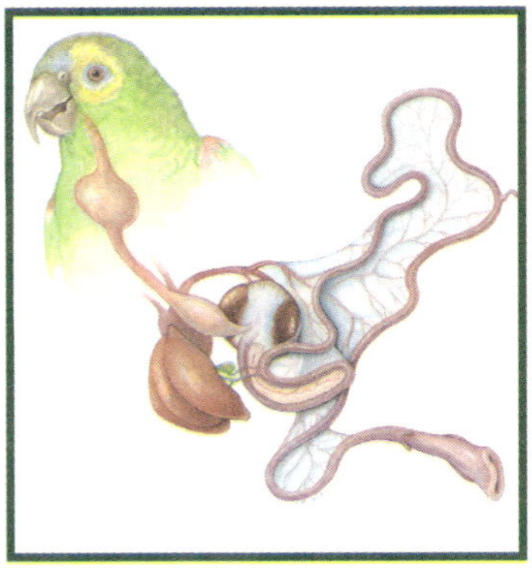

LARGE INTESTINES

The large intestines of psittacines consist of **paired ceca** (absent in budgerigars and rudimentary in most psittacines) and a straight, short, small diameter **colorectum** (comparable to the mammalian rectum). This last structure is often more commonly referred to as the colon.

The colon extends from the ileocecal junction to the cloaca and is located in the dorsal part of the left caudal quadrant of the coelomic cavity. The primary function of the colon is the reabsorption of water and electrolytes. This is carried out by a continuous antiperistalsis unique to avian species. Antiperistalsis arises in the cloaca and moves orad fading either at the ileocolic junction or the ceca. This antiperistalsis allows for water and electrolyte reabsorption to occur in the colon and ceca (if present) by moving urine from the cloaca into the intestines.

Ceca contain the largest microbial and protozoal populations of the avian GIT. Proximal in the ceca are the **cecal tonsils** with well-developed lymphatic tissue which helps in monitoring the microenvironment of the ceca. Cellulose digestion by bacterial fermentation and bacterial vitamin synthesis are two important processes that occur in the ceca. Additionally, ileal contents in the colon can be moved into the ceca for further digestion by fermentation. Histologically, ceca are very similar to the small intestines.

The presence of ceca within the various avian species varies greatly. They are absent in budgerigars and only rudimentary in other psittacines, passerines, and diurnal raptors. They are present in gallinaceous species, waterfowl, owls, and ratites. Within ratites, ostriches have large sacculated ceca while emus, cassowaries, and rheas have only vestigial ceca.

CLINICAL ADVISORY

Common clinical disorders of the ceca include parasitism, impaction, and typhlitis. Bacterial colitis frequently diagnosed in psittacines may or may not be associated with colon prolapse. It is important to differentiate between a colon and cloacal prolapse since colon prolapses are much more amenable to surgical correction than are cloacal prolapses.

THE CLOACA

The **cloaca** is the termination site for the digestive and urogenital systems (see illustration on this page) and is formed by three compartments. The **coprodeum**, the most cranial and usually largest of the compartments, is where the rectum empties. The **urodeum** is dorsal to the coprodeum and has openings from the ureters and genital ducts. The **protodeum** receives contents from both the coprodeum and urodeum and provides an exit to the outside via the vent. The **vent** (equivalent to the mammalian anus) is controlled by a striated sphincter muscle.

The coprodeum, as an extension of the colon, is an important absorptive organ as well as the last part of the digestive system. When a bird defecates, the **coprourodeal fold,** which separates these two compartments, protrudes through the vent to prevent fecal contamination of the urodeum and proctodeum.

The Cloaca

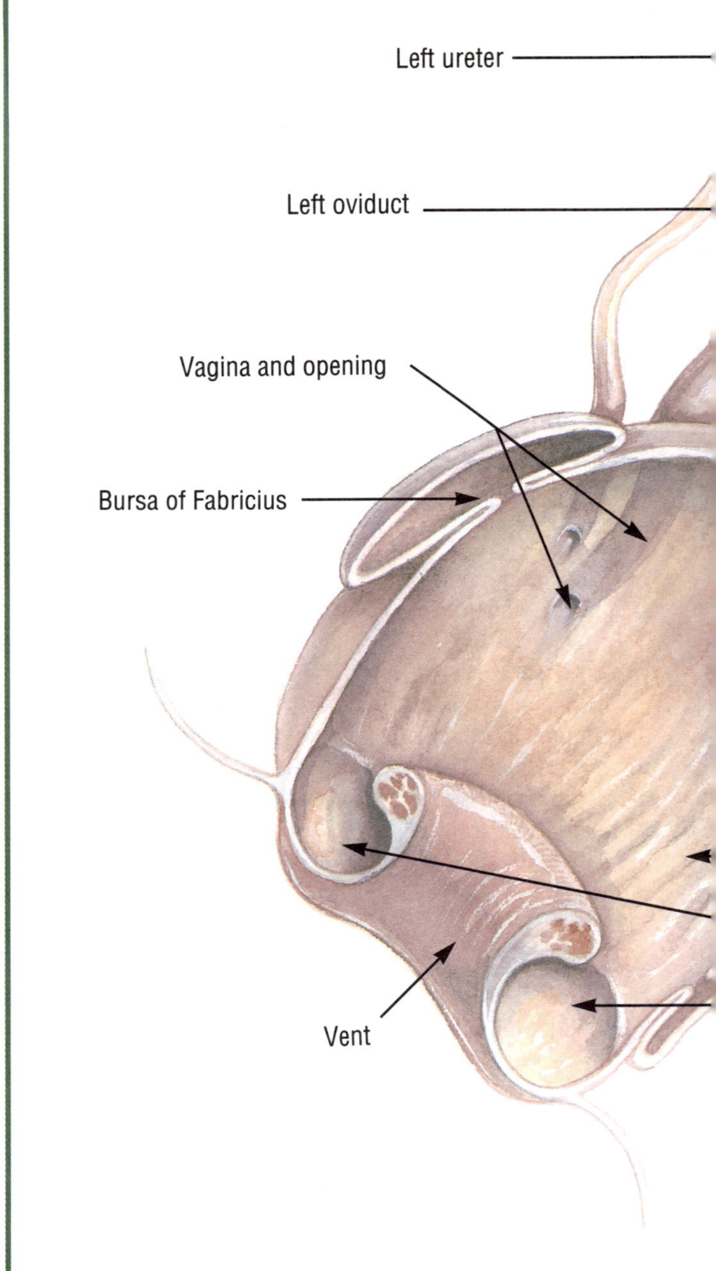

CLINICAL ADVISORY

Cloacal disorders are a common problem in avian gastroenterology. Clinical signs that should alert the clinician to cloacal problems are flatulence, tenesmus, a soiled perivent area, protruding tissue through the vent, and foul smelling feces. Some of the more commonly diagnosed problems of the cloaca and vent are sphincter laceration, tear, blunt trauma, stenosis; cloacal stricture; cloacal impaction; prolapse of the cloaca; cloacal papillomas; and cloacitis. Surgical procedures such as cloacal prolapse amputation or replacement and papilloma resection require a thorough understanding of the anatomy.

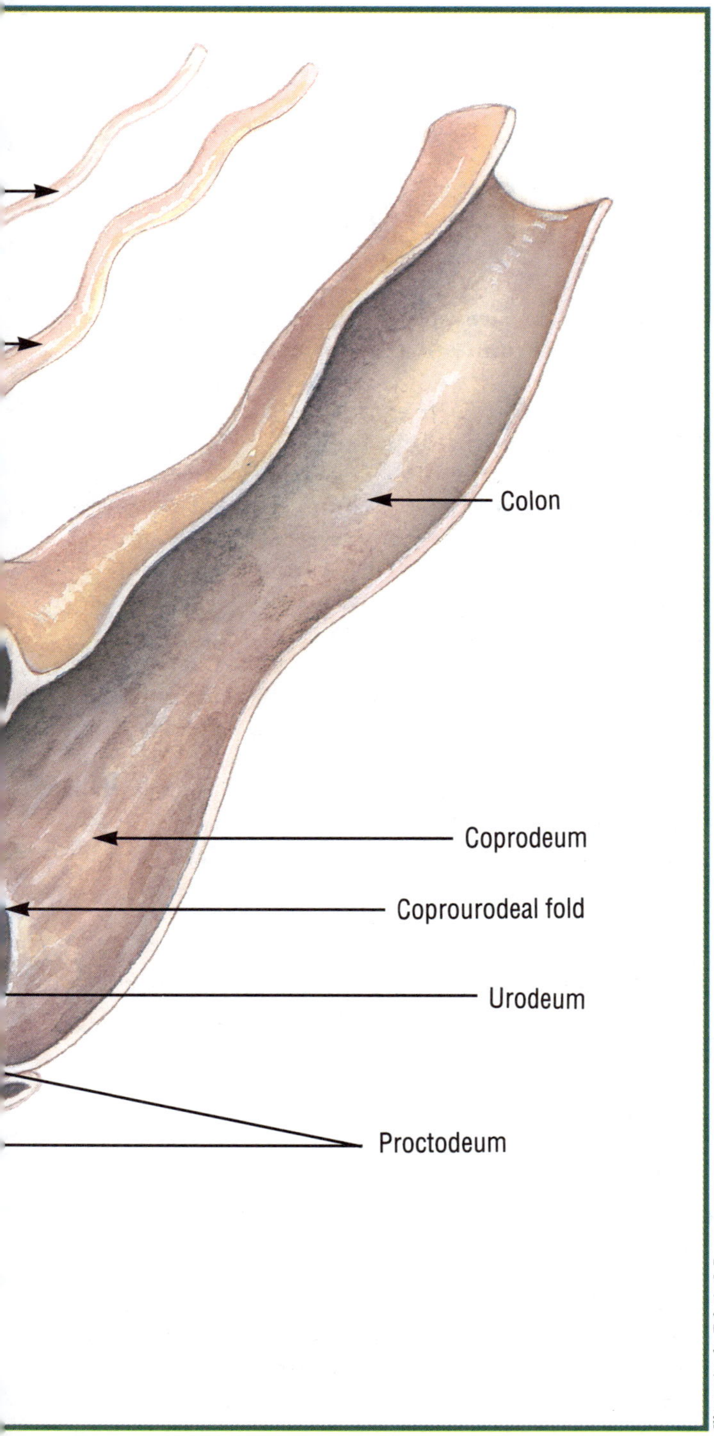

The **bursa of Fabricius**, located in the dorsal median wall of the cloaca (urodeum), is the site of B-cell lymphocyte differentiation. Clinical disorders of the bursa occasionally seen in young birds are hypoplasia, lymphoid depletion, and necrosis (usually associated with infectious bursal disease or papovavirus).

CONCLUSION

The gastrointestinal system of birds is distinct from that of mammals in ways that specifically support its adaptation for flight and reflect variations in the avian diet. The normal flora of psittacines is different from mammals in that it is primarily composed of gram positive organisms.

An understanding of the basic anatomy and physiology of the avian gastrointestinal system is vital for the clinician approaching an avian patient that exhibits signs suggestive of gastrointestinal disease. A systematic approach to diagnosis and treatment, however, is frequently rewarded with a positive outcome.

About the Authors

Dr. Deem and Dr. Bennett are on the staff of the Wildlife and Zoological Medicine Service, Department of Small Animal Clinical Sciences, University of Florida, Gainesville, Florida.

References

Duke GE: Alimentary canal: Anatomy, regulation of feeding, and motility, in Sturkie PD (ed): *Avian Physiology* (ed 4). New York, Springer-Verlag, 1986, pp 269–288.

Duke GE: Alimentary canal: Secretion and digestion, special digestive functions, and absorption, in Sturkie PD (ed): *Avian Physiology* (ed 4). New York, Springer-Verlag, 1986, pp 289–302.

King AS, McLelland J: Coelomic cavities, in *Birds - Their Structure and Function*. Philadelphia, Bailliere Tindall, 1984, pp 79–83.

King AS, McLelland J: Digestive system, in *Birds - Their Structure and Function*. Philadelphia, Bailliere Tindall, 1984, pp 84–109.

Lumeij JT: Gastroenterology, in Ritchie BW, Harrison GJ, Harrison LR (eds): *Avian Medicine: Principles and Application*. Lake Worth, Florida, Wingers Publishing, 1994, pp 482–521.

McKibben JS, Harrison GJ: Clinical anatomy (with emphasis on the Amazon parrot), in Harrison GJ, Harrison LR (eds): *Clinical Avian Medicine and Surgery*. Philadelphia, WB Saunders Co, 1986, pp 31–66.

McLelland J: Digestive system, in *A Color Atlas of Avian Anatomy*. Philadelphia, WB Saunders Co, 1991, pp 47–65.

McLelland J: Peritoneum and peritoneal cavities, in *A Color Atlas of Avian Anatomy*. Philadelphia, WB Saunders Co, 1991, pp 65–88.

RESOURCES

Association of Avian Veterinarians
P.O. Box 811720
Boca Raton, Florida 33481
Phone: (407)393-8901

Avian Gastrointestinal Radiography

Marjorie C. McMillan, DVM
The Windhover Veterinary Center
Walpole, Massachusetts

The Windhover Bird Clinic
Walpole, Massachusetts

Contrast studies of the avian gastrointestinal tract may be necessary for a complete evaluation of gastrointestinal disturbances.

Medical Considerations and Indications for a Gastrointestinal Barium Examination

Since infectious diseases, parasites, toxins, and metabolic disturbances associated with kidney and liver diseases are common causes of gastrointestinal signs in birds, a complete history, thorough physical examination, survey radiographs, and laboratory data are indicated prior to contrast radiography. The primary indications for a gastrointestinal barium examination in birds are acute, chronic, or nonresponsive regurgitation, vomition, or diarrhea; palpation of an abnormal crop or abnormal abdomen; hemorrhagic diarrhea; or abnormal survey radiographic findings such as an obstructive pattern or organ displacement.

When clinically evaluating avian gastrointestinal problems, differentiation between physiologic and pathologic regurgitation and between diarrhea and polyuria is important. Physiologic regurgitation is associated with courtship feeding or affection toward an owner. These birds are healthy, and sexual display often precedes the regurgitation. The regurgitated material contains undigested food and does not have a foul odor. Pathologic regurgitation is not associated with sexual behavior and often has a foul or abnormal odor. These birds regurgitate undigested food or tenacious mucus, often have weight loss, and appear unhealthy.

Polyuria is a more common cause of loose droppings than diarrhea. The fecal portion of the dropping is well formed and surrounded by a clear or opaque, watery urate (Figure 1, A and B). Determination of renal function by uric acid levels and liver involvement by serum aspartate aminotransferase (SAST; SGOT) rather than barium examination is indicated. Change in color of the fecal portion is more common than change in consistency.

Lime green or mustard green feces are associated with hepatic disease and impaired excretion of biliverdin.[1] Brown or hemorrhagic feces usually indicate enteric problems. However, determining whether bloody droppings originate from gastrointestinal or renal problems can be difficult.

Infectious diseases such as psittacosis, colibacillosis, candidiasis, and Pacheco's viral hepatitis are frequent causes of alimentary tract distur-

Originally published in Volume 5, Number 4, April 1983

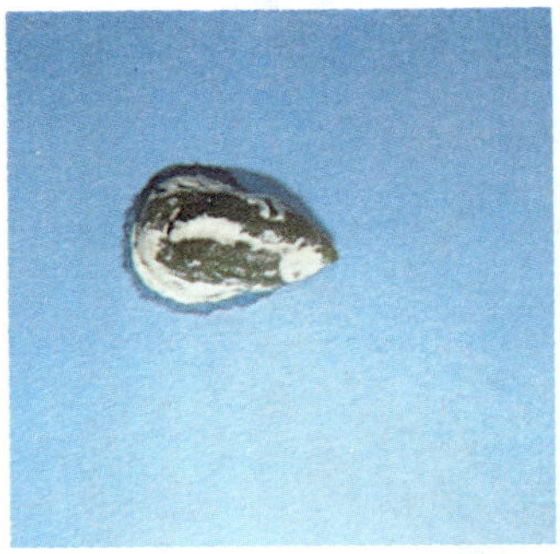

Figure 1A—Normal droppings from an Amazon parrot.

Figure 1A

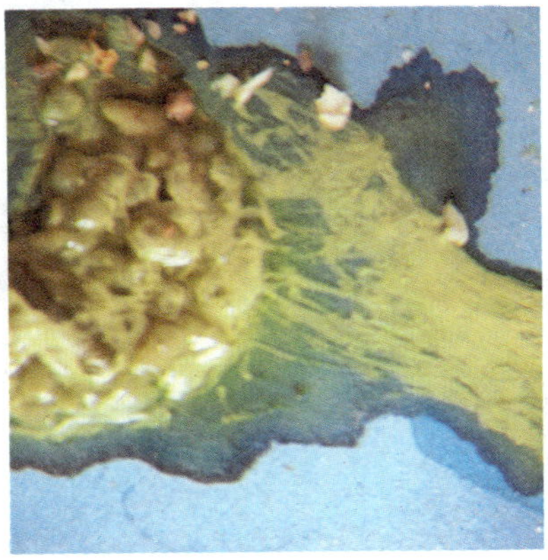

Figure 1B—Lime green droppings associated with abnormal liver and kidney functions.

Figure 1B

bances in newly acquired birds. A crop or cloacal culture helps to identify abnormal bacteria, yeast, and chlamydia. Survey radiographs in these instances show a distended, fluid-filled crop and intestines, hepatomegaly, and enlarged kidneys. Radiographs of an Amazon parrot showing enlarged kidneys and liver secondary to *Escherichia coli* infection are shown in Figure 2.

Ingestion of toxic materials such as heavy metal or plants may produce gastrointestinal signs as well as neurological signs. Lead poisoning due to ingesting paint chips from any source can cause regurgitation, diarrhea, and neurologic signs.[2] Plants, wood, and other foreign material causing local irritation can result in enteritis. Overeating grit, improper hand rearing techniques, or ingesting thread and wool from cage coverings can cause impacted crops.

Gastrointestinal parasites are uncommon in pet birds because many birds are wormed in quarantine stations or aviaries. However, since ascarids, tapeworms, and coccidia are occasionally seen, fecal examination is recommended in birds with gastrointestinal signs. Crop washings in birds with chronic regurgitation can demonstrate parasites as well as fungus and bacteria.

Kidney and liver diseases cause secondary gastrointestinal signs. Infections, neoplasia, and metabolic disorders (lipidosis[3] and hemochromatosis[4]) produce serious impairment of these organs.

Iodine deficiency resulting in thyroid enlargement, which impairs normal crop emptying, is a common cause of regurgitation in the budgerigar as a result of extrinsic crop compression (Figure 3).

Radiographic Technique

Prior to contrast examination, evaluation of survey radiographs for proper radiographic technique, location of the abdominal viscera, presence of gas and fluid, bowel distention, and foreign material is important. The presence of large amounts of gas and/or fluid in the crop often indicates gastrointestinal problems unless respiratory-induced aerophagia is present or the bird is being tube fed. Birds normally do not have gas in the intestinal tract, so that the presence of gas with or without distention is abnormal. Distended fluid-filled intestinal loops indicate gastrointestinal problems except in mynahs and toucans. Because of the high water content in their diet, these birds normally have slightly distended fluid-filled intestinal loops. Any abnormal location of the gastrointestinal tract is noted.

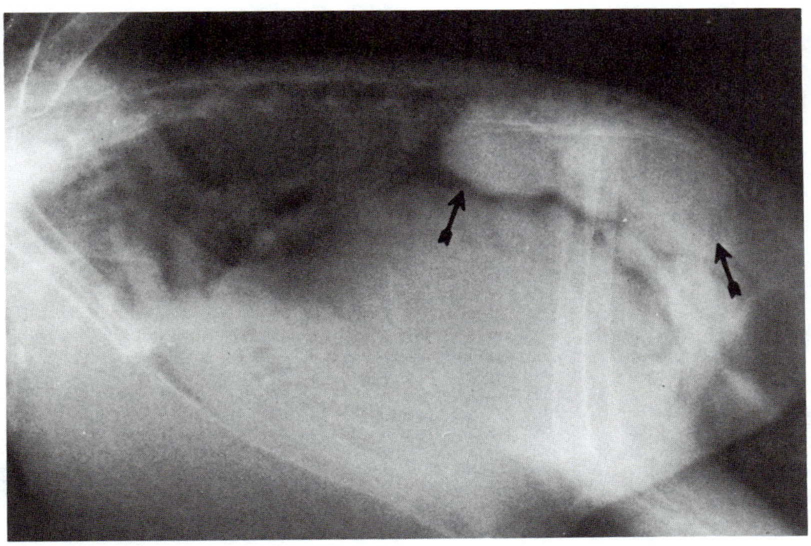

Figure 2A

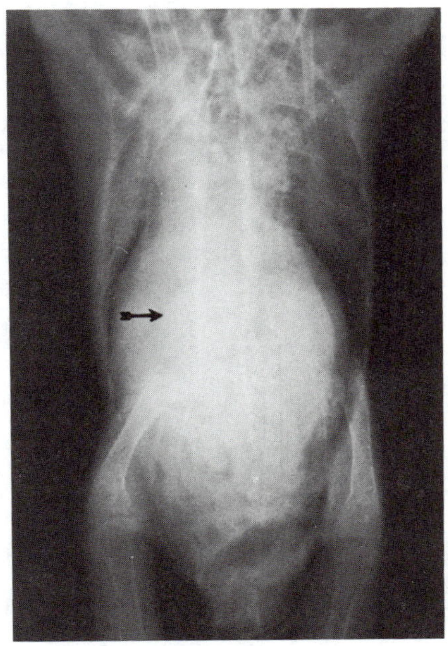

Figure 2B

Figure 2—**(A)** Lateral radiograph of an Amazon parrot showing enlarged kidneys *(arrows)* and liver secondary to *E. coli* infection. **(B)** Ventrodorsal view of the same parrot.

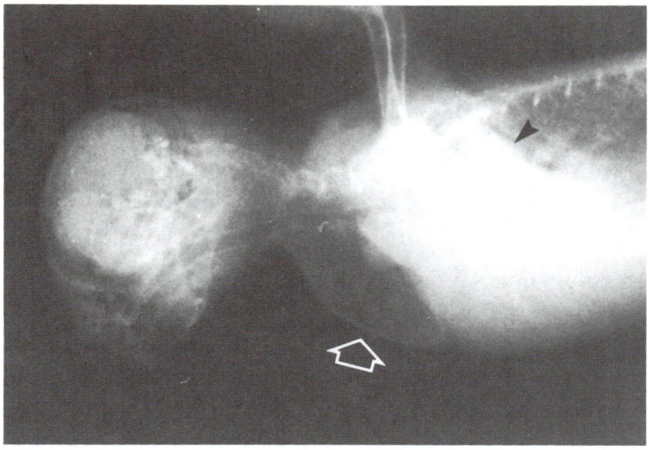

Figure 3—Lateral radiograph of the cranial thoracic area of a budgerigar showing an enlarged thyroid gland *(closed arrow)* and distended crop *(open arrow)*. The soft-tissue density visualized at the thoracic inlet extending into the crop may represent an enlarged thyroid or soft tissue displaced anteriorly by a larger caudal thyroid mass.

Displacement may be due to extrinsic masses or organ enlargement. Radiopaque material is normally present in the gizzard if the bird is receiving grit. Proper positioning[5] and at least two views, lateral and ventrodorsal, are necessary for evaluation. Because exposure factors vary with the size of the bird, film-screen combinations, and radiographic equipment, it is difficult to recommend a specific kilovolt peak, milliamperage, and time. For average parrots (weighing 350 to 500 g) a technique comparable to feline radiographic studies is appropriate. Parakeets require 5 to 10 kvp less and canaries and finches need a 15 kvp decrease. Larger parrots (macaws and large cockatoos) require about the same kilovolt peak setting as cats.[6] For par speed film-screen combinations, a tabletop technique at 100 mA for 1/60 second at 40 in. provides diagnostic radiographs.

Currently, a rare-earth ultradetailed film-screen[a] combination provides the most satisfactory avian radiographs. This film-screen combination requires a fivefold increase in the milliampere seconds over the par speed combination. Single-screen mammography packs with single-emulsion film can be substituted for the cassette system.

Tranquilizers and anesthetics are usually not necessary for radiographic procedures. Since the effects of these agents on gastrointestinal motility in birds is not thoroughly known, it is better not to use such agents when evaluating the gastrointestinal tract. A Plexiglas device[b] in combination with sandbags and tape provides adequate restraint and eliminates the need for personnel in the room during an exposure.

Procedure

The barium study is often tailored to the individual bird according to the history and clinical signs. If the crop is the area of concern, a double-contrast examination is indicated. Food and water are withheld for about four hours. Sometimes small amounts of seeds may remain in the crop or proventriculus. If the quantity is small, the study is still undertaken, though it is best to have the gastrointestinal tract empty. Barium sulfate suspension is administered orally into the crop[d] via a stomach tube (Figure 4). The size of the bird determines the volume of barium and whether an oral speculum is necessary (Table I). When the tube is palpated in the crop, a volume of barium is slowly given to gently distend the crop. If a double-contrast study of the crop is performed, half the amount of barium is given and the remainder of the volume is given as air.

Radiographs are made in the ventrodorsal and lateral planes immediately after administration of contrast medium and 30 minutes, 60 minutes, 2 hours, 4 hours, and 24 hours later. Timing of the radiographs may vary

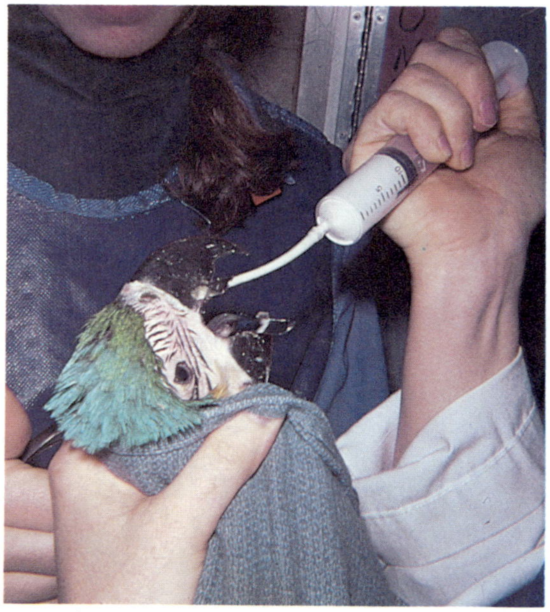

Figure 4—Administration of barium to a blue and gold macaw using a nasal speculum.

[a]Kodak Lanex fine single or Kodak Ortho M-1, Eastman Kodak Co., Rochester, NY 14650.

[b]B.D. Creations, Lindenhurst, NY 11757.

[c]Liquid Polibar 55% W/W, E-Z-M Co., Inc., Westbury, NY 11590.

[d]In birds without crops, such as canaries, finches, and mynahs, the barium is given into the esophagus or proventriculus.

TABLE I

VOLUME OF BARIUM SULFATE IN AVIAN GASTROINTESTINAL RADIOGRAPHY[6]

Bird	*Volume (ml)*	*Tube (French)*	*Type of Speculum*
Canary, finch	0.25–0.5	5	None
Parakeet	1.0–3.0	5	None
Cockatiel, conure, lovebird	3.0–5.0	8	Hemostat
Smaller parrots	10.0	10	Nasal
Larger parrots	15.0	12	Nasal

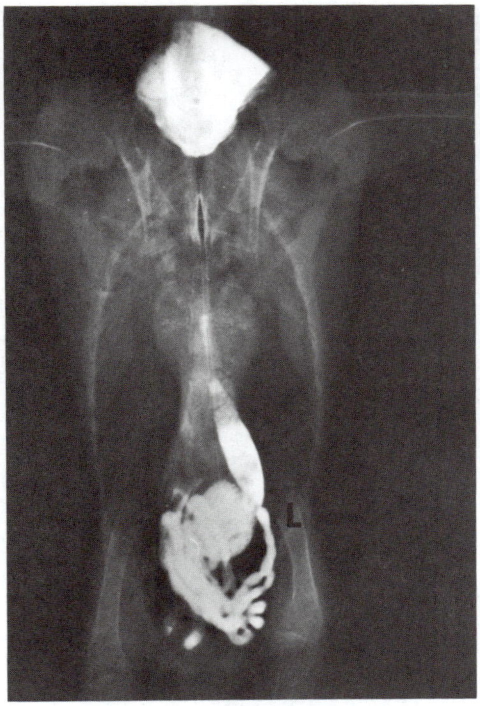

Figure 5A

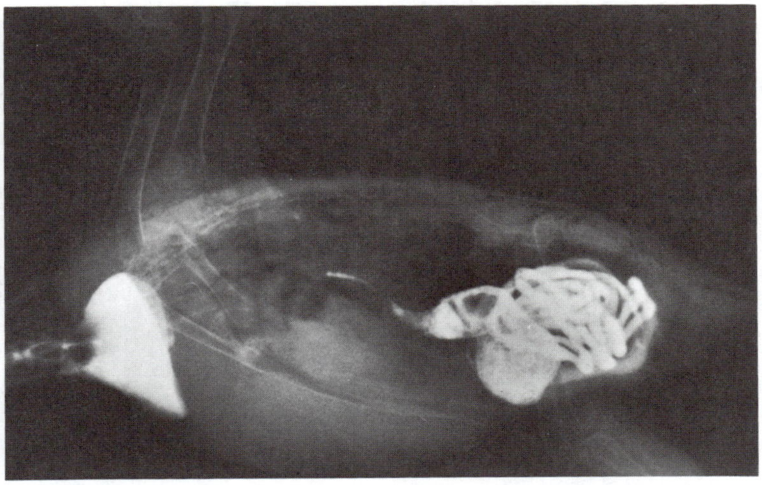

Figure 5B

Figure 5 (**A** and **B**)—A normal barium series. One-hour radiographs show filling of the crop, proventriculus, gizzard, and small intestines with barium. The radiolucent area in the proventriculus is a gas bubble.

depending on whether the upper gastrointestinal tract or lower region is of concern. Results of radiographs during the study may also alter the scheduling.

In normal studies in the immediate radiographs, the crop is filled with barium and a small amount of barium may be present in the esophagus and proventriculus (Figure 5). In 15 to 30 minutes, the proventriculus and gizzard and about half of the small intestines are filled. There is a decrease in the amount of contrast in the crop. By one hour the barium has filled the gastrointestinal tract. In four hours, the crop should be completely empty, although varying amounts of barium may remain in the proventriculus, gizzard, and intestines.

Radiographic Interpretation

Changes in transit time, thickening and/or irregularity of mucosal lining, distention, displacement of the gastrointestinal tract, and filling defects are radiographic signs associated with gastrointestinal disorders. When evaluating the significance of radiographic changes in contrast examinations, persistence of a lesion in subsequent radiographs is important. Motility in a dynamic system such as the gastrointestinal tract causes normal anatomic variation, which when visualized on only one radiograph leads to misinterpretation.

Delay in transit time results from functional or mechanical ileus. Mechanical ileus from extraluminal lesions or intraluminal masses such as foreign bodies is unusual in birds (Figure 6).

Functional ileus associated with severe gram-negative gastroenteritis is a more common cause of delayed transit of barium. Distention of the entire gastrointestinal tract is observed with severe gram-negative infections rather than obstruction (Figure 7). In addition to infection, lead toxicity, parasites, and egg peritonitis are associated with functional ileus. An increase in transit time has not been observed.

Thickening and irregularity of the crop and esophagus (Figure 8) are associated with candidiasis. Mucosal irregularity from neoplasia is difficult to distinguish from gastrointestinal fungal infections (Figures 9 and 10). Pathologic filling defects are unusual but do occur with neoplasia and fungal granuloma (Figure 11). Commonly, residual seed coated with barium is mistaken for filling defects. Thickening of the proventriculus, gizzard, and intestines has not been visualized radiographically.

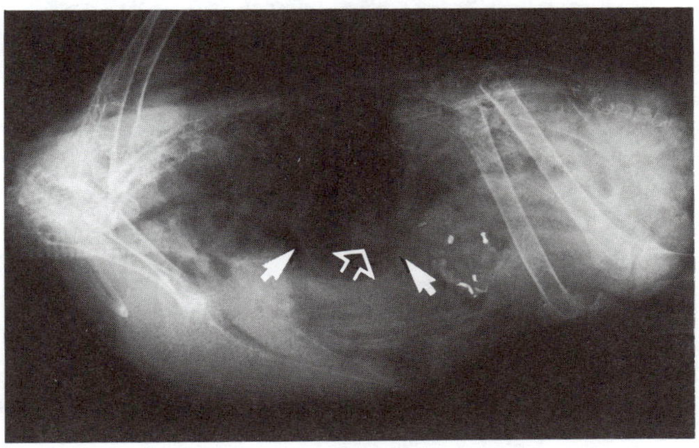

Figure 6—Distention of the proventriculus *(closed arrows)* with gas secondary to obstruction in a greater sulfur crested cockatoo. This parrot had ingested electric wire. If the type of heavy metal cannot be determined through historical information, the possibility of heavy-metal intoxication such as lead poisoning, in addition to obstruction, should also be considered. Foreign material *(open arrow)* is present in the lumen. Metallic foreign material is present in the gizzard.

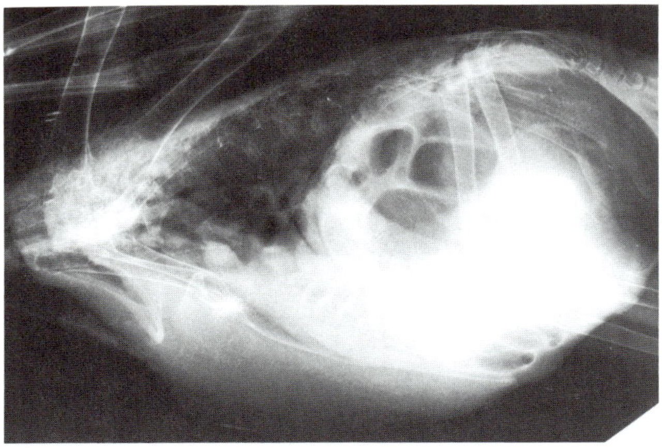

Figure 7A

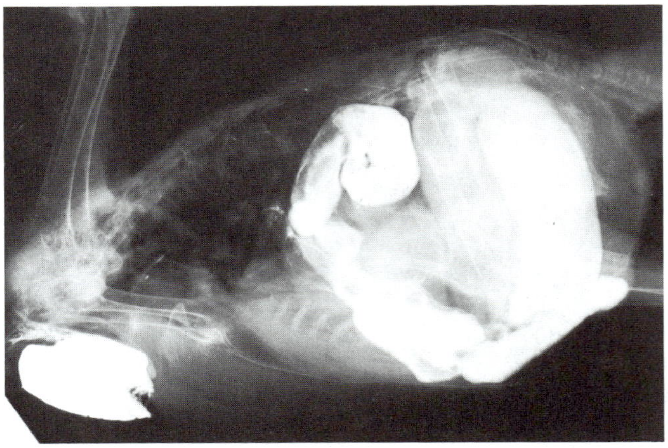

Figure 7B

Figure 7—**(A)** Survey radiographs of a blue and gold macaw showing marked distention of the gastrointestinal tract with gas. **(B)** In the one-hour radiograph, there is displacement of the duodenum and distention of the loops of intestines with barium. On autopsy, there was no evidence of obstruction. Serositis and associated gram-negative infection produced a functional ileus.

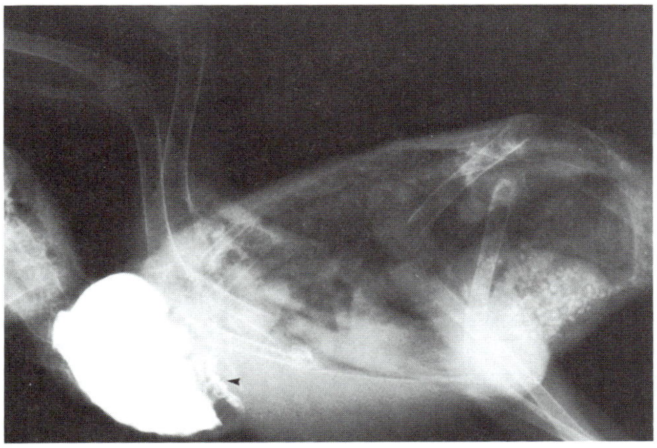

Figure 8A

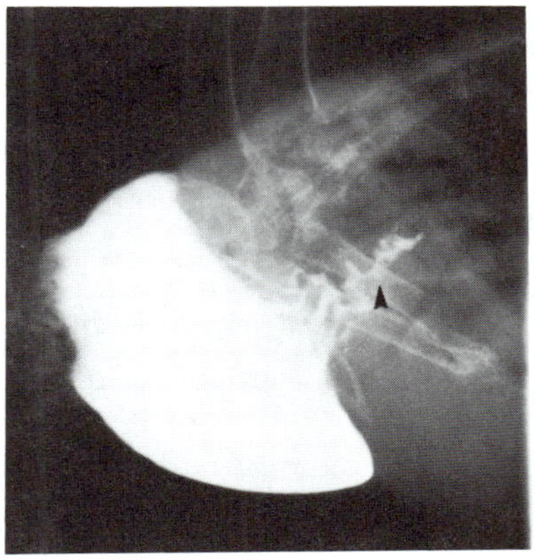

Figure 8B

Figure 8—**(A)** A double-contrast study of the crop showing thickening and irregularity of the crop wall due to candidiasis *(arrow)*. **(B)** Esophageal abnormality in same bird also due to candidiasis *(arrow)*.

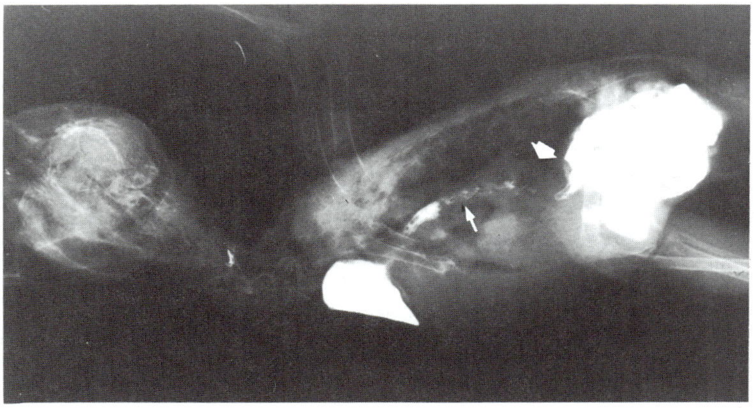

Figure 9—Squamous cell carcinoma causing a nodular mass *(large arrow)* and mucosal irregularity *(small arrow)* in the esophagus and proventriculus of a 47-year-old Amazon parrot.

Localized distention of the crop occurs secondary to enlarged thyroids, lead toxicity, and obstruction in the proventriculus, gizzard, or upper intestines. Distended atonic cloacae can occur secondary to spinal trauma and neoplastic involvement of sacral nerves.

Displacement of the gastrointestinal tract due to extrinsic mass or organ enlargement may be visualized by barium contrast examination. Viewing the direction

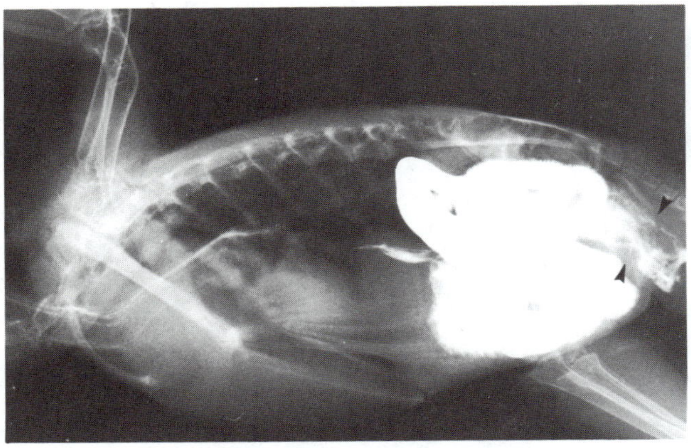

Figure 10—Filling defects and mucosal abnormality *(arrows)* in the rectum of a mynah with an adenocarcinoma.

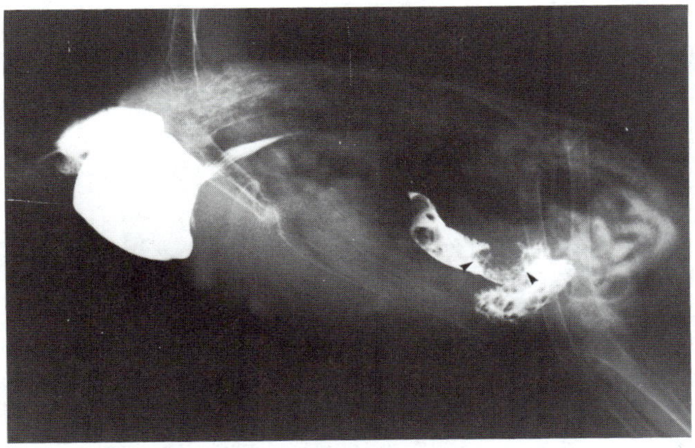

Figure 11—*Aspergillus* granuloma in an Amazon parrot *(arrows)* causing a large filling defect in the proventriculus.

in which the gastrointestinal tract is displaced will aid in determining which organ or organs may be involved (Figure 12).

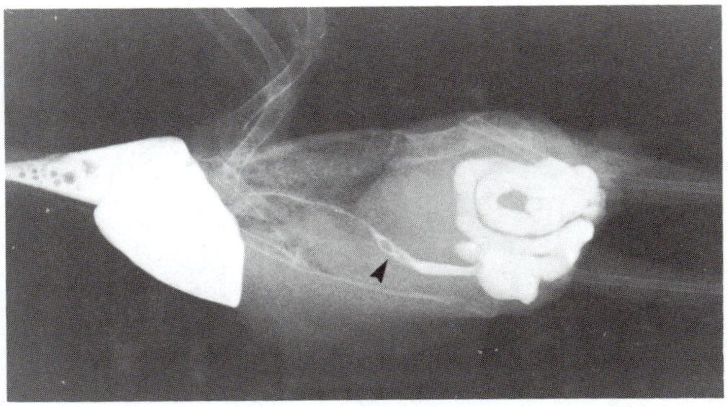

Figure 12—Ventral displacement of the esophagus and proventriculus *(arrow)* in a budgerigar from a renal tumor.

Summary

Barium contrast examination is indicated for thorough evaluation of avian gastrointestinal disturbances. An appropriate diagnostic workup should precede radiographic examination. Findings on survey radiographs suggest that gastrointestinal problems can be pursued with a barium study. In the author's experience, the most common finding on survey radiographs indicating a gastrointestinal abnormality is distention of the gastrointestinal tract with gas and fluid. Obstructive ileus causing this pattern is unusual, and other causes such as infection and toxicity should be considered. Delayed transit time, distention of intestines, and mucosal irregularities are common lesions observed during the barium series.

REFERENCES

1. McDonald SE, Bayer EV: Psittacosis in pet birds. *Calif Vet* 4:6-17, 1981.
2. Woerpel RW, Rosskopf WJ: Heavy-metal intoxication in caged birds. Part 1. *Compend Contin Educ Pract Vet* 4:729-738, 1982.
3. Leav I, et al: A naturally occupying lipidosis in shell parakeets, *Melopsittacus undulatus. Lab Invest* 18(4):433-437, 1968.
4. Lowestine LJ, Petrak ML: Iron pigment in the livers of birds, in Montali RJ, Migaki G (eds): *The Comparative Pathology of Zoo Animals.* Washington, DC, Smithsonian Institute Press, 1980, pp 127-135.
5. Evans SM: Avian radiographic diagnosis. *Compend Contin Educ Pract Vet* 3:660-666, 1981.
6. McMillan MC: Avian radiology, in Petrak ML (ed): *Diseases of Cage and Aviary Birds.* Philadelphia, Lea & Febiger, 1982, pp 329-360.

Radiographic Diagnosis of Avian Abdominal Disorders

Marjorie C. McMillan, DVM
The Windhover Veterinary Center
Walpole, Massachusetts

Many avian diseases create radiographic abnormalities, and failure to recognize them may lead to misdiagnoses and inappropriate treatment. Radiographic examination, however, must complement an accurate history, thorough physical examination, and clinical laboratory data. It is not a substitute for these procedures. The interpretation and significance of certain radiographic abnormalities vary with species, age, sex, and duration in captivity. In addition, the frequency of certain radiographic findings varies with the species of bird under consideration. For example, traumatic injury to the extremities and skull predominates in raptors, whereas infectious diseases and nutritional deficiencies are common in exotic birds.

The radiographic technique used for birds as well as the normal radiographic anatomy of birds are reported in the literature[1,2]; specifically, birds and mammals differ in that birds lack an omentum, well-developed mesenteric attachments, and a falciform ligament. Because of short mesenteric attachments, the abdominal organs of birds remain relatively fixed in position. Fat deposits between organs are minimal, and thus differentiation of specific organ margins is more difficult in birds than it is in dogs and cats. Because only a rudimentary, incomplete diaphragm is present, the cardiac silhouette and bilobed liver blend into a homogeneous soft tissue that has an hourglass appearance on ventrodorsal radiographs. The soft tissue density of abdominal viscera contrasts with the radiolucent surrounding air sacs.

Radiographic findings associated with abdominal disorders are:

1. Changes in the size, shape, position, and density of specific organs
2. Homogeneous abdominal density
3. Loss of abdominal air sac space
4. Visualization of a mass.

Radiographic Abnormalities

Hepatomegaly is a common radiographic finding in psittacines. In a lateral radiograph, the liver normally does not extend beyond the sternum. If the bird is positioned properly for a ventrodorsal view, the liver normally does not extend laterally beyond a line parallel to the sternum connecting the scapula and acetabulum (Figure 1).

Originally published in Volume 8, Number 9, September 1986

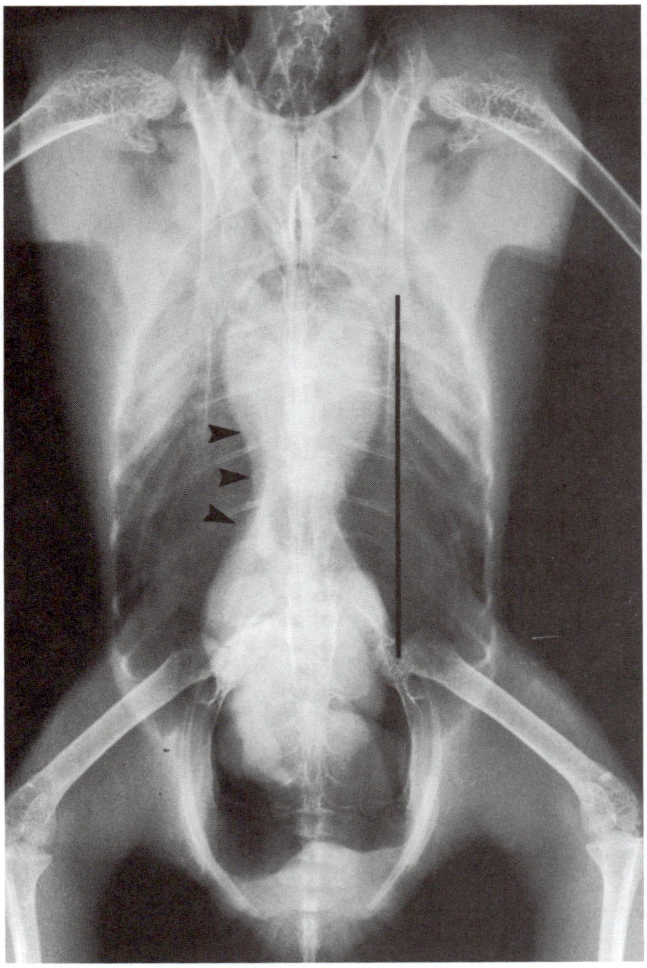

An enlarged liver may cause cranial displacement of the cardiac silhouette, dorsal displacement of the proventriculus, and caudodorsal displacement of the ventriculus. The hourglass configuration of the cardiohepatic silhouette is altered, and the liver is visualized as bulging into the abdominal air sacs. Many viral diseases[3-6] (such as Pacheco's disease, REO [respiratory enteric orphans] disease, Newcastle disease virus, and papovavirus) and bacterial infections (particularly gram-negative organisms, mycobacteria,[7,8] and chlamydia) may result in hepatomegaly (Table I). Often, splenomegaly also is present (Figure 2). Parasites are an uncommon cause of liver disease, although toxoplasmosis in mynahs (*Acridotheres* spp.)[9] and liver flukes in a sulphur-crested cockatoo (*Kakatoe galerita*)[10] have been reported. Such metabolic abnormalities as hemochromatosis in mynahs (*Gracula religiosa*),[11,12] lipidosis in parakeets (*Melopsittacus undulatus*),[13] fatty degeneration, and gout may involve the liver, spleen, kidneys, and heart. Primary and metastatic neoplasia occur most commonly in parakeets; while lymphoma[14,15] (Figure 3), biliary adenocarcinoma, hepatocellular carcinoma,[16] and meta-

Figure 1—Ventrodorsal radiograph of a normal Amazon parrot demonstrates the hourglass appearance of a cardiohepatic silhouette (*arrows*) and the lateral extent of liver (*solid line*). Loss of hourglass configuration or extension of liver lobes beyond the solid line indicates hepatomegaly.

Figure 2—Lateral radiograph of a blue and gold macaw shows splenomegaly *(large arrows)* and kidney enlargement *(curved arrow)* associated with psittacosis.

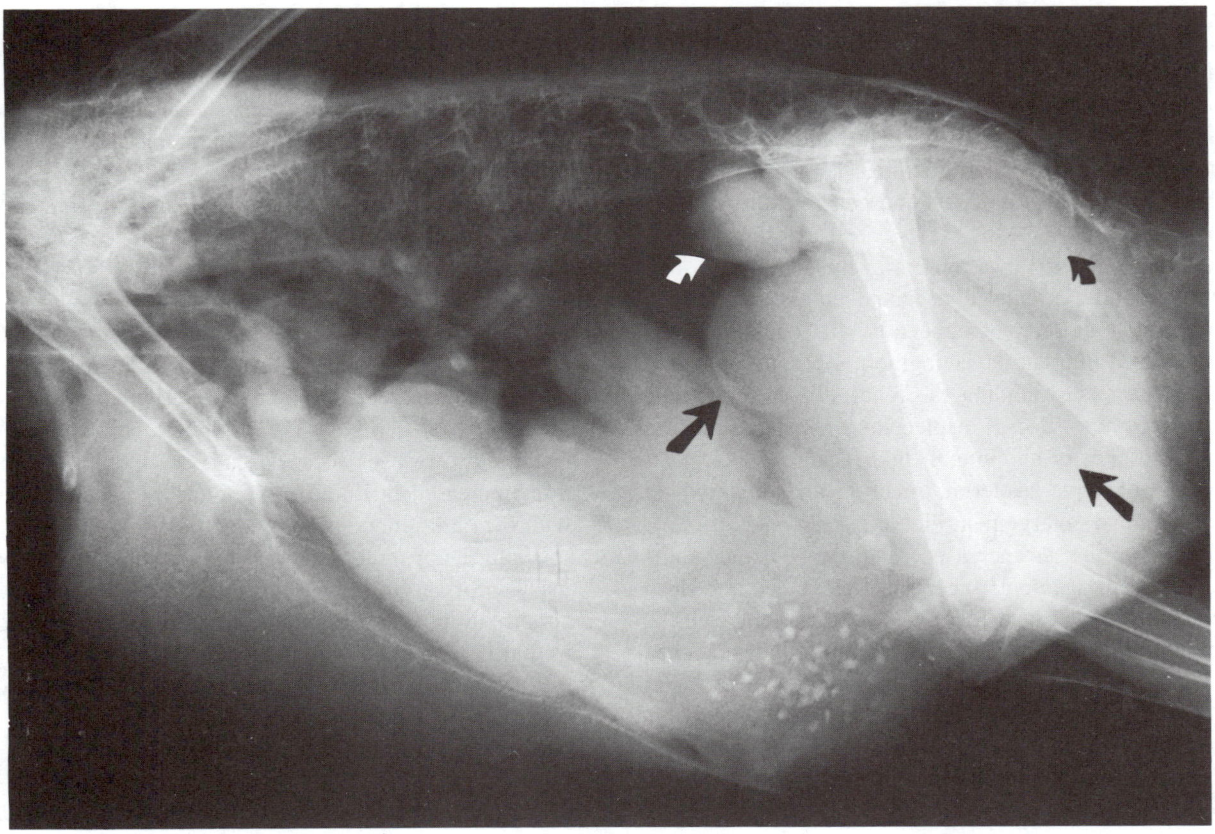

TABLE I
Causes of Hepatomegaly, Splenomegaly, and Nephromegaly

Hepatomegaly	*Splenomegaly*	*Nephromegaly*
Infectious	**Infectious**	**Infectious**
Viral	Viral	Bacterial
Bacterial	Bacterial	Chlamydial
Chlamydial	Chlamydial	
Mycobacterial	Mycobacterial	**Neoplastic**
Fungal		Adenocarcinoma
	Neoplastic	Embryonal nephroma
Neoplastic	Lymphoma	
Primary	Hemangiosarcoma	**Metabolic**
Hepatocellular carcinoma	Fibrosarcoma	Gout
Biliary adenocarcinoma	Leiomyosarcoma	Dehydration
Fibrosarcoma		Lipidosis
Hemangiosarcoma	**Metabolic**	
Hepatoma	Lipidosis	**Cystic**
Lymphoma	Hemochromatosis	
Metastatic		**Toxic**
Adenocarcinoma		Lead
Fibrosarcoma		
Melanoma		
Parasitic		
Toxoplasmosis		
Flukes (cestodes)		
Metabolic		
Hemochromatosis		
Lipidosis		
Fatty degeneration		
Gout		

static adenocarcinoma[16] have been reported in larger psittacines. In mynahs, hepatomas occur in association with hemochromatosis.[17]

The spleen usually is not apparent radiographically (Figure 4). Splenomegaly, often in combination with hepatomegaly, occurs in systemic infections, neoplasia, and such metabolic disorders as lipidosis and hemochromatosis (Table I).

The kidneys are firmly adherent to the synsacrum, have smoothly rounded cranial and caudal poles, are flattened dorsoventrally, and are surrounded by air. The kidneys are best visualized in a lateral radiograph. Obliteration of normal air density surrounding the renal silhouette indicates renal enlargement, dorsal displacement of abdominal viscera, or presence of abdominal fluid (Figure 5). Nephritis from gram-negative bacterial infection and chlamydiosis may cause renal enlargement (Table I).

Dehydration causes increased renal density and, sometimes, renal enlargement. Incomplete clearance and flushing of renal tubules lead to "renal constipation," with an accumulation of uric acid crystals in the kidneys.[18] Theoretically, any condition resulting in impaired renal clearance of uric acid crystals could result in nephromegaly and increased renal density. In addition, changes in kidney size and density are seen in psittacines in association with acute hemolysis caused by lead toxicity.[19] These changes probably are caused by hemoglobin blockage of kidney tubules, with resultant decreased renal tubular function. In contrast to generalized nephromegaly observed in the conditions mentioned, kidney tumors usually cause enlargement of only the cranial or caudal pole with ventral displacement of the ventriculum[2,20] (Figure 6).

Hormonal changes result in cyclic atrophy and recrudescence of the gonads. Hypertrophied testicles are visualized as symmetric enlargements in the ventrodorsal view and as superimposed circular soft tissue masses, cranial and ventral to the kidneys, in the lateral radiograph (Figure 6). An enlarged oviduct results in loss of air sac density below the kidneys and increased soft tissue density in the dorsal abdominal region (Figure 7). Pathologic enlargement of the testicles and ovaries occurs because of neoplasia.[21] In addition, increased medullary bone density occurs in females with ovarian tumors[22] and oviduct abnormalities.

Changes apparent on survey radiographs provide preliminary information for certain disease processes; however, abnormalities of the gastrointestinal tract are best evaluated by barium-contrast examination.[23] As an example, gas in the gastrointestinal tract of birds is abnormal. If an external source of gas (such as tube feeding or aerophagia) is eliminated, a gastrointestinal abnormality is the most likely cause.

Proventricular dilatation,[24] also called *blue and gold ma-*

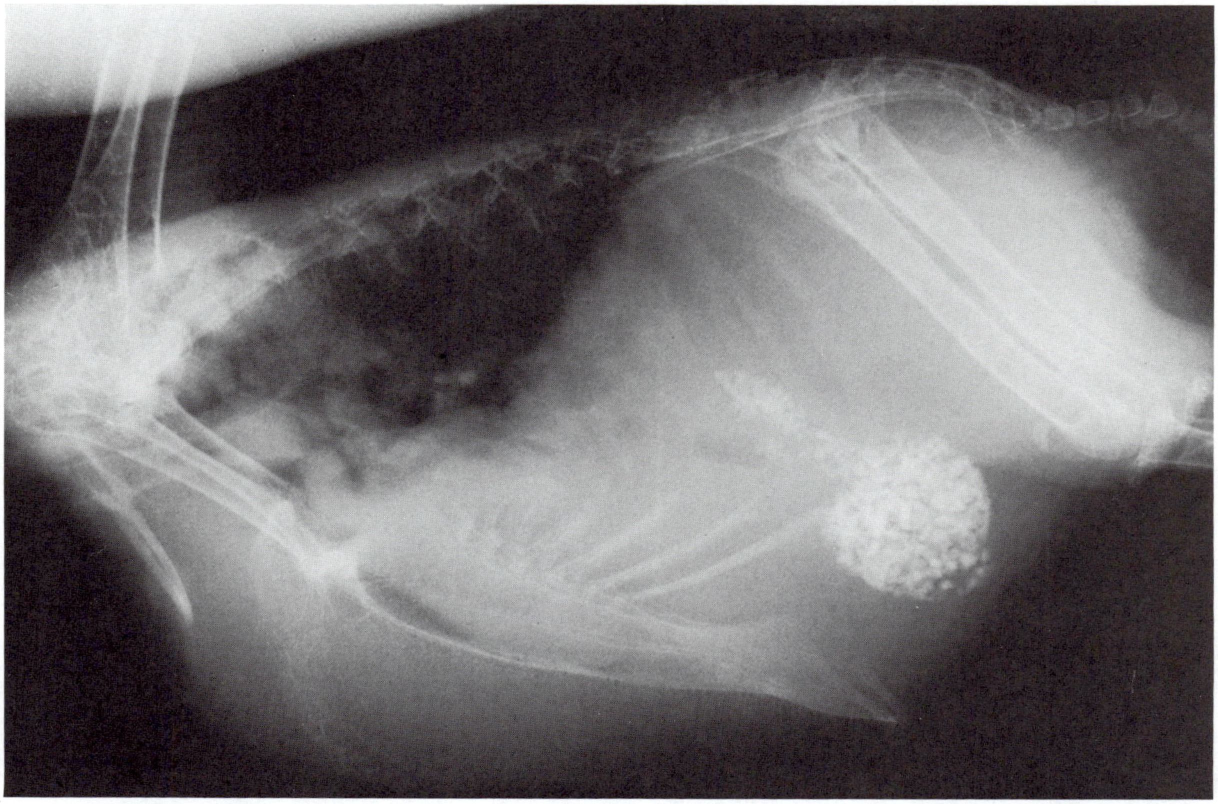

Figure 3A

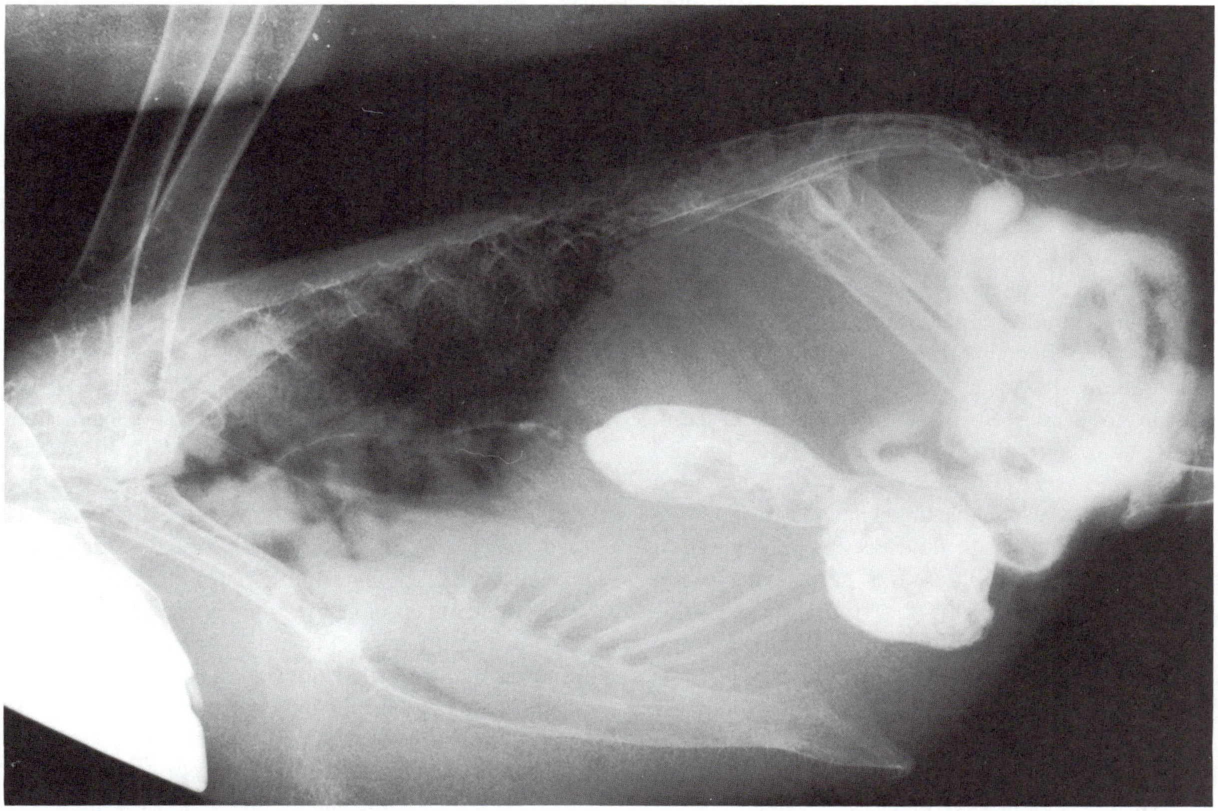

Figure 3B

Figure 3—(**A**) Survey lateral radiograph of an African gray parrot shows dorsal displacement of the proventriculus and caudodorsal displacement of the ventriculus by an enlarged liver. The homogeneous soft tissue mass in the dorsal abdomen obliterates the air sac space below the kidneys and between the lungs and viscera. (**B**) After one hour, the barium-contrast series indicated that the intestines were displaced caudally by a dorsal mass, which was an enlarged spleen. Hepatic and splenic enlargement were caused by lymphosarcoma.

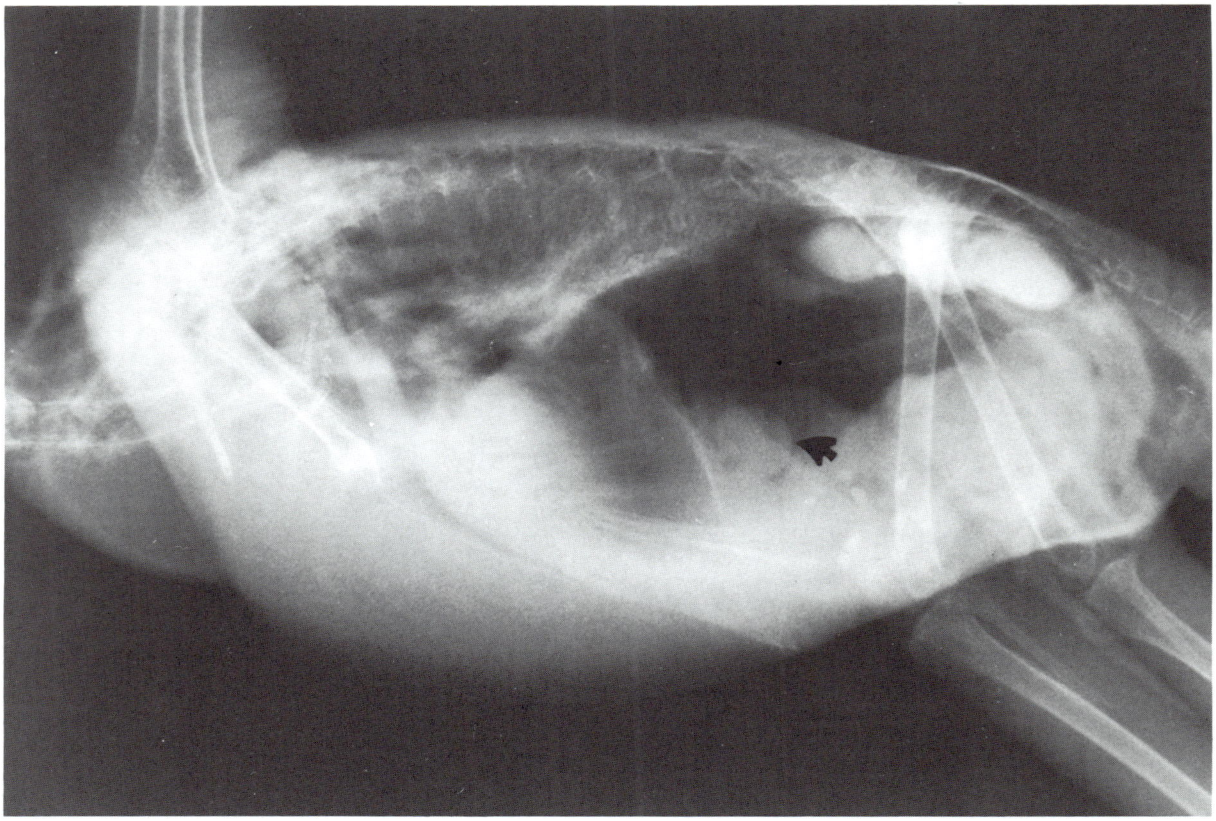

Figure 4—The normal size, shape, and location of the spleen (*arrow*) are apparent in this lateral radiograph of an African gray parrot. Peribronchial infiltrate is present in the hilar and mid region of the caudal lung.

caw syndrome[25] or *infiltrative splanchnic neuropathy*,[3] causes functional ileus resulting in marked gastrointestinal distention. Birds are presented with weight loss, uncontrollable regurgitation, history of passing undigested seeds, and dehydration. In all except a few cases, the disease is fatal. Radiographic changes range from slight distention of the proventriculus with gas to marked distention of the gastrointestinal tract (Figure 8). Barium may persist in the intestinal tract up to 72 hours after administration. The proventriculus is massively distended and may contain food or gas. The ventriculus also is distended and thin walled. The crop is usually distended with fluid. Histologically there is diffuse mononuclear cell infiltration of intrinsic and extrinsic splanchnic nerves supplying the crop, proventriculus, ventriculus, and duodenum. Although most commonly reported in the blue and gold macaw (*Ara ararauna*), the disease occurs in other macaws (e.g., the green-winged macaw [*Ara chloroptera*] and hyacinth macaw [*Hyacinthinus anodorhynchus*]) as well as in cockatoos, conures, and African gray parrots (*Psittacus erithacus*).

Functional ileus also occurs in association with inflammatory processes involving the abdomen. In birds with egg peritonitis, a generalized increased fluid density obscures abdominal detail and dilated gas-filled bowel loops may be apparent. Intestinal serosal adhesions associated with egg peritonitis also result in decreased intestinal motility (Figure 9). Gas-distended loops of intestine are also visualized in conjunction with the massive ascites commonly seen in mynahs with liver failure from hemochromatosis.

Gas and fluid distention of the intestinal tract caused by mechanical ileus can occur from a foreign body obstruction (Figure 10); stricture; neoplasia; and extrinsic masses involving the thyroid gland, oviduct, and spleen. Impaction of the ventriculus with grit results in upper gastrointestinal obstruction (Figure 11). Often these birds have been fed inappropriately sized grit, allowed to eat freely after being deprived of grit for a long period, or have a deprived appetite because of an underlying illness. Radiographs show an increased amount of grit firmly compressed in the ventriculus. Grit also may be visualized in the proventriculus and crop. Barium-contrast examination shows delayed emptying of the crop. Small amounts of barium may pass from the crop, through the ventriculus, and into the intestinal tract.

Atonic distention of the cloaca occurs with spinal trauma and infiltrative neoplastic processes involving the sacral nerves (Figure 12). Obstruction caused by cloacal polyps, papillomas, or adenocarcinoma also causes distention. Laying hens normally have a more dilated cloaca to facilitate passage of eggs; this should not be considered pathologic.

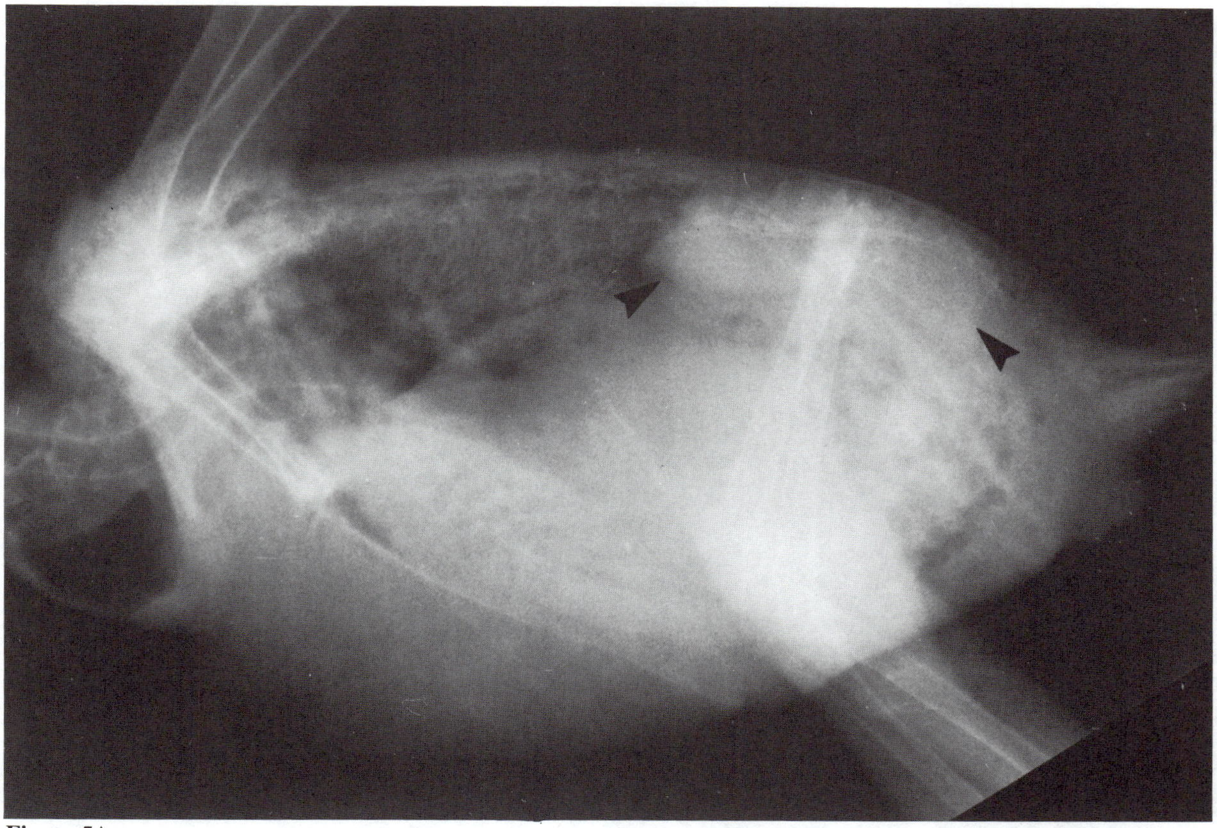

Figure 5A

Figure 5—(**A**) Kidney enlargement (*arrows*) with loss of air sac space ventral and cranial to kidneys is best demonstrated in a lateral radiograph. (**B**) Enlarged cranial kidney pole (*arrows*) is apparent in this ventrodorsal view. Nephromegaly in this Amazon parrot was caused by nephritis from *Escherichia coli* infection.

Additional Imaging Techniques

Urography,[2,26] ultrasonography,[27] and gastrointestinal barium-contrast studies[23] may aid in evaluating abdominal masses.

Urography outlines the kidneys, ureters, and cloaca. Radiographs taken at 10 seconds, 60 seconds, and 2 minutes after administration of contrast material provide the most useful information.[26] Irregularity of kidney size and shape and distention of the cloaca associated with renal neoplasia may be visualized by this means (Figures 6 and 12).

The presence of air sacs makes ultrasound examination difficult in birds. When abdominal fluid obliterates the air sacs, however, abdominal masses may be detected.

A gastrointestinal barium-contrast series helps the veterinarian localize abdominal masses and evaluate mechanical and functional ileus. Displacement of portions of the gastrointestinal tract by extrinsic masses, intraluminal masses, and hypomotility has been reported.

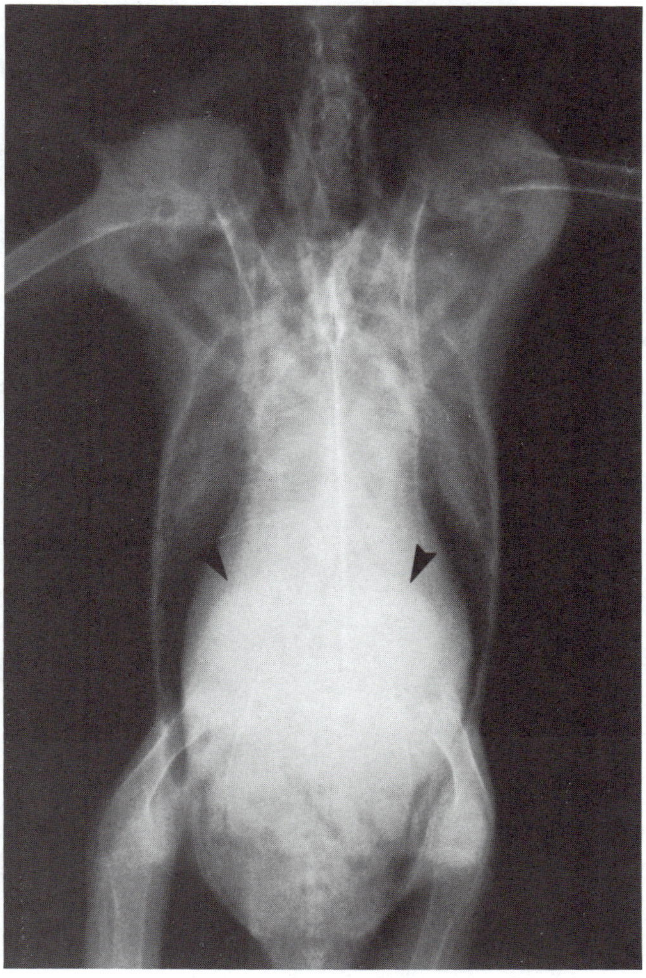

Figure 5B

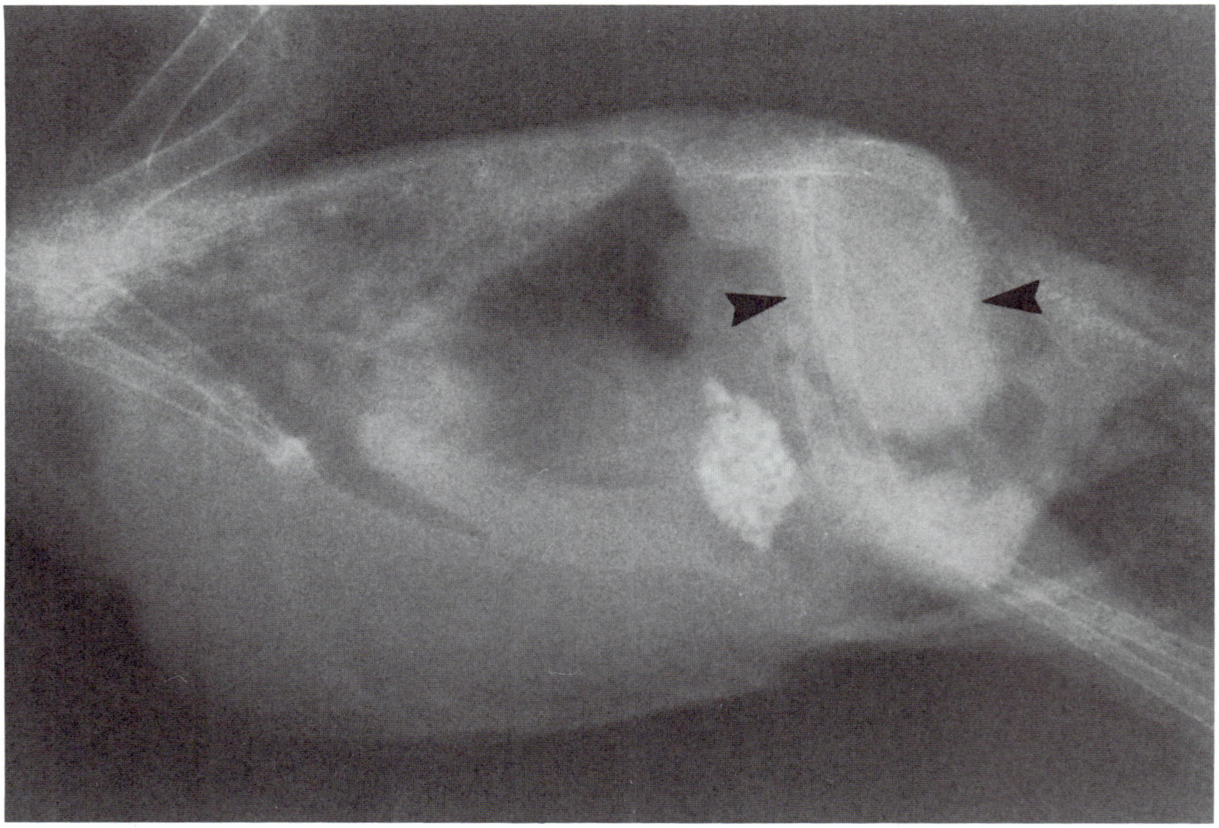

Figure 6A

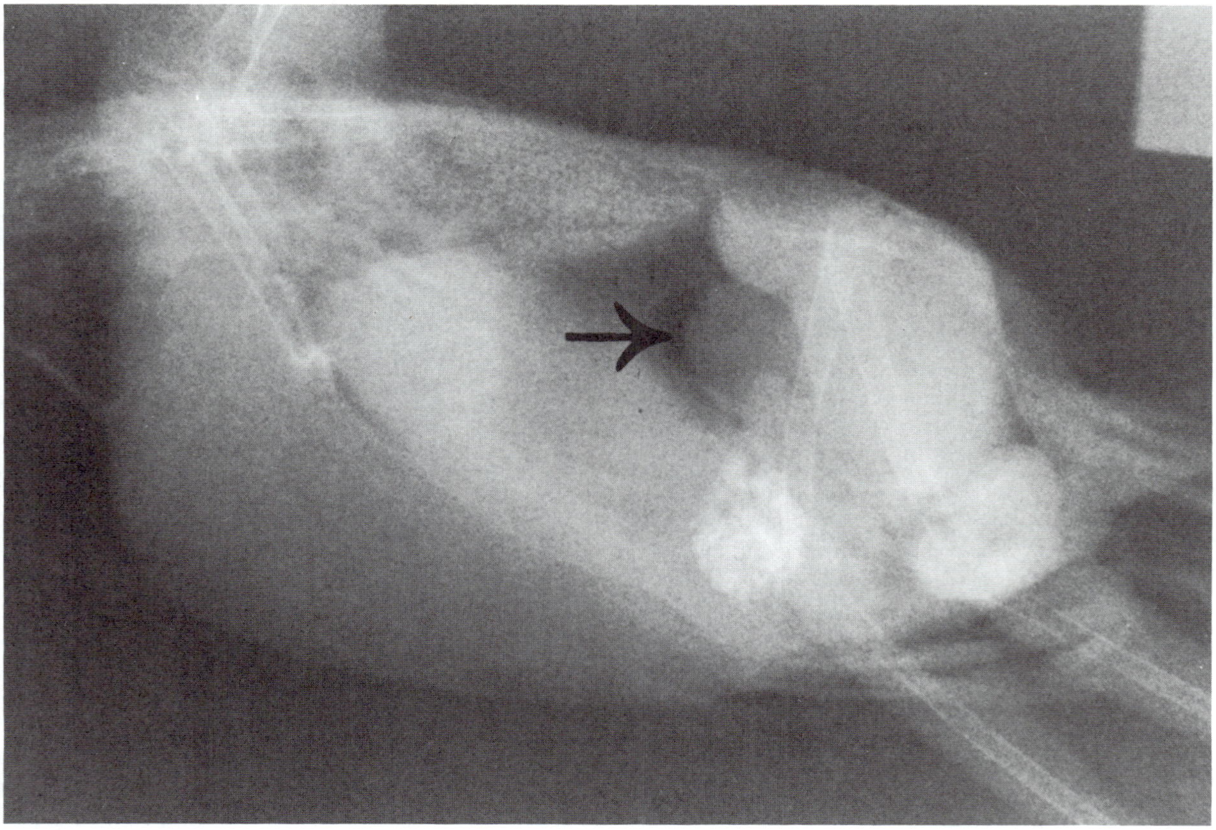

Figure 6B

Figure 6—(**A**) Renal adenocarcinoma (*arrows*) in this budgerigar is producing a large irregular mass from the caudal pole of a kidney. (**B**) The intravenous excretory urogram is enhancing the caudal pole renal adenocarcinoma in another budgerigar. The normal testicle (*arrow*) is ventral to the cranial kidney pole.

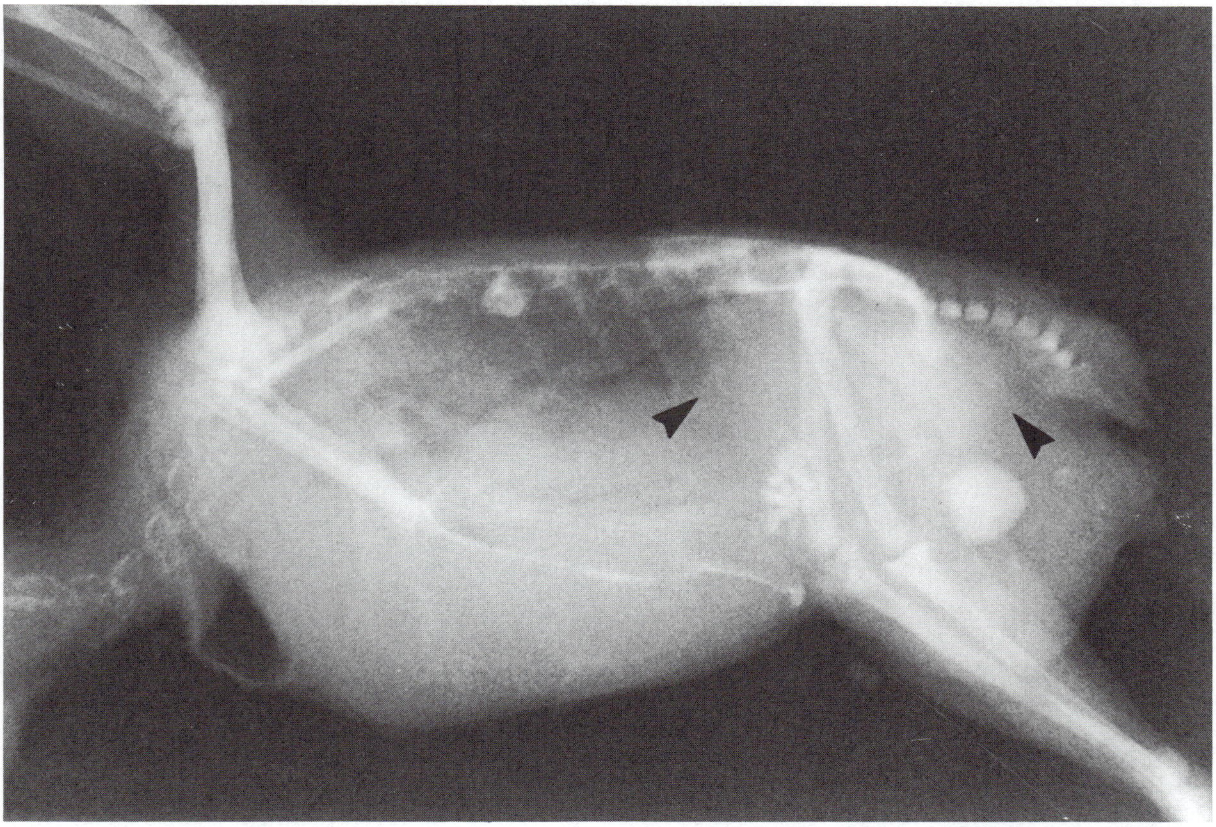

Figure 7A

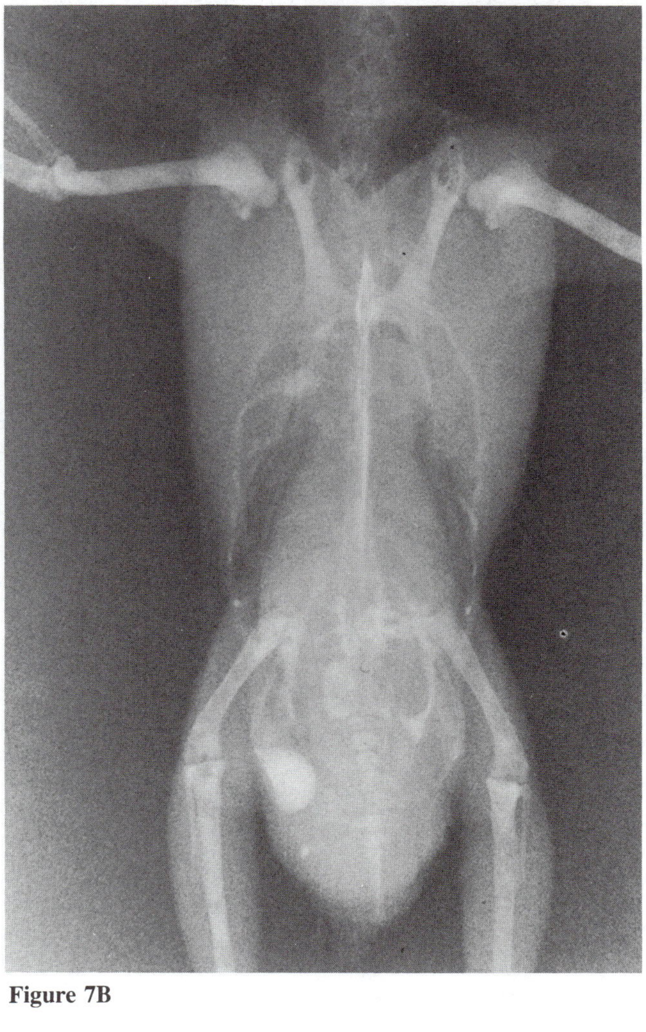

Figure 7B

Figure 7—(**A**) The soft tissue mass (*arrows*) in the dorsal abdomen obscuring visualization of the kidneys is an enlarged oviduct. The ventriculus is displaced cranially, and an abdominal hernia is apparent. (**B**) Mottled increased medullary bone density and well-defined circular regions of increased bone density involve the left pubis and ribs. These changes in budgerigars result from increased estrogen levels.

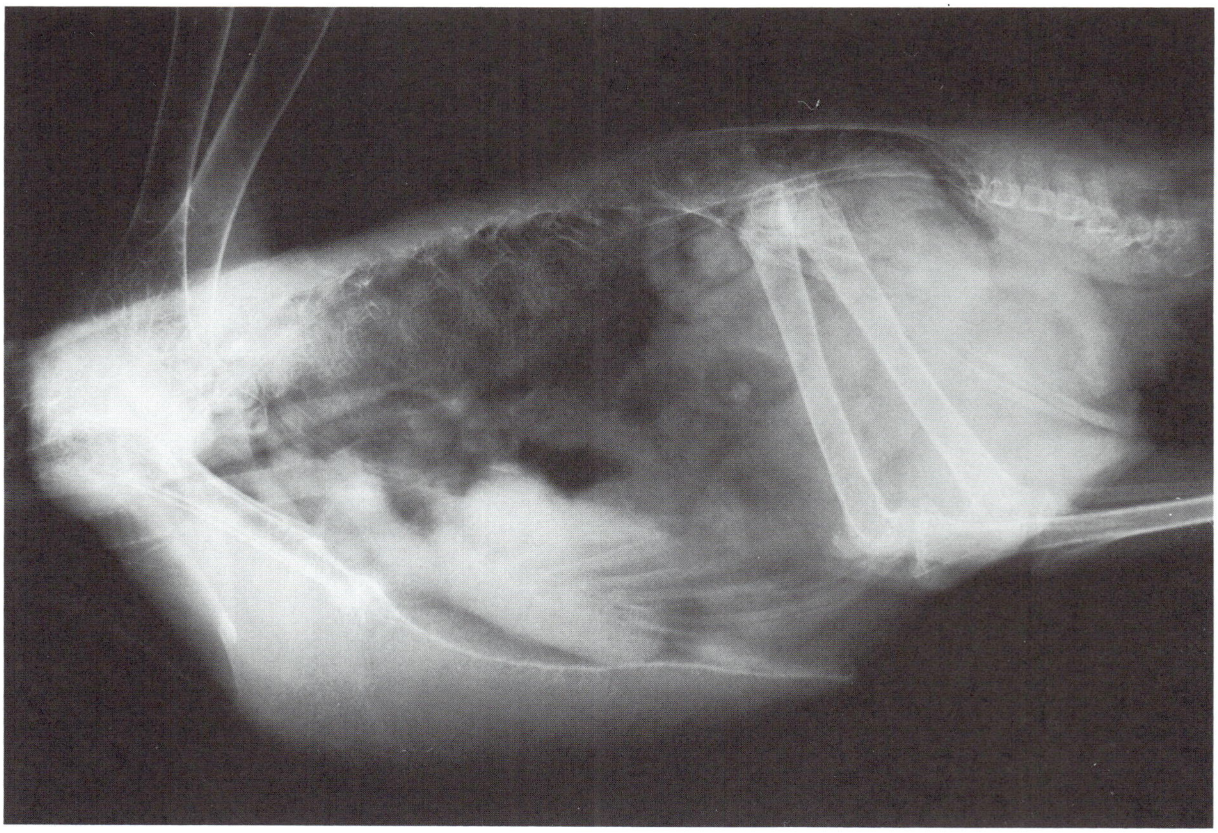

Figure 8A

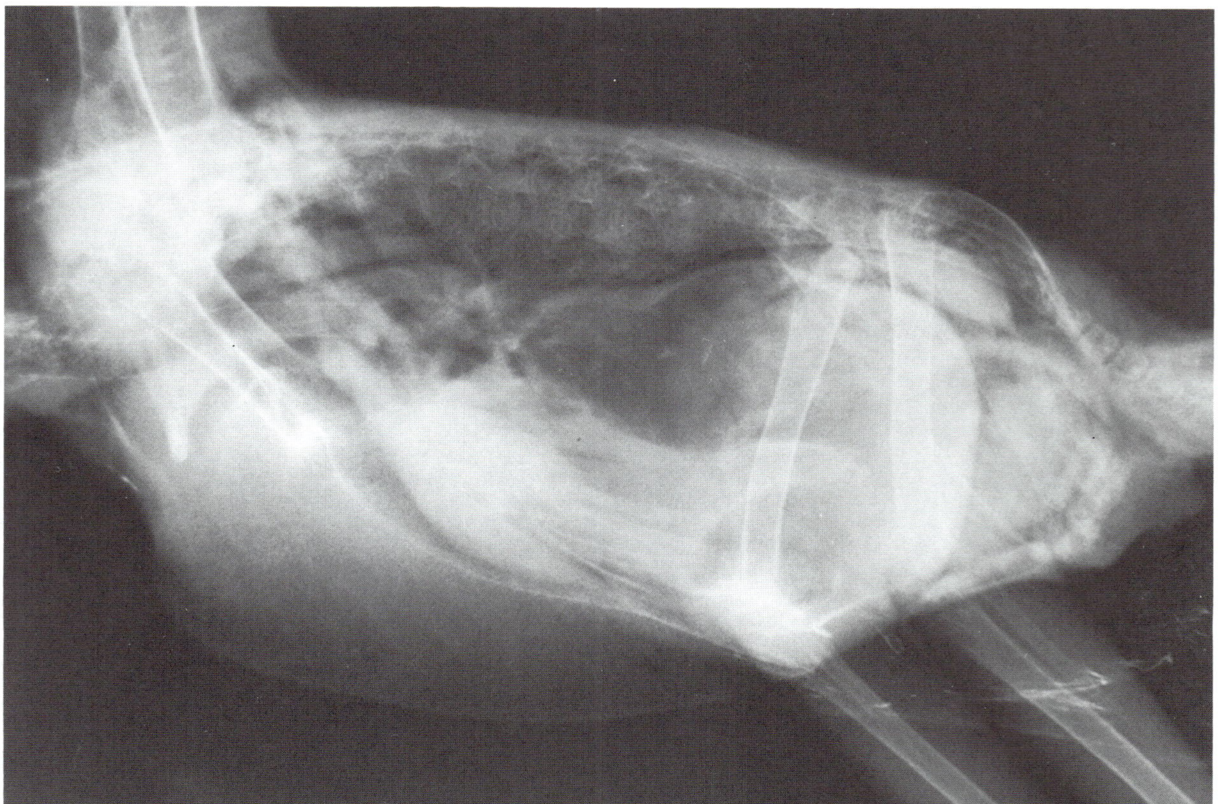

Figure 8B

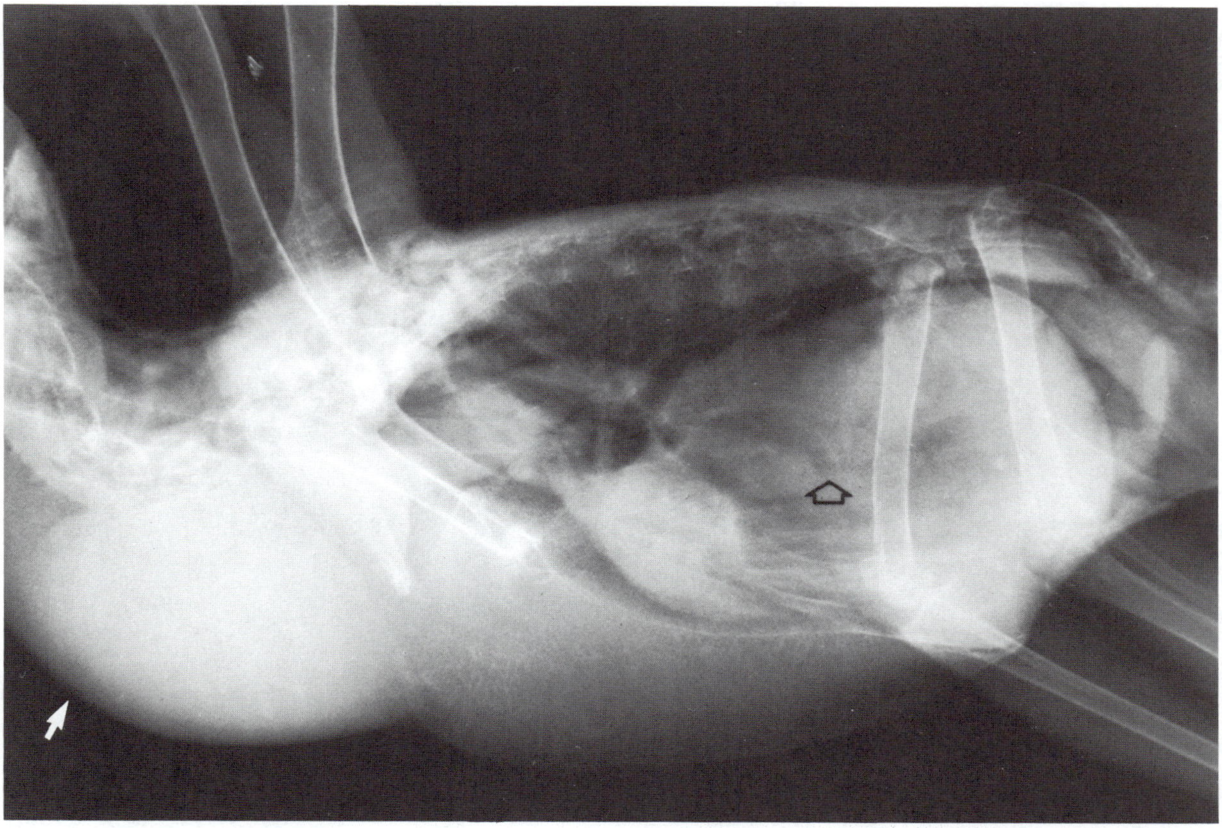

Figure 8C

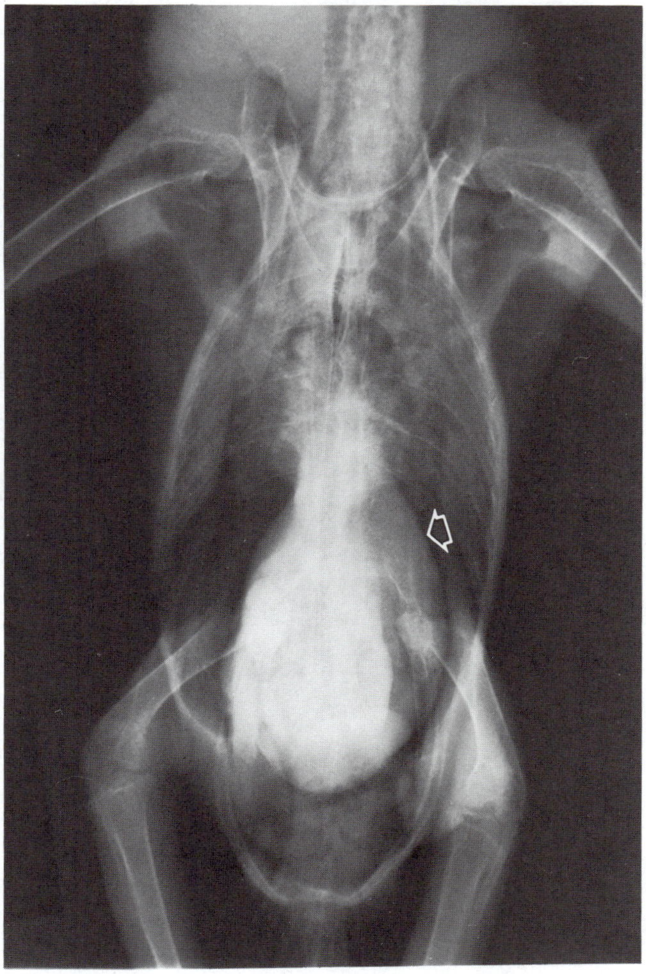

Figure 8D

Figure 8—(**A** through **F**) Radiographic changes associated with infiltrative splanchnic neuropathy. The radiographs are of blue and gold macaws. (**A**) Small amounts of gas and fluid are present in the proventriculus, ventriculus, and intestines. (**B**) Marked distention from the proventriculus and ventriculus being filled with gas and fluid. (**C**) Fluid-filled dilated proventriculus (*open arrow*) and ventriculus. The crop (*closed arrow*) is distended with fluid. (**D**) Ventrodorsal view of the parrot shown in **C**. The distended proventriculus (*open arrow*) could be mistaken for an enlarged liver lobe. (*Figure 8 continues next page*)

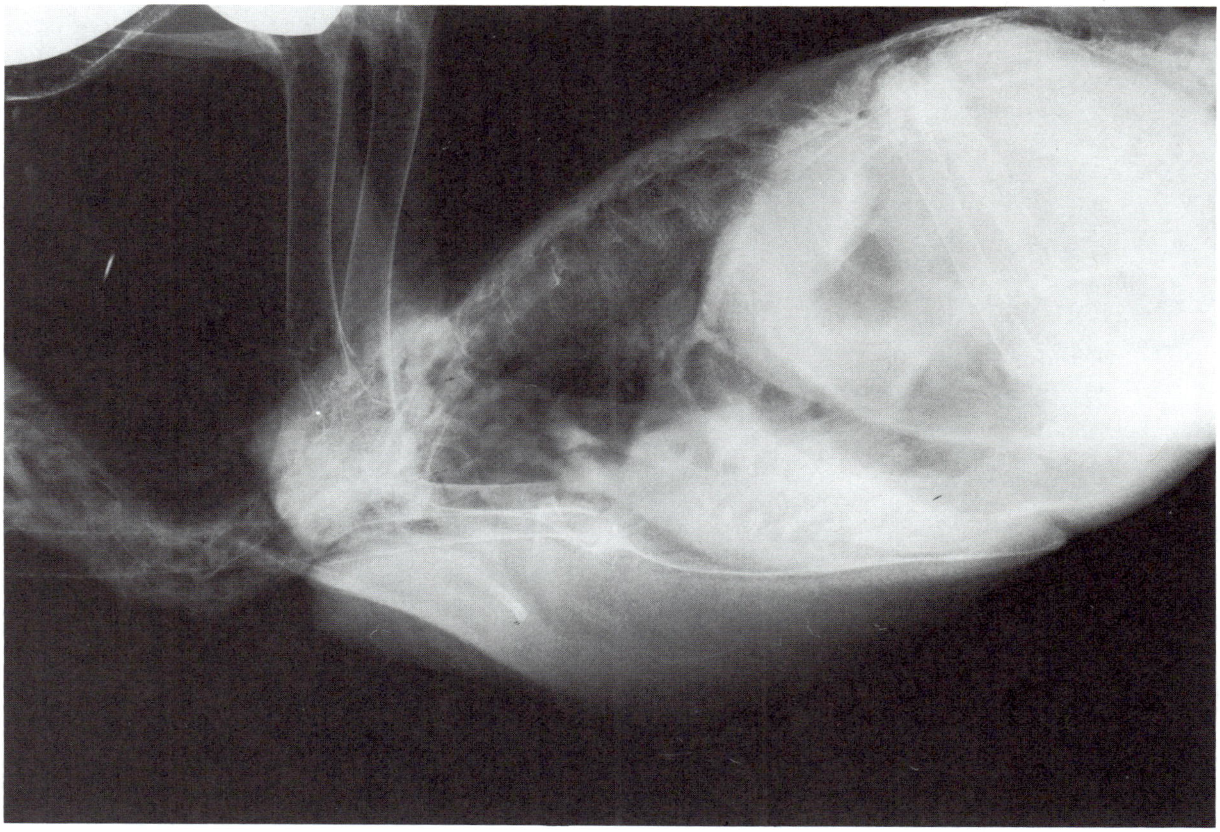

Figure 8E

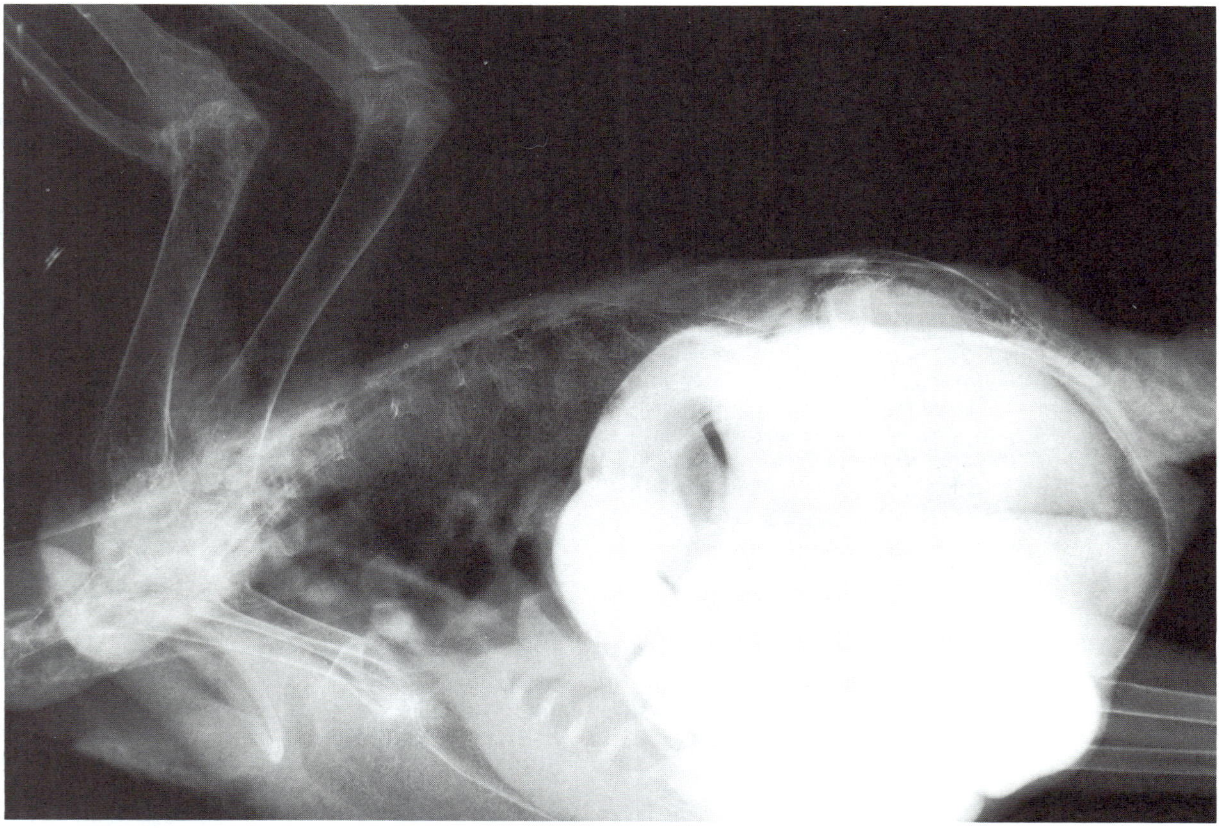

Figure 8F

Figure 8 continued—(**E**) Massive distention from the intestines being filled with gas and fluid because of functional ileus. (**F**) This radiograph shows retention of barium in dilated intestines eight hours after a barium-contrast series.

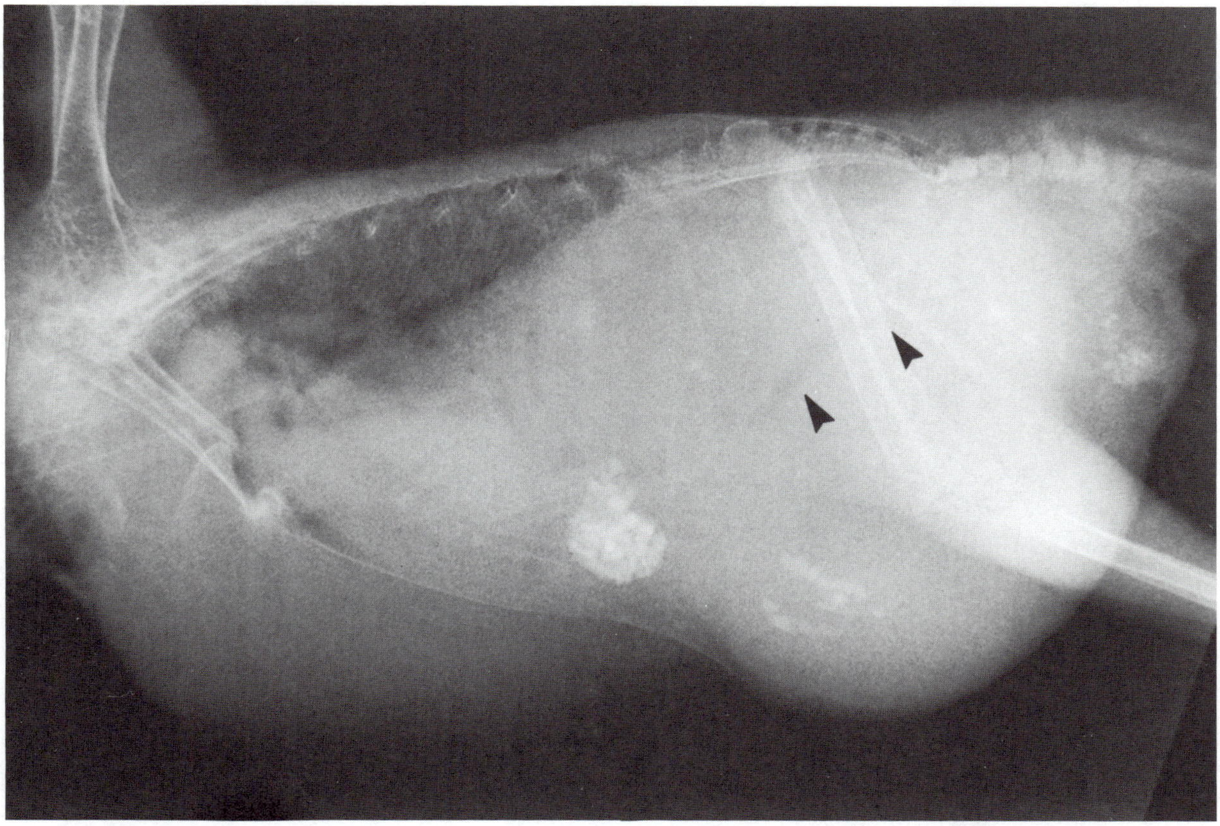

Figure 9A

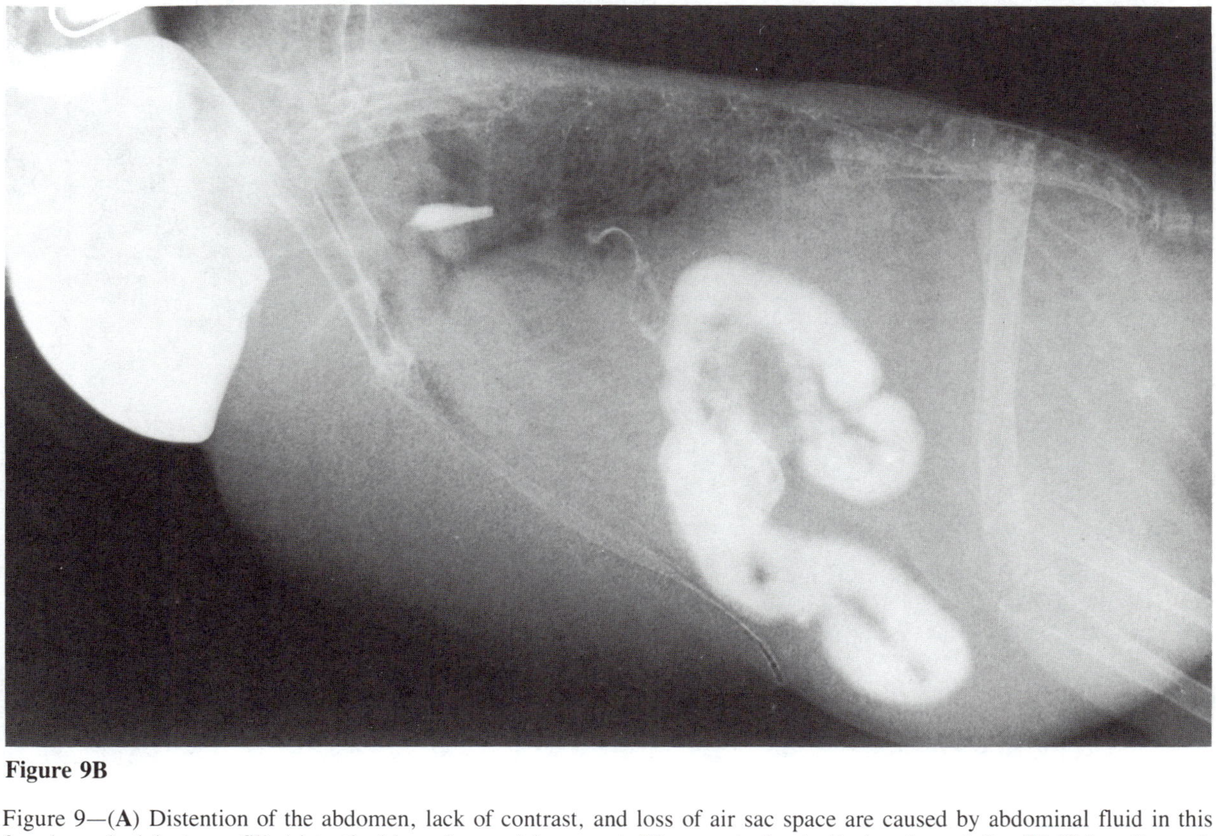

Figure 9B

Figure 9—(**A**) Distention of the abdomen, lack of contrast, and loss of air sac space are caused by abdominal fluid in this female cockatiel. A gas-filled intestinal loop (*arrows*) is present. The ventriculus is displaced cranially. (**B**) This radiograph shows abnormal positioning of the proventriculus, ventriculus, and intestines 30 minutes after a barium-contrast series. The intestines are dilated. Egg peritonitis with abdominal fluid and adhesions is present.

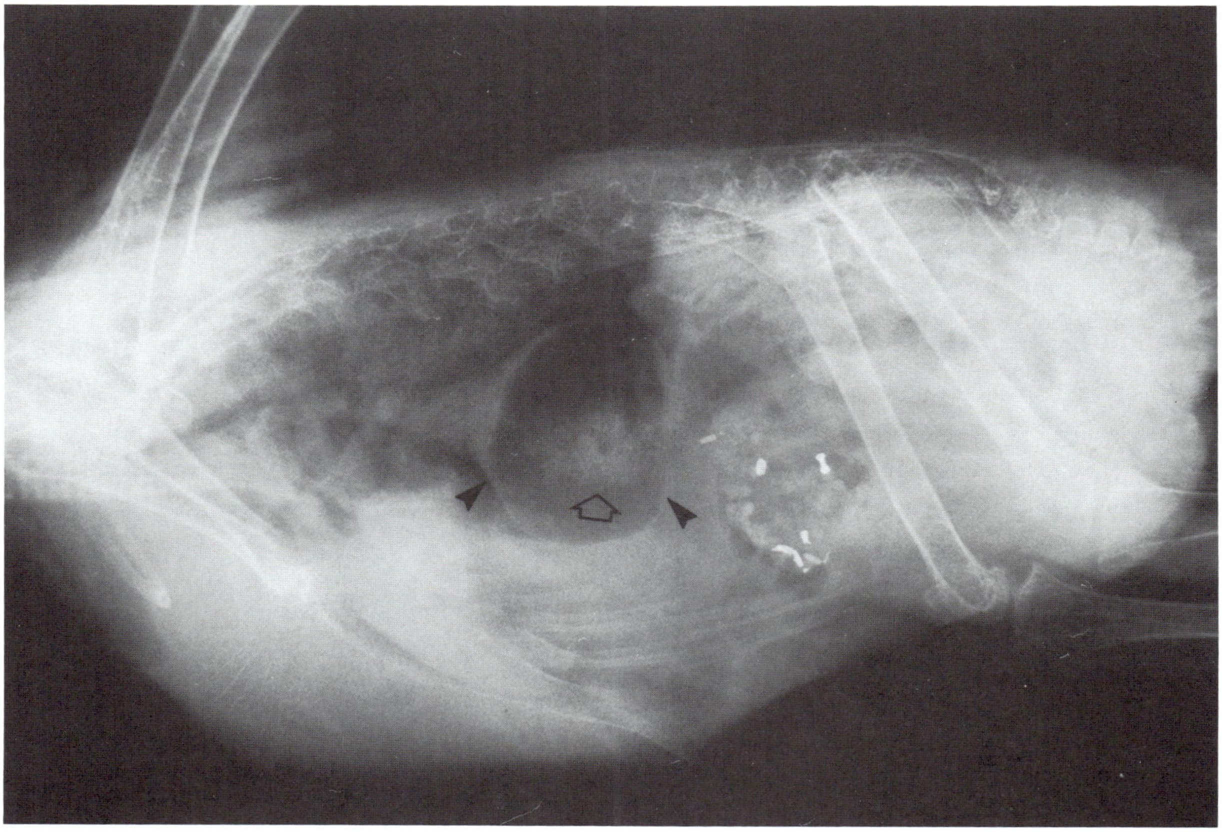

Figure 10A

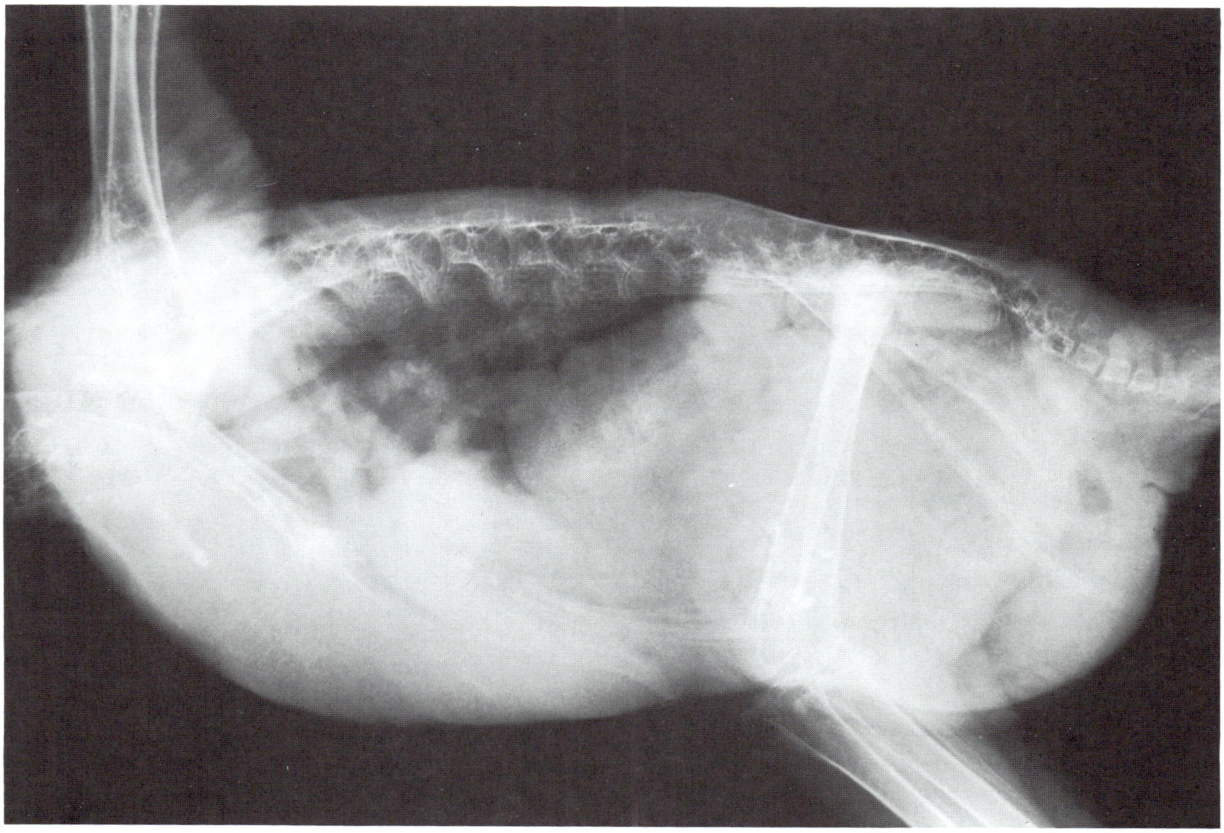

Figure 10B

Figure 10—(**A**) Gaseous distention of the proventriculus (*closed arrows*) and intraluminal foreign material (*open arrow*). Metallic foreign material is present in the ventriculus. (**B**) Radiograph taken 36 hours later shows that the foreign material still persists. Lack of abdominal contrast and mild abdominal distention are attributable to the presence of fluid. This cockatoo ingested a toy that perforated the gastrointestinal tract, causing peritonitis.

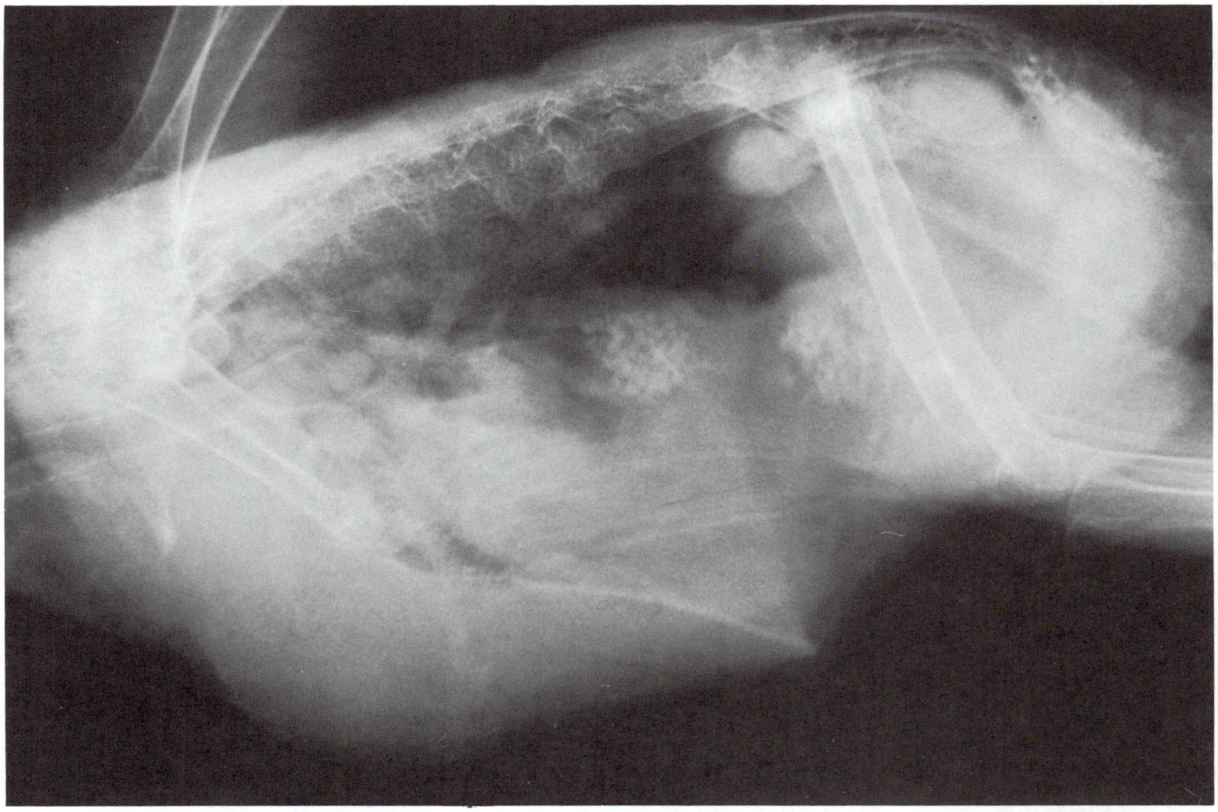

Figure 11A

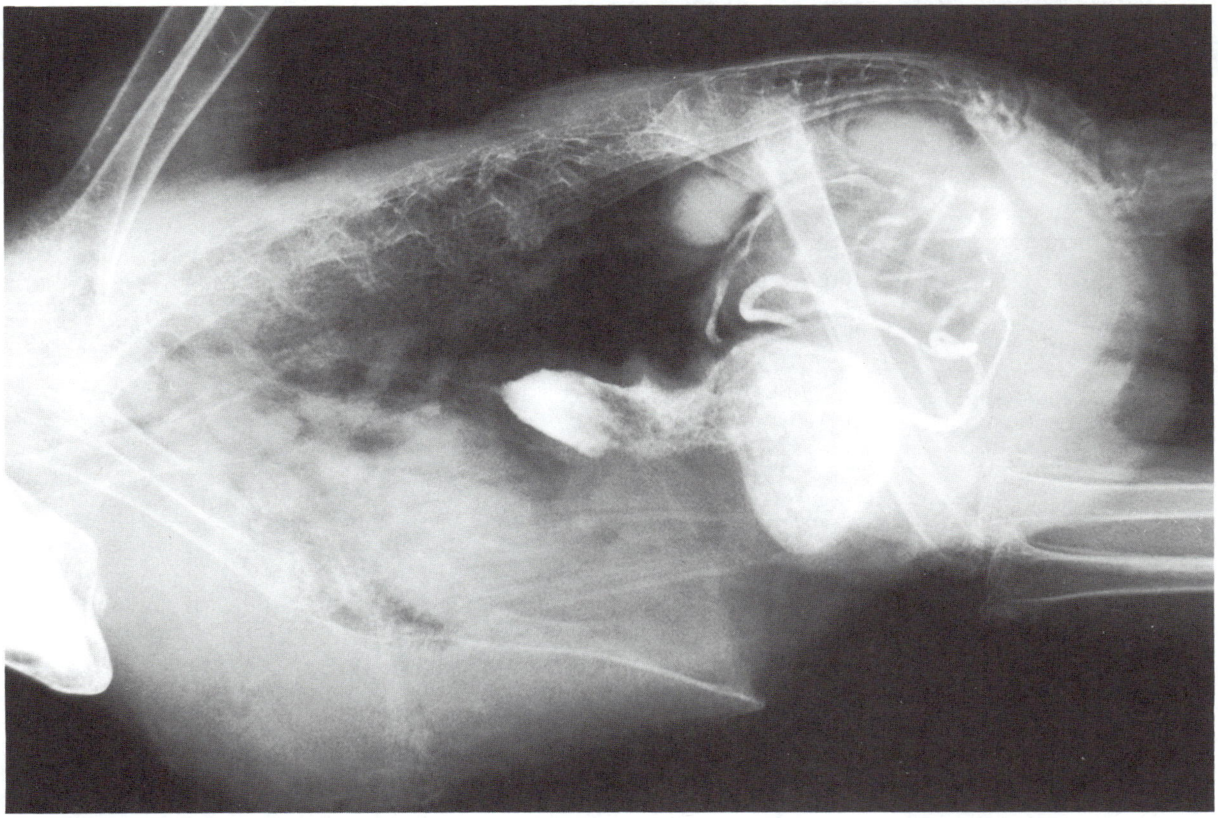

Figure 11B

Figure 11—(**A**) The presence of grit in the proventriculus is unusual. (**B**) A radiograph taken 36 hours after a barium-contrast series shows the barium still present in the crop, proventriculus, and ventriculus. Only small amounts of barium entered the intestines. This Amazon parrot was allowed to consume a large amount of grit after years of no access to grit. The impaction was removed surgically, and the parrot recovered uneventfully.

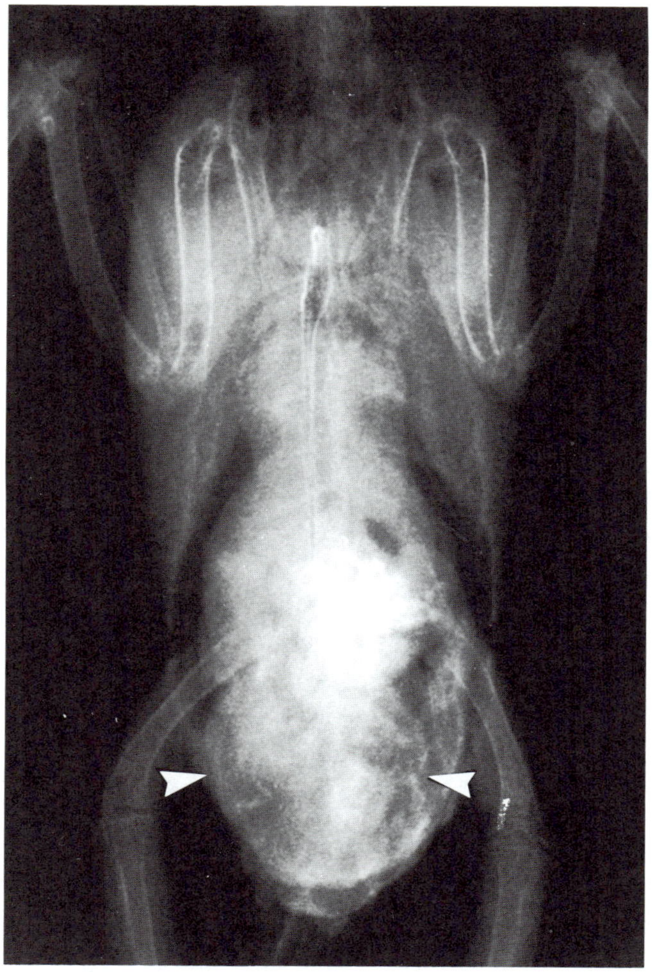

Figure 12—Intravenous excretory urogram shows irregularity in the kidney and distended cloaca (*closed arrows*). On autopsy, this budgerigar had a renal adenocarcinoma with involvement of sacral nerves.

REFERENCES

1. Evans SM: Avian radiographic diagnosis. *Compend Contin Educ Pract Vet* 3(7):660-666, 1981.
2. McMillan MC: Avian radiology, in Petrak ML (ed): *Diseases of Cage and Aviary Birds*. Philadelphia, Lea & Febiger, 1982, pp 329-360.
3. Graham DL: An update on selected pet bird virus infections. *Proc Annu Meet AAV*:267-280, 1984.
4. Gerlach H: Virus diseases in pet birds. *Proc Annu Meet AAV*:87-109, 1983.
5. Clubb SL: Infectious diseases. *Proc Annu Meet AAV*:91-101, 1982.
6. Simpson CF, Hanley JE: Pacheco's parrot disease in psittacine birds. *Avian Dis* 21(2):209-219, 1976.
7. Rosskopf WJ, Woerpel RW, Yanoff SR, et al: Tuberculosis in a parrot. *Mod Vet Pract* 62(10):777-778, 1981.
8. Dolphin RE, Olsen DE, Gallina AM: Tubercular infection in a sulfur-crested cockatoo. *VM SAC* 74(6):833-835, 1979.
9. Dhillon AS, Thacker HL, Winterfield RW: Toxoplasmosis in mynahs. *Avian Dis* 26(2):445-449, 1982.
10. Minsky L, Petrak ML: Diseases of the digestive system, in Petrak ML (ed): *Diseases of Cage and Aviary Birds*. Philadelphia, Lea & Febiger, 1982, pp 432-448.
11. Lowenstine LJ, Petrak ML: Iron pigment in the livers of birds, in Montali R, Migaki G (eds): *The Comparative Pathology of Zoo Animals*. Washington DC, Smithsonian Press, 1978, pp 127-135.
12. Randell MG, Patnaik AK, Gould WJ: Hepatopathy associated with excessive iron storage in mynah birds. *JAVMA* 179(11):1214-1217, 1981.
13. Leav I, Crocker AC, Petrak ML, et al: A naturally occurring lipidosis in shell parakeets, *Melopsittacus undulatus*. *Lab Invest* 18(4):433-437, 1968.
14. Palmer GH, Stauber E: Visceral lymphoblastic leukosis in an African gray parrot. *VM SAC* 26(9):1355-1356, 1981.
15. Petrak ML: Unpublished case material, Angell Memorial Animal Hospital, Boston, MA, 1983.
16. Petrak ML: Case presentations, AFA, Las Vegas, NV, 1980.
17. McMillan MC: Unpublished case material, Angell Memorial Animal Hospital, Boston, MA, 1978.
18. Knox DW: Gout in reptiles and birds, with observations on a comparable syndrome in man, in Montali R, Migaki G (eds): *The Comparative Pathology of Zoo Animals*. Washington DC, Smithsonian Press, 1978, pp 137-141.
19. Woerpel RW, Rosskopf WJ: Heavy metal intoxication in caged birds. Part I. *Compend Contin Educ Pract Vet* 4(10):729-738, 1982.
20. McMillan MC, Petrak ML: The clinical significance of abdominal enlargement in the budgerigar (*Melopsittacus undulatus*). *Compend Contin Educ Pract Vet* 3(10):898-904, 1981.
21. Petrak ML, Gilmore CE: Neoplasms, in Petrak ML (ed): *Diseases of Cage and Aviary Birds*. Philadelphia, Lea & Febiger, 1982, pp 606-637.
22. Schlumberger HG: Polyostotic hyperostosis in the female parakeet. *Am J Pathol* 35(1):1-23, 1959.
23. McMillan MC: Avian gastrointestinal radiography. *Compend Contin Educ Pract Vet* 4(5):273-284, 1983.
24. Ridgway RA, Gallerstein GA: Proventricular dilatation in psittacines. *Proc Annu Meet AAV*:228-230, 1983.
25. Woerpel RW, Rosskopf WJ, Hughes E: Proventricular dilatation and wasting syndrome: Mysenteric ganglioneuritis and encephalomyelitis of psittacines: An update. *Proc Annu Meet AAV*:25-28, 1984.
26. McNeel SV, Zenoble RD: Avian urography. *JAVMA* 178(4):366-368, 1981.
27. Peterson ME, Rantanen NW, Stauber E: Ultrasonic imaging in diagnosis of an abdominal mass in a pigeon. *Mod Vet Pract* 64(10):825-826, 1983.

Radiology of Avian Respiratory Diseases

Marjorie C. McMillan, DVM
The Windhover Veterinary Center
Walpole, Massachusetts

Angell Memorial Animal Hospital
Boston, Massachusetts

The anatomy and physiology of the avian respiratory system result in changes in radiographic patterns that are different from the interstitial, alveolar, peribronchial, and vascular patterns described in mammals. Because birds lack a true pleural space, pneumothorax and pleural effusion do not occur. Pleural fluid is usually attributed to extension from abdominal disease. Avian lungs are firmly attached to the thoracic wall, and thus atelectasis is not associated with thoracic problems. Lung volume remains constant during the respiratory cycle. Because the bronchial tree consists of an interconnecting network of tubules, air bronchograms are not a feature of consolidating pulmonary change. The interstitium is poorly developed so that marked interstitial patterns do not occur radiographically.

Indications

Birds with signs of upper respiratory disease (e.g., sneezing, nasal discharge, and/or infraorbital and periorbital swelling) but that otherwise are healthy may not require radiographic examination on initial presentation. If signs persist or recur after proper medical management, radiographs are indicated. Dyspnea, open-mouthed breathing, wheezing, tail bobbing, coughing, oral abscesses, loss of vocalization, exercise intolerance, abdominal distention, weight loss, and auscultatory abnormalities are indications for radiographic examination.

Preradiographic Considerations

Birds with severe respiratory problems may tolerate only a cursory examination. If respiratory distress is severe or the patient is debilitated, supportive treatment with oxygen and fluids is necessary before physical or radiographic examination. Rapid intramuscular injection of fluids and stabilization in an atmosphere of 40% oxygen before beginning diagnostic procedures may be indicated. In stable patients, an oral speculum allows visualization of the choanal slit, pharynx, glottis, and tongue. Auscultation in a quiet area with a pediatric stethoscope placed over the pectoral region, back, and trachea may reveal abnormal clicks, wheezes, and fluid sounds as well as cardiac murmurs and arrhythmia. Differences in air flow, harshness of sounds, or lack of air flow may be detected if the nostrils are auscultated.

Because abdominal masses or fluid can compromise the respiratory system by extending into the lung or air sacs or by cranial displacement of viscera, abdominal palpation may suggest a cause of respiratory distress.

Originally published in Volume 8, Number 8, August 1986

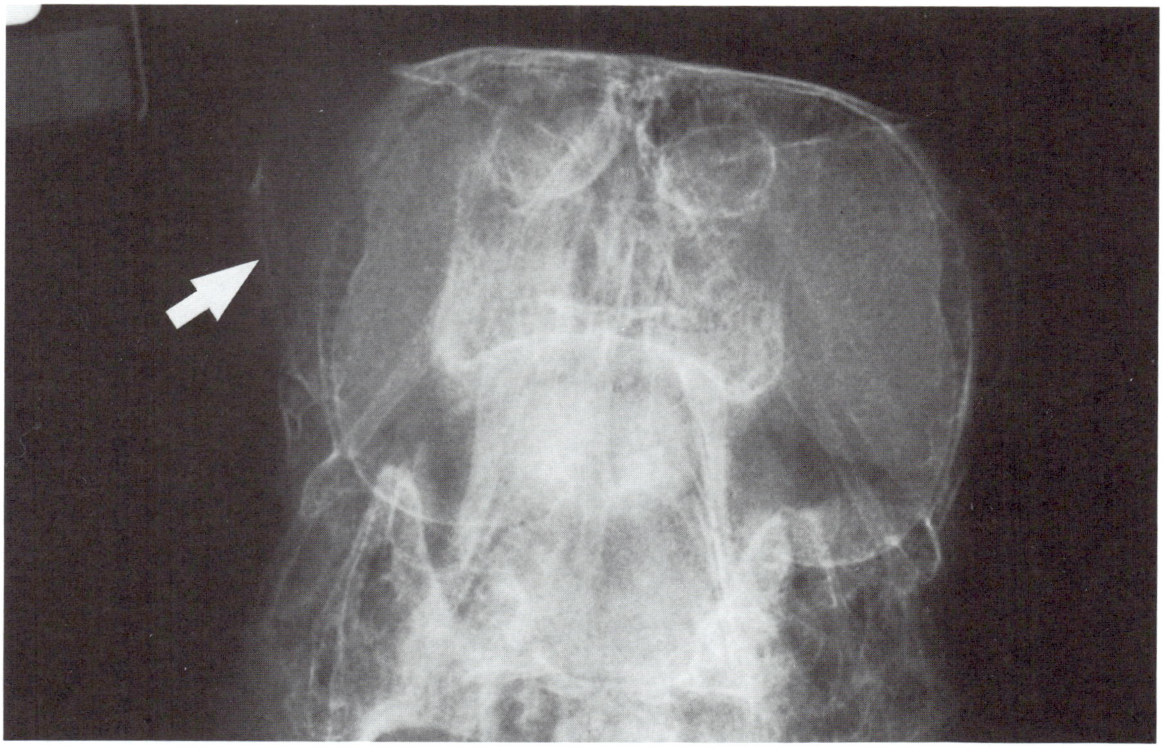

Figure 1—Rostrocaudal view of an Amazon parrot's skull shows a supraorbital abscess displacing scleral ossicle (*arrow*) with no bone erosion.

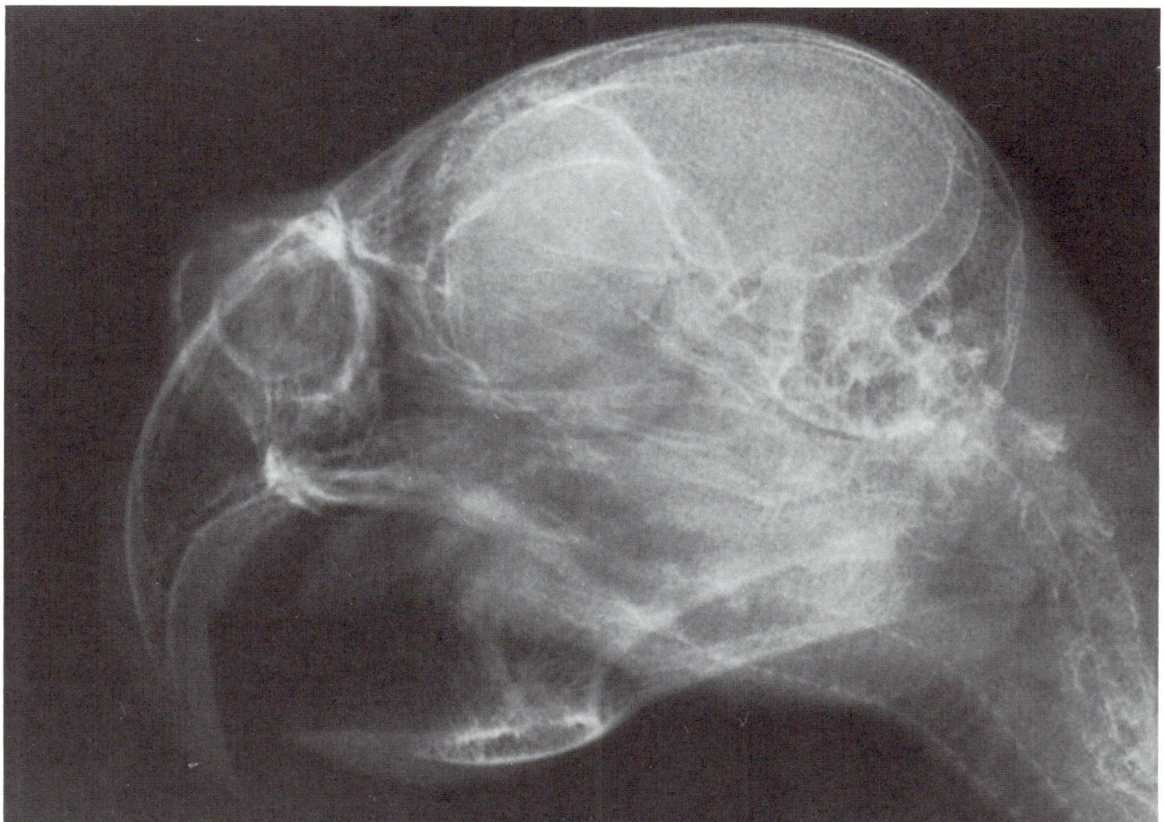

Figure 2—Lateral view of a Senegal parrot's skull demonstrates mineralization within a mass that involved the right nostril. Aspergillosis was diagnosed by biopsy and culture.

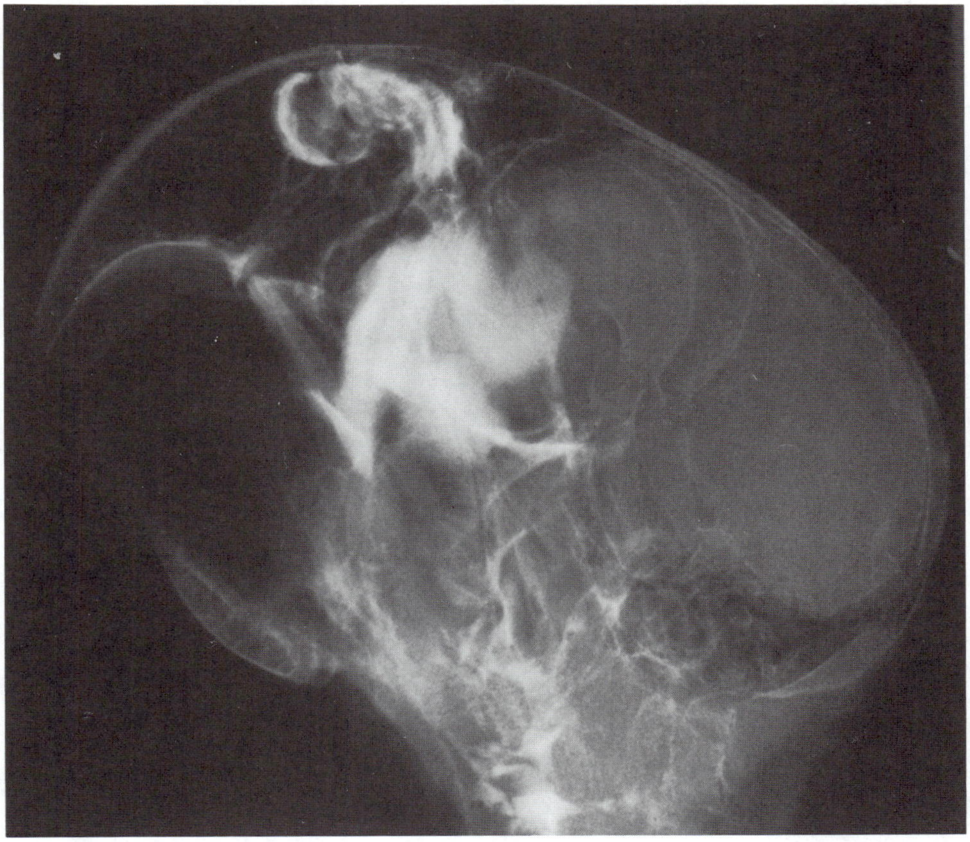

Figure 3A

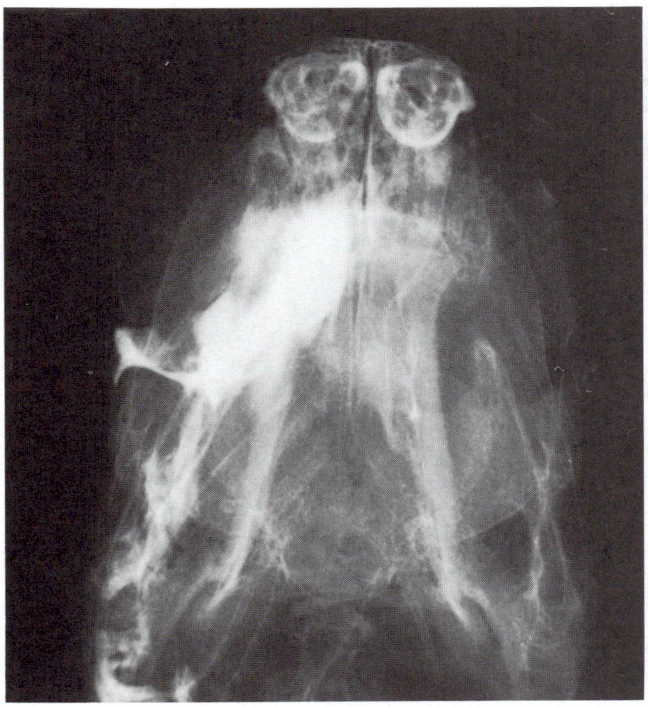

Figure 3B

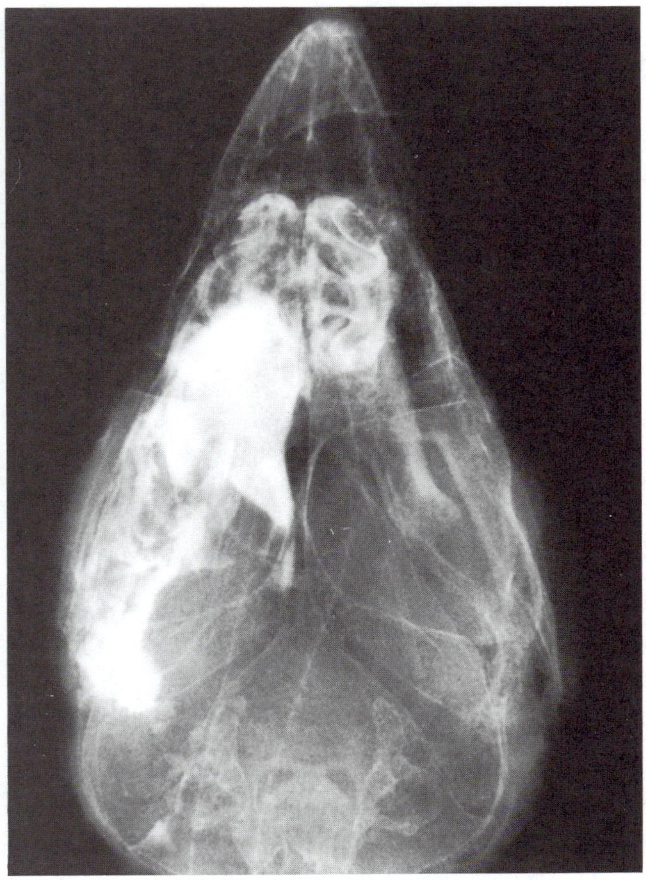

Figure 3C

Figure 3—Positive-contrast sinography of a normal parrot demonstrates the flow of contrast material into the contralateral sinus, nasal cavity, and periorbital and auricular regions. Contrast agent was injected into the right infraorbital sinus. (**A**) Right lateral, (**B**) rostrocaudal, and (**C**) ventrodorsal views.

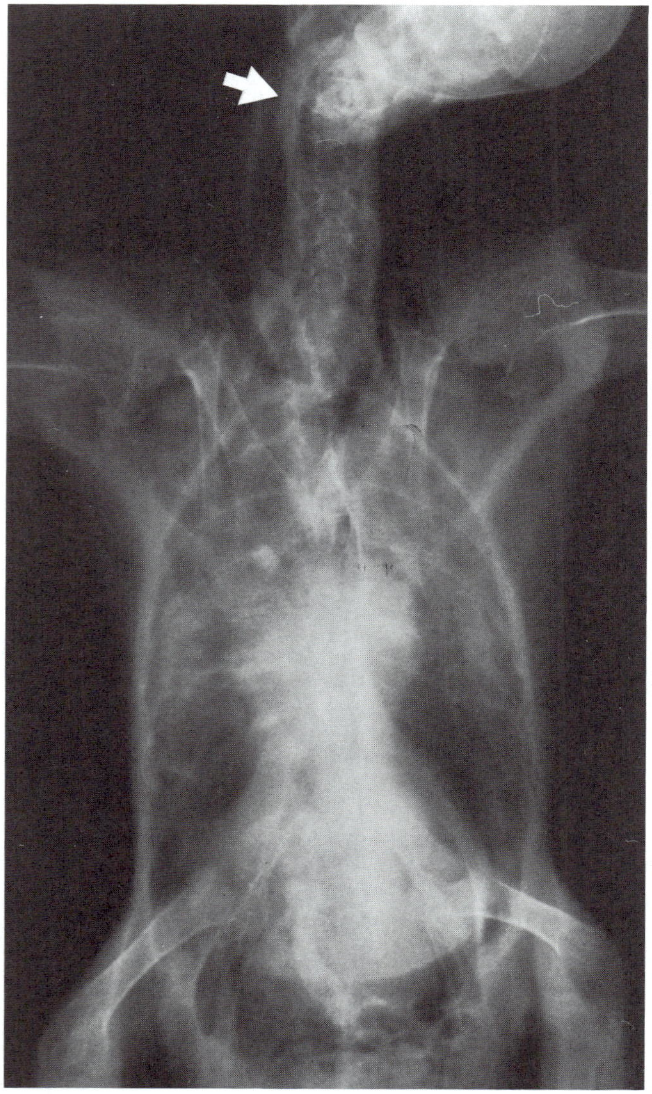

Figure 4—Increased parabronchial pulmonary density is present in the mid portion of both lungs of this parrot. The *arrow* points to a tracheal mass. Aerophagia is apparent. Pneumonia and tracheal abscess were secondary to hypovitaminosis A.

Radiographic Abnormalities

Diseases involving the upper respiratory tract, nasal cavity, infraorbital sinuses, cervicocephalic air sacs, and trachea may show no radiographic abnormalities.

Localized soft tissue densities are often abscesses (Figure 1) and may involve the nasal and oral cavities, periorbital region, or trachea. They are most commonly associated with hypovitaminosis A. Neoplasia is infrequent, but squamous cell carcinoma with bone involvement has been reported.[1] Fibrosarcomas often invade the beak and cause a significant soft tissue mass. Granulomas are the result of chronic rhinitis of bacterial[2] or fungal infection (Figure 2). Parasitic granulomas[3] are infrequent. Localized subcutaneous air pockets and granulomas are reported in association with disease of the cervicocephalic air sac system.[4]

Positive-contrast rhinography and sinography may aid in radiographic evaluation[5] (Figure 3). Studies of normal radiographic patterns in psittacines demonstrate communication between the infraorbital sinus and the nasal cavity, beak, opposite sinus, periorbital region, and tympanic region. This communication helps explain the beak deformities and massive swelling evident around the ocular and aural regions and associated with some of the upper respiratory diseases.

Radiographic changes commonly are caused by lower respiratory tract disorders. These include changes in normal reticular pulmonary pattern, bronchial thickening, abnormal air sac density, subcutaneous emphysema, aerophagia, and discrete masses.

Parabronchial infiltrates cause a blotchy appearance to the usually uniform pulmonary pattern. This change is seen frequently in birds with avian pneumonia along the caudal midlateral aspects of the lungs[6] and is best visualized in ventrodorsal radiographs (Figure 4). Aerodynamics in the

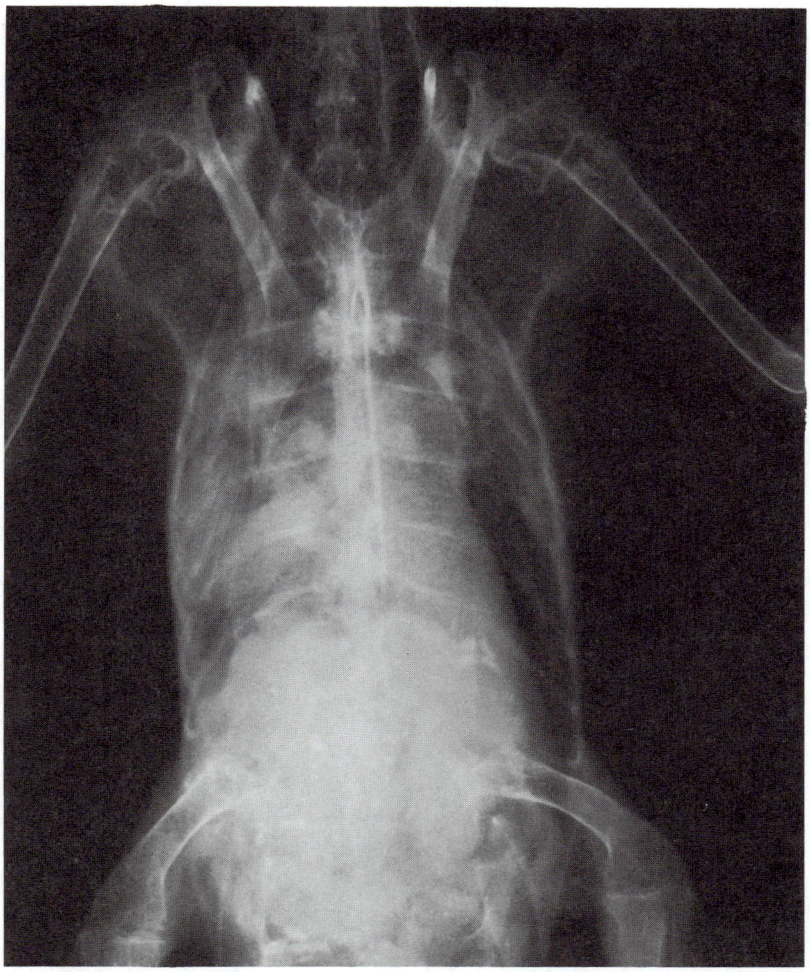

Figure 5—Consolidation present in the right lung of this mynah bird obliterated the normal reticular pattern. The lesion was caused by aspergillosis.

neopulmo contribute to the depositing of pathogens in this region. Focal areas of consolidation obliterate the parabronchial pattern so that, instead of a pronounced parabronchial wall with an air-filled center, the air is replaced by a soft tissue density. Caseous exudate or fluid, such as hemorrhage or edema, also may obliterate the parabronchi. Abscesses, fungal granulomas, or tumors also may cause discrete, well-defined, soft tissue masses that replace the normal pulmonary pattern (Figure 5). In ventrodorsal radiographs, the peripheral portions of the avian lung normally have greater density than the central portions. With the development of the neopulmo, the lateral portion of the lung increases,[7] causing increased soft tissue density. Infiltration around the bronchi results in an ability to visualize parallel walls of the air-filled bronchi. This infiltration occurs within the pulmonary parenchyma and extends into the air sacs (Figure 6).

Air sac disease may cause a barrel-shaped appearance to the avian thorax (Figure 7). Thickened and consolidated air sacs do not change in size as much as normal air sacs do during expiration, thus resulting in relatively fixed dimensions of the chest that mimic full inspiration. The abdominal air sacs become blunted, and lines across the air sacs become apparent. The normal air density becomes a subtle, gray, soft tissue density that may be homogeneous or irregular. Sharply demarcated soft tissue lines and obscured abdominal detail are present in lateral radiographs (Figure 8). Bacterial infections, hypovitaminosis A complicated by bacterial infection, and such fungal diseases as aspergillosis and mucormycosis[8] cause consolidating air sacculitis. Because viral diseases with secondary bacterial involvement play a significant role in pulmonary disease in other species, a similar situation probably exists in birds. Viruses interfere with the bactericidal action of the lung and cause direct cell damage, which may result in bacterial complications between Days 6 and 10 of infection.[9] Chlamydiosis also may cause primary air sacculitis; but it is usually a systemic disease associated with multiple-organ

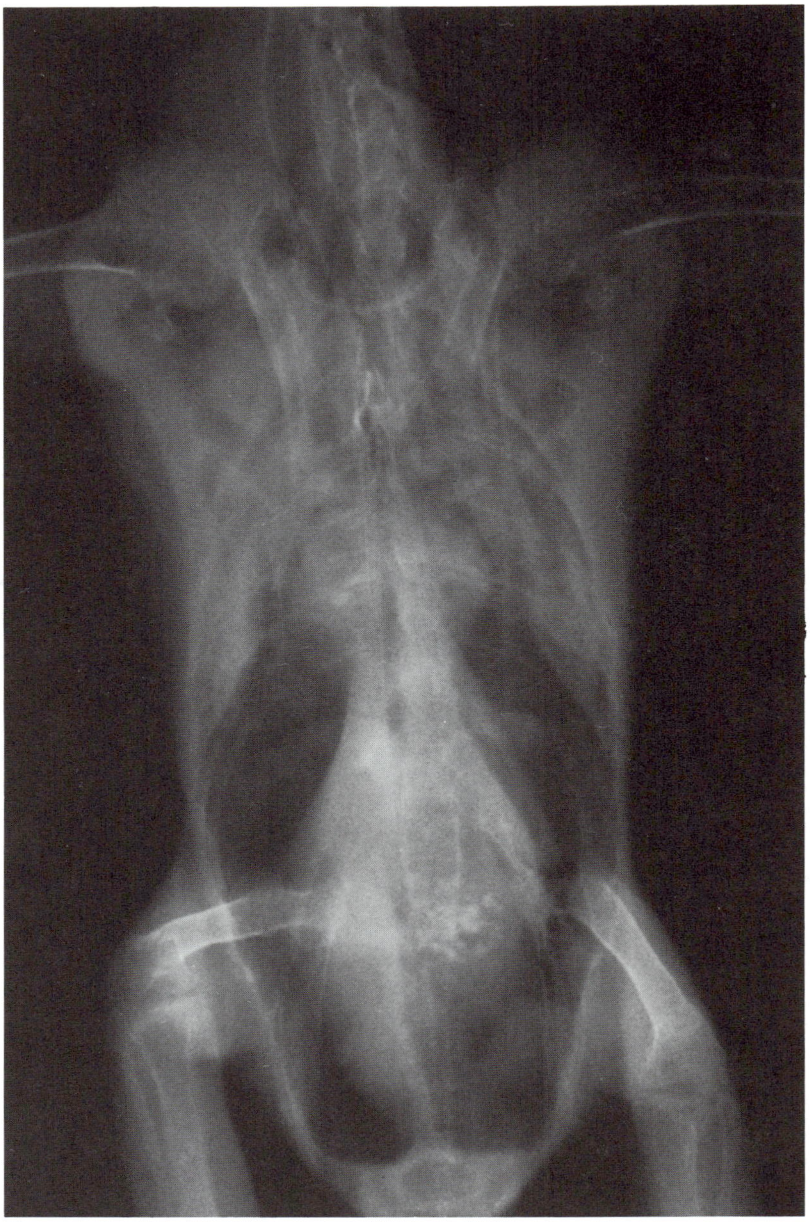

Figure 6—This view shows increased air sac density and blunting of abdominal air sacs, which were caused by air sacculitis. Prominent bronchi from wall thickening extend to clavicular air sacs.

involvement and, often, concurrent gram-negative infection.

Gas is not normally found in the gastrointestinal tract of birds. Radiographically detectable aerophagia often accompanies significant respiratory problems. In such cases, the air is uniformly distributed throughout the intestinal tract with no evidence of distention or localization (Figure 9). Subcutaneous emphysema may occur in association with traumatic air sac rupture.

Pulmonary masses are uncommon. When they do occur, they are usually abscesses or granulomas rather than neoplasms.

Summary

Radiographic changes associated with avian respiratory disorders often are subtle. The ventrodorsal view is most helpful for assessment of lung and air sac lesions. Pneumonia and air sacculitis are the most commonly encountered lower respiratory tract abnormalities. Prominence or obliteration of pulmonary reticular pattern, visualization of intrapulmonary bronchi, increased air sac density, blunted air sacs, and fixed appearance to air sacs are the radiographic changes that may be apparent. Radiographic lesions are uncommon with upper respiratory disease; but localized soft tissue masses, usually abscesses, may be apparent.

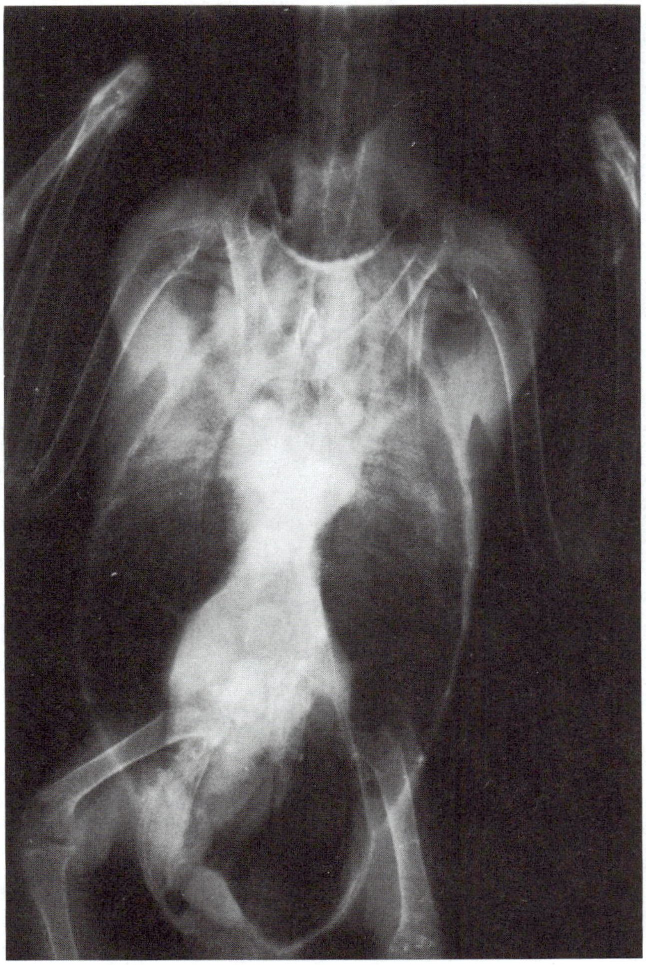

Figure 7—A barrel-shaped appearance, prominent lines across the air sacs, and increased parabronchial pattern indicate air sacculitis and pneumonia.

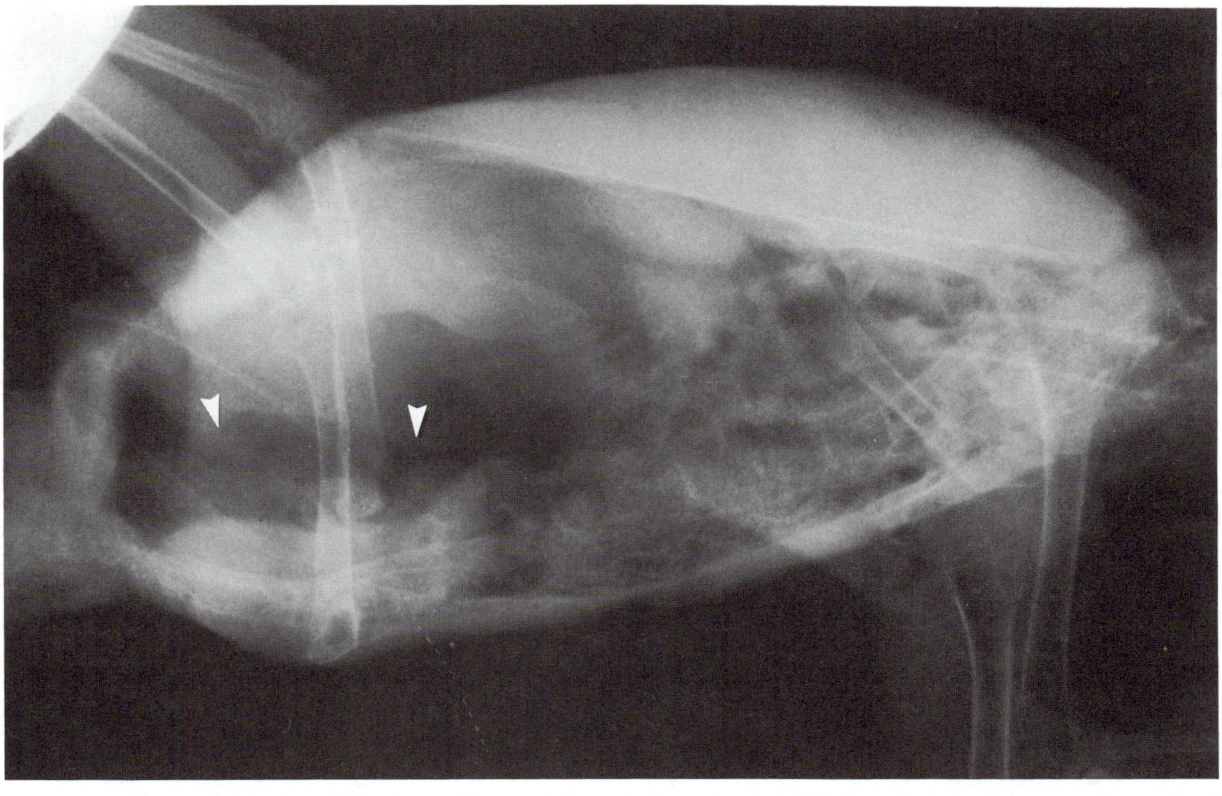

Figure 8—Ventral abdominal detail is obscured by overlying soft tissue density. Soft tissue lines in air sacs are the result of consolidating air sacculitis (*arrows*).

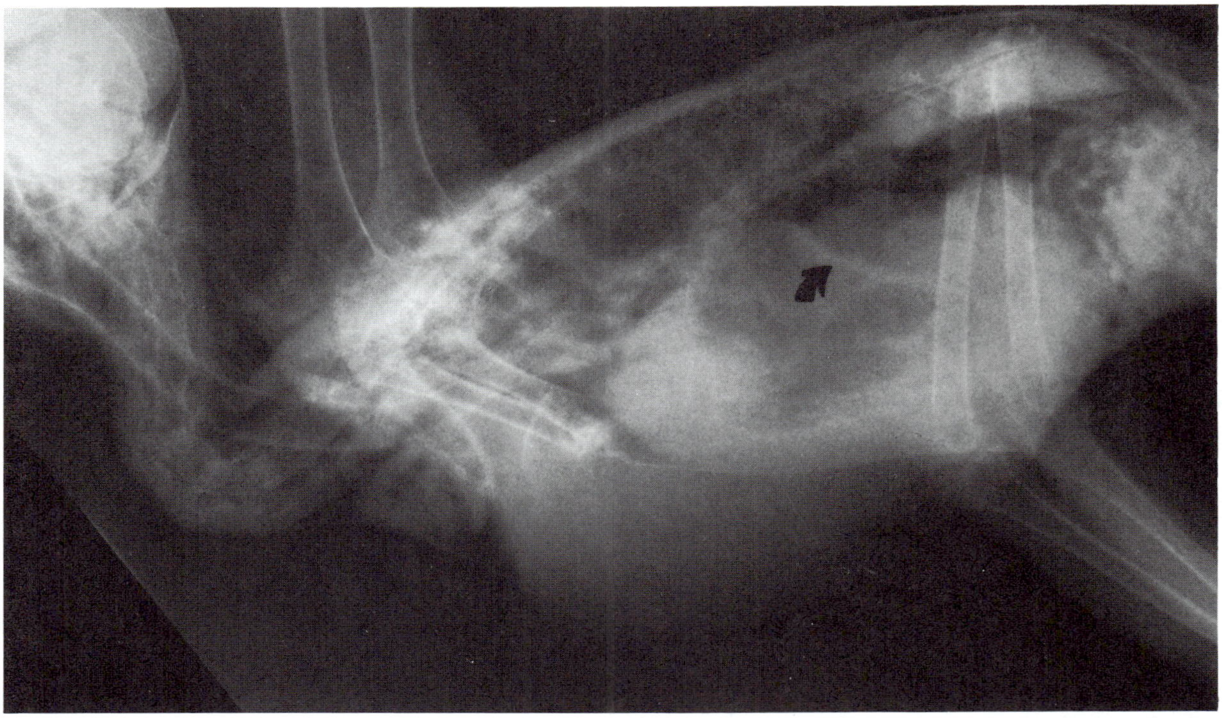

Figure 9—Gas is uniformly distributed throughout the small intestine. Air sac changes are present (*arrow*). Aerophagia is secondary to respiratory distress.

REFERENCES

1. Altman RB: Respiratory diseases of psittacine birds. *Small Anim Vet Med [Update Series]* 10:1-7, 1978.
2. Crane SW, Jacobson E, Shields RP: Cryosurgical removal of an intranasal granuloma from an African gray parrot. *VM SAC* 75(3):499-501, 1980.
3. McMillan MC: Avian radiology, in Petrak ML (ed): *Diseases of Cage and Aviary Birds*. Philadelphia, Lea & Febiger, 1982, pp 329-360.
4. Walsh MT, Mays MC: Clinical manifestations of cervicocephalic air sacs of psittacines. *Compend Contin Educ Pract Vet* 6(9):783-792, 1984.
5. McMillan MC: Unpublished radiographic studies, Angell Memorial Animal Hospital, Boston, MA, 1979.
6. Lowenstine LJ: Avian anatomy and its relation to disease processes. *Proc Annu Meet AAV*:1-9, 1984.
7. Duncker H: Structure of the avian respiratory tract. *Respir Physiol* 22:1-19, 1974.
8. Dawson CO, Wheeldon EB, McNeil PE: Air sac and renal mucormycosis in an African gray parrot (*Psittacus erimacus*). *Avian Dis* 20(3):593-600, 1976.
9. Green GM: Lung defense mechanisms. *Med Clin North Am* 57(3):547-562, 1973.

Avian Emergency Medicine and Critical Care

The Animal Medical Center
New York, New York
James K. Morrisey, DVM

KEY FACTS

- ❑ A significant portion of avian patients present as emergencies or are in need of intensive care.
- ❑ Fluids should be given by intravenous or intraosseous route at a maintenance rate of 50 ml/kg/day.
- ❑ Transfusions and the use of colloidal compounds are necessary in many cases of chronic, debilitating disease.
- ❑ Nutritional support through a gavage tube, esophagostomy tube, or intraduodenal catheter is often necessary for treatment of critically ill birds.

An understanding of avian emergency medicine and critical care is an important component to the successful treatment and management of pet birds in practice. Although many anatomic and physiologic differences exist between birds and mammals, most of the elements involved in critical care management of mammals hold true for avian critical care. This article reviews the important aspects of critical care and emergency medicine that are unique to avian species.

INITIAL EXAMINATION

The examination of critical care patients should be done rapidly in an effort to gain as much pertinent information as possible. Observing a bird in a cage environment provides immediate information on respiratory status, patient attitude, and other routine clinical signs. Placing a severely stressed bird in a warm oxygen cage also can be beneficial in obtaining a more concise history. The physical examination, diagnostic evaluation, and initial treatment may need to be conducted in stages to allow the patient time to recover before being subjected to continued human handling.

It is preferable to gather certain diagnostic data before treatment, including a complete blood count (CBC), biochemical profiles, and culture specimens. The patient's stability, however, dictates the extent of data that can be gathered before initial therapy. A facemask can be used to administer oxygen while handling anemic or dyspneic birds. If anemia is suspected, a toenail clip can be used for quick determination of packed cell volume (PCV), total solids, and blood glucose levels before complete blood work is performed.

FLUID THERAPY

Fluid therapy is indicated for dehydrated, anorectic, or weak birds and for birds suffering from hemorrhage or shock. Hydration status can be assessed by evaluating skin turgor around the eye and hydration of mucous membranes. In birds with 5% dehydration, the skin returns slowly to normal position. The skin of birds with 7% to 10% dehydration does not return to normal position, and the mucous membranes are tacky; ropy saliva may be observed in the mouth.

The route of fluid replacement depends on several factors: severity of dehydra-

First-time publication

tion, severity of disease, and condition of the patient. Subcutaneous fluids are adequate in minor cases of dehydration or in anorectic birds that can be tube-fed. Intravenous catheters can be placed by using short, small-gauge catheters (22 to 26 gauge by 19 mm) in the right jugular (Figure 1), brachial (Figure 2), or medial metatarsal vein. I prefer using the metatarsal vein, if large enough, because the reptile-like skin of the feet helps to hold the catheter securely in place. Birds must be of sufficient size (heavier than 90 grams if jugular catheters are used) for catheter placement and should not be so ill as to suffer from vascular fragility or collapse.[1]

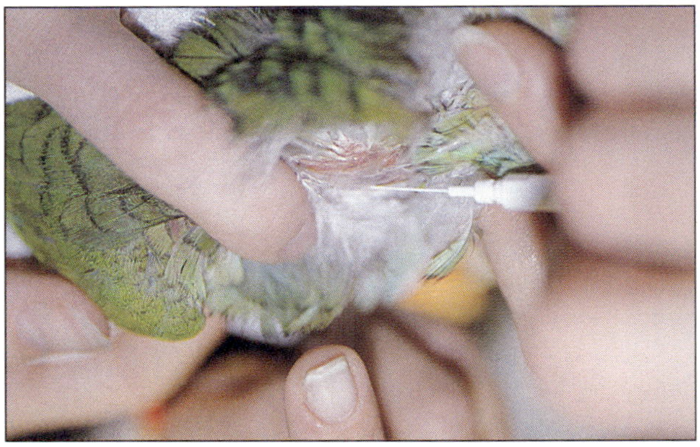

Figure 1—A 24-gauge catheter is being placed in the right jugular vein of a spectacled Amazon parrot.

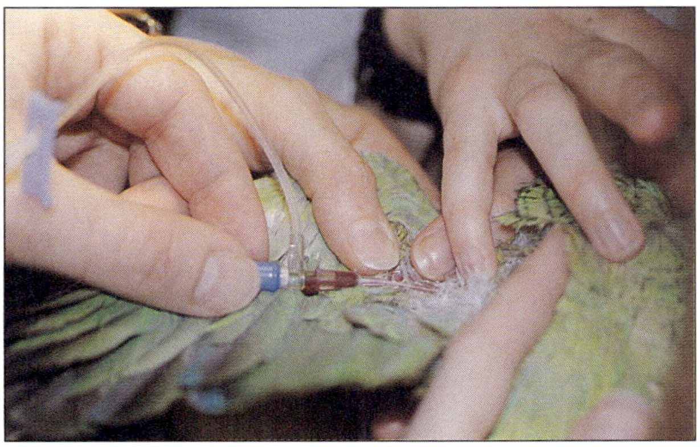

Figure 2—A 26-gauge catheter is placed in the brachial vein of an Amazon parrot. A figure-of-eight wing wrap is used to keep the catheter in place. Blood is being collected in heparinized capillary tubes for analysis.

Intraosseous catheters can be placed in small birds or in large birds with poor vascular quality. The usual sites of placement are the distal ulna and proximal tibiotarsus. Short spinal needles (20 to 22 gauge by 3.1 cm) can be used in large birds, while 22- to 25-gauge injection needles should be used in smaller patients. Intraosseous catheters can cause pain on injection and subsequent lameness if placed in the leg. These effects are temporary and are generally outweighed by the benefits of the catheter. Continuous-rate infusion pumps are ideal for fluid administration; however, some birds have a tendency to chew on the extension tubing. In such cases, fluids can be administered in boluses three to five times per day. Because the intraosseous space is finite, boluses must be given slowly over several minutes with steady pressure. For more information, see the article entitled A Technique of Intraosseous Cannulation for Intravenous Therapy in Birds by Branson Ritchie.

The fluid requirement for maintenance and fluid deficits can be calculated for birds as follows:

$$\text{Maintenance} = 50 \text{ ml/kg/day}$$
$$\text{Fluid deficit (ml)} = \text{weight (kg)} \times \% \text{ of dehydration}$$

Thus, a 500-kg bird that is 10% dehydrated would need 25 ml of maintenance fluids and an additional 5 ml (0.5 kg × 10) to correct dehydration. During the initial 24 hours, maintenance fluids and one half of the fluid deficit should be given. The remainder of the fluid deficit should be given during the next 48 hours.[2,3] Lactated Ringer's solution or other polyionic solutions are used. Dextrose can be added to fluids to make a 2.5% to 5% solution. A 10% solution can be used in severely debilitated birds. A 2.5% solution has been used subcutaneously in birds without the complications observed in mammals.[2] Although clinical studies are sparse, colloidal compounds, such as hetastarch, are apparently beneficial for increasing osmotic pressure caused by hypoproteinemia.[4] The dose is 10 to 15 ml/kg three times a day for up to four doses. Colloids are often used if serum protein levels are lower than 2.0 mg/dl and if pulmonary edema is suspected.

TRANSFUSIONS

Anemia is a common clinical finding in birds presented as emergencies. The anemia may be caused by acute blood loss or associated with chronic disease. Blood volume is estimated at 10% of the body weight in kilograms (i.e., 10 ml per 100 g of weight). An otherwise healthy bird can lose approximately 30% of its blood volume with minimal effects.[5] Common causes of acute blood loss include trauma, gastrointestinal and genitourinary bleeding, hemolysis, and idiopathic hemorrhage.[2] Chronic anemia associated with decreased production can be caused by any chronic debilitating disease, especially hepatic or renal disease, toxins, nutritional deficiencies, or chronic viral or bacterial infection. Anemic birds should be given iron dextran at an intramuscular dose of 10 mg/kg repeated weekly if needed, regardless of whether a transfusion is given.

A study involving acute anemia in pigeons suggested that fluid replacement with lactated Ringer's solution was more effective than iron dextran or homologous or heterologous transfusions.[5] In birds with chronic anemia or anemia caused by chronic disease, homologous or heterologous transfusions can, however, have clinical benefit. Most studies suggest transfusions when the packed cell volume is 20% or less.[2,3,5,6]

Transfusions should be taken from healthy birds of the same species or from species as closely related as possible. The sample should be drawn in 0.9% citrate using 0.1 ml of citrate per 0.9 ml of blood. A small amount of heparin can be substituted if citrate is not available.

The amount transfused is 10% to 20% of the patient's blood volume. This amount can be expected to increase the packed cell volume by 2% to 5%. A rough cross-match can be performed by using donor red cells and recipient serum. An absence of gross agglutination or hemolysis suggests compatibility.[3] Currently, no studies involving transfusion viabilities have been performed in psittacines; therefore, the goal of a transfusion is to stabilize the patient so that further diagnostic testing can be done to determine the cause of the anemia.

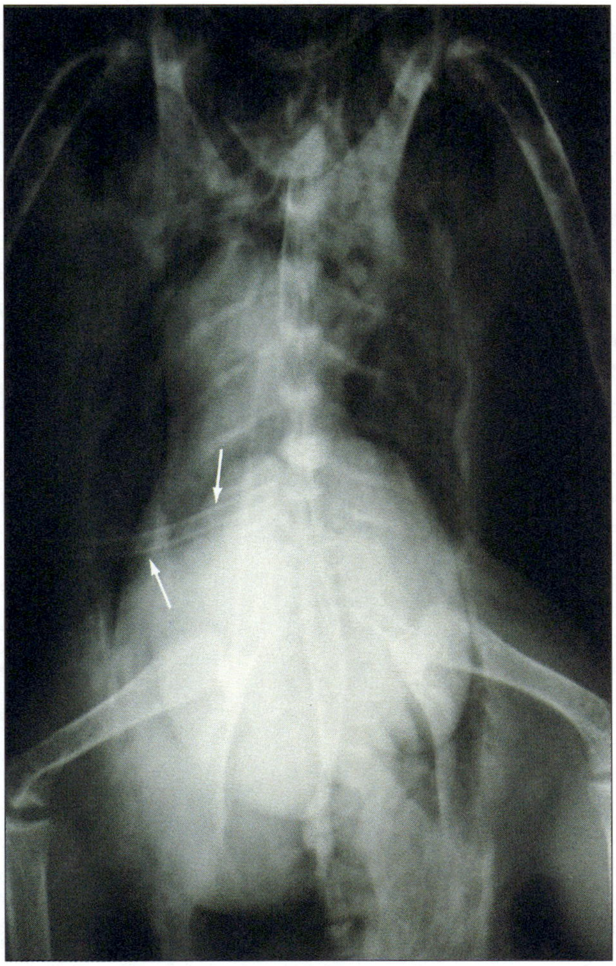

Figure 3—This radiograph shows placement of an air sac cannula (*arrows*) in the right abdominal air sac of a domesticated duck.

OXYGEN THERAPY AND RESPIRATORY DISTRESS

Dyspneic birds should be placed in a warm oxygen cage on presentation. A brief physical examination can be performed after the bird has been stabilized. Several commercial oxygen cages for birds have controlled heat and humidity levels. A human or small animal incubator attached to an oxygen source is often adequate. A facemask can be used to deliver oxygen during handling and diagnostic testing if necessary. Prolonged periods of oxygen elevation can cause oxygen toxicity in birds, as occurs in mammals. In studies, budgerigars showed lethargy and depression when kept on 68% to 87% oxygen for longer than four days.[7] Therefore, oxygen levels greater than 40% should be of limited duration.

Birds presenting with severe obstructive respiratory patterns should have an air sac cannula placed immediately (Figure 3). An inhalant anesthetic should be administered through a facemask until the tube is placed. The bird can be positioned in lateral recumbency with the leg pulled in a caudal direction. An incision should be made in the skin caudal to the last rib (in the same site used for surgical sexing), and blunt dissection should be used to expose the abdominal air sac. A small knick should be made and a shortened tracheal tube inserted into the air sac. The surrounding skin and musculature should be sutured around the tube to hold it in place. If a cuffed tube has been placed, the cuff can be inflated to help retain the tube within the air sac. Oxygen can be attached directly to the tube, or the bird can be placed in an oxygen-rich environment during recovery. The air sac cannula also can be used to deliver nebulized antibiotics to specific air sacs in cases of severe air sacculitis.

NUTRITIONAL SUPPORT

Patients suffering from anorexia, malnutrition, maldigestion, or weight loss (despite an adequate appetite) need nutritional support. Most often, tube feeding or gavage feeding is used. A curved metal feeding needle with a balled tip is recommended. Rubber feeding tubes can be used; however, considerable care should be taken to ensure the bird does not bite the feeding tube and swallow the end.

Several enteric feeding formulas on the market offer from <1.0 kcal/ml to 2.0 kcal/ml. Hand-feeding formulas for baby birds also can be used. The feed should be warmed in hot water to body temperature in order to avoid gut stasis and curdling. The volume is estimated at 3 cc per 100 grams of weight. Baby birds can be fed up to 5 cc per 100 grams of weight, as they have a greater crop capacity. Regurgitating birds should be fed smaller amounts to decrease the likelihood of regurgitation. Birds experiencing persistent regurgitation may need to have a feeding tube placed into the proventriculus. An esphagostomy incision can be made at the base of the mandible and a red rubber feeding tube passed through the crop directly into the proventriculus. The tube should then be sutured into place and food given by slow bolus. The amount given should be roughly half of the amount that would be given into the crop. If it is necessary to bypass the crop and proventriculus, a Foley catheter can be placed directly into the duodenum through an incision made through the lower abdominal wall.[2] An easily absorbed liquid diet should be given with a continuous-rate infusion pump or in multiple small boluses.

The nutritional requirements for avian patients may be calculated by using the basal metabolic rate (BMR) and minimum energy requirement (MER). The basal metabolic rate is the minimum energy required for life, while the minimum energy requirement is the basal metabolic rate plus the energy required for normal physical activity, digestion, and absorption. The additional stress of hospitalization and illness may increase the basal metabolic rate one- or twofold beyond normal. The formulas for determining the basal metabolic rate and minimum energy requirement are:

$$\text{BMR} = \text{K}\ (\text{wt}_{\text{kg}}{}^{0.75})$$

where

K = 129 for passerines (e.g., finches, canaries)
K = 78 for nonpasserines (e.g., parrots)

and

$$\text{MER} = 1.5 \times \text{BMR}$$

Therefore, for a 300-gram Amazon bird, the formula for the basal metabolic rate would read BMR = 78 ($0.3^{0.75}$) = 32 kcal/day. The average minimum energy requirement for a hospitalized bird is 1.5 × BMR = 1.5 × 32 = 48 kcal/day. The additional stress of hospitalization and illness increases the minimum energy requirement by 1.5; therefore 48 × 1.5 = 72 kcal/day. If the feeding formula has 2 kcal/ml, then 36 ml of tube feed are needed per day or 9 ml given four times daily.

The use of total parenteral nutrition (TPN) is possible in birds. Preliminary studies have shown some success in maintaining catheters and vascular access devices for administration of total parenteral nutrition.[2,8] This option should be considered in cases of severe regurgitation, gastrointestinal stasis, orofacial trauma, certain gastrointestinal surgeries, and maldigestion/malabsorption problems. Difficulties are encountered with maintenance of catheters or vascular access devices, contamination of materials resulting in sepsis, and metabolic complications associated with administration of total parenteral nutritional solutions. Considerably more work is needed to determine appropriate formulas and delivery methods to minimize the complications associated with these nutritional products.

Vitamin supplementation should be considered in birds with poor dietary history. Vitamins A, D, and E are available in an injectable combination and are often used in birds with calcium deficiency or other nutritional deficiencies. B-complex vitamins are often given to anorectic birds orally, in subcutaneous fluids, or by direct injection.

ANTIMICROBIAL AGENTS

Antimicrobial agents should be considered for any severely debilitated bird. Septicemia may be a primary or secondary problem in many critically ill birds. Birds that are immunosuppressed from noninfectious causes also may benefit from antimicrobial treatment. Birds with simple closed fractures, uncomplicated heavy-metal toxicity, hypocalcemia, and other noninfectious problems may not require or benefit from the use of antimicrobials.[2] The agent used should depend on several factors: spectrum of the agent, toxicity of the drug, and severity of illness. The routine use of stronger antibiotics and antifungals is discouraged, as doing so may be selective for resistance and make less pathogenic organisms more pathogenic.

When antibiotics are used, they should be given as a complete course, generally 7 to 14 days, unless the antibiotic is changed because of culture and sensitivity test results. Samples for culture should be taken before any antibiotics are administered, if possible, so that the bacterial population can be accurately identified and treated accordingly.

The route of administration depends on type of antibiotic, severity of illness of the patient, and affected organ. Many antibiotics are only available as injectable forms, such as piperacillin, enrofloxacin, and the aminoglycosides. The injectable form of enrofloxacin may be given orally, although it has a very bitter taste. Mixing with juices or cherry flavoring facilitates patient acceptance.

Parenteral administration is preferred initially, as it allows rapid onset of therapeutic blood levels. Any patient with an intravenous or intraosseous catheter in place probably warrants administration of intravenous or intraosseous antibiotics. In cases of severe gastrointestinal disease, oral administration may prove more beneficial and may be given in addition to or instead of parenteral antibiotics.

Nebulization of antimicrobials is useful in cases of lower respiratory disease, such as pneumonia, tracheitis, and air sacculitis. For example, nebulization of amphotericin is an excellent means of delivery in cases of aspergillosis. The solvent (e.g., saline, sterile water) used for nebulization varies with drug selection. In general, the same solvent used for drug rehydration is used for nebulization. Mixing antibiotics or antifungals in the same solution usually is not recommended, as the drugs may precipitate. Upper respiratory disease warrants use of intranasal ophthalmic forms of antibiotics or nasal flushes with antibiotics diluted in warm saline or sterile water.

CORTICOSTEROIDS

The use of corticosteroids in avian emergency medicine is a subject of much debate. The use of single-injection or very short-term corticosteroid therapy has clinical merit. Steroids are most beneficial in cases of shock (especially when accompanied by hypoglycemia) and in cases of acute trauma (especially head trauma). Only short-acting preparations, such as methylprednisolone sodium succinate and dexamethasone sodium phosphate, should be used. Although published doses vary, I use methyprednisolone sodium succinate at a one-time dose of 20 to 30 mg/kg intravenously or intraosseously in patients with head trauma. In cases of shock from other causes, the dose can be lowered to 10 mg/kg intravenously, intraosseously, or intramuscularly. Shock doses of dexamethasone sodium phosphate vary from 0.5 to 4 mg/kg intravenously, intraosseously, or intramuscularly.

SHOCK

The state of shock manifests in birds as severe weakness, pale mucous membranes, minimal response to stimuli, and poor peripheral perfusion. Peripheral perfusion can be estimated by weak pulses at the metatarsal and ulnar arteries and poor refill of the ulnar vein following blanching. Reduced vascular volume is indicated by poor filling (0.5 seconds) of the ulnar vein if occluded proximally.[2] Birds presented in shock should be treated quickly and aggressively. An intravenous or intraosseous catheter should be placed immediately. Because placing an intravenous catheter in poorly perfused vessels may be difficult, an intraosseous catheter may be more advantageous to place. Usually the intravenous catheter can be placed without administering anesthesia. If placement of an intraosseous catheter is necessary, low levels of isoflurane can be administered through a facemask, unless the bird is severely debilitated.

Samples for packed cell volume, total solids, and blood glucose should be estimated from blood collected in the catheter hub, by venipuncture using an insulin needle, or by clipping a toenail. Several drops of blood should be used to make slides for estimated white blood cell and differential counts. The slides of collected blood also give information on toxic changes, number of immature red and white cells, and presence of hemoparasites.

Once the catheter is in place, a shock dose of 25 mg/ml can be given as a slow bolus through the catheter. Polyionic fluids, such as lactated Ringer's solution, are used initially. The bird should then be placed on a continuous-rate infusion pump or slow-drip fluids if possible. To combat hypovolemia, it is beneficial to give continuous fluids immediately following shock doses of fluids, as the fluids shift to extravascular spaces.

Rapidly acting corticosteroids can be used in cases of shock. I prefer methylprednisolone sodium succinate at a dose of 10 mg/kg intravenously or intraosseously. If methylprednisolone sodium succinate is unavailable, dexamethasone sodium phosphate can be used at a dose of 2 to 4 mg/kg intravenously, intraosseously, or intramuscularly.

Young birds with acute disease and old birds with chronic disease are often hypoglycemic as a result of whole-body energy depletion. Intravenous or intraosseous boluses of 50% dextrose using 1 to 2 cc/kg mixed 1:2 with warm lactated Ringer's solution or saline should be given if blood glucose is less than 200 mg/dl. The bird should then be placed on fluids with 7.5% to 10% dextrose. If sepsis is suspected, bacteriocidal antibiotics should be given intravenously.

Unless they are actively bleeding, critically ill birds with anemia (packed cell volume of 20%) should be given a transfusion after shock treatment has been concluded and the patient has stabilized. Colloidal therapy is indicated for volume expansion if the bird is hypoproteinemic. Hetastarch (or other colloidal compounds) can be given intravenously or intraosseously at a slow rate of 10 to 15 ml/kg. The dose can be repeated up to three more times during the next 24 hours if necessary.

Diagnostic tests may have to wait until the bird has stabilized, as many treatment measures (e.g., intramuscular injection and fluid administration) can alter diagnostic parameters.

About the Author

Dr. Morrisey is a second-year resident in avian and exotic animal medicine at The Animal Medical Center, New York, New York.

REFERENCES

1. Bond MW, Downs D, Wolf S: Intravenous catheter therapy. *Proc Assoc Avian Vet*:8–14, 1993.
2. Quesenberry KQ, Hillyer EV: Supportive care and emergency therapy, in Ritchie BW, Harrison GJ, Harrison LR (eds): *Avian Medicine: Principles and Applications.* Philadelphia, WB Saunders, 1994, pp 382–416.
3. Quesenberry KQ, Hillyer E: Hospital management of the critical avian patient. *Proc Assoc Avian Vet*:365–369, 1989.
4. Stone EG, Redig PT: Preliminary evaluation of hetastarch for the management of hypoproteinemia and hypovolemia. *Proc Assoc Avian Vet*:197–199, 1994.
5. Bos JH: Treatment of anemic birds with iron dextran therapy, homologous, and heterologous blood transfusions. *Proc Assoc Avian Vet*:221–225, 1990.
6. Rosskopf WJ: Pet avian emergency care. *Proc Assoc Avian Vet*:341–356, 1991.
7. Stauber E: Effects of increased concentration of inspired oxygen. *Proc Eur Assoc Avian Vet*:105–114, 1991.
8. Degernes L: Administration of total parenteral nutrition in pigeons. *Am J Vet Res* 55(5):660–665, 1994.

Egg Binding, Hormonal Control, and Therapeutic Considerations

Tuscon Wildlife Rehabilitation Center
Tucson, Arizona
Stormy Hudelson, DVM   Paul Hudelson, MA

KEY FACTS

- Egg binding is a life-threatening situation that requires immediate attention.
- Egg binding is most commonly seen in cockatiels, finches, canaries, and budgerigars.
- The hen usually is presented with half-closed eyes and fluffed feathers and may show hypocalcemic tetany.
- Quiet, a heated cage, and correction of hypocalcemia are the most important aspects of therapy.
- In finches, egg binding must be resolved within one hour.

An understanding of how oviposition occurs is necessary to be able to intervene successfully when the mechanism fails, that is, when egg binding (i.e., retention of an egg in the uterus or oviduct) occurs. Under normal conditions, oviposition in birds is a controlled event culminating in strong and rapid uterine (shell gland) muscle contractions in conjunction with relaxation of the uterovaginal sphincter. If either of these events does not occur, the egg will not be laid. Egg binding is a significant cause of mortality in the poultry and pet bird industries. With the assumption that all avian species hormonally control oviposition in the same manner,[a] we propose treatment of the egg-bound pet bird through use of prostaglandins to stimulate uterine contractions and simultaneously relax the uterovaginal sphincter.[1]

CAUSES

Egg binding is seen most often in cockatiels, finches, canaries, and budgerigars.[2] It usually is seen in unmated birds; however, it can be a cause of death in older hens.[2] Egg-bound birds often lack muscle tone because of exercise-restricted life-styles and may be obese. Genetic factors may contribute to egg binding in birds (as in mammals with dystocia), but no information is available to support this assertion. Rosskopf,[3] however, found that budgerigar flocks with lipomatosis have a higher incidence of egg binding. Peritonitis or oophoritis from any of several causes may effectively block enough of the prostaglandin released or produced by the follicles to cause egg binding. A similar situation to that found by Kelly et al[4] may be induced: ligation of the largest and second largest preovulatory follicles (F_1 and F_2) delayed oviposition.

Any scarring,[5] neoplasia, cysts,[6] or inflammation of the oviduct,[7] vagina, or cloaca could potentially cause an egg not to be passed. Any debilitating condition—whether infectious, metabolic, or nutritional[7]—could cause egg

[a]Etches RJ: Personal communication, Department of Animal Sciences, University of Guelph, 1992.

Updated from original publication in Volume 15, Number 3, March 1993 retention or malformation. A malformed egg or one that is too large may be retained. If eggs are ectopic, they obviously cannot pass and require surgical intervention. Ectopic eggs may result from uterine rupture or reverse movement of the egg up the oviduct. Failure of the ova to enter the infundibulum can cause yolk peritonitis. Interestingly, the hysterectomies commonly done in cockatiels have not been shown to produce ectopic ova; this is most likely because of the hormonal control the uterus shares in ovulation (to be discussed later).

The most common cause of egg binding is hypocalcemia.[5] Estrogen, produced by the primary follicle, causes development of external sexual characteristics, such as browning of the cere of budgerigars and reddening of the comb of chickens. Estrogen also stimulates medullary bone production and causes the liver to produce yolk precursors. Calcium from the bone (usually the femur, although any bone can supply calcium) is then liberated and carried to the uterus to be deposited on the shell. Calcium also is vital in muscle contraction. If a bird is unable to consume an adequate amount of calcium, thus causing a drop in blood calcium, uterine inertia and egg binding can occur. If hypocalcemia is severe, hypocalcemic tetany and occasionally fractured bones can occur. Birds on a seed diet are nearly guaranteed to be calcium deficient because of the poor calcium–to–phosphorus ratio of grains.

Another consideration is an inadequate amount of calories. A bird producing eggs has an increased caloric requirement and should be fed an ample amount of good-quality food to prevent a catabolic state.[3] If the owner removes eggs as they are laid, the hen may continue to produce many more eggs than its normal clutch size and become exhausted. A deficiency of vitamin E or arginine vasotocin and prostaglandin precursors may also cause problems. Further causes can include administration of antiprostaglandins as therapeutic agents, influx of adrenalin[8] from administration or stress (e.g., a sudden drop in environmental temperature),[2,3] and use of some of the sulfonamide antibiotics (e.g., trimethoprim-sulfamethoxazole), which cause a decrease in calcium carbonate to be laid down for the shell because of interference of the agents with carbonic anhydrase.[2]

HORMONAL CONTROL OF OVIPOSITION

When a bird becomes competent to reproduce, the ovary must become activated. Once the ovary is activated, follicular maturation occurs with several ovum reaching maturity in sequential order. After the largest follicle ovulates, the ovum travels along the oviduct to become a complete egg before being passed. In domestic hens, this process occurs within 24 to 26 hours after ovulation. For most of this time (approximately 20 hours), the egg is in the uterus.[9]

Ovulation, with or without oviposition, is preceded by uterine contraction.[10] Oviposition, except for the last occurrence in a sequence, is followed by ovulation within one hour.[11] In a study of follicular control of oviposition in hens, Kelly et al[4] showed that the largest and second largest preovulatory follicles (F_1 and F_2) and the largest postovulatory follicle (R_1) were able to produce products that can induce oviposition without the endocrine events that precede ovulation. It was concluded that the physiologic events that control oviposition and ovulation can be independent of each other. Olson and Hertelendy[12] supported this view during a study in which arginine vasotocin was injected into a chicken before predicted oviposition and resulted in premature oviposition; however, ovulation still occurred at the appropriate time.

Although ovulation may not be necessary for oviposition, the follicles are. Follicles mature and become enlarged as they sequester yolk precursors.[9] Follicular hierarchy is established through the largest follicle being the first to ovulate. According to a study by Etches et al,[13] when a follicle reaches a size large enough to be part of the follicular hierarchy, it is capable of producing prostaglandins. Hertelendy and Hammond[14] found that prostaglandins do not affect steroidogenesis and are not produced in response to luteinizing hormone. Etches et al[13] also found evidence to support the theory, but when they incubated granulosa cells with ovine luteinizing hormone and then with A23187 (calcium ionophore), a 15- to 20-fold increase in prostaglandin $F_2\alpha$ ($PGF_2\alpha$) was seen. The induced increase in prostaglandin $F_2\alpha$ and the fact that oviposition occurs prematurely when ovulation is induced prematurely[15,16] led Etches et al[13] to suggest that preovulatory surges of protein and steroid hormones may be involved in initiation of prostaglandin production of oviposition. The article also demonstrated that each follicle increases its ability to produce prostaglandin $F_2\alpha$ as it ages and moves through the hierarchy.

The fact that the F_1 produces the most prostaglandin has also been confirmed by several other studies.[17–19] Prostaglandins are oxytocic substances that have been shown to cause uterine contractions and oviposition.[9,10,20] This, as well as the large increase in prostaglandin concentration shortly before oviposition, indicates that prostaglandins are a main influence in oviposition. The increase in prostaglandin $F_2\alpha$ from F_1 also is seen during the preovulatory uterine contractions with the first ovulation of a sequence.[10] The last oviposition of a sequence is not directly followed by ovulation although the usual increase in prostaglandin occurs. Olson et al[11] suggested in their study that R_1 and F_2 are the major contributors to the increase in prostaglandin. They also found that prostaglandin E_2 (PGE_2) concentration is increased in the plasma from F_1 at terminal oviposition. The investigators cautiously suggest that prostaglandin E_2 may therefore be important at this time.

A lesser amount of prostaglandins is synthesized in the uterus by the conversion of arachidonate,[21] but this is probably insignificant because the venous drainage of the uterus is not as high as that of F_1. The prostaglandins in the myometrium and mucosa follow a similar cycle as the follicular prostaglandins: increasing before oviposition and then dramatically dropping at the time of oviposition. Nevertheless, once the prostaglandins are produced they must interact with the uterus to induce contractions.

It is believed that increased intracellular calcium ions (Ca^{++}) and decreased intracellular cyclic 3',5'-adenosine monophosphate (cAMP) may be able to induce uterine smooth muscle contractions.[22] Prostaglandin $F_2\alpha$ apparently binds to a single class of binding sites in the uterus.[23] Once the prostaglandin $F_2\alpha$ reaches these sites, it causes a time- and dose-dependent mobilization of cellular calcium.[22] Molnar et al[22] demonstrated no influence by prostaglandin $F_2\alpha$ on cAMP. Both prostaglandin E_1 and prostaglandin E_2 have, however, been demonstrated to be associated with a low- and high-affinity binding site in the myometrium.[1]

At the nanomolar range, prostaglandin E_1 and prostaglandin E_2 caused a suppression of cAMP; but at the macromolar range, there was a dose-related increase of cAMP.[23] Prostaglandin E_2 was less effective than was prostaglandin E_1 for causing uterine muscle contractions.[22] When prostaglandin E_2 and prostaglandin $F_2\alpha$ are present together, Wechsung and Houvenaghel[24] found an increase in uterine pressure and a simultaneous decrease in vaginal pressure. In contrast to prostaglandin $F_2\alpha$, prostaglandin E_1 and prostaglandin E_2 have been demonstrated to cause relaxation of the hen vagina.[24]

Once uterine contractions begin, arginine vasotocin reaches a maximum level and then rapidly declines. Arginine vasotocin is an oxytocinlike substance of the neurohypophysis. During oviposition, a depletion of arginine vasotocin in the neurohypophysis and a simultaneous transient increase in the plasma was demonstrated by Tanaka and Nakajo.[25] Koike, Shimada, and Cornett[26] found a single receptor in the hen uterus for arginine vasotocin. Once it arrives at the uterus, arginine vasotocin induces prostaglandin production in the uterine tissue and then works synergistically to potentiate the uterine contractions.[27]

To determine the stimulus for arginine vasotocin release, Saito et al[18] treated hens with indomethacin (prostaglandin inhibitor), which delayed oviposition and uterine contractions. Arginine vasotocin was not released until the uterus was injected with prostaglandin E_2, after which contractions occurred. Because ovulation and increased plasma levels of prostaglandins did not occur, it seems that uterine contractions are the stimulus for arginine vasotocin release. Saito et al[18] also demonstrated that an egg in the uterus is not necessary for uterine contractions by finding that uterine contractions and increased arginine vasotocin levels occur at the expected time of oviposition after induced premature oviposition. In addition, when premature oviposition is induced by arginine vasotocin injection, there is no increase in prostaglandin levels, thereby suggesting that arginine vasotocin does not stimulate prostaglandin production.[12]

These data suggest that the follicles produce prostaglandins and release them to be transported to the uterus, where they cause contraction of the uterus and relaxation of the uterovaginal sphincter. This, in turn, stimulates release of arginine vasotocin, which also affects uterine contraction.

CLINICAL SIGNS

Clinical signs can range from weakness with mild, occasional abdominal contractions[2] to sudden death.[3] The history may include recent egg laying,[28] nest activity, or previous problems with egg laying. Birds experiencing egg binding often show signs of illness, that is, fluffed feathers, half-closed eyes, and weakness. Signs of straining to pass the egg may be absent.[29] In more advanced cases, the hen might move to the floor of the cage and show signs of hypocalcemic tetany. Occasionally, fractures also may be present. In severe cases, egg yolk peritonitis, which is indicated by a fluid-filled abdomen, must be considered. On abdominocentesis, the fluid usually is cellular; and, if the yolk has not become inspissated, obvious yolk material may be revealed.[7]

If the egg is firmly lodged in the pelvic area, secondary problems from arterial, venous, and nerve compression can occur[30] and might result in circulatory shock, swollen or cold feet, and lameness. In addition, retention of feces and water can cause renal damage or autointoxication (or both) as a result of gut blockage causing bacterial overgrowth.[3]

According to Hasholt,[30] canaries may present with hanging wings and tail as well as swelling around the base of the tail. Budgerigars may sit on the tail with legs extended in a ventral direction and abducted, with the wings and body erect.[30] Budgerigars and other small passerines evidently have acute onset of signs and rapid progression to death if not treated promptly. In finches, the egg should be removed within an hour of the time distress is first noted.[2] Larger psittacines may have a slower progression of problems, which may be unnoticed by their owners for several days. Nonetheless, by the time any bird experiencing egg binding is presented to the veterinarian, an emergency situation is occurring and must be handled promptly.

DIAGNOSIS

Diagnosis usually is accomplished by the history and clinical signs. Palpation of the egg usually is possible unless it is high in the oviduct, the bird is obese, or the egg has a very soft shell. A decision must be made whether the egg higher in the oviduct is retained or coursing the tract normally. If the hen is stable, time will answer that dilemma. Radiographs can be helpful in making a diagnosis, but soft-shelled eggs may be difficult to appreciate.

TREATMENT

When the bird is presented, a complete physical examination should be done carefully to prevent undue stress to the bird. If it is alert and not showing signs of shock or toxicity, the hen should be placed in a warm (85°F to 90°F [30°C to 33°C]), quiet environment after being given 50 mg of calcium gluconate and 50 g calcium lactate/10 ml intramuscularly at 0.5 to 1.0 ml/kg.[2] Most eggs will pass in two to three hours. Some veterinarians also give a multivitamin injection at this time.[2] If the bird is dehydrated or in shock and showing hypocalcemic tetany, intravenous fluids (with or without glucose) should be given. Maintenance fluids should be administered at approximately 50 ml/kg/day. The maximum intravenous bolus for a cockatiel is 2 ml.

Many birds experiencing egg binding may be acidotic; thus, glucose should not be given at first unless at a concentration of 2.5% or if bicarbonate is given simultaneously because glucose is an acidifying agent.[2] Ten percent calcium gluconate at 50 to 100 mg/kg can be given intravenously at a slow rate to effect if venous access is possible.[1] If not, calcium should be given at a rate of up to 0.5 mg/g intramuscularly. Gentle massaging of the uterine area may stimulate contractions. The bird should then be returned to the heated cage. If it still fails to pass, the egg should be collapsed by creating a longitudinal crack and involution of the egg through digital pressure or by passing a needle through the dilated cervix or through the abdominal uterine wall[3,7,31]; contents of the egg are then aspirated. An 18-gauge needle is used for larger psittacines, and a 22-gauge needle is used for smaller birds.[2] The hen is returned to the heated cage. The egg is most often passed in 30 minutes, but according to one reference it may take one to two days.[3]

Pieces of shell may occasionally be retained and need to be removed with forceps through the cervix. Care must be taken not to tear the uterus. Oxytocin administered after one hour at 0.00625 units/g may be considered,[3] but another more appropriate choice may be to apply prostaglandin E_2 vaginal gel to the cervix. Prostaglandin E_2, as opposed to oxytocin, has the combined effect of inducing uterine contractions and relaxing the uterovaginal sphincter.[1] In addition, prostaglandin E_2 may have a built-in safety mechanism because it causes an increase in cAMP and thus uterine muscle relaxation when given in larger doses.[18] If the clinician is presented with a finch or canary, aggressive methods usually are required because these birds cannot tolerate egg binding for more than an hour.[2,3] Prophylactic antibiotics, such as the cephalosporins, may be considered.

If medical treatment is not successful or if the uterus has torn during the procedures, surgery is required. If egg yolk peritonitis is apparent (abdominal swelling), a ventral midline approach is required and care must be taken not to rupture the abdominal air sacs; if the air sacs are ruptured, abdominal fluid and yolk material enter the respiratory system. The only type of suction we use is manual removal of the fluid by a sterile syringe. Evisceration may (and has) occurred during use of suction devices.

The fluid should be sent for culture and sensitivity testing as well as cytologic examination. The uterus is incised over the egg, and the egg and any shell remnants are removed. The uterus should be closed with an inverting suture pattern. If no abdominal fluid is present, a lateral laparotomy may be useful, especially if a hysterectomy is going to be done. For an excellent description of these surgical approaches, the reader is encouraged to consult other literature.[2]

PREVENTION

Exercise by free flying or, if wings are clipped, by moving the bird up and down on a perch to encourage wing flapping; a good nutritional plan; and proper lighting (unfiltered sunlight) are mandatory for prevention of egg binding. Avoiding positive reinforcement of sexual behavior[32] and removing other breeding stimuli, such as nest boxes and male birds, might help. Sometimes changing the bird's location or altering the light schedule (or both) is enough.

If absolutely necessary, progesterone (3 mg/100 g intramuscularly every four to six weeks) can suppress ovulation; however, side effects, such as lethargy, obesity, polydipsia, and polyuria, can occur. If chronic egg laying is a problem, hysterectomy may be the best option.

About the Authors

Dr. Hudelson, who is a Diplomate of the American Board of Veterinary Practitioners (Avian Specialty), and Mr. Hudelson are currently affiliated with the Tucson Wildlife Rehabilitation Center in Tucson, Arizona.

REFERENCES

1. Asboth G, Todd H, Toth M, Hertelendy F: PGE_2 binding, synthesis, and distribution in hen oviduct. *Am J Physiol* 248:E80–E88, 1985.
2. Harrison G, Harrison L: *Clinical Avian Medicine and Surgery*, ed 1. Philadelphia, WB Saunders Co, 1986, pp 344, 372–373, 588–590.
3. Rosskopf WI, Woerpel RW: Egg binding in caged and aviary birds. *Mod Vet Pract* 65(6):437–440, 1984.
4. Kelly JD, Etches RJ, Guemene D: Follicular control of oviposition in the hen. *Poult Sci* 69:288–291, 1990.
5. McMillan MC: Imaging of avian urogenital disorders. *AAV Today* 2(2):74–80, 1988.
6. Hochleithner T, Lechner C: Egg binding in a budgerigar *(Melopsittacus undulatus)* caused by a cyst of the right oviduct. *AAV Today* 2(3):136–138, 1988.
7. Rosskopf WJ, Woerpel RW: Pet avian obstetrics. *Proceedings of the First International Conference on Zoological and Avian Medicine.* Oahu, Hawaii, AAV/AAZV, 1987, pp 213–231.
8. Prasad A, Davis LE, Dale HE: Adrenergic response of the avian uterus. *Poult Sci* 43:192–197, 1964.
9. Shimada K, Saito N: Control of oviposition in poultry. *Crit Rev Poult Biol* 2(3):235–253, 1989.
10. Shimada K, Olson DM, Etches RJ: Follicular and uterine prostaglandin levels in relation to uterine contraction and the first ovulation of a sequence in the hen. *Biol Reprod* 31:76–82, 1984.
11. Olson DM, Shimada K, Etches RJ: Prostaglandin concentrations in peripheral plasma and ovarian and uterine plasma and tissue in relation to oviposition in hens. *Biol Reprod* 35: 1140–1146, 1986.
12. Olson DM, Hertelendy F: Plasma levels of 13,14-dihydro-15-keto prostaglandin F_2a in relation to oviposition and ovulation in the domestic hen *(Gallus domesticus). Biol Reprod* 24:496–504, 1981.
13. Etches RJ, Kelly JD, Anderson-Langmuir CE, Olson DM: Prostaglandins production by the largest pre-ovulatory follicles in the domestic hen *(Gallus domesticus). Biol Reprod* 43:378–384, 1990.
14. Hertelendy F, Hammond RW: Prostaglandins do not affect steroidogenesis and are not being produced in response to oLH in chicken granulosa cells. *Biol Reprod* 23:918–923, 1980.
15. Wilson SC, Sharp PJ: The effects of progesterone on oviposition and ovulation in the domestic fowl. *Br Poult Sci* 17: 163–173, 1976.
16. Etches RJ, Cunningham FJ: The effect of pregenolone, progesterone, deoxycorticosterone or corticosterone on the time of ovulation and oviposition in the hen. *Br Poult Sci* 17:637–742, 1976.
17. Shimada K, Olson DM, Etches AI: The effect of indomethacin on ovarian prostaglandin release in hens. *Biol Reprod* 35:1147–1153, 1986.
18. Saito N, Shimada K, Koike TI: Interrelationship between arginine vasotocin, prostaglandin, and uterine contractility in the control of oviposition in the hen (*Gallus domesticus*). *Gen Comp Endocrinol* 67:342–347, 1987.
19. Saito N, Sato K, Shimada K: Prostaglandin levels in peripheral and follicular plasma, the isolated theca and granulosa layers of pre- and postovulatory follicles, and the myometrium and mucosa of the shell gland (uterus) during a midsequence-oviposition of the hen (*Gallus domesticus*). *Biol Reprod* 36:89–96, 1987.
20. Olson DM, Bieller HV, Hertelendy F: Shell gland responsiveness to prostaglandin $F_{2\alpha}$ in relation to oviposition in the domestic hen (*Gallus domesticus*). *Biol Reprod* 24:496–503, 1978.
21. Toth M, Asboth G, Hertelendy F: Turnover of lipid-bound arachidonate and biosynthesis of prostanoids in the endometrium and myometrium of the laying hen. *Arch Biochem Biophys* 226:27–36, 1983.
22. Molnar M, Asem E, Hertelendy F: Differential effects of prostaglandin $F_{2\alpha}$ and of prostaglandins E_1 and E_2 on cyclic 3',5'-monophosphate production and intracellular calcium mobilization in avian uterine smooth muscle cells. *Biol Reprod* 36:384–391, 1987.
23. Toth M, Olson DM, Hertelendy F: Binding of prostaglandin $F_{2\alpha}$ to membranes of shell gland muscle of laying hens: Correlations with contractile activity. *Biol Reprod* 20: 390–398, 1979.
24. Wechsung E, Houvenaghel A: Effect of prostaglandins on oviduct tone in the domestic hen *in vivo*. *Prostaglandins* 15:491–505, 1978.
25. Tanaka K, Nakajo S: Participation of neurohypophysial hormone in oviposition in the hen. *Endocrinology* 70:453–458, 1962.
26. Koike TI, Shimada K, Cornett LE: Plasma levels of immunoreactive mesotocin and vasotocin during oviposition in chickens: Relationship to oxytocic action of the peptides *in vitro* and peptides interaction with myometrial membrane binding sites. *Gen Comp Endocrinol* 70:119–126, 1988.
27. Rzasa J: The effect of arginine vasotocin on prostaglandin production on the hen uterus. *Gen Comp Endocrinol* 53: 260–267, 1984.
28. Rich GA: Ovariohysterectomy in an egg bound cockatiel. *Companion Anim Pract* 1(2):48–49, 1987.
29. Stunkard JA: *Diagnosis Treatment and Husbandry of Pet Birds*, ed 1. Edgewater, MD, Stunkard Publishing Co, 1984, pp 49–50.
30. Hasholt J: Diseases of the female reproductive organs of pet birds. *J Small Anim Pract* 7:313–320, 1966.
31. Rosskopf WJ, Woerpel RW: Egg binding in an Amboina king parrot. *VM SAC* 77(2):231–232, 1982.
32. Amand W: *Zoo and Wildlife Medicine*, ed. 1. Philadelphia, WB Saunders Co, 1978, p 306.

UPDATE

CLARIFICATION OF TREATMENTS

Currently there is some confusion over which type of prostaglandin is appropriate to use when an egg-bound bird is presented. In the presence of extracellular calcium, prostaglandin $F_{2\alpha}$ ($PGF_{2\alpha}$) can cause powerful shell-gland (uterus) contractions. As with oxytocin, $PGF_{2\alpha}$ is unable to relax the uterovaginal sphincter (cervix) and may cause uterine rupture. If $PGF_{2\alpha}$ is administered parenterally, it may cause systemic reactions, such as increased blood pressure, bronchoconstriction, and general smooth-muscle contractions.[1] If $PGF_{2\alpha}$ is used when the cervix is not dilated, it could cause dilation from the constant pressure being applied, reverse peristalsis, or uterine rupture. With these considerations, there apparently is no justification for using $PGF_{2\alpha}$ instead of oxytocin.

When presented with an egg-bound bird, we conduct a physical examination followed by the administration of fluids (crystalloids without lactate), which must be supplied concomitantly with calcium to prevent renal disease. The calcium can be delivered intramuscularly or diluted in a slow intravenous drip to effect if the bird is in tetany. The patient should then be placed in a heated cage.

If a small bird has been egg bound for more than an hour or if a large bird has been egg bound for more than three to five hours, then PGE_2 gel should be applied to the cervix at a dose of about 1 ml/kg of body weight. A much lower dose may be adequate. Researchers found that one microgram of PGE_2 injected into the uterus of chickens can induce oviposition within five minutes.[2] PGE_2 gel can be ordered through an obstetrics and gynecology physician and frozen in small aliquots.

If the uterus is free of adhesions or other pathologic findings, the egg usually is laid within 15 minutes of PGE_2 application. An excess of PGE_2 causes smooth muscle relaxation. If no contractions occur after PGE_2 application, the clinician should identify whether the cervix is dilated. In the presence of dilation, intervention can include gentle manual pressure to push the egg out, collapsing of the egg by ovocentesis, or (assuming that the egg is not too large) a low dose of oxytocin. If adhesions, neoplasia, or other pathologic findings are present, this protocol may fail and surgery will be required.

Additional information on the role of prostaglandins in avian reproduction and on environmental manipulations to control oviposition is available in the literature.[3–5]

REFERENCES

1. Darling L, Talbot RB: *Veterinary Pharmaceuticals and Biologics.* Kansas, Veterinary Medicine Co, 1993.
2. Murakami Y, Fujihara N, Koga O: Plasma levels of arginine vasotocin in the hen before and immediately after premature oviposition induced by prostaglandins and arachidonic acid. *Jpn Poult Sci* 27: 346–355, 1990.
3. Hudelson KS, Hudelson PM: A brief review of the female avian reproductive cycle with special emphasis on the role of prostaglandins and clinical application. *J Avian Med Surg*, in press.
4. Hudelson KS: A review of the mechanisms associated with avian reproduction and their clinical application. *Sem Avian Exotic Pet Med*, in press.
5. Etches RJ: *Reproduction in Poultry*. Toronto, Canada, Oxford University Press, 1995.

A Technique of Intraosseous Cannulation for Intravenous Therapy in Birds

KEY FACTS

- **Substantial fluid imbalances or deficits require intravenous fluid therapy for quick, accurate, reliable expansion of the peripheral circulation.**
- **An alternative approach to avian intravenous catheterization, based on intraosseous access to the peripheral circulation, was adapted from techniques used in human pediatrics.**
- **Intraosseous cannulas have been successfully used to administer drugs, fluids, and parenteral nutritional supplements to many avian patients.**

University of Georgia
Branson W. Ritchie, DVM
Cynthia M. Otto, DVM
Kenneth S. Latimer, DVM, PhD
Dennis T. Crowe, Jr., DVM

SUSTAINING LIFE in a dehydrated or traumatized patient frequently depends on rapid establishment of an appropriate fluid balance. Avian patients presented for medical evaluation, particularly in emergency situations, are often severely dehydrated or in a state of metabolic compromise. Such compromise can be caused by septicemia, prolonged anorexia, acute trauma with excessive blood loss, chronic diarrhea, regurgitation, or major organ failure resulting in acid–base imbalances.[1-3]

Many mild cases of dehydration can be conservatively managed with subcutaneous or oral fluid administration. In critically ill birds, oral or subcutaneous fluid replacement does not provide the rapid expansion of intracellular or extracellular fluid spaces essential for proper perfusion of major organs. As in mammalian patients, substantial fluid imbalances or deficits require intravenous fluid therapy for fast, accurate, reliable expansion of the peripheral circulation.

Intravenous fluid therapy in conscious patients is generally avoided by avian practitioners because of the many difficulties associated with effective management of fluid delivery. Maintenance of peripheral indwelling catheters is complicated by small and fragile vessels, lack of dermal tissue for catheter stabilization, and patient temperaments refractory to the necessary bandaging and manipulation. Repeated boluses of intravenous fluids or drugs (via the jugular, median ulnar, or tibiotarsal veins) have been recommended for avian patients. This technique is stressful and requires frequent restraint or anesthesia for repeated venipuncture of the peripheral vessels.[3]

Because of the difficulty of maintaining continuous access to the peripheral circulation of birds, the documented benefits (in human and veterinary practice) of administering intravenous drugs, fluids, and parenteral nutritional supplements have remained largely unavailable to avian practitioners. For this reason, intraosseous access to the peripheral circulation was adapted from techniques currently used in human pediatrics as an alternative approach to avian intravenous catheterization.

Originally published in Volume 12, Number 1, January 1990

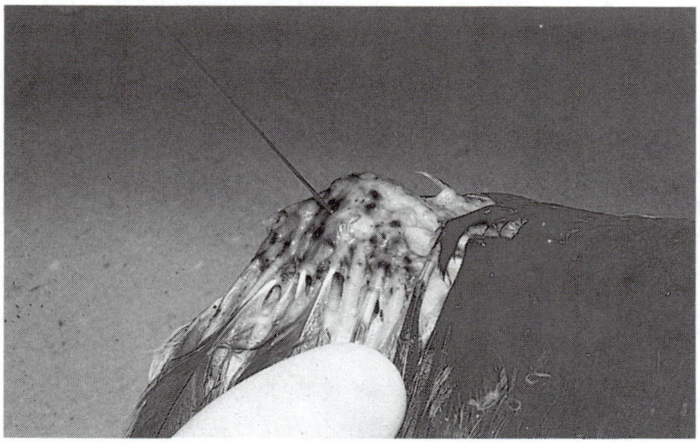

Figure 1—The distal end of the ulna is located, the feathers are removed, and the area is aseptically prepared. The needle is positioned in the center of the bone parallel to the median plane of the ulna.

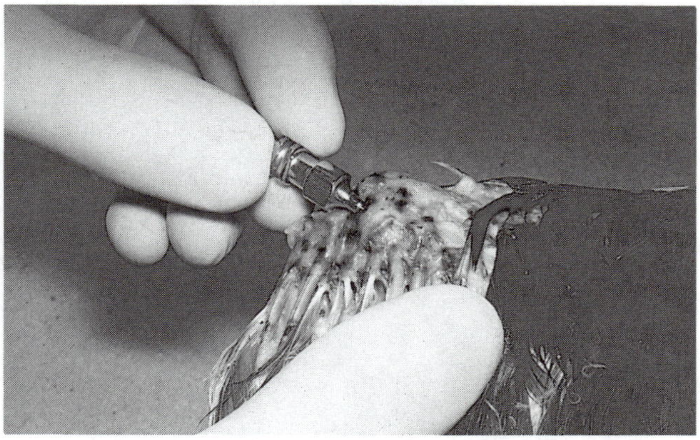

Figure 2—The practitioner supports the patient's wing with one hand while applying firm pressure in a rotating motion to allow the cannula to penetrate the cortex.

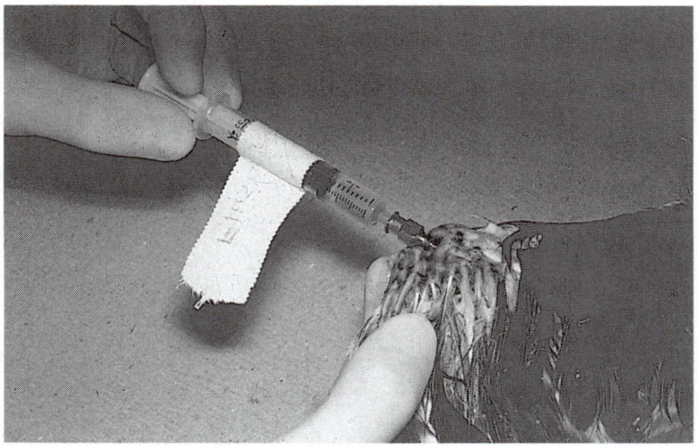

Figure 3—The cannula is flushed with heparinized saline. Proper positioning and patency are checked by gentle aspiration of bone marrow.

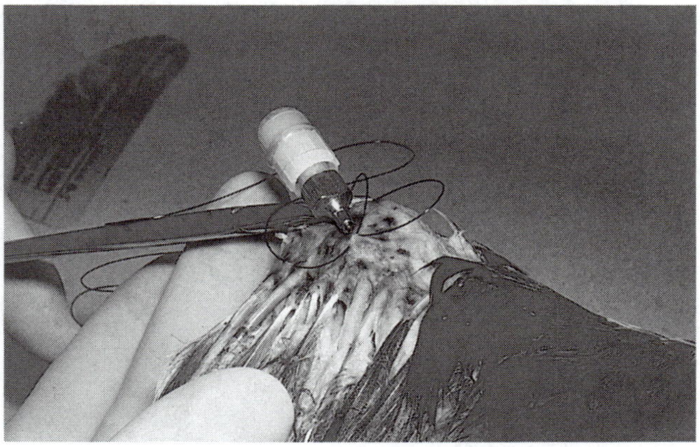

Figure 4—The cannula is secured by being sutured to the soft tissue of the distal ulna.

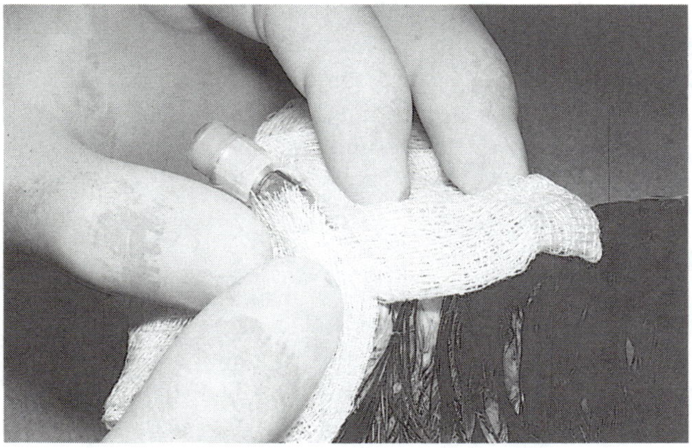

Figure 5—Antibiotic ointment is applied to the base of the catheter, and a slit 2 × 2-inch patch of gauze is used to pad the needle hub.

INTRAOSSEOUS CANNULATION

In birds, the most accessible and easily maintained site for intraosseous cannula placement is the distal end of the ulna. In patients the size of Amazon parrots or larger, 18- to 22-gauge spinal needles are ideal. In smaller species and neonates, 25- to 30-gauge hypodermic needles are effective. As dictated by the patient's size, the chosen cannula should be long enough to penetrate to the midpoint of the ulna.

Depending on the temperament and condition of the patient, anesthesia (with isoflurane) can be used during cannula placement or the cannula can be inserted without anesthesia. In most of the clinical cases in which we have placed intraosseous cannulas, the patients were so depressed that the cannula was easily introduced without chemical restraint.

BEFORE CANNULA PLACEMENT, the feathers are removed from the patient's carpus and the area is aseptically prepared. The needle is positioned at the center of the distal end of the ulna and parallel to the median plane of the bone (Figure 1). This placement ensures that the can-

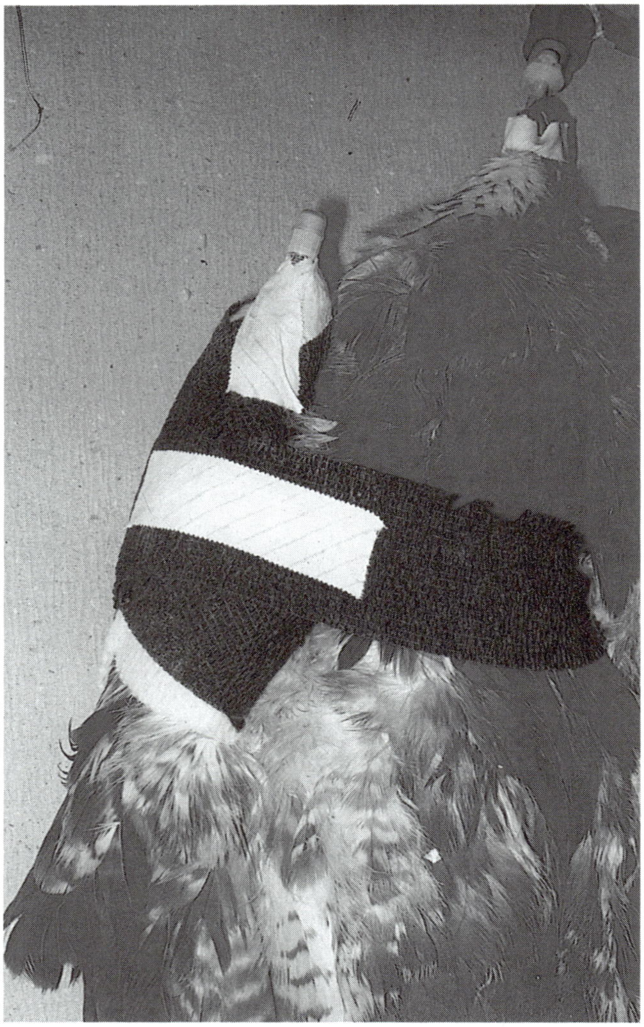

Figure 6—The wing is immobilized with a standard figure-of-8 bandage.

nula will be situated in the center of the medullary canal. To advance the cannula, the practitioner supports the patient's ulna with one hand and applies firm pressure to the cannula with a slight rotating movement (Figure 2).

The process is the same as that used to position a retrograde intramedullary pin. After the needle penetrates the cortex, the needle should pass without resistance deep into the marrow cavity (Figure 2). If there is further resistance, a second cortex is probably being engaged; redirection of the needle tip is recommended. After placement, the wing is palpated to ensure that the cannula has not exited the bone. Aspiration by syringe usually produces a small amount of bone marrow. The needle is then flushed with heparinized saline, which should flow freely (Figure 3).

The cannula is secured by wrapping a small strip of tape around the hub of the needle and suturing the strip to the soft tissue of the distal ulna (Figure 4). The insertion site is coated with antibiotic ointment and is padded with a 2 × 2-inch patch of gauze slit to fit around the needle hub (Figure 5). The wing is placed in a standard figure-of-8 bandage in order to prevent unnecessary tension or trauma to the cannula (Figure 6).

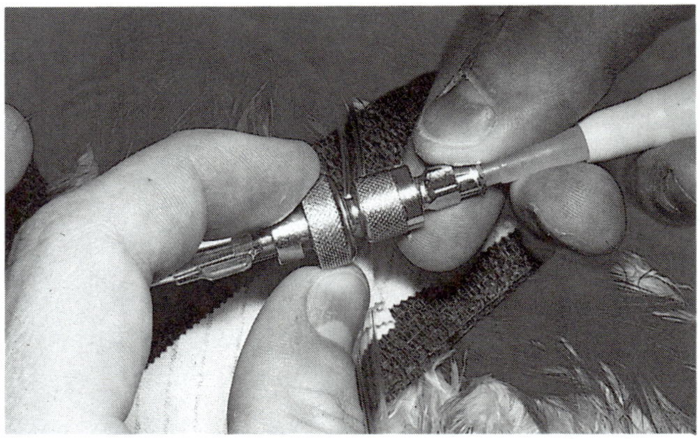

Figure 7—Continuous fluid delivery is provided by connecting the cannula to a pediatric drip intravenous administration set. An intravenous swivel facilitates maintenance and prevents tangling of the lines.

For continuous fluid administration, the cannula can be connected to a standard intravenous administration set. A catheter swivel can facilitate maintenance (Figure 7). For intermittent use, the cannula can be maintained with an intravenous catheter plug. Although we have maintained patent cannulas for 72 hours without flushing, the cannula should be flushed twice daily with heparinized saline (10 units/ml).

EVALUATION

In order to evaluate the potential problems caused by the use of this technique in birds, three permanently injured raptors scheduled for euthanasia were maintained with intraosseous cannulas for 72 hours. The cannulas remained patent and easily accessible throughout the study.

After the investigation period, blood was collected and submitted for analysis by complete blood count, avian chemistry profile, and aerobic and anaerobic cultures on blood agar at 37 °C (98.6 °F). The cannulas were removed; samples from the tips were streaked onto blood agar and placed in aerobic and anaerobic conditions at 37 °C. The birds were euthanatized, and complete sets of tissue (including the ulnae) were submitted for histologic evaluation.

NONE OF THE PATIENTS demonstrated significant deviations from reference laboratory values in the complete blood count. All three birds had slightly elevated lactate dehydrogenase levels attributable to bone marrow penetration by the catheter. The aerobic and anaerobic cultures from the blood and catheter tips were negative. At necropsy, none of the patients had discernible gross lesions in the carpal joint.

Histologic evaluation of the soft tissue was unremarkable. Histologic evaluation of the ulnae indicated that cannula placement produced mild, localized intramedullary hemorrhage as well as subsequent hemosiderosis, heterophilic inflammation, intramedullary fibrosis, discrete intramarrow fat necrosis, and focal osteoblast proliferation with reactive bone formation. Minute particles of necrotic cortical bone, presumably displaced during cannula placement, were occasionally observed. These changes were considered to be minimal in light of the size and length of the cannulas used.

CONCLUSIONS

Further investigations should more fully determine the attributes and limitations of intraosseous cannulation. The technique has already proven to be a safe, rapid, practical method of delivering therapeutic materials to the systemic circulation of birds. Intraosseous cannulas are quickly and easily placed and have been successfully used to administer drugs, fluids, and parenteral nutritional supplements to numerous avian patients.

In mammals, fluids and drugs administered through intraosseous cannulas rapidly reach the peripheral circulation via sinusoid-rich bone marrow.[4-6] The clinical responses to therapeutic agents administered to birds by the intraosseous route suggest equally rapid access to the peripheral circulation. Placement of an intraosseous cannula can be completed in minutes, even by a novice. The necessary equipment is readily available in most veterinary practices.

REPEATED RESTRAINT OR ANESTHESIA, as is necessary for intermittent intravenous boluses using peripheral veins, is not required with the intraosseous technique. The cannula provides continuous intravenous fluid therapy and can be used for intermittent dosing of intravenous drugs with minimal stress to the patient. The technique also preserves the peripheral veins for the blood samples necessary in monitoring rehydration or treatment parameters.

About the Authors

Drs. Ritchie, Otto, and Crowe are affiliated with the Department of Small Animal Medicine and Dr. Latimer is with the Department of Pathology, College of Veterinary Medicine, University of Georgia, Athens, Georgia.

REFERENCES

1. Harrison GJ: What to do until a diagnosis is made, in Harrison GJ, Harrison LR (eds): *Clinical Avian Medicine and Surgery*. Philadelphia, WB Saunders Co, 1986, pp 356–361.
2. Harrison GJ, Woerpel RW, Rosskopf WJ, Karpinski LG: Symptomatic therapy and emergency medicine, in Harrison GJ, Harrison LR (eds): *Clinical Avian Medicine and Surgery*. Philadelphia, WB Saunders Co, 1986, pp 362–375.
3. Redig PT: Fluid therapy and acid-base balance in the critically ill avian patient. *Proc Assoc Avian Vet*:59–73, 1984.
4. Hodge D: Intraosseous infusions: A review. *Pediatr Emerg Care* 1:215–218, 1985.
5. Tocantins LM: Rapid absorption of substances injected into the bone marrow. *Proc Soc Exp Biol Med* 45:292–296, 1940.
6. Papper EM: The bone marrow route for injecting fluids and drugs into the general circulation. *Anesthesiology* 3:307–313, 1942.

Comparative Avian and Mammalian Cytodiagnosis—Part I

KEY FACTS

- **Cytologic evaluation of tissue or fluid from mammals and birds can provide a quick presumptive or definitive diagnosis.**
- **Cytologic techniques and interpretations used for birds are basically identical to those used for domestic mammals.**
- **Mammalian and avian inflammatory responses can be divided into three categories: neutrophilic/heterophilic, mixed-cell, and macrophagic inflammation.**
- **Neoplasms can be classified as carcinomas, sarcomas, or discrete-cell neoplasms.**
- **Abnormal body effusions from birds or mammals can be classified as transudative, modified transudative, exudative, hemorrhagic, malignant, or chylous.**

Colorado State University
Fort Collins, Colorado
Terry W. Campbell, DVM, PhD

CYTOLOGY is a valuable in-house diagnostic tool that is often performed by veterinarians involved in the care of domestic mammals. Cytodiagnosis can also be a useful diagnostic aid in the evaluation of avian patients. The aim of this article is to review the basic principles of veterinary diagnostic cytology and demonstrate the similarities between interpretation of mammalian and avian cytologic specimens.

Various methods of sample collection for cytologic evaluation are available. The choice of the sample collection procedure depends on the location of the tissue or fluid to be sampled, the animal species, and the preference of the cytologist. The basic sample collection techniques (i.e., fine-needle aspiration biopsy, contact [impression] smears, and wash samples) and sample processing procedures used in mammalian cytodiagnosis also apply to birds. Several publications describe these sampling techniques.[1-3]

Various staining procedures can be used for cytologic diagnosis. Many veterinary cytologists prefer Romanovsky techniques (i.e., Wright's and quick Romanovsky stains) for routine procedures because they can provide adequate staining for hematologic and cytologic evaluation. The Romanovsky stains are simple, rapid procedures that make them easily adaptable to the clinical laboratory.

Before a proper cytologic interpretation can be made, the cytologist must first be familiar with the normal cytology of the tissue or fluid being examined. By knowing which cells are normally present, the cytologist can detect cells not normally present. Also, a strong background in pathology and clinical medicine enables the veterinarian to make proper cytodiagnostic interpretations. An advantage in being able to use cytology as a diagnostic tool is that a presumptive (or sometimes definitive) diagnosis can often be obtained quickly.

The same approach to interpretation of the cellular response is made regardless of the source of the sample. The cytologist examines the stained slide containing the sample and determines what types of cells predominate. The three primary diagnoses made from cytologic examination are inflammation, neoplasia, and cellular hyperplasia (benign neoplasia).[1-3]

INFLAMMATION

A diagnosis of inflammation is made if inflammatory cells predominate. The inflammatory cells of most mammals include neutrophils, eosinophils, lymphocytes, plasma cells, monocytes, and macrophages. The inflammatory cells of birds include the same cell types except that neutrophils are replaced by heterophils.

Although eosinophils are considered to be inflammatory

Originally published in Volume 12, Number 5, May 1990

TABLE I
Comparison of Avian and Mammalian Inflammation

Types and Characteristics of Inflammation	*Avian*	*Mammalian*
Inflammatory cells	Heterophils, eosinophils, lymphocytes, plasma cells, monocytes, and macrophages	Neutrophils, eosinophils, lymphocytes, plasma cells, monocytes, and macrophages
Neutrophilic/heterophilic inflammation	Predominately heterophils (more than 70% of inflammatory cells)	Predominately neutrophils (more than 70% of inflammatory cells)
Mixed-cell inflammation	Mixture of granulocytes and mononuclear leukocytes; more than 50% of inflammatory cells are heterophils	Mixture of granulocytes and mononuclear leukocytes; more than 50% of inflammatory cells are neutrophils
Macrophagic inflammation	Predominately mononuclear leukocytes (more than 50% of inflammatory cells)	Predominately mononuclear leukocytes (more than 50% of inflammatory cells)

cells in birds, their presence in inflammatory lesions is rare. This finding may be attributable to their rare involvement in inflammatory processes or their changes in appearance in inflammatory lesions; these changes may make the eosinophils difficult to differentiate from heterophils. An eosinophilic inflammatory response is occasionally found in mammals and suggests a hypersensitivity response to a certain antigenic stimulation (i.e., parasites and allergens).

INFLAMMATORY lesions can be divided into the subclassification of neutrophilic/heterophilic (acute), mixed-cell (chronic active [subacute]), and macrophagic (chronic) inflammation (Table I). Neutrophilic/heterophilic inflammation is characterized by the predominance of mammalian neutrophils or avian heterophils (Figure 1). Thus, more than 70% of the inflammatory cells are neutrophils (in mammals) or heterophils (in birds) in lesions with this type of inflammation. There may also be a mixture of mononuclear leukocytes (i.e., monocytes, macrophages, lymphocytes, or plasma cells).

The neutrophils or heterophils may appear degenerated depending on the cause of the inflammation. Degenerative changes of these cells vary from mild changes indicated by nuclear swelling and hyalinization of the nuclear chromatin (appearing as a homogeneously pink nucleus) to severe changes resulting in nuclear rupture. Slow progressive degeneration of neutrophils or heterophils in a nontoxic environment results in nuclear pyknosis and hypersegmentation. These changes represent the natural aging of these cells.

In areas of mixed-cell inflammation, more than 50% of the mammalian inflammatory cells are neutrophils and more than 50% of the avian inflammatory cells are heterophils (Figure 2). The number of mononuclear leukocytes (monocytes, macrophages, lymphocytes, and plasma cells), however, is increased. The presence of reactive lymphocytes and plasma cells indicates localized antigenic stimulation.

The neutrophils or heterophils are typically nondegenerative in this type of inflammation, thus suggesting that the causative agent has low toxicity. Mixed-cell inflammation in mammals and birds usually indicates an inflammatory response that is not as severe as neutrophilic/heterophilic inflammation.

Macrophagic inflammation in mammals and birds is represented by a predominance of mononuclear leukocytes (Figure 3). Therefore, more than 50% of the inflammatory cells are monocytes, macrophages, lymphocytes, and plasma cells. Macrophagic inflammation is often caused by mild agents that tend to be persistent irritants, such as foreign bodies and infections caused by *Mycobacterium* species, *Chlamydia* organisms, and fungi.

Macrophages often coalesce into mutinucleated giant cells, especially if large-sized foreign material is present (i.e., fungal elements or foreign bodies). Macrophages and giant cells do not necessarily indicate chronicity and can occasionally be present in lesions with neutrophilic/heterophilic inflammation.

TISSUE HYPERPLASIA OR BENIGN NEOPLASIA

Once the cytologist has determined that the cellular response is neither an inflammatory response nor representative of normal cellularity, a decision may be made between a diagnosis of tissue hyperplasia or malignant neoplasia.

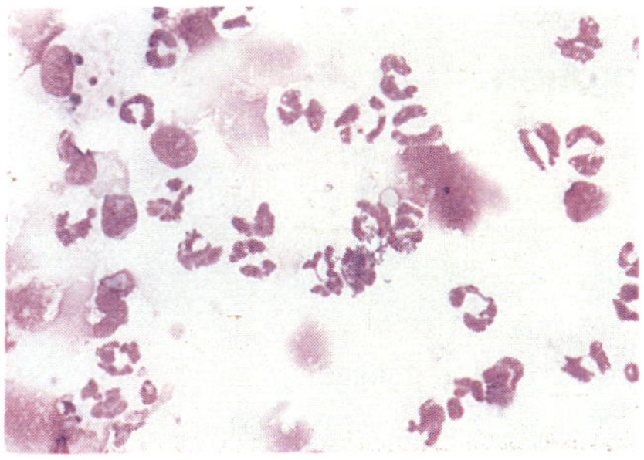

Figure 1—Neutrophilic inflammation. A predominance of degenerated neutrophils in the transtracheal aspirate from a horse with tracheobronchitis. (Diff-Quik®)

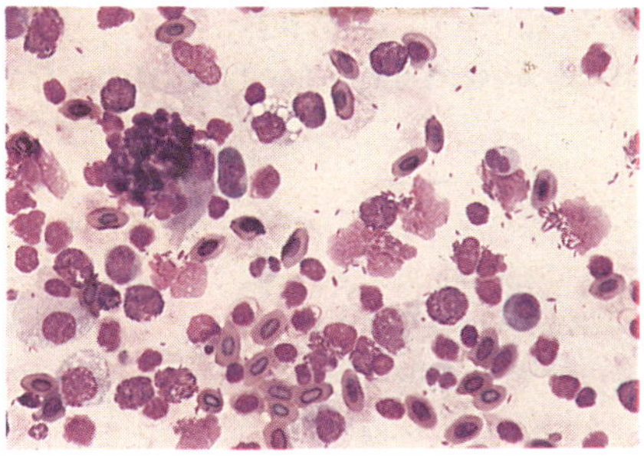

Figure 2—Mixed-cell inflammation. A predominance of nondegenerated heterophils with occasional macrophages, lymphocytes, and plasma cells in a sinus aspirate from a green-cheeked Amazon parrot (*Amazona viridigenalis*) with macrophagic sinusitis. (Diff-Quik®)

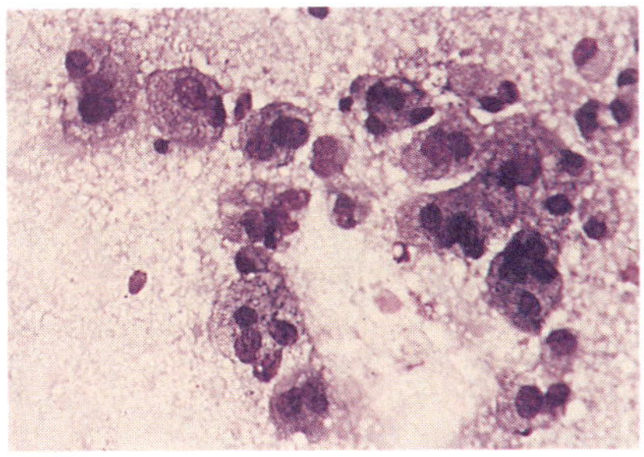

Figure 3—Macrophagic inflammation. A predominance of macrophages and multinucleated giant cells in a biopsy imprint of cutaneous xanthomatosis from a green-winged macaw (*Ara chloroptera*). (Diff-Quik®)

Tissue hyperplasia is a proliferative process in tissue that is usually responding to cellular injury or chronic stimulation (i.e., glandular tissue).

The cell morphology of tissue hyperplasia is usually indistinguishable from that of benign neoplasia. Cells from hyperplastic tissue may appear immature, exhibit cytoplasmic basophilia, and have pale vesicular nuclei. Cells from hyperplastic tissue may have a high mitotic index with normal-appearing mitotic figures. The cells have a uniform nucleus-to-cytoplasm ratio. Fibrous or epithelial-cell hyperplasia is common in lesions with macrophagic inflammation.

Unlike malignant neoplasia, cellular hyperplasia in mammals and birds is uniform. Malignant cells tend to be highly polymorphic.

MALIGNANT NEOPLASIA

The cytomorphologic criteria for malignant neoplasia involve information concerning the general features of cells sampled from the lesion. The general cellular features refer to the cellularity and overall appearance of the cell population in the smear. Malignant neoplasms often provide highly cellular samples because the cells have lost their normal cell-to-cell interactions and tissue alternation creates greater cellular exfoliation.

Malignant neoplasms from mammals or birds often provide cellular samples that contain a polymorphic population of cells that appear to have a common origin; however, a uniform population of cells that are foreign to the location from which they were taken may also suggest malignant neoplasia (metastatic lesion). Circumstantial evidence for neoplasia may include the presence of hemorrhage in an area without a history of trauma. This finding suggests a possible erosive neoplastic mass that has resulted in hemorrhage. A common location for such hemorrhage is a spontaneous hemoperitoneum resulting from an abdominal neoplasm. Thus, chronic hemorrhage in the abdominal cavity of a bird or mammal with radiographic evidence of an abdominal mass suggests abdominal neoplasm even if there is no direct evidence (i.e., neoplastic cells in the abdominal fluid) of malignant neoplasia.

The nuclear features represent the most significant cytologic criteria for malignant neoplasia. Cells derived from malignant neoplasms of birds or mammals tend to have moderate to marked variations in nuclear size (nuclear anisocytosis) and in nucleus-to-cytoplasm ratios. Other nuclear features of malignancy include variable nuclear shapes (nuclear polymorphism), abnormal nucleoli (multiple, large, or irregular), irregular chromatin (i.e., coarse, hypochromatic, and irregularly clumped), multinucleation, and a high mitotic index.

MULTINUCLEATION AND increased mitotic index can also be features of tissue hyperplasia or benign neoplasia in mammals and birds; however, abnormal mitotic figures (i.e., multipolarity) and multinucleated cells with polymorphic or uneven nuclei suggest malignancy. Nuclear molding resulting from compression by adjacent cells or from a second nucleus within the same cell also suggests malignancy. Some malignant cells have small satellite nuclei adjacent to a large nucleus or in the cytoplasm.

Cytoplasmic features of malignant cells are less helpful than are nuclear characteristics. For example, cytoplasmic basophilia (indicating increased cytoplasmic RNA attributable to increased metabolic activity) is a feature of immaturity and can be found in malignant cells and cells taken from areas of tissue hyperplasia or benign neoplasia. Other cytoplasmic features suggesting malignancy include variations in staining quality, abnormal vacuolation of inclusions, and variable cytoplasmic margins.

Finally, the structural features of malignant cells can aid in the classification of neoplasms of birds and mammals. Malignant neoplasms can be classified cytologically as epithelial (carcinomas), mesenchymal (sarcomas), or discrete-cell (round-cell) neoplasms. Carcinomas of animals are characterized by abnormal-appearing epithelial cells (Fig-

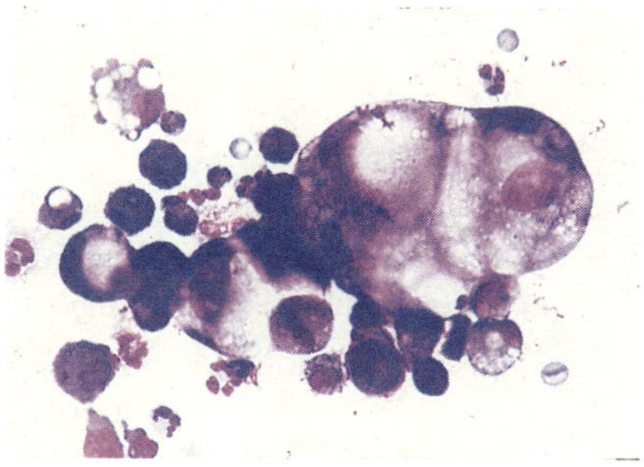

Figure 4—Carcinoma. Epithelial cells demonstrating features of neoplasia from an aspiration biopsy of a mammary adenocarcinoma in a cow. (Diff-Quik®)

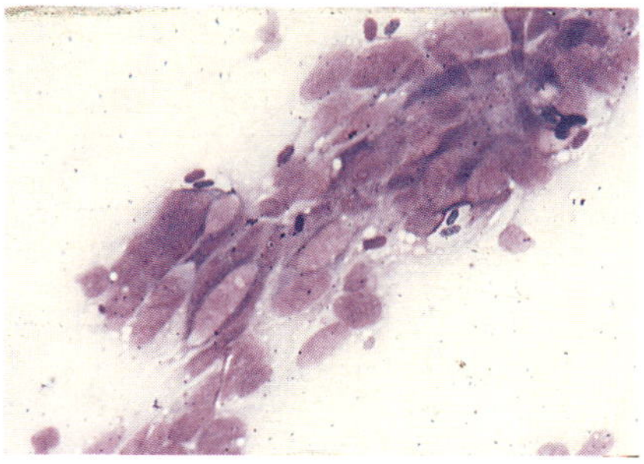

Figure 5—Sarcoma. A cluster of polymorphic spindle-shaped cells in a contact smear from a fibrosarcoma of a budgerigar (*Melopsittacus undulatus*). (Diff-Quik®)

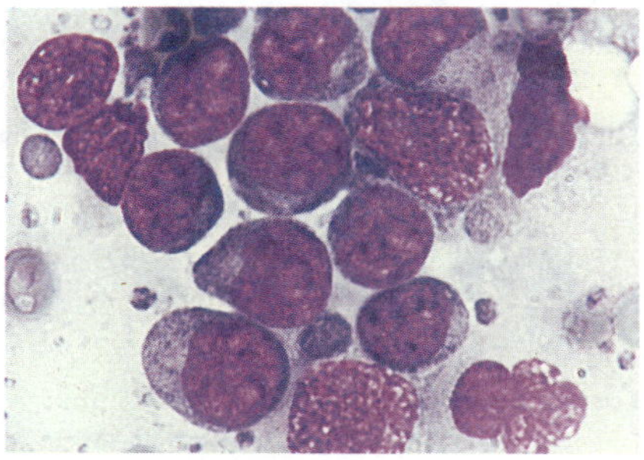

Figure 6—Round-cell neoplasm. Large, immature lymphocytes in a lymph-node aspirate from a dog with lymphoid neoplasia. (Wright's stain)

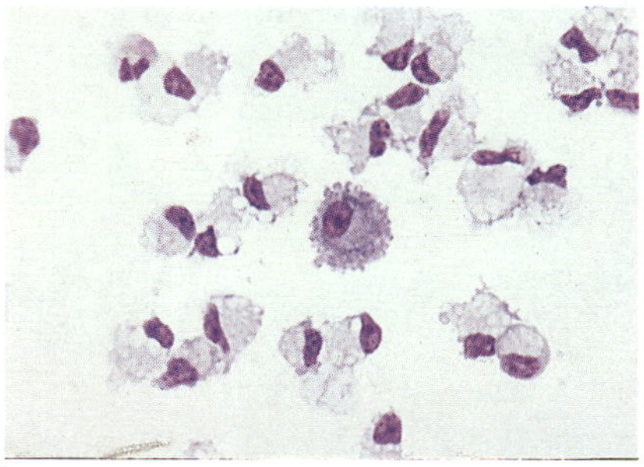

Figure 7—Modified transudate. Macrophages and mesothelial cell (*center*) in the abdominal fluid from a mynah (*Gracula religiosa*). (Diff-Quik®)

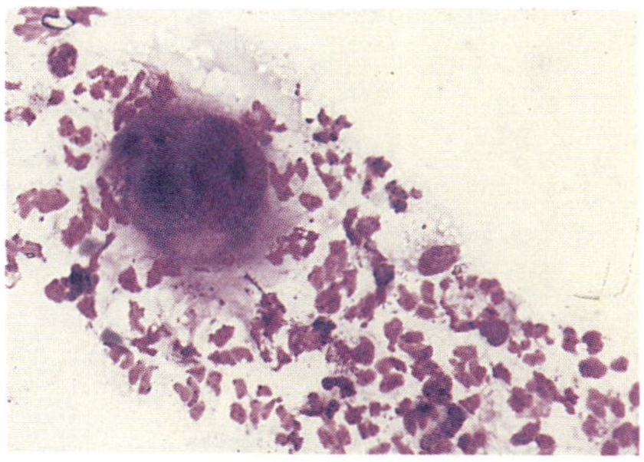

Figure 8—Exudative or malignant effusion. A marked number of degenerated neutrophils and an abnormal squamous epithelial cell in the peritoneal fluid of a horse with gastric squamous cell carcinoma. (Diff-Quik®)

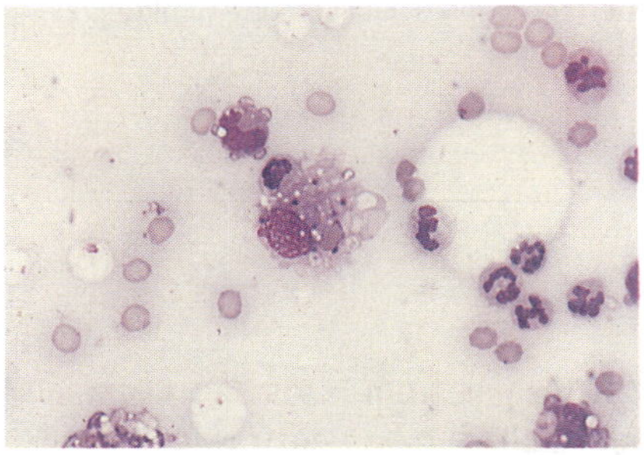

Figure 9—Hemorrhagic effusion. Erythrocytes, nondegenerated neutrophils, and a macrophage demonstrating erythrocytophagy in the thoracic fluid from a dog with a hemothorax. (Diff-Quik®)

ure 4). These cells tend to exfoliate well and often appear in cellular aggregates (cell clustering must be differentiated from clumping as seen in highly cellular samples). Cells from carcinomas tend to be round to polyhedral with distinct cytoplasmic margins; however, multinucleated giant cells may form as one cell blends into the next with loss of distinct cytoplasmic margins.

SARCOMAS TEND TO produce poorly cellular samples because the cells are embedded within an extracellular matrix. Therefore, traumatic exfoliation by scraping the tissue is often required to improve the cell yield.

In birds and mammals, cells from sarcomas tend to be spindle shaped with poorly defined cytoplasmic margins. Unlike epithelial cells, they tend to exfoliate as single cells or in small clusters. The fusiform shape may vary with the type of sarcoma. For example, fibrosarcomas produce elongated to spindle-shaped cells that are thinner than the broader fusiform cells of osteogenic sarcomas (Figure 5). The extracellular matrix (i.e., osteoid or collagen) produced by some sarcomas may be seen in the noncellular background.

Discrete-cell neoplasms produce a highly cellular sample that is composed of round cells. These cells exfoliate as individual cells because they are derived from cells that have no normal cell-to-cell interaction. Examples of mammalian discrete-cell neoplasms are lymphosarcomas, mast-cell neoplasms, histiocytomas, and transmissible venereal tumors of dogs (Figure 6). A common discrete-cell neoplasm reported to occur in birds is lymphoid neoplasia.

EFFUSIONS

The abnormal accumulation of fluids in the body cavities of mammals can result from increased vascular permeability, a decrease in the osmotic pressure of plasma (i.e., hypoalbuminemia), an increase in intravascular hydrostatic pressure, or interruption of normal fluid drainage attributable to obstruction of lymphatic flow. The same mechanisms may also be involved in the accumulation of body fluids in birds; such accumulation is mainly confined to the abdominal cavity. Two common causes of ascites in birds are inflammatory and neoplastic processes.

TABLE II
Comparison of Effusions from Birds and Mammals

	Type of Effusion			
Characteristics	*Transudate*	*Exudate*	*Hemorrhagic*	*Malignant*
Appearance	Thin, watery, clear, odorless	Thick, cloudy, may have odor	Resembles peripheral blood	Thick and cloudy or resembles peripheral blood
Color	Colorless to pale straw color	White, red, or yellow	Red	White, red, or yellow
Specific gravity	Less than 1.015	Greater than 1.020	Greater than 1.020	Greater than 1.020
Protein content	Less than 3.0 g/dl	Greater than 3.0 g/dl	Greater than 3.0 g/dl	Greater than 3.0 g/dl
Coagulation	None	Frequent	Occasional	Occasional
Cellularity	Poor (leukocytes are rare)	Marked (numerous leukocytes)	Moderate to marked (erythrocytes and macrophages showing erythrocytophagy)	Moderate to marked (leukocytes, erythrocytes, and/or malignant cells)

Effusions from birds and mammals can be classified as transudates, modified transudates, exudates, hemorrhagic effusions, malignant effusions, or chylous effusions (Table II). Although they are important in mammals, chylous effusions have not been reported to occur in birds and therefore are not discussed in this article.

Transudates result from abnormal accumulation of normal body fluid. Mammalian and avian transudates are characterized by low cellularity (i.e., less than 1000 cells/μl in dogs, cats, and birds or 3000 cells/μl in horses), low specific gravity (less than 1.015), and low total protein (less than 2.5 g/dl). Transudates may be colorless to a pale straw color and are clear to slightly turbid.

Transudates have a mixture of leukocytes and mesothelial cells. Most of the cells are mononuclear cells (monocytes, macrophages, and mesothelial cells). Occasional nondegenerated neutrophils (in mammals) or heterophils (in birds) are present. Normal mesothelial cells, which are the large squamous cells that line serosal surfaces of organs, become reactive when the serous membranes are irritated (i.e., in long-standing effusions). Reactive mesothelial cells are round to oval, exfoliate singly or in small clusters, may have scalloped or villuslike eosinophilic cytoplasmic margins, and may demonstrate multinucleation, mitotic activity, or cytoplasmic vacuolation.

Modified transudates resemble normal transudates but have a higher cellularity (1000 to 5000 cell/μl in dogs, cats, and birds) and protein content (2.5 to 3.0 g/dl). Mononuclear cells (macrophages, monocytes, and mesothelial cells) are the predominate cells in this type of effusion (Figure 7). Occasional nondegenerated neutrophils (in mammals) or heterophils (in birds) may be present.

EXUDATIVE EFFUSIONS result from inflammatory processes within body cavities. They are characterized by high cellularity (greater that 5000 cells/μl in dogs, cats, and birds or 10,000 cells/μl in horses). Exudates vary in color and turbidity, are often viscous, may have a foul odor, and frequently clot during sample collection.

The cellular characteristics of exudates vary by cause, host response, and duration (Figure 8). Neutrophilic/heterophilic inflammatory effusions show a predominance of neutrophils (mammalian) or heterophils (avian). Septic effusions may contain intracellular bacteria and degenerated neutrophils or heterophils. Mononuclear leukocytes may predominate among the cells of exudates caused by nonseptic, mild irritation in the body cavity. Reactive mesothelial cells are common in exudates.

Erythrocytes are the predominant cell of hemorrhagic effusions (Figure 9). Acute hemorrhagic effusions resemble peripheral blood except that the total cell counts and total protein content are usually lower. Mammalian platelets or avian thrombocytes disappear quickly and may not be present, even in acute hemorrhagic effusions. Chronic hemorrhagic effusions are characterized by macrophages with varying degrees of erythrocytophagy.

Malignant effusions may have the features of modified transudates, exudates, or hemorrhagic effusions. These effusions are identified by the presence of malignant cells; however, these cells are not always present because the neoplasm may not have begun to shed cells or because it exfoliates poorly (i.e., sarcomas). If neoplastic cells are present, their characteristics may allow the cytologist to determine the type of neoplasm involved (e.g., carcinoma, sarcoma, or lymphosarcoma).

CONCLUSION

Cytologic evaluation of tissue or fluid from mammals and birds can provide a quick presumptive or definitive diagnosis. Cytologic techniques and interpretations used in avian medicine are basically the same as those of domestic mammalian medicine.

About the Author

Dr. Campbell is an Associate Professor in Zoological Medicine in the Department of Clinical Sciences at Colorado State University in Fort Collins, Colorado.

REFERENCES

1. Perman V, Alsaker RD, Riis RC: *Cytology of the Dog and Cat*. Denver, CO, American Animal Hospital Association, 1979.
2. Rebar AH: *Handbook of Veterinary Cytology*. St Louis, MO, Ralston Purina Co, 1978.
3. Campbell TW: *Avian Hematology and Cytology*. Ames, IA, Iowa State University Press, 1988.

Comparative Avian and Mammalian Cytodiagnosis—Part II*

KEY FACTS

- Cytologic evaluation of avian and mammalian lymphoid tissue specimens is similar.
- The cytology of transtracheal aspirates of birds and mammals is similar.
- Hepatic cytology of birds and mammals is similar except for the frequent occurrence of hematopoiesis in the avian liver.
- Despite the presence of feathers on birds and hair on mammals, cutaneous and subcutaneous lesions from birds and mammals often resemble each other cytologically.

Colorado State University
Fort Collins, Colorado
Terry W. Campbell, DVM, PhD

CYTOLOGIC ANALYSIS is often used to make a presumptive or definitive diagnosis of disease in mammals and is also useful for avian patients. Part I of this two-part presentation discussed the similarities between birds and mammals in the cellular responses of inflammation, tissue hyperplasia (benign neoplasia), and malignant neoplasia. This part compares avian and mammalian cytology of the lymphoid tissue, respiratory tract, liver, and skin.

LYMPHOID TISSUE

Mammalian lymph nodes are frequently sampled for the cytologic evaluation of lymphoid tissue. Alterations in the cells of lymph nodes can reflect systemic or localized disease. Most avian species have no lymph nodes; however, lymphoid aggregates occur in the walls of the gastrointestinal tract, abdominal organs (i.e., the liver), serous membranes, and skin (i.e., the comb of galliform birds). Cecal tonsils (which occur in the proximal cecum of some birds), the bursa of Fabricius, and the spleen are large lymphoid aggregates in birds but are difficult to sample in the living bird.

More than 90% of the cell population of normal lymphoid tissue of birds and mammals consists of small mature lymphocytes. These lymphocytes resemble those found in peripheral blood. They have a high nucleus-to-cytoplasm (N–C) ratio, a condensed nucleus with heavy chromatin clumping, and a scant amount of basophilic cytoplasm. Normal lymphoid tissue also contains a low percentage of other cells (less than 10% of the cell population), including lymphoblasts, prolymphocytes, macrophages, plasma cells, and granulocytes. The background of lymphoid tissue from birds and mammals contains pale blue cytoplasmic fragments of varying shapes and sizes.

Hyperplasia of lymphoid tissue may be associated with enlargement of the lymphoid organ (i.e., lymph nodes of mammals or the spleen in birds). Cytologic study reveals an increased number of immature lymphocytes (lymphoblasts and prolymphocytes); but small mature lymphocytes predominate. Lymphoblasts are large lymphocytes with large vesicular nuclei, prominent nucleoli, and deeply basophilic cytoplasm. A prolymphocyte resembles a lymphoblast but lacks a prominent nucleolus. Hyperplastic lymphoid tissue may also be reactive; this condition is represented by an increase in the number of macrophages and plasma cells (Figure 1).

Inflammation of lymphoid tissue (lymphadenitis) is easier to detect in the lymph nodes of mammals than in the

Originally published in Volume 12, Number 6, June 1990

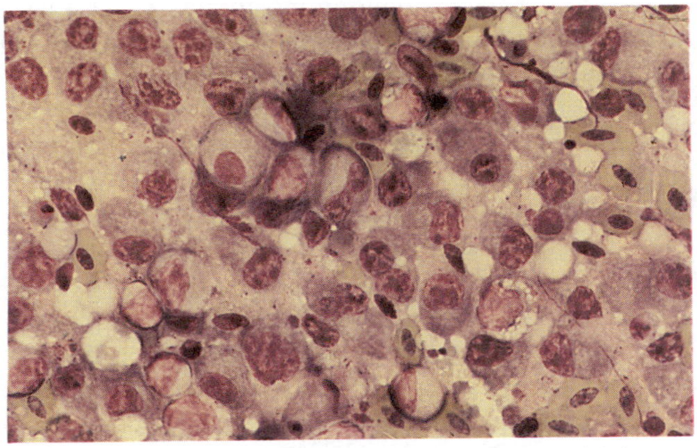

Figure 1—Reactive lymphoid tissue in a splenic imprint from a yellow-naped Amazon parrot (*Amazona ochrocephala auropalliata*). Note the marked increase in the number of plasma cells. (Diff-Quik®)

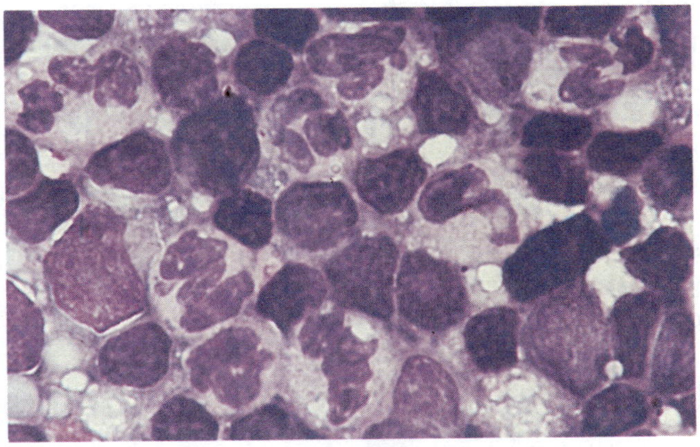

Figure 2—A lymph node aspiration biopsy from a domestic cat reveals numerous neutrophils indicative of lymphadenitis. (Diff-Quik®)

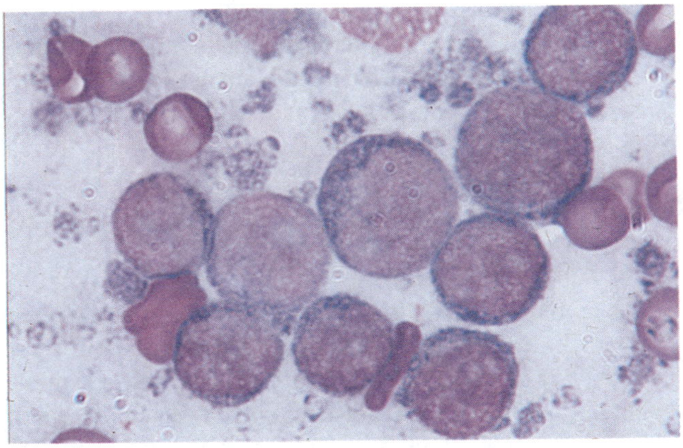

Figure 3—A lymph node aspiration biopsy from a dog shows a predominance of immature lymphocytes indicating lymphoid neoplasia. In the background are cytoplasmic fragments that are typical in lymphoid cytology. (Diff-Quik®)

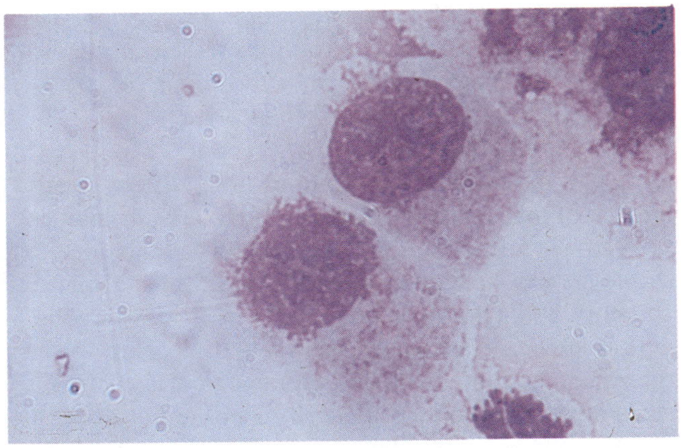

Figure 4—Two goblet cells in a transtracheal aspirate from a horse. (Diff-Quik®)

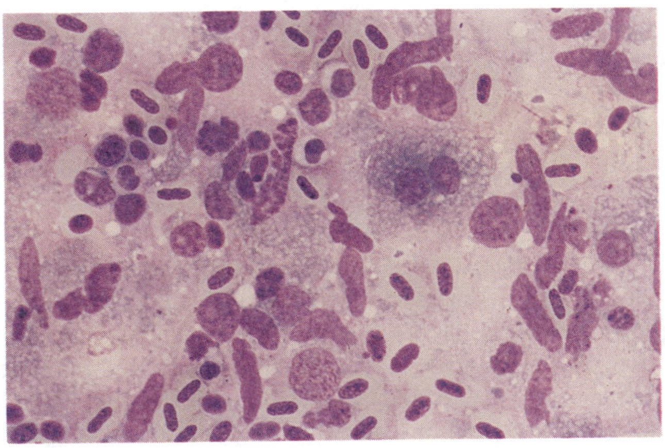

Figure 5—A marked number of spindle-shaped free nuclei and few intact cells in a liver imprint from a budgerigar (*Melopsittacus undulatus*) with a histologic diagnosis of a metastatic fibrosarcoma involving the liver. The spindle-shaped nuclei and cells suggest an increase in the connective tissue elements of the liver and could represent a cirrhotic change or neoplasia of the connective tissue. (Diff-Quik®)

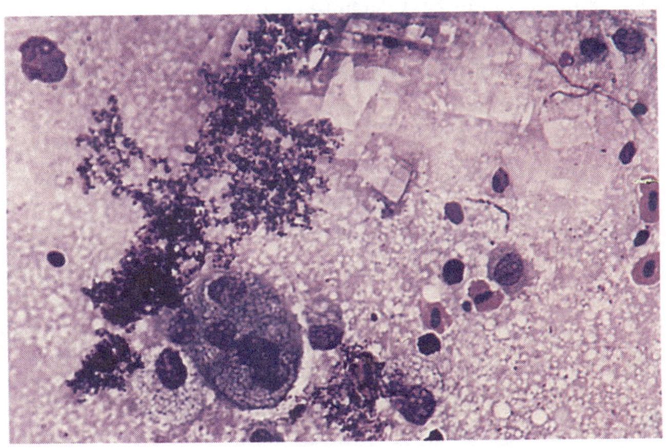

Figure 6—An imprint of cutaneous xanthomatosis from a green-winged macaw (*Ara chloroptera*) reveals macrophages, multinucleated giant cells, and cholesterol crystals. (Diff-Quik®)

lymphoid tissue of birds. Because avian lymphoid aggregates are a part of other tissues and organs, inflammation of the nonlymphoid tissue may also be associated with the lymphoid components in the cytologic specimen. Lymphadenitis in mammals is identified by an increase in the number of inflammatory cells (i.e., neutrophils, eosinophils, and macrophages) (Figure 2). Reactive lymphoid hyperplasia is often associated with lymphadenitis. The causative agent of lymphadenitis may be present in the cytologic specimen.

LYMPHOID NEOPLASIA can affect birds and mammals. This condition is usually represented by a monotonous, monomorphic population of lymphocytes. Most of the lymphocytes (more than 90% of the cell population) are lymphoblasts or prolymphocytes. The neoplastic lymphocytes may occasionally reveal nuclear pleomorphism; multiple, large nucleoli; and cytoplasmic vacuolation. The number of mitotic figures is usually increased in samples obtained from patients with lymphoid neoplasia (Figure 3).

RESPIRATORY TRACT

Although the respiratory system of birds differs greatly from that of mammals, the cytology is remarkably similar. Transtracheal aspirates from birds and mammals yield a variable number of respiratory epithelial cells. The ciliated respiratory epithelial cells are columnar cells with abundant basophilic, granular cytoplasm; the cilia are at the large end of the cell. An eccentric, round to oval nucleus is located at the small pole of the cell (opposite the cilia).

Goblet cells resemble the ciliated respiratory epithelial cells but lack cilia (Figure 4). The cytoplasm of goblet cells often contains prominent metachromatic granules and vacuoles. The number of macrophages present in normal avian and mammalian transtracheal aspirates varies.

Cytologic samples from patients with tracheobronchitis have numerous neutrophils (in mammals) or heterophils (in birds) as well as macrophages. Septic tracheobronchitis is confirmed by the presence of leukocytic phagocytosis of bacteria. Degenerative changes in epithelial cells (e.g., loss or clumping of cilia, cytoplasmic vacuolation, cellular fragmentation, and karyolysis) may be evident in samples from patients with various disorders involving the trachea and bronchi. The number of goblet cells in the samples also increases with irritation and inflammation of the trachea and bronchi.

LIVER

Samples for cytologic evaluation of the liver of birds or mammals can be obtained by fine-needle aspiration biopsy or by contact smears made from specimens of excised tissue. The normal liver of birds and mammals provides highly cellular specimens that often contain a variable amount of contamination by peripheral blood. Normal hepatocytes from these two types of animals are large, round to polyhedral cells with one or two round to oval, eccentric nuclei. The nuclei are uniform in appearance and usually contain a prominent nucleolus. The abundant cytoplasm of the hepatocytes is usually basophilic and granular.

Hepatocellular degeneration is usually indicated by the presence of swollen hepatocytes with cytoplasmic vacuolation, which suggests fatty change. Unstained smears made from livers with fatty degeneration appear greasy during gross inspection of the slide.

The cytology of hepatic inflammation (hepatitis) reveals numerous inflammatory cells. The number of inflammatory cells present is greater than that expected as a result of contamination by peripheral blood in animals with marked leukocytosis of peripheral blood. The type of inflammatory cells that predominate may indicate the category of inflammation and suggest a possible cause. In birds, hepatic inflammation must be differentiated from ectopic granulocytopoiesis. This is easily accomplished by determining whether developing granulocytes are present. In samples from birds with hepatic inflammation, the heterophils appear mature.

Primary and metastatic neoplasia involving the liver of birds and mammals can occasionally be detected by cytodiagnosis. Primary neoplasms contain cells with various features of neoplasia. Metastatic lesions may simply reveal the presence of cells foreign to the liver (Figure 5). These cells may or may not have features of malignant neoplasia.

SKIN AND SUBCUTIS

The cytologic evaluation of cutaneous lesions is common in avian and mammalian medicine. The skin of birds and mammals is composed of keratinized stratified squamous epithelium; however, the presence of feathers in avian skin and hair in mammalian skin is an obvious difference. The cellular characteristics of various cutaneous lesions are similar. For example, inflammatory lesions involving the skin are similar in the two types of animal—the avian heterophil replacing the mammalian neutrophil. Chronic inflammatory lesions of the skin in both types of animal are often associated with superficial squamous epithelial hyperplasia and fibrous hyperplasia surrounding the lesion.

EPIDERMAL inclusion cysts of mammals are benign cystic lesions that are filled with cornified squamous epithelial cells and debris. Cholesterol crystals may also be present. Feather cysts of birds resemble the epidermal inclusion cyst of mammals and reveal numerous cornified squamous epithelial cells and debris on cytologic examination. Acute feather cysts are highly vascularized, and the sample may be heavily contaminated with peripheral blood. Long-standing epidermal inclusion cysts of mammals and feather cysts of birds often reveal an inflammatory response because of the antigenic nature of keratin.

Cutaneous xanthomatosis is a common disorder of birds but is rarely reported to occur in mammals. This condition is frequently associated with cutaneous hemorrhage (e.g., hemorrhage associated with feather cysts) or necrosis of

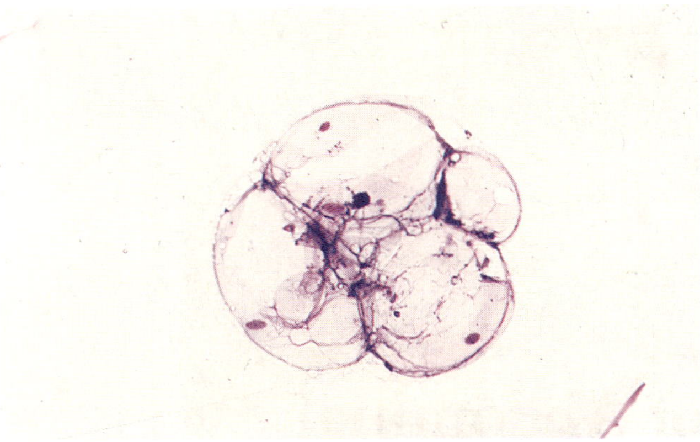

Figure 7—A small cluster of lipocytes from a fine-needle aspirate of a lipoma from a dog. (Diff-Quik®)

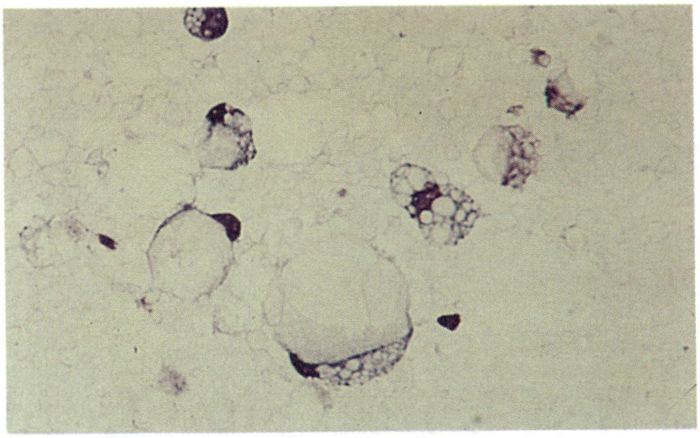

Figure 8—Lipocytes from a lipoma from a budgerigar (*Melopsittacus undulatus*). (Diff-Quik®)

the epithelium. The cytologic findings are characterized by the presence of numerous macrophages, multinucleated giant cells, and cholesterol crystals (Figure 6).

SUBCUTANEOUS lipomas are common in dogs and certain species of birds (i.e., budgerigars). Unstained smears made from lipomas have a greasy appearance, and the stained smear reveals a large amount of fat droplets. The number of lipocytes varies. In mammals, the lipocytes are large mononuclear cells with an eccentric nucleus that is pushed to the cell margin (Figure 7). The cytoplasm is abundant and clear. Lipocytes of birds resemble those of mammals; however, the cytoplasm tends to be foamy and usually contains numerous large vacuoles (Figure 8). Lipocytes from avian or mammalian lipomas tend to exfoliate as single cells or in small clusters.

Subcutaneous hematomas or seromas of birds and mammals resemble each other cytologically, except for the presence of the avian nucleated erythrocytes. Numerous erythrocytes are present in early lesions. With resolution of the hematoma, there is an increasing number of leukocytes—primarily macrophages showing a variable amount of erythrocytophagy. Seromas may develop from resolving hematomas or independently from them. Seromas are characterized by poorly cellular, serumlike fluid that is rich in protein.

CONCLUSION

Cytologic evaluation of samples obtained from lymphoid tissue, the respiratory tract, the liver, and cutaneous or subcutaneous lesions are common in avian and mammalian medicine. Both types of animal show similar cellular responses; therefore, the cytologist who is well versed in mammalian cytodiagnosis can easily evaluate avian cytologic specimens.

About the Author

Dr. Campbell is an Associate Professor in Zoological Medicine in the Department of Clinical Sciences at Colorado State University in Fort Collins, Colorado.

BIBLIOGRAPHY

Campbell TW: *Avian Hematology and Cytology*. Ames, IA, Iowa State University Press, 1988.

Perman V, Alsaker RD, Riis RC: *Cytology of the Dog and Cat*. South Bend, IN, American Animal Hospital Association, 1979.

Rebar AH: *Handbook of Veterinary Cytology*. St. Louis, MO, Ralston Purina Co, 1978.

The Clinical Significance of Abdominal Enlargement in the Budgerigar (*Melopsittacus undulatus*)

Marjorie C. McMillan, DVM
The Windhover Veterinary Center
Walpole, Massachusetts

Margaret L. Petrak, VMD
Angell Memorial Animal Hospital
Boston, Massachusetts

Abdominal enlargement is a common physical finding in domestic middle-aged and older budgerigars (three years and older). Many veterinarians believe that this finding indicates a tumor and they recommend euthanasia without further consideration. Although budgerigars have a high incidence of neoplasia,[1] other more treatable causes of abdominal distention should not be disregarded in making a diagnosis. The definitive diagnosis should be based on age, sex, history, physical examination, significant clinical findings, and ancillary diagnostic testing.

It is helpful to divide the causes of abdominal enlargement into nonpathologic and pathologic entities (Table I).

Depending on whether the cause is nonpathologic or pathologic, and whether the duration is acute or chronic, the bird may present with *sick bird syndrome* (fluffing, anorexia, and lethargy) or it may be asymptomatic except for an observable abdominal swelling.

History and Causes of Illness

Since many causes of abdominal enlargement are related to the female genital tract, it is important to determine the bird's sex. This is easy with many budgerigars. The cere in birds over six months of age is usually blue in males and tan to brown in females. However, a small percentage of female budgerigars have blue ceres. This can cause problems when speculating whether an abdominal enlargement in a bird with a blue cere is pathological or due to physiological hypertrophy of the oviduct (Figure 1).

Knowing the bird's age may be helpful in limiting the differential diagnosis. Since the average life expectancy of the budgerigar in captivity is about six years, birds over age three are past middle age and are at high risk for neoplasia. Liver disease with hepatomegaly also tends to occur in middle-aged and older birds, although neoplasia and liver disease have been observed in budgerigars as young as six months of age. Liver disease from a variety of causes is a common clinical finding in budgerigars; however, certain breeds may have an inherited predisposition to lipidosis[2] resulting in fatty degeneration of the liver and other organs (Figure 2). Recognizing these breeds may help in diagnosing the abdominal problem.

Originally published in Volume 3, Number 10, October 1981

TABLE I

Causes of Abdominal Enlargement

Nonpathologic
1. Laying female (hen)
2. Obesity—subcutaneous lipomas and intra-abdominal fat
3. Pseudocoprostasis
4. Aerophagia

Pathologic
1. Neoplasia
2. Hepatomegaly
3. Egg binding
4. Cysts—oviduct, ovarian, and renal
5. Hernia
6. Peritonitis—egg and other causes
7. Ascites

Liver Disease

Liver disease is one of the commonest clinical problems encountered in budgerigars. The causes are categorized as either viral, bacterial, chlamydial, toxic, metabolic, or neoplastic.

Pacheco's parrot disease, caused by a herpesvirus, can be induced in budgerigars by IM inoculation of the virus, but it has not been reported in the literature as a naturally occurring disease. A parrot adenovirus and a chicken strain of adenovirus[11] have both produced hepatitis in budgerigars inoculated IM. Lymphoid leukosis, which is known to be caused by a virus in chickens, has been seen in budgerigars, but it has not yet been proven to be viral in origin.

Toxic material from the intestines passes into the liver and can cause liver damage. Because the liver functions as a filter for the intestine, it is subjected to toxic assault. The percentage of liver disease in budgerigars due to toxins is unknown. Contaminated seeds are conjectured to be a source of toxins. Mycotoxins are known to have produced liver disease in budgerigars, causing the liver to have a *hobnailed* appearance. The possibility of fungicides contaminating seed supplies should not be overlooked.

Lipidosis almost always affects the liver. Cholesterol occurs in the liver, as well as in other organs, in abnormal amounts and histiocytes attempt to remove it. The liver is often moderately enlarged and pale.

Fatty degeneration of the liver occurs commonly in obese birds and produces an enlarged yellow or yellow brown liver. Diet and abnormal metabolism of fat may both be involved in its occurrence.

Adenocarcinomas of the bile ducts and liver cells have been seen in budgerigars, including one only four months old. It is not uncommon for fibrosarcomas and malignant kidney tumors to metastasize to the liver.

Depending on the acuteness or chronicity, the liver may be larger or smaller than normal in almost any of the aforementioned diseases.

Historical information regarding diet may yield some clues as to the source of the problem. Hypocalcemia is implicated in egg binding. Many budgerigars are fed an all-seed diet with no vitamin or mineral supplementation. Seed mixtures are low in calcium and vitamin D_3, resulting in low blood calcium levels. There are also hypotheses that certain types of liver disease may be diet related. Information concerning past egg binding, recent clutches, and soft-shelled eggs may also be useful when considering egg binding and egg peritonitis problems.

Past episodes of illness with fluffing, anorexia, lethargy, and abnormal dark brown droppings, followed by spontaneous recovery are often reported in budgerigars with liver disease. Many of these birds develop epistaxis or hemorrhagic droppings. Overgrown beaks and toenails with brown streaking usually indicate liver problems.

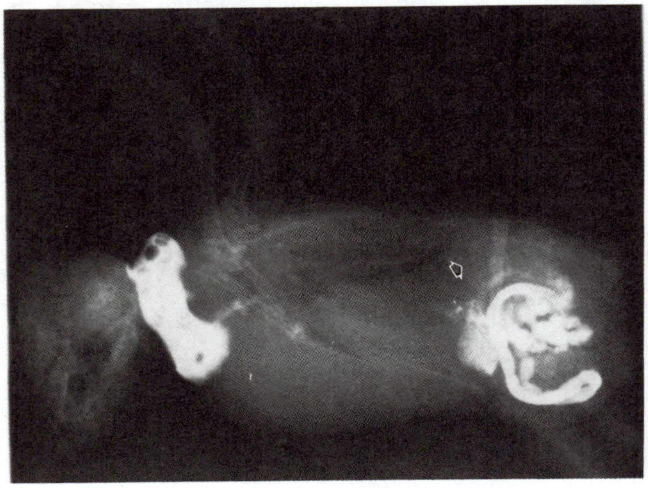

Figure 1—Lateral abdominal radiograph showing ventral and caudal displacement of barium-filled intestinal loops by enlarged oviduct *(arrow)*.

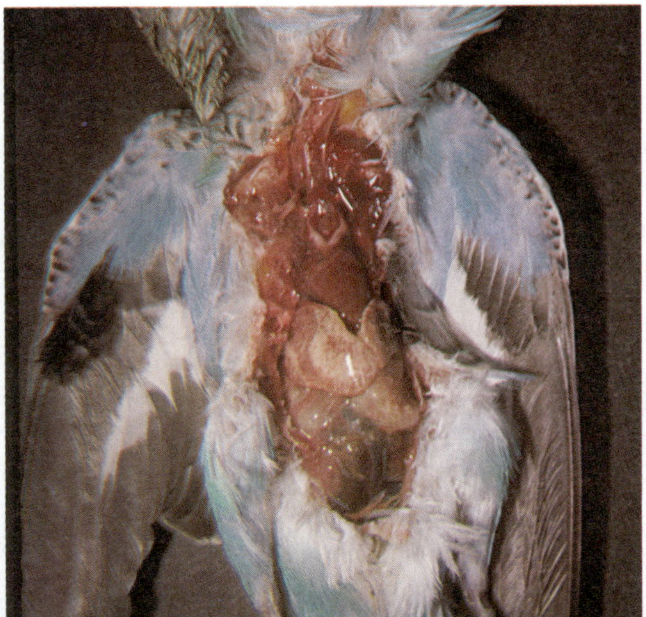

Figure 2—Gross autopsy specimen with enlarged, pale liver from lipidosis.

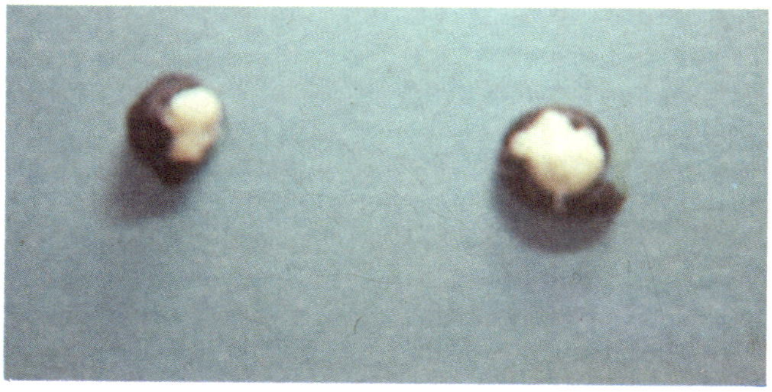

Figure 3A

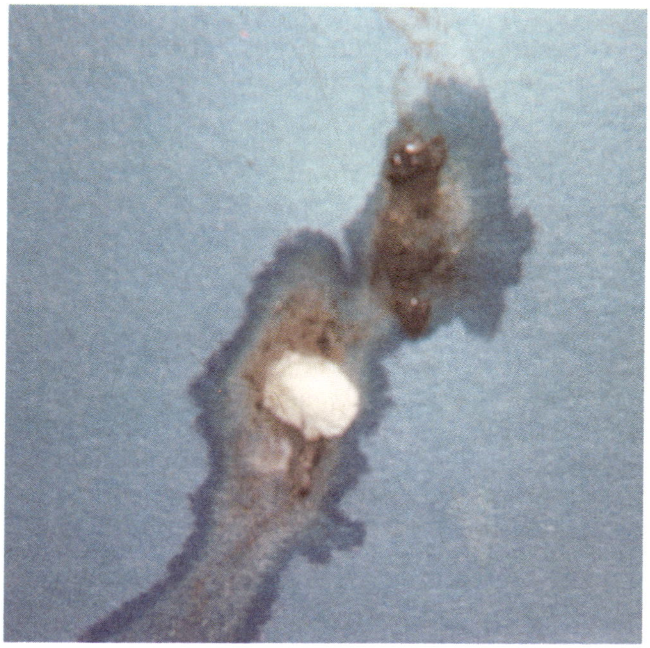

Figure 3B

Figure 3 (A and B)—Normal droppings (A) and loose gray droppings from budgerigar with lipidosis (B).

Birds with voracious appetites and weight loss usually have neoplasia or liver disease.

Physical Examination and Clinical Signs

Observation of the bird in the cage prior to handling may reveal subtle abnormalities that are not obvious when restraining the animal. *Tail bobbing,* often associated with respiratory problems, is common in abdominal disorders. Since birds lack a true diaphragm, masses often result in organ displacement, causing pressure on the lungs, air sacs, or heart. Abdominal fluid can also accumulate around the heart and lungs and cause respiratory distress. Changes in posture such as a *penguinlike* stance are often the result of egg binding. Unilateral paresis or paralysis is associated with renal tumors involving the sciatic nerve.

Regurgitation movements may be observed, or there may be regurgitated material on the cage floor. Regurgitation occasionally occurs in birds with liver disease and kidney neoplasia.

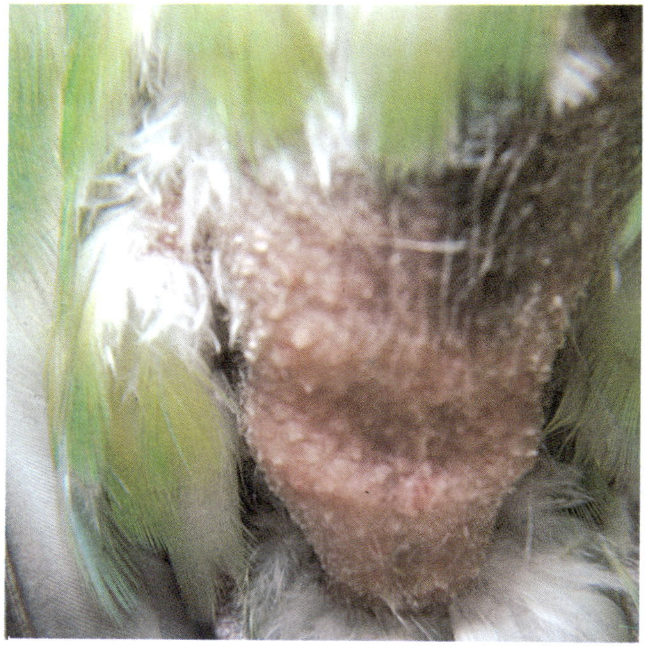

Figure 4A

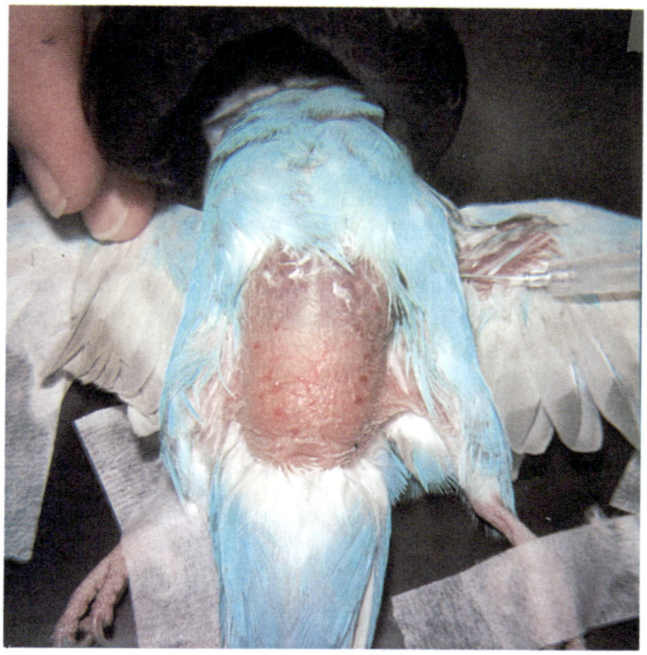

Figure 4B

Figure 4 (A and B)—Normal abdominal space measuring about 5 mm (A). Enlarged abdomen in budgerigar with abdominal mass (B).

The droppings should be evaluated for change in size, color, and consistency (Figure 3). Laying hens will normally develop large, bulky, slightly loose droppings. Dilute, voluminous urate may be seen with renal tumors, and occasionally a hemorrhagic urate portion occurs. There may be a dark brown fecal portion due to upper gastrointestinal hemorrhage or a lime green dropping with yellow urate in liver disease. Bright red blood around the droppings or streaked within the droppings

TABLE II

SUMMARY OF CLINICAL SIGNS

1. Abdominal enlargement—firm or fluctuating abdomen
2. *Tail bobbing*
3. Change in droppings—size, color, consistency
4. Postural change
5. Tenesmus
6. Unilateral paresis or paralysis
7. Regurgitation
8. Weight change

may occur with egg binding. Tenesmus and difficulty passing droppings may be the result of a lesion in the abdominal cavity. Extremely obese birds may have difficulty passing droppings or may have pasting around the vent due to accumulation of large amounts of subcutaneous adipose tissue around the cloaca.

A complete physical examination[a] should be performed unless the bird cannot tolerate the stress incurred because of its weakened condition.[b] The sternum and pectoral muscles should be palpated to determine weight loss. The normal abdominal space between the terminal portion of the sternum and pubic bones is about 5 mm (Figure 4). An increase in this distance or a lack of compressibility indicates the possibility of an abdominal problem. The consistency of the abdominal enlargement should be considered. A firm, hard swelling is usually due to organ enlargement, a displaced gizzard, a tumor, or an egg, whereas soft, fluctuant swelling is often the result of fluid, a cyst, or a hernia. If physical findings confirm an abdominal problem, additional diagnostic tests should be performed to more specifically localize the lesion.

[a]Since the scope of this paper is abdominal disease, emphasis is placed on this region and description of abnormal physical findings referable to abdominal problems. Discussion of a complete physical examination can be found elsewhere.[3]

[b]If the bird cannot tolerate a physical examination, supportive treatment such as fluids and oxygen should be started prior to examination.

Diagnosis

When an abdominal disorder is suspected, radiography often provides additional diagnostic information. Proper positioning and technique are essential for diagnostic radiographs.[4,12] Radiographic signs suggestive of abdominal disease include gizzard displacement, loss of abdominal air sac space, homogeneous abdominal density, and a mass. The grit-filled gizzard normally lies between the acetabula and to the left of the midline in the ventrodorsal radiograph. Hepatomegaly tends to cause caudal and dorsal gizzard displacement. Renal masses cause ventral displacement of the gizzard and, depending on in which pole the mass is located, they can cause cranial or caudal displacement as well. Kidney tumors are the abdominal neoplasm most commonly seen in The Windhover Bird Clinic. Because of the location of the kidneys, the tumors are not amenable to surgical removal. Oviduct enlargement usually causes ventral and caudal dislocation of the gizzard. Masses and/or fluid can cause loss of normal symmetry to the abdominal air sacs. Because the abdominal cavity is surrounded by the vertebrae, sternum, and pubic bones, there is little room for expansion, so abdominal organs tend to be compressed when a space-occupying lesion is present. This results in loss of distinction between organs and impingement on normal air sac space, making the abdomen appear to be a homogeneous density (Figure 5). In small birds it is difficult to distinguish between fluid and a mass. In larger birds this distinction is easier.

Egg peritonitis can cause loss of contrast and a functional ileus with stagnant, gas-filled loops. Normally calcified eggs are easily visualized, but soft-shelled eggs can be difficult to diagnose. Abnormal attempts at egg production can be seen and increased bone density suggestive of polyostotic hyperostosis[5] can be recognized (Figure 6).

A barium study helps demonstrate displacement of the intestinal tract and draping of the intestines over a mass when the exact location cannot be determined from survey radiography (Figure 1). Other contrast

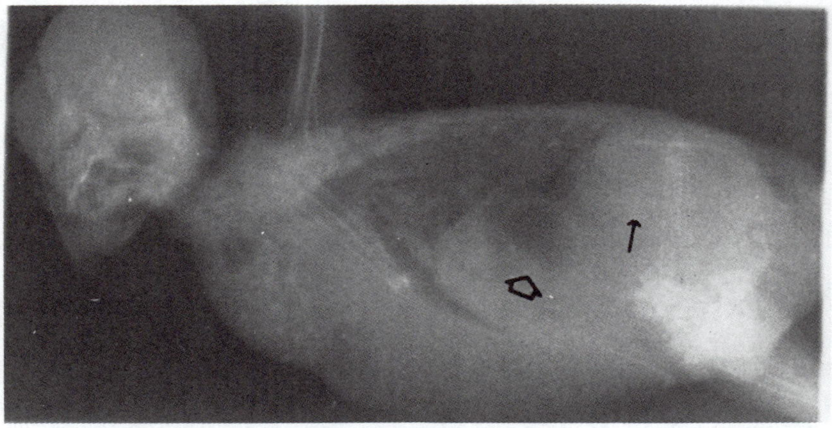

Figure 5—Lateral abdominal radiograph showing homogeneous abdominal density and displacement of gizzard ventral and caudal by renal cyst *(closed arrow)*. Air is present in the proventriculus *(open arrow)* from partial obstruction.

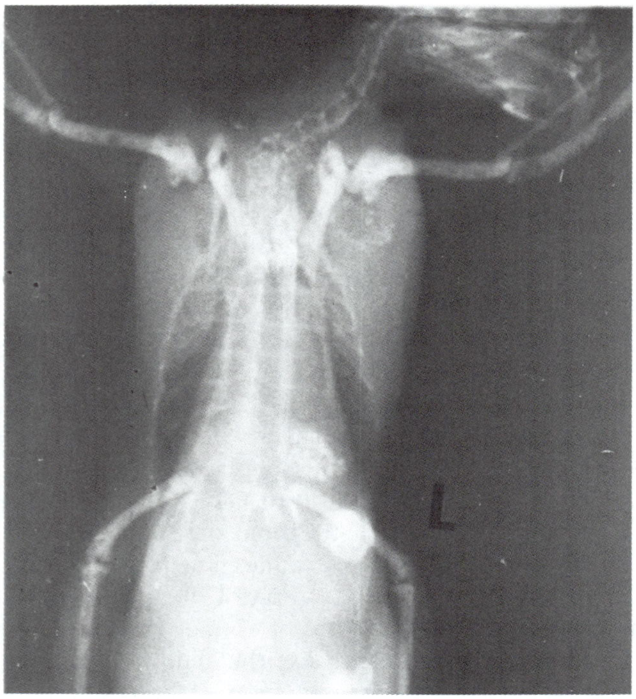

Figure 6—Polyostotic hyperostosis, abnormal calcific densities in oviduct, abdominal fluid, and cranial gizzard displacement are present in the ventrodorsal radiograph.

examinations have not proved useful in the budgerigar, and additional clinical research must be performed to determine their value.

If fluid is present, abdominocentesis and fluid analysis should be performed. The abdominal skin, from the sternum to vent, is prepared aseptically, and a 25-gauge needle is gently inserted into the abdominal cavity about 2 mm cranial to the vent and off the midline. Obvious subcutaneous blood vessels are avoided. As much fluid as possible is aspirated since this will alleviate any dyspnea associated with the fluid accumulation. The type of fluid most commonly aspirated is a clear yellow hypocellular, modified transudate that is often associated with cystic oviduct enlargement and possibly hyperestrogenism.

Yellow floccular fluid or dark brown fluid has been seen in cases of egg peritonitis. A hemorrhagic fluid is associated with bleeding secondary to liver rupture from liver disease. A clear, watery transudate is suggestive of cirrhosis or heart failure. These fluid descriptions are just guidelines, though; all fluids must be submitted for analysis and culture and correlated with clinical and radiographic findings.

Much research is currently being conducted on serum microchemistries and their clinical significance in cage birds. It appears that LDH, SGOT, GGTP, and SGPT are present in high levels in the liver of larger psittacines and they become elevated in liver disease.[6] In the authors' experience, budgerigars have shown significant elevation in SGPT correlated with serious liver disease on autopsy; however, other authors believe that SGOT and GGTP are more reliable indicators of liver problems. Uric acid levels rise in renal disease, and values greater than 15 mg/dl are considered significant.[7] The significance of hematocrits and serum total protein levels has been reported by Lafeber.[8] Changes in blood glucose levels may be useful in monitoring response to treatment. Many ill birds quickly become hypoglycemic. Chronic illness, liver problems, and starvation can result in hypoglycemia. Hyperglycemia can occur with stress, diabetes mellitus, and renal disease. Normal blood glucose values range from 210 to 520 mg/dl with a mean of 390 mg/dl.[9]

Treatment[c]

Once the cause of abdominal enlargement is determined, appropriate treatment can be recommended. In some instances exploratory surgery may be necessary to confirm what is suspected from the clinical workup or to remove a neoplasm. However, since budgerigars do not tolerate extensive surgery well and abdominal exposure is difficult, exploratory procedures are only considered after more conservative methods have been exhausted. If surgery is to be done, care must be taken to prepare the bird for the procedure to increase the chances of success. Supportive fluid therapy should be started 24 hours prior to surgery. A dose of 0.25 to 0.30 ml 2.5% dextrose and 0.45% sodium chloride/30 g body weight IM every 8 to 12 hours is helpful. If there is liver disease, 0.01 ml vitamin K can be injected IM 24 hours prior to surgery and on the day of surgery—this seems to aid in hemostasis. Food is not withheld before surgery. Halothane anesthesia is used,[10] and heat must be supplied to maintain body temperature. After induction, a 25-gauge needle is inserted into the brachial vein so that fluids and/or blood can be administered as needed during the surgery (Figure 7). If extensive blood loss is anticipated either because of underlying liver problems or because of the extent of the procedure, fresh blood for transfusion is taken from a donor colony. An ophthalmic cautery[d] is useful for maintaining hemostatis during the procedure. The bird is placed in an incubator for recovery, and fluids and oxygen are administered as necessary.

Egg and Oviduct

Egg-bound birds can usually be treated fairly easily by manually removing the egg. This can often be done in the exam room. One squeezes gently just cranial to the egg with the thumb and first finger, gradually working the egg out of the cloaca. If the egg cannot be easily extruded, placing the bird in an incubator to provide heat, administering 10% calcium gluconate orally, and injecting warm mineral oil or another lubricant around the egg with a lacrimal cannula may help in removing it or may allow the bird to pass the egg naturally. Since hypocalcemia is linked to egg binding, 10% calcium

---

[c]Dosages are based on empirical use until blood and tissue levels of drugs used in pet birds are determined.

[d]Comcept ACCU-TEMP Cautery®, Concept Inc., Clearwater, FL 33516.

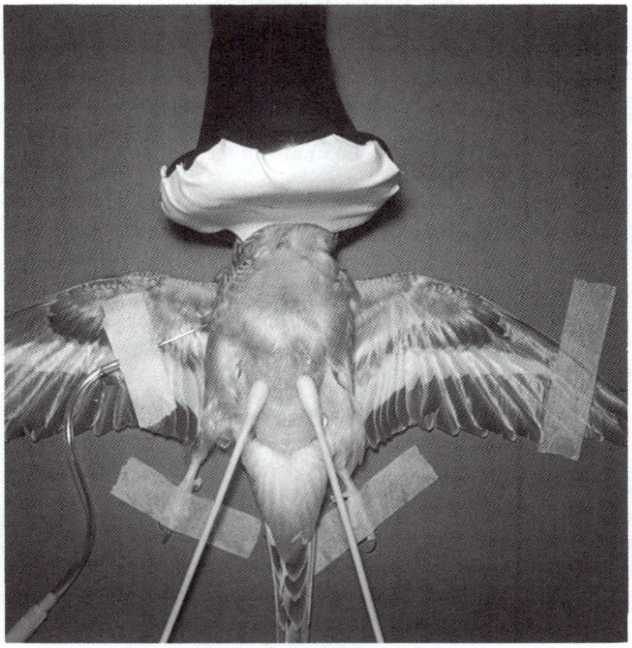

Figure 7—Administration of blood and fluid during surgery improves the chances for success.

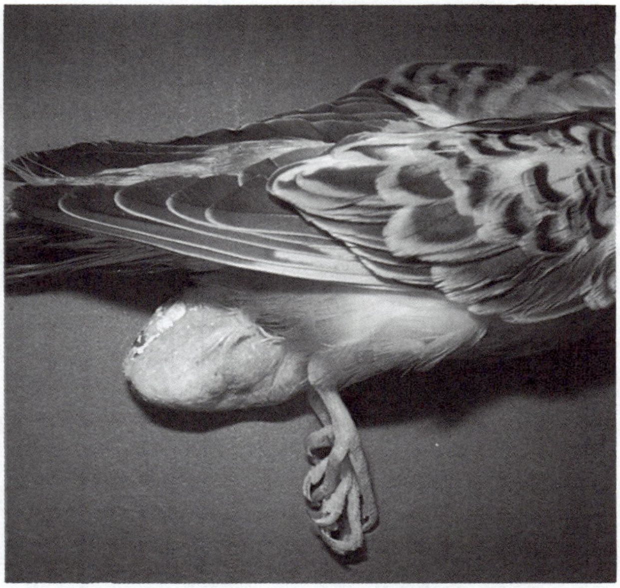

Figure 8—Abdominal hernia associated with hyperestrogenism.

gluconate is given orally at a rate of 2 drops/30 minutes for up to one to two hours or until the egg is passed. The bird's condition is carefully monitored and if it worsens, more invasive procedures should be instituted. In some instances anesthesia may be necessary to facilitate the procedure, especially if the egg is unusually large. In rare instances, surgical opening of the oviduct may be indicated. If the bird is in shock because of the egg binding, its condition should be stabilized by administering fluids and keeping the bird warm prior to any manipulation.

If the egg is broken during the procedure, the abdomen is gently massaged cranially to caudally so that the egg shell and contents can be extruded through the cloaca. If the egg shell does not pass, 48 hours are allowed for the broken shell to pass naturally before considering surgical removal. If much manipulation is necessary and the procedure is prolonged, antibiotics and fluids are indicated.

Egg peritonitis, often a chronic debilitating illness, carries a guarded prognosis. The diagnosis can be elusive and, perhaps because many cases are advanced by the time a definitive diagnosis is reached, the treatment is rarely successful. The selection of antibiotic should be based on culture results of abdominal fluid (if obtainable) and on any bacterial growth. In some instances there is only minimal fluid or a thick, tenacious exudate which defies aspiration and coats the abdominal organs. Systemic antibiotics, intraperitoneal infusion with antibiotics in small volume so as not to drown the bird, supportive fluid therapy, and gavage feeding are recommended. Despite intensive therapy, though, results are frequently unrewarding. If the bird recovers, hormone therapy (methyltestosterone 5 mg/oz drinking water daily for 7 to 10 days) is recommended to suppress ovarian activity.

Oviduct enlargement with a secondary abdominal hernia and fluid in the abdominal cavity and oviduct can be reduced with diuretics and methyltestosterone. Methyltestosterone 5 mg is given in 1 oz drinking water daily for 7 to 10 days and is gradually decreased to administration once or twice a week to control fluid and hernia size. The dosage is titrated to the individual bird's need, so recommendations may vary in different circumstances. Mibolerone[e] has not been as useful as methyltestosterone in the authors' experience. Furosemide syrup, one drop orally every other day, may aid in controlling fluid accumulation if methyltestosterone alone is not successful.

Hernias are difficult to surgically repair because of birds' scanty abdominal muscles. Birds that chronically bind eggs or that are excessive egg layers can also be controlled with methyltestosterone.

Liver Disease

Psittacosis was the great scourge of budgerigar breeders until chlortetracycline was discovered. Feeding of medicated seed has helped control this disease, but it is wise to bear in mind that budgerigars are susceptible. Psittacosis is a systemic disease, and the liver is seriously involved. Diagnosis is made by elementary bodies seen by electron microscopy in the liver, spleen, or air sacs or by injection of infective material into mice.

Since there are many causes of liver disease, a biopsy is necessary to make a sure diagnosis as a basis for proper therapy. Although the authors have sometimes done biopsies through laparotomies or surgery, as discussed previously, these are critical procedures in smaller birds. Therapy also depends on the clinical severity of

[e]Cheque®, The Upjohn Co., Kalamazoo, MI 49001.

the problem. Antibiotics, fluid therapy, and glucose are frequently given for liver problems. If there is hemorrhaging, injectable vitamin K is given IM. For neurologic manifestations, neomycin given at a rate of 1 drop twice a day has been clinically helpful. Glucocorticoids have also been administered (in critically ill birds that are not responding to other therapy), but this is a questionable procedure when the exact type of liver disease is not known, since steroids exacerbate some liver problems. Dietary changes, lipotrophic agents, and glucose can be given to aid management in chronic cases.

Conclusion

Abdominal enlargement in the budgerigar can be the result of many disease processes. Neoplasia and liver problems are common and are responsible for the majority of abdominal problems. Egg binding and cystic oviducts are easily diagnosed and are usually amenable to conservative medical management. Only through physical examination, radiography, and laboratory testing can a diagnosis be reached and appropriate therapy instituted. A rational approach to avian patients will result in better, more successful treatment.

REFERENCES

1. Petrak ML, Gilmore CE: Neoplasms, in Metrak ML (ed): *Diseases of Cage and Aviary Birds.* Philadelphia, Lea & Febiger, 1969, pp 459-489.
2. Leav I, et al: A naturally occurring lipidosis in shell parakeets, *Melopsittacus undulatus. Lab Invest* 18(4):433-437, 1968.
3. Soifer FK: Physical examination and medication of cage birds. *Vet Clin North Am* 3(2):143-158, 1973.
4. Silverman S: Avian radiographic technique and interpretation, in Kirk RW (ed): *Current Veterinary Therapy VI.* Philadelphia, WB Saunders Co, 1977, pp 671-674.
5. Schlumberger HG: Polyostotic hyperostosis in the female parakeet. *Am J Pathol* 35(1):1-23, 1959.
6. Galvin C: Laboratory diagnostic aids in pet bird practice. *1980 Scientific Proceedings of the 47th Annual Meeting of American Animal Hospital Association,* pp 41-52.
7. Altman RB: Diseases of the avian urinary system, in Kirk RW (ed): *Current Veterinary Therapy VI.* Philadelphia, WB Saunders Co, 1977, pp 703-705.
8. Lafeber TJ: Respiratory diseases. *Vet Clin North Am* 3(2):199-227, 1973.
9. Altman RB, Kirmayer AH: Diabetes mellitus in the avian species. *JAAHA* 12(4):531-537, 1976.
10. Altman RB: Avian anesthesia. *Compend Contin Educ Pract Vet* II(1):38-43, 1980.
11. Hirsch AS: Report of research in progress: a three part study. *Systemic Pathology Produced in the Budgerigar (Melopsittacus undulatus) following Virus Inoculation.* Dept. of Microbiology, Pathology and Public Health, School of Veterinary Medicine, Purdue University, West Lafayette, IN.
12. Evans SM: Avian radiographic diagnosis. *Compend Contin Educ Pract Vet* 3:660-666, 1981.

KEY FACTS

- The incidence of reported human disease from known avian zoonotic pathogens is low.
- There is a greater chance of encountering zoonotic organisms in recently imported birds.
- Clean aviary settings and sound personal hygiene reduce exposure to potential zoonotic agents.
- Many potential avian zoonotic diseases have not been thoroughly investigated in commonly maintained pet birds.

Avian Zoonoses: Proven and Potential Diseases Part I. Bacterial and Parasitic Diseases

Branson W. Ritchie, DVM
Department of Small Animal Medicine

David W. Dreesen, DVM, MPVM
Department of Medical Microbiology

College of Veterinary Medicine
University of Georgia
Athens, Georgia

An estimated 45 million to 70 million birds are maintained as pets or in aviary settings in the United States. Birds intended for the global pet markets are collected from numerous geographic locations and, after a brief quarantine period, are placed in direct contact with their new owners. Of 345 birds examined in one study, 24% had at least one known zoonotic organism.[1] In a Canadian quarantine station, 207 of 269 (77%) birds examined at postmortem were found to have some type of zoonotic infection.[2] The stresses associated with shipping, diet manipulation, and new environments enhance the chances of a bird shedding zoonotic microorganisms. Despite the number of potential pathogenic organisms, the close human association with birds, and the increasing quantity of avian species maintained in captivity, the incidence of human disease caused by recognized avian zoonotic pathogens is low. Nonetheless, veterinary practitioners dealing with commonly maintained captive birds should be aware of these potential diseases.

Chlamydia

Chlamydia psittaci, an obligate intracellular organism with worldwide distribution, is a well-known pathogen of humans and animals. Based on infectivity characteristics in birds, several strains are believed to exist. In humans, chlamydia organisms have been associated with clinical syndromes varying from a flulike illness to death. Diseases caused by chlamydia have been exhaustively reviewed in the literature.[3-8]

In general, the frequency of reported *C. psittaci* infections in both humans and birds has been on the increase in the past several decades. Clinical manifestations in birds are extremely variable, ranging from inapparent infection to severe septicemia and acute death.[4] Presenting signs are highly variable and depend on age; species; and general condition, including poor feathering, listlessness, depression, anorexia, weight loss, conjunctivitis, nasal discharge, dyspnea, diarrhea, torticollis, tremors, convulsions, and green- or yellow-stained urates.[4,6-8] Estimates of infectivity in the captive avian population vary from 20% to 50%, with disease isolation most commonly occurring in recently purchased birds.[4] The incidence of chlamydiosis in wild psittacine populations is reported to be about 1%.[6] Parrots, parakeets, and

Originally published in Volume 10, Number 4, April 1988

pigeons are believed to be the natural reservoirs of disease; while young birds of most species and the large South American parrots are most susceptible to infections.[5,6]

Incubation of *C. psittaci* varies with the infected avian species and the strain of chlamydia but may range from 40 days to 1 1/2 years.[6] Transmission may occur by direct contact with feces or respiratory secretions or by aerosolization of feather or fecal dust.[5-8] During the acute phase of infection, fecal shedding is extensive and infected carriers may intermittently shed the organism for months. Diagnosis can be accomplished by fecal culturing or by serologic methods, including latex agglutination, direct complement fixation, hemagglutination inhibition, and ELISA testing.[5-8] Some species, notably the African grey parrot, cockatiel, and budgie, may remain serologically negative despite active infections.[4] The tetracyclines have proven to be the most reliable form of therapy because they interfere with the synthesis of chlamydial proteins.[6]

Salmonella

Salmonellosis has been reported in a number of avian species, including poultry, pigeons, doves, sparrows, lories, finches, parakeets, cockatiels, Amazon parrots, cockatoos, macaws,[9-11] turkeys, ducks, geese, pheasant, quail, canaries, titmice, gulls, starlings,[12-15] roseate spoonbills, umbrella birds, hornbills, ravens, blue-crowned parrots,[16] black-crowned night herons, common egrets, little blue herons, cattle egret, snowy egret, Louisiana heron,[17] barn owls, falcons, red-tailed hawks,[18-20] and African grey parrots.[12,21] Salmonella infections can be peracute, acute, chronic, or subclinical, depending on the number of organisms encountered; their serotype; and the age, species, and condition of the host.[22-25] In the avian host, clinical manifestations associated with salmonellosis include depression, lethargy, anorexia, weight loss, shivering, diarrhea, pasty vent, lameness, abscess formation, convulsions, and sudden death.[12,22-27,28] The only sign of disease in breeding birds with subclinical infections may be poor hatching or excessive fledgling mortality.[12] Osteomyelitis and arthritis caused by a *Salmonella* species were diagnosed in a crow.[29]

Reports on the frequency of salmonellosis in avian hosts vary with the population sampled, for example, 18.2% of all species examined at a Canadian quarantine station,[2] 10% of free-flying pigeons in Germany, 25 of 270 mixed psittacine birds,[30] 2 of 16 finches, 4 of 93 parakeets, 1 of 38 cockatiels, 2 of 16 small parrots, 7 of 86 medium-sized parrots, 2 of 18 macaws,[9] 4 of 39 canaries,[12] 4 of 133 doves, 1 of 29 pigeons, 6 of 79 sparrows,[10] 2 of 105 free-flying raptors,[20] and 53 of 266 sparrows.[25] *Salmonella* organisms could not be isolated from any fecal samples in a study involving scarlet macaws, double yellow-headed Amazon parrots, green-cheeked Amazon parrots, nanday conures, quaker parakeets, cockatiels, peach-faced lovebirds, and budgies.[31] An outbreak of salmonellosis in a zoo aviary was attributed to infected African grey parrots being added to the collection.[21]

The ability of *Salmonella* serotypes to penetrate the mucosal barrier separates the primary pathogens from secondary invaders. The noninvasive serotypes are believed to be responsible for carrier syndromes.[11] *Salmonella* can survive extended periods in organic matter, feces, and dirt, living up to 28 months in avian feces.[25] Transmission may occur through ingestion of contaminated food or water or through direct contact by aerosolization of fecal or feather dust.[11,27] Salmonellosis in birds is associated with variable morbidity and mortality, depending on the age, condition, and species infected. Mortality in young birds is usually 100%.[23,26] Lories and African grey parrots are considered to be highly susceptible to *Salmonella* infection, suffering high mortality rates even with the noninvasive serotypes.[11] *Salmonella* caused the death of 2000 of 4400 (45%) and 60 of 170 canaries (35.3%) following a four- to five-day incubation period and two to four days after clinical signs developed.[25,28] *Salmonella* infection is responsible for the high mortality of greenfinches and house sparrows during the spring in Britain.[32,33] Any bird surviving an infection may become an asymptomatic carrier and shed infective organisms in the stool.[22,25]

Salmonellosis is one of the most commonly reported zoonotic diseases, with a number of human outbreaks traced to avian species.[10,23,34-36] Examples include a child with bloody diarrhea, vomiting, and fever who was found to be infected with the same *Salmonella* serotype that was isolated from a pet bird that died following an episode of diarrhea.[37] A human case of salmonellosis was reported following handling of an injured gull.[38] Individuals handling wild avian species should be particularly careful, as asymptomatic carriers may actively shed salmonella when stressed.[17,19,24-27]

Diagnosis of salmonellosis is based on isolation of the organism from infected tissues or feces. *Salmonella* organisms are excreted intermittently, even during active infection; thus, a single negative fecal culture is usually inconclusive.[39] Fecal cultures of asymptomatic carriers often yield false-negative results.[11]

Antibiotic sensitivity varies widely with each *Salmonella* serotype; thus, therapy should be based on cultures and sensitivity testing.[22,23,25] Successful therapy may require three to eight weeks, and a bird should not be considered free of *Salmonella* infection until three consecutive weekly fecal cultures are negative.[27] Even repeated therapy has failed to eliminate carriers in some cases.[25] Most common disinfectants rapidly kill *Salmonella* organisms. Preventive measures should include several negative fecal cultures of all new arrivals in an aviary, purchase and storage of food in sealed rodent-proof containers, exclusion of wild birds or rodents from the aviary, and strict caretaker hygiene.

Mycobacteria

In humans, tuberculosis is primarily caused by *Mycobacterium tuberculosis*. Two other typical species, *M. bovis* and *M. avium*, cause most avian infections and have, on occasion, caused clinical signs consistent with true tuberculosis in humans. For purposes of this discussion, the term *tuberculosis* is used to define the disease caused by any one of these three strains. Infections caused by typical strains of *Mycobacterium* are usually associated with a chronic debilitating disease typified by granulomatous host reactions. Incubation of mycobacteria may require weeks to months and is governed by the degree of exposure and the host condition.[39] During this prolonged incubation period, infected humans and animals are usually asymptomatic and can be responsible for rapid dissemination of mycobacterial organisms.[40]

The most consistent clinical indications of tuberculosis in birds are weight loss and severe muscle atrophy. Other clinical manifestations include sudden death, depression, abdominal enlargement, hemorrhagic diarrhea, hemoptysis, darker than normal feathers, follicle atrophy, sinusitis, dyspnea, oral plaques, and lameness associated with arthritis or osteomyelitis.[41–48] Parrots have been reported to develop proliferative nodular or diffuse keratinous skin lesions around the mucocutaneous junction of the eyes and beak.[49,50]

The pathogenesis of tuberculosis in birds is not entirely clear. It is hypothesized that the organism localizes primarily in the gastrointestinal tract following chronic ingestion of contaminated food or water. The lack of lymph nodes in birds is considered instrumental in allowing systemic hematogenous distribution to the lymphatics, liver, spleen, kidneys, skeletal system, heart, lungs, gonads, skin, thyroid, and adrenal glands secondarily infected.[39,51–56] Primary pulmonary disease from aerogenic transmission is rare.[49,54,57] Avian tuberculosis transmitted to a parrot via contaminated tatoo ink resulted in cutaneous lesions at the injection site.[48]

Mycobacteria have been isolated from a large number of birds in the following orders: Galliformes, Anseriformes, Gruiformes, Charadriiformes, Columbiformes, Falconiformes, Strigiformes, Coconiiformes, and Passeriformes.[43,48,53,58–65] Tuberculosis has also been diagnosed in canaries, finches, macaws, grey-cheeked parakeets, canary-wing parakeets, blue-headed pionus, spectacled Amazon parrots, blue-fronted Amazon parrots, toco toucans,[48,66,67] a sulfur-crested cockatoo,[68] green-cheeked Amazon parrots,[47] and dwarf parrots.[69]

Tuberculosis in birds is primarily caused by *M. avium*. Like humans, however, psittacine birds are also susceptible to *M. tuberculosis* and *M. bovis*.[54,70–73] Domestic fowl seem to be the primary hosts of avian tuberculosis and are relatively resistant to infection, while parrots and related species are apparently highly susceptible.[50,70] Psittacine birds are more resistant to *M. avium* than to the other mycobacteria strains and are apparently the only avian order susceptible to *M. tuberculosis*.[42,74,75] From several reports, *Brotogeris* parakeets, Amazon parrots, and pionus may be more susceptible than other psittacines to mycobacterial infections.[42,76,77]

Numerous surveys have indicated a relatively high degree of *M. avium* present in the global avian population. Various studies involving wild birds have indicated a 3.9% to 40% infectivity, depending on the species tested and the geographic location.[41,61,65,78] In a survey of parrots in England, 56 of 154 (36.4%) birds were positive for *M. avium*.[71] At the Philadelphia Zoo, tuberculosis was isolated in 217 of 3505 (6.2%) avian necropsies.[49] Necropsy records at the National Zoo showed tuberculosis infectivity in 11 of 22 orders of avian species maintained in the collection; 4% was the highest annual mortality reported. During one year, the susceptible population was found to have a 14.2% infectivity rate, with finches being most commonly infected. Ratites, birds of prey, and psittacines were rarely positive.[43,54] In a private practice serving a large bird-owning clientele, 30 parakeets belonging to the *Brotogeris* genus were cultured positive for *M. avium*; while during a six-year period, only 12 other cases of avian tuberculosis were diagnosed.[66]

Avian species are rarely implicated in human disease despite the relatively large number of captive birds reported with tuberculosis.[79] Because of the protracted incubation period, however, it is often difficult to establish the source of exposure. Although humans are considered to be relatively resistant to *M. avium* infection, naturally occurring avian tuberculosis can be a secondary source of human disease.[61,79–82] A person could potentially transmit tuberculosis to a pet (or vice versa) if exchanging of food by mouth is routinely practiced.[81] Avian tuberculosis exhibits a high degree of natural resistance to standard antitubercle drugs, and this refractivity to therapy has resulted in fatal infections in humans.[39,56,66,81] The source of initial infection could not be determined in four men infected with *M. avium*.[81] A three-year-old girl died 30 days after developing a fever coupled with vomiting, diarrhea, and mesenteric lymphadenitis; *Mycobacterium avium* was isolated from her lymph nodes.[81] A 60-year-old man died with avian tuberculosis after two years of chronic disease; *Mycobacterium avium* was isolated from a canary that was housed in the man's bedroom.[81] Avian tuberculosis has also been isolated from bird ticks; however, the potential of arthropod transmission is yet to be studied.[83]

Antemortem diagnosis of avian tuberculosis remains difficult and unreliable. The results of acid-fast stains of cloacal or tracheal material are inconsistent.[39,42,66] Radiographs are considered inadequate, as avian tubercles are not known to calcify. The use of intradermal tuberculin, which is used in mammals and chickens, has proven unreliable in other avian species.[84] The slide agglutination test developed for poultry, although better than the intradermal tuberculin test, has poor sensitivity in other avian species. A modification of this test using citrated plasma in a rapid agglutination test may be beneficial in diagnosing *M. avium* infection.[85] Experimentally, hematologic parameters are inconsistent in detecting avian infections, although elevated total serum protein was a nonspecific finding in one tuberculosis study.[43,54] Biopsies of affected tissue and postmortem examinations remain the most accurate way of diagnosing tuberculosis.

Treatment for tuberculosis in birds has been discussed in the literature.[49,66] Therapy in the avian patient should be discouraged, however, because an effective avian antitubercule drug is not available for use in humans and tuberculosis in birds is usually a consistent, shedding, open infection.[39] Once present, tuberculosis bacilli can survive in a bird facility for several years and are resistant to typical physical and chemical destruction.[39,56,81,83] Prevention of tuberculosis depends on sound hygienic practices and protection of aviary collections from free-ranging birds.[40] Subcutaneous administration of killed decapsulated bacilli was found to provide 100% immunity for natural and artificial infection in some avian species. The vaccine, however, has not been properly studied for use in common captive species.[86]

Yersinia

Yersinia pseudotuberculosis and *Y. enterocolitica* are responsible for causing a variety of disease syndromes in humans and animals. These gram-negative, non-spore–forming rods have a species-dependent geographic distribution pattern.

Yersinia enterocolitica occurs worldwide, with isolations in Northern Europe, Canada, the United States, and South Africa.[87] Infected geese, ducks, robins, canaries, pigeons, and gulls with clinical signs that include listlessness, anorexia, weight loss, and diarrhea have been reported and death has occurred.[87–89] The animal reservoir, means of transmission, and epidemiology of *Y. enterocolitica* are not well understood; however, investigators have linked serotypes found in robins and other animals with serotypes producing disease in humans.[90–92] The frequent recovery of this species from the gastrointestinal tract and excreta of animals suggests a fecal–oral transmission.[87,88] Unlike *Y. pseudotuberculosis, Y. enterocolitica* infection evidently is less common in animals than in humans.[87]

Yersinia pseudotuberculosis occurs primarily in Northern Europe and is endemic in the Scandinavian countries and France. Isolates from other geographic locations may occur through importation of diseased animals.[87] Clinical manifestations reported in birds are inconsistent but include listlessness, ruffled feathers, anorexia, diarrhea, respiratory distress, incoordination, and sudden death.[93] Infections are usually fatal in birds by producing fulminating septicemia. *Yersinia*-caused granulomas have been reported in budgies and canaries.[2] Epizootics associated with increased stress from severe winter conditions, reproductive activity, and overheating have been reported in turkeys, ducks, pigeons, doves, canaries, magpies, grackles, and finches.[87,94–96] Sporadic infections have been described in more than 50 species of birds, including coots, goldfinches, jackdaws, flycatchers, puffins, rooks, starlings, skylarks, sparrow hawks, thrushes, swallows, warblers, blackbirds, eiders, woodpeckers, martins, oystercatchers, partridges, pheasants, swifts, wrens, owls, swans, grackles, canaries, finches, pigeons,[97,98] crows, martins,[89] toucans,[99] king penguins,[100] red-vented parrots, gannets, parakeets,[101] amadarats, fingerfinches, butterfly finches, caban finches, snow buntings,[93] lady gouldian finches,[102] cockatoos, toucans, and owls.[94] In a 1974 avian mortality report from the London Zoo, *Yersinia pseudotuberculosis* was the most common bacterial agent isolated from acclimatized birds. Recoveries were made from speckled pigeons, barbets, Indian shama, maroon tanager, wood quail, touraco, and black-crowned motmot.[103] In the United Kingdom, *Y. pseudotuberculosis* was isolated from 21 species of wild birds.[87] In North America, sporadic isolations of *Y. pseudotuberculosis* from domestic and wild birds have been documented.[104]

Birds and rodents are considered the principal reservoirs of *Y. pseudotuberculosis.* Transmission of the organism from animal to animal and from animal to human is believed to occur by fecal and urine contamination of food and water supplied by infected wild birds or rodents.[87] Avian fecal secretions containing *Yersinia* have been shown to be infective to other birds, mammals, and humans.[87,96]

Strong circumstantial evidence suggests that human disease follows exposure to infected animals, as the same strains of *Y. pseudotuberculosis* infect both animals and humans. Further evidence for animal-to-human transmission includes chronologic peaks of infectivity in both hosts, animal contact in the histories of human patients, and sequential increases in human and animal infections from endemic rural areas.[87] A person was found to have acute mesenteric lymphadenitis caused by *Y. pseudotuberculosis* following exposure to contaminated feces from a pet canary.[105,106]

Antemortem diagnosis of *Y. pseudotuberculosis* infection is difficult because of variations in the type of environmental stress, virulence of the agent, and susceptibility of the host. Various wild birds are known to be refractory to natural infection; in avian species, however, acquired immunity to *Y. pseudotuberculosis* infection remains largely unstudied.[94] Diagnosis is based on laboratory isolation using a cold enrichment technique and subsequent identification. *Yersinia* is difficult to isolate, and a diligent laboratory pursuit is often necessary for positive results.

Campylobacter

Campylobacter organisms are gram-negative, motile, non-spore–forming, curved, spiral rods that have been implicated in enteric disease of humans and animals. *Campylobacter fetus, C. intestinalis,* and *C. jejuni* have all been shown to be enteric avian pathogens; but only *C. intestinalis* and *C. jejuni* have been reported to cause human disease. *Campylobacter jejuni* is the most common subspecies isolated from avian species.[107] Infected birds may be asymptomatic or show signs of anorexia, somnolence, diarrhea, and emaciation; fledgling mortality is common.[108] *Campylobacter* has been isolated from chickens, turkeys, pheasants, geese, pigeons, Pekin robins, nandus, finches, canaries,[109] ducks, sparrows, starlings, and blackbirds.[110,111] The prevalence of *C. jejuni* in the intestinal flora of asymptomatic avian species may be substantial. In two studies, 83 of 94 free-ranging ducks[112] and 35% of migrating ducks[109] tested were found to be harboring *C. jejuni*.

Campylobacter jejuni can be transmitted by direct fecal or aerosol contact, contaminated fomites, or infected vectors; and consumption of contaminated poultry is considered to rival *Salmonella* in zoonotic importance.[113,114] The avian strains of *C. jejuni* are not serologically uniform, and details on human cross-infectivity from birds other than poultry have not been sufficiently studied.[12] Some avian *Campylobacter* species are believed to be distinct biotypes and may not be involved in human disease.[111] In a pilot study, captive birds were found to play at least a minor role in non-food–borne human infections.[115]

A presumptive diagnosis of campylobacteriosis can be made by examining stools for motile, curved, spiral rods using phase-contrast microscopy. Confirmation is by isolation of the organism, usually within a microaerophilic environment.

Giardia

Giardia is a protozoan parasite that has a wide geographic and host distribution. Infection occurs by ingestion of infective cysts that contaminate the environment after being passed via the infected host feces. Avian species reported with giardiasis include herons, turkey vultures, house sparrows, bitterns, egrets, western meadowlarks, cockatiels, budgerigars, conures, Amazon parrots, cockatoos, and macaws.[116,117] Clinical findings in birds may include weight loss, depression, ruffled feathers, chronic diarrhea, neonatal mortality, cachexia, muscle weakness, eosinophilia, hypoproteinemia, persistent feather picking, pruritus, and occasionally gastrointestinal erosions.[30,117,118] In one study of 77 parakeets from several sources, 66% were actively shedding *Giardia*.[119] *Giardia* was isolated in 70% of cockatiels; 55% of parakeets; 25% of lovebirds; 5% of grey-cheeked parakeets and conures; and 1% of Amazon parrots, cockatoos, and macaws examined.[117]

Giardia cysts are highly virulent. Only a few cysts can cause severe pathogenic gastrointestinal changes. The parasite withstands moderate temperature ranges and survives standard chlorination of drinking water.[120,121] Historically, numerous host-specific species of *Giardia* were considered to exist worldwide; but it is now recognized that they are morphologically similar. Some *Giardia* species are highly host specific, while others are capable of infecting a broad host range.[120-124] Even though human infections from companion animals, including pet birds, have not been proven, evidence supports the contention that direct transmission of *Giardia* from numerous animal species to humans can occur.[30,120,125,126] The relatively high rate of *Giardia* infections reported in some avian species leads one to ponder the public health significance of infected pet birds.[119,127]

Infections are typically more severe in the young and immunocompromised.[127-129] *Giardia* infection was most commonly diagnosed in young birds, and an inverse relationship between infection and age appeared to exist. Infections resolved as the birds reached maturity. When uninfected or recovered birds were placed with infected birds, however, active shedding was induced, indicating a lack of host immunity. Infection rates increased during periods of confinement and overcrowding.[119]

There is no clinical sign considered pathognomonic for giardiasis, and positive diagnosis depends on recovering trophozoites or cysts from the host.[125] Asymptomatic avian hosts can harbor and intermittently shed *Giardia*, thus complicating the identification of infected individuals.[117,130] *Giardia* is usually missed on routine fecal examinations because commonly used sugar and salt flotation solutions destroy cysts.[131] Satisfactory diagnosis in the avian patient can be augmented by using multiple, fresh, direct-mount smears; using the zinc sulfate centrifugation method; or fixing avian feces in polyvinyl alcohol and preparing a slide with trichrome stain.[117,125,132] High numbers of false-negative results occur if fecal samples are more than 5 to 10 minutes old when evaluated.[117] In contrast to diagnostic sensitivity in humans and dogs, fecal smears from parakeets properly identified 83% of infected birds; while mucosal scrapings identified only 25% of those infected.[119,130,132] A number of immunologic tests, including an ELISA test and precipitin test, have been developed and have proven reliable for detecting *Giardia* in humans.[133,134] These procedures have not been evaluated in birds but may prove more reliable than current diagnostic methods for detecting *Giardia* infections.

Because of the potential of *Giardia* transmission from birds to humans, any bird shedding the parasite should be treated. Administering 20 to 30 mg/kg of metronidazole once a day for two days is the currently recommended avian therapy.[117] Transmission of the parasite can be prevented by adhering to sound personal and aviary hygiene. Several fecal examinations should be conducted during quarantines of new additions to an aviary. Water supplies should be periodically examined for *Giardia*, particularly in breeding aviaries where a high degree of unexplained neonatal mortality has occurred.

Cryptosporidia

Cryptosporidium is considered to be a primary protozoan pathogen capable of causing disease alone or in association with bacterial, viral, or other parasitic pathogens.[135] Infection occurs by ingestion of infective sporulated oocysts. The persistence of clinical signs in some hosts is currently considered to be the result of the oocyst's ability to excyst within the host, causing immediate reinfection.[136] *Cryptosporidium* most commonly localizes in the small and large intestines but has also been associated with pathologic invasion of the stomach, bile ducts, pancreatic ducts, and gallbladder of various host species.[136-138] In addition to gastrointestinal involvement in birds, the organism has been associated with respiratory tract, conjunctival sac, and bursal lesions.[136] Avian species harboring cryptosporidia may be asymptomatic or, depending on whether the gastrointestinal or respiratory tract is involved, may show signs of depression, dehydration, pyrexia, anorexia, persistent diarrhea, malabsorption, abdominal pain, vomiting, convulsions, coughing, sneezing, and nasal discharge.[135,139-142] Species of *Cryptosporidium* have been isolated from chickens, quails, pheasants, peafowl, peacocks, geese, ducks, budgerigars, canaries,[136,143,144] turkeys,[139,140] red-lored Amazon parrots,[145] and finches.[146]

Cryptosporidium is classified with the enteric coccidian protozoan parasites and was originally believed to be host specific.[136,147,148] Recent studies have shown that cross-transmission exists among a wide range of host species.[149] Isolates from mammals and birds have been transmitted to homologous and heterologous species; however, studies have demonstrated that the species of *Cryptosporidium* infecting quail, pheasants, and chickens were only transmissible to other avian species and not to mammals. Likewise, isolates from humans and guinea pigs were only infective for other mammals and not for birds.[136,148,150] One *Cryptosporidium* species isolated from a red-lored Amazon parrot was considered to be morphologically similar to that identified in other animal species.[145] Cryptosporidial infections in avian species tend to be subclinical, and shedding rates may be so low that cryptosporidia pose little threat to humans.[143] Further information on the infectivity and zoonotic potential of *Cryptosporidium* isolation from pet avian species is needed, however.

The small size of the organisms (4 to 6 μ) and low excretion rates in infected individuals make cryptosporidia difficult to detect in routine fecal examinations under low magnification.[143] Diagnosis is enhanced by centrifugation flotation of feces in a high-gravity salt solution. Smears of the supernate can be stained with Giemsa, carbolfuchsin, periodic acid-Schiff, or nigrosin to aid in identification of oocysts.[151,152]

Cryptosporidia oocysts have sporulated and are infectious at the time of excretion.[143,149] Cleaning fecal material from housing every two to three days to reduce infection rates, a preventive measure used to control other coccidia, is thus of no benefit.[135] Oocysts are resistant to many commonly used disinfectants. Household ammonia appears to provide an adequate killing effect, as does heating contaminated materials to 65 °C for 30 minutes.[153,154] No treatment has proven effective for eliminating the organism in the host.[135,136]

REFERENCES

1. Keymer IF: The unsuitability of non-domesticated animals as pets. *Vet Res* 91:373–381, 1982.
2. Rigby CE, Pettit JR, Papp-Vid G, et al: Isolation of salmonella, Newcastle disease virus and other infectious agents from quarantined imported birds in Canada. *Can J Comp Med* 45:366–370, 1981.
3. Butcher GD, Panigrahy B, Grimes JE, et al: Chlamydiosis: Avian host spectrum. *Southwest Vet* 37:33–36, 1986.
4. Mohan R: Epidemiologic and laboratory observations of *Chlamydia psittaci* infection in pet birds. *JAVMA* 184:1372–1374, 1984.
5. Grimes JE: Latex agglutination: A rapid serologic diagnostic aid for psittacine chlamydiosis. *Proc Assoc Avian Vet*:249–253, 1985.
6. Gerlach H: Chlamydia, in Harrison GJ, Harrison LR (eds): *Clinical Avian Medicine and Surgery*. Philadelphia, WB Saunders Co, 1986, pp 457–463.
7. Paster MB: Chlamydiosis: A review of current literature, treatment, control. *Proc Assoc Avian Vet*:215–248, 1985.
8. Fudge AM: Update on chlamydiosis, in Harrison GJ (ed): *Veterinary Clinics of North America: Small Animal Practice*, vol 14. Philadelphia, WB Saunders Co, 1984, pp 201–221.
9. Mohan R: Salmonella infection in pet birds. *Proc Assoc Avian Vet*:78, 1983.
10. Sambyal DS, Sharma VK: Screening of free-living animals and birds for *Listeria*, *Brucella*, and *Salmonella* infections. *Br Vet J* 127:50–53, 1972.
11. Gerlach H: Bacterial diseases, in Harrison GJ, Harrison LR (eds): *Clinical Avian Medicine and Surgery*. Philadelphia, WB Saunders Co, 1986, pp 434–453.
12. Panigrahy B, Gilmore WC: Systemic salmonellosis in an African grey parrot and salmonella osteomyelitis in canaries. *JAVMA* 183:699–700, 1983.
13. Jungherr E: Paratyphoid infections in birds. *Vet Med* 35:112–116, 1940.
14. Glickman LT, McDonough PL, Shin SJ, et al: Bovine salmonellosis attributed to *Salmonella anatum*-contaminated haylage and dietary stress. *JAVMA* 178:1268–1272, 1981.
15. Coulson JC, Butterfield PL, Thomas C: The herring gull *Larus argentatus* as a likely transmitting agent of *Salmonella monterideo* to sheep and cattle. *J Hyg* 91:437–443, 1983.
16. Sedgwick CJ, Robinson PT, Lochner FK: Zoonoses: A zoo's concern. *JAVMA* 167:828–829, 1975.
17. Locke LN, Ohlendorf HM, Shillenger RB, et al: Salmonellosis in a captive heron colony. *J Wildl Dis* 10:143–145, 1974.
18. Locke LN, Newman JA: Paratyphoid in a barn owl. *Chesapeake Sci* 11:67–68, 1970.
19. Sykes GP, Murphy C, Hardaswick V: Salmonella infection in a captive peregrine falcon. *JAVMA* 179:1269–1271, 1981.
20. Kirkpatrick CE, Calvin BA: *Salmonella* sp. in nestling common barn owls (*Tyto alba*) from southwestern New Jersey. *J Wildl Dis* 22:340–343, 1986.
21. Komorowski RA: Epizootic salmonellosis in an open zoo aviary. *Arch Environ Health* 27:110–111, 1973.
22. Meir JE: Salmonellosis and other bacterial enteritides in birds, in Kirk RW (ed): *Current Veterinary Therapy VIII*. Philadelphia, WB Saunders Co, 1983, pp 637–640.
23. Williams JE: Paratyphoid infections, in Hofstead MS, et al (eds): *Diseases of Poultry*, ed 7. Ames, IA, Iowa State University Press, 1978, pp 117–176.
24. Wallach JD, Boever WJ: *Diseases of Exotic Animals*. Philadelphia, WB Saunders Co, 1983, pp 852, 853, 905, 940, 941.
25. Fiennes RN: Diseases of bacterial origin, in Petrak ML (ed): *Diseases of Cage and Aviary Birds*, ed 2. Philadelphia, Lea & Febiger, 1982, pp 497–515.
26. Arnall L, Keymer IF: *Bird Diseases*. New Jersey, THF Publications, 1976, pp 113–121.
27. Ryan TP: Salmonellosis in caged birds. *Mod Vet Pract* 66:383–384, 1985.
28. Keymer IF: Specific diseases of the canary and other passerine birds. *Mod Vet Pract* 40:32–35, 1959.
29. Daoust PY: Osteomyelitis and arthritis caused by *Salmonella typhimurium* in a crow. *J Wildl Dis* 14:483–485, 1978.
30. Panigrahy B, Grimes JE, Rideout MS, et al: Zoonotic diseases of psittacine birds: Apparent increased occurrence of chlamydiosis, salmonellosis, giardiasis. *JAVMA* 175:359–361, 1979.
31. Bowman TA, Jacobson ER: Cloacal flora of clinically normal captive psittacine birds. *J Zoo Anim Med* 11:81–85, 1980.
32. MacDonald JW, Cornelius LW: Salmonellosis in wild birds. *Br Birds* 62:28–30, 1969.
33. Wilson JE, MacDonald JW: Salmonella infection in wild birds. *Br Vet J* 123:212–219, 1967.
34. Nikitiuk NM: The role of animals and birds as sources of salmonella infections in man. *Zh Mikrobiol Epidemiol Immunobiol* 47:123–130, 1970.
35. Steele JH: Salmonellosis: A major zoonosis. *Arch Environ Health* 19:871–875, 1969.
36. Wobeser GA, Finlayson MC: *Salmonella typhimurium* infection in house sparrows. *Arch Environ Health* 19:882–884, 1969.
37. Anderson HD: Salmonellosis—Washington. *Morbid Mortal Weekly Rep* 4(15), 1971.
38. MacDonald JW, Brown DD: Salmonella infection in wild birds in Britain. *Vet Rec* 94:321–322, 1974.
39. Gerlach H: Bacterial disease, in Harrison GJ, Harrison LR (eds): *Clinical Avian Medicine and Surgery*. Philadelphia, WB Saunders Co, 1986, pp 438–439.
40. Karlson G: Avian tuberculosis, in Montali RI (ed): *Mycobacterial Infections of Zoo Animals*. Washington, DC, Smithsonian Institute Press, 1978, pp 21–24.
41. Poulding RH: Tuberculosis in gulls: A preliminary investigation. *Bull Br Ornithol* 77:144, 1957.
42. Britt JO, Howard EB, Rosskopf WJ: Psittacine tuberculosis. *Cornell Vet* 70:218–225, 1980.
43. Ensley PK, Montali RJ, Smith E, Bush M: Avian tuberculosis at the

National Zoological Park. *Proc Am Assoc Zoo Vet*:203–205, 1975.
44. Woerpel RW, Rosskopf WJ: Retro-orbital *Mycobacterium tuberculosis* infection in a yellow-naped Amazon parrot. *Avian/Exotic Practice* 1:7–10, 1984.
45. Clark FD: Mycobacteriosis in a red-tailed hawk. *Southwest Vet* 37:200–201, 1986.
46. Peavy GM, Silverman S, Howard EB, et al: Pulmonary tuberculosis in a sulfur-crested cockatoo. *JAVMA* 169:915–919, 1976.
47. Petrak ML: A possible case of *Mycobacterium tuberculosis* in a parrot. *Proc Assoc Avian Vet*:165–166, 1984.
48. Van Derheyden N: Avian tuberculosis: Diagnosis and attempted treatment. *Proc Assoc Avian Vet*:203–211, 1986.
49. Fox H: *Diseases in Captive Wild Mammals and Birds*. Philadelphia, JB Lippincott, 1923, pp 503–510.
50. Gale NB: Tuberculosis, in Davis JW, et al (eds): *Infections and Parasitic Diseases of Wild Birds*. Ames, IA, Iowa State University Press, 1971, pp 89–93.
51. Scott HH: Tuberculosis in man and lower animals. *Spec Rep Ser Med Res Council [Lond]*:149, 1930.
52. Harrison JM, Harrison JG: Plumage changes in wild tubercular wood pigeons. *Bull Br Ornithol* 76:76, 1966.
53. Karlson AG, Davis CL, Cohn ML: Skotochromogenic *Mycobacterium avium* from a trumpeter swan. *Am J Vet Res* 23:575, 1962.
54. Montali RJ, Bush M, Thoen CO, Smith E: Tuberculosis in captive exotic birds. *JAVMA* 169:920–927, 1976.
55. Harrison JM: Tuberculosis in a wild sparrow hawk. *J Pathol Bacteriol* 60:583, 1948.
56. Karlson AG: Tuberculosis, in Hofstead MS, et al (eds): *Diseases of Poultry*, ed 6. Ames, IA, Iowa State University Press, 1972, pp 252–271.
57. Petrak ML: *Diseases of Cage and Aviary Birds*. Philadelphia, Lea & Febiger, 1969, p 284.
58. Sulton JB, Gibbes H: Tuberculosis in birds. *Trans Pathol Soc [Lond]* 35:477, 1984.
59. Sibley WK: Further observations on tuberculosis in fowls and other birds. *Trans Pathol Soc [Lond]* 41:332, 1980.
60. Brickford AT, Ellis GH, Moses HE: Epizootiology of tuberculosis in starlings. *JAVMA* 149:312–317, 1966.
61. Plum N: Studies on the occurrence of avian tuberculosis among wild birds, especially gulls, sparrows, rats, and hares. *Abstract Vet Bull* 13:28–32, 1942.
62. Jennings AR, Soulsby EJ: Disease in wild birds. *Bird Study* 4:216, 1957.
63. MacDonald JW: Mortality in wild birds with observations on weights. *Bird Study* 9:147, 1962.
64. Garden EA: Tuberculosis in eiders. *Wildfowl Trust 12th Annu Rep*:165, 1960.
65. Mitchell CA, Duthie RC: Tuberculosis in the common crow. *Can J Comp Med* 14:109, 1950.
66. Rosskopf WJ, Woerpel RW, Lane R, Blake WR: Avian tuberculosis in the grey-cheeked parakeet and other related *Brotogeris* parakeets. *Proc Assoc Avian Vet*:219–236, 1986.
67. Fudge AM, McEntee L: Cutaneous and systemic tuberculosis in a grey-cheeked parakeet. *Proc Assoc Avian Vet*:215–218, 1986.
68. Dolphin RE, Olsen DE, Gallina AM: Tubercular infection in a sulfur-crested cockatoo. *VM SAC* 74:833–835, 1979.
69. Riddell C, Atkinson DR: Two cases of mycobacteriosis in psittacine birds. *Can Vet J* 22:145–147, 1981.
70. Thoen CO, Richards WD, Jarnagin JL: Tuberculosis in captive exotic birds. *JAVMA* 169:920–927, 1976.
71. Moore VA: The morbid anatomy and etiology of avian tuberculosis. *J Med Res* 11:521–536, 1904.
72. Cheville NF, Richard WD: The influence of thymic and bursal lymphoid systems in avian tuberculosis. *Am J Pathol* 97:122, 1971.
73. Feldman WH: Tuberculosis of poultry, in Biester HH, Schwartz LH (eds): *Diseases of Poultry*, ed 4. Ames, IA, Iowa State University Press, 1965, pp 287–315.
74. Griffith AS: Tuberculosis in captive wild animals. *J Hyg* 28:198, 1928.
75. Merchant IA, Packer RA: *Veterinary Bacteriology and Virology*. Ames, IA, Iowa State University Press, 1968.
76. Ackerman LJ, Benbrook SC, Walton BC: *Mycobacterium* tuberculosis infection in a parrot (*Amazona farinosa*). *Am Rev Respir Dis* 109:388–390, 1974.
77. Rosskopf WG: Tuberculosis in a parrot. *Mod Vet Pract* 62:777–778, 1981.
78. Gordon RF, Gasside JS, Dobson N, Reid J: An extensive outbreak of tuberculosis in ducks. *Vet Rec* 53:575, 1941.
79. Falk GA, Hadley SJ, Sharkey FE, et al: *Mycobacterium avium* infections in man. *Am J Med* 54:801–810, 1973.
80. Kleeburg HH: Tuberculosis and other mycobacterioses, in Hubbert WT, et al (eds): *Diseases Transmitted from Animals to Man*, ed 6. Springfield, IL, Charles C Thomas, 1975, pp 345–348.
81. Kubin M, Kruml J, Horak J, et al: Pulmonary and non-pulmonary diseases in humans due to avian mycobacteria. *Am Rev Respir Dis* 94:20–30, 1966.
82. Crawford AB: Studies in avian tuberculosis. *Am Rev Tuberculosis* 37:594–597, 1938.
83. Blagodarnyi RA, et al: Isolation of atypical mycobacteria from spontaneously infected bird ticks (*Argus persicus*). *Probl Tuberk* 49:75–77, 1971.
84. Spears HN, Dobson N: The avian tuberculin test and its specificity. *Vet Rec* 53:365, 1941.
85. Gotz K: Studies for recognition and control of avian tuberculosis in zoological parks using citrate plasma in a rapid agglutination test. University of Munich, PhD dissertation, 1984.
86. Ross L: Immunizing potency of inactivated and living *Mycobacterium avium* and *Mycobacterium* intracellular vaccines against tuberculosis of domestic fowl. *Acta Vet Brno* 43:133–138, 1974.
87. Mair NS: Yersiniosis in wildlife and its public health implications. *J Wildl Dis* 9:65–71, 1973.
88. Langford EV: *Yersinia enterocolitica* isolated from animals in the Fraser Valley of British Columbia. *Can Vet J* 13:109–113, 1972.
89. Hacking WA, Sileo L: *Yersinia enterocolitica* and *Yersinia pseudotuberculosis* from wildlife in Ontario. *J Wildl Dis* 10:452–457, 1974.
90. Ahvonen P, Thal E, Vasenius H: Occurrence of *Yersinia enterocolitca* in animals in Finland and Sweden. *Yersinia, Pasteurella,* and *Francisella*. *Contrib Microbiol Immunol* 2:135–136, 1973.
91. Krogstad O, Teige J, Lassen J: *Yersinia enterocoliticia* type 2 associated with disease in goats. *Acta Vet Scand* 13:594–596, 1972.
92. Toma S: Survey on the incidence of *Yersinia enterocolitca* in the province of Ontario. *Can J Public Health* 64:477–487, 1973.
93. Keymer IF: Specific diseases of the canary and other passerine birds. *Mod Vet Pract* 40:32–35, 1959.
94. Wetzler TF: Pseudotuberculosis, in Davis JW, et al (eds): *Infections and Parasitic Diseases of Wild Birds*. Ames, IA, Iowa State University Press, 1971, pp 75–88.
95. Clark GM, Locke LN: Observations on pseudotuberculosis in common grackles. *Avian Dis* 6:506–510, 1962.
96. Stovell PL: Epizootological factors in three outbreaks of pseudotuberculosis in British Columbia canaries. University of British Columbia, Vancouver, Masters thesis, 1983.
97. Mair NS, Harbourne JF, Greenwood MT, White G: *Pasteurella pseudotuberculosis* infection in the cat: Two cases. *Vet Rec* 81:461–462, 1967.
98. Harshfield GS: Fowl chlorea, in Biester HE, Schwartz LH (eds): *Diseases of Poultry*, ed 5. Ames, IA, Iowa State University Press, 1965, pp 359–373.
99. Urbain A, Nowel J: Epidemic de pseudotuberculose chez de toucans de curier et des toucans ariel. *Bull Acad Vet Fr* 90:188–190, 1937.
100. Fiennes RN T-W: Report of the pathologist for the year 1960. *Proc Zool Soc [Lond]* 137:173–196, 1961.
101. Fiennes RN T-W: Report of the society's pathologist for the year 1962. *Proc Zool Soc [Lond]* 143:53–78, 1964.
102. Dhillon AS: A veterinarian's role as a detective tracking *Yersinia pseudotuberculosis*. *VM SAC* 29:1288–1289, 1984.
103. Keymer IF: Report on deaths at the London Zoo from 1974–1975. *J Zool* 184:296–313, 1978.
104. Hubbert WT: Yersinosis in mammals and birds in the United States: Case report and review. *Am J Trop Hyg* 21:458–463, 1972.
105. Huatko SI, Rodin AE: *Pasteurella pseudotuberculosis* infection in man. *Can Med Assoc J* 88:1108–1112, 1963.
106. Daniels JJ HM: Enteral infection *Pasteurella pseudotuberculosis*. Isolation of the organism from human feces. *Br Med J* 2:997–998, 1961.
107. Blaser MJ: Epidemiology of *Campylobacter* infections, in Butzler JP (ed): *Campylobacter Infection in Man and Animals*. Ames, IA, Iowa State University Press, 1984.
108. Dorrenstein GM, vander Hage MH, Cornelisse JL: *Campylobacter* infection in cage birds—Clinical, pathological, and bacteriological aspects, in *Proceedings of the Joint Meeting of Veterinary Pathologists*. Utrecht, Netherlands, Organization of Veterinary Patholo-

gists, 1984.

109. Luechtefeld NAW, Bluser MJ, Reller LB, et al: Isolation of *Campylobacter fetus* subsp *jejuni* from migratory waterfowl. *J Clin Microbol* 12:406–408, 1980.
110. Smibert RM: *Vibrio fetus* var *intestinalis* isolated from the intestinal content of birds. *Am J Vet Res* 30:1437–1442, 1969.
111. Evans RH, Carey DP: Zoonotic diseases, in Harrison GJ, Harrison LR (eds): *Clinical Avian Medicine and Surgery*. Philadelphia, WB Saunders Co, 1986, pp 537–540.
112. Prescott JF, Bruin-Misch CW: Carriage of *Campylobacter jejuni* in healthy and diarrheic animals. *Am J Vet Res* 42:164–165, 1981.
113. Franco DA: An evaluation of the public health significance of *Campylobacter* sp. as a food borne pathogen: Consideration for prevention and control. Emory University, Atlanta, GA, Masters thesis, 1986.
114. Karmali MA, Fleming PC: *Campylobacter enteritis* in children. *J Pediatr* 94:527–533, 1979.
115. Communicable Disease Control Section, Seattle-King County Department of Public Health: Surveillance of the Flow of *Salmonella* and *Campylobacter* in a Community, August 1984.
116. Kudla J, Nohynkova E: Flagellates of the human intestine and of the intestines of other species, in Krier J (ed): *Parasitic Protozoa*, vol II. New York, Academic Press, 1978, pp 1–138.
117. Fudge A: Avian giardiasis: Syndromes, diagnosis and therapy. *Proc Assoc Avian Vet*:155–164, 1986.
118. Panigraphy B, Elissalde G, Grumbles LC, Hall CF: Giardiasis in parakeets. *Avian Dis* 22:815–818, 1978.
119. Scholtens RG, New JC, Johnson S: Nature and treatment of giardiasis in parakeets. *JAVMA* 180:170–173, 1982.
120. Davies RB, Hibler CP: Animal reservoirs and cross species transmission of *Giardia*, in Jakubowski W, Hoff JC (eds): *Water-Borne Transmission of Giardiasis*. Cincinnati, OH, U.S. Environmental Protection Agency, 1978, pp 104–125.
121. Grant DR, Woo PTK: Comparative studies of *Giardia* spp. in small mammals in southern Ontario: Host specificity and infectivity of stored cysts. *Can J Zool* 56:1360–1366, 1978.
122. Center for Disease Control: Annual summary 1975. *Morbid Mortal Weekly Rep* 24:33, 1976.
123. Center for Disease Control: Annual summary 1976. *Morbid Mortal Weekly Rep* 25:34, 1977.
124. Center for Disease Control: Annual summary 1977. *Morbid Mortal Weekly Rep* 26:39, 1978.
125. Kirkpatrick C, Farrell J: Giardiasis. *Compend Contin Educ Pract Vet* 4:367–376, 1982.
126. Visvesvara GS, Healy GR, Meyer EA: Comparative antigenic analysis of *Giardia* from the human, the cat, and the guinea pig. *J Protozool* 27:38A, 1980.
127. Barlough JE: Canine giardiasis: A review. *J Small Anim Pract* 20:613–623,1979.
128. Wolf MS: Giardiasis: Current concepts in parasitology. *N Engl J Med* 298:319–321, 1978.
129. Finneman HH, Kaplan AP: The association of giardiasis with reduced intestinal secretory immunoglobulin A. *Dig Dis Sci* 17:793–797, 1972.
130. Pitts RP, Twedt DC, Mallie KA: Comparison of duodenal aspiration with fecal flotation for diagnosis of giardiasis in dogs. *JAVMA* 182:1210–1211, 1983.
131. Levine ND: *Giardia lamblia*: Classification, structure, identification, in Jakubowski W, Hoff JC (eds): *Water-borne Transmission of Giardiasis*. Cincinnati, OH, U.S. Environmental Protection Agency, 1979, pp 1–8.
132. Roudebush P, Delivorius MH: Duodenal aspiration via flexible endoscope for diagnosis of giardiasis in a dog. *JAVMA* 187:162–163, 1985.
133. Greene EL: Immunodiagnostic detection of *Giardia* antigen in feces by a rapid visual enzyme-linked immunosorbent assay. *Lancet* 2:691–693, 1985.
134. Vinayak VK, Jain P, Naik SK: Demonstration of antibodies in giardiasis using immunodiffusion technique with *Giardia* cysts as antigen. *Ann Trop Med Parasitol* 72:581–582, 1978.
135. Moon HW, Woodmansee DB: Cryptosporidiosis. *JAVMA* 189:643–646, 1986.
136. O'Donoghue PJ: *Cryptosporidium* infections in man, animals, birds, and fish. *Aust Vet J* 62:253–258, 1985.
137. Kovatch RM, White JD: Cryptosporidiosis in two juvenile Rhesus monkeys. *Vet Pathol* 9:426–440, 1972.
138. Snyder SP, England JJ, Mchesney AE: Cryptosporidiosis in immunodeficient Arabian foals. *Vet Pathol* 15:12–17, 1978.
139. Fletcher OJ, Munnell JF, Page RK: Cryptosporidiosis of the bursa of fabricius in turkeys. *Avian Dis* 19:630, 1975.
140. Hoerr FJ, Ranck FM, Hastings TF: Respiratory cryptosporidiosis in turkeys. *JAVMA* 173:1591–1593, 1978.
141. Tham VL, Kniesberg S, Dixon BR: Cryptosporidiosis in quails. *Avian Pathol* 11:619–626, 1982.
142. Slavin D: *Cryptosporidium meleagridis*. *J Comp Pathol* 65:262–266, 1955.
143. Angus KW: Cryptosporidiosis in man, domestic animals, and birds. A review. *J Royal Soc Med* 76:62–70, 1983.
144. Proctor SJ, Kemp RL: *Crytosporidium anserinium* in a domestic goose from Iowa. *J Protozool* 21:664–666, 1974.
145. Doster AR, Mahaffey EA, McClearen JR: Cryptosporidia in the cloacal coprodeum of red-lored parrots (*Amazona autumalts*). *Avian Dis* 23:654–660, 1979.
146. Barnes JH: Parasites, in Harrison GJ, Harrison LR (eds): *Clinical Avian Medicine and Surgery*. Philadelphia, WB Saunders Co, 1986, pp 472–485.
147. Pohlenz JH, Moon W, Cheville NF, Bemrick WT: Cryptosporidiosis as a probable factor in neonatal diarrhea of calves. *JAVMA* 172:452–457, 1978.
148. Vetterling JM, Jarvis HR, Merrill TG, Sprinz H: *Cryptosporidium wrairi* sp. from the guinea pig, *Cavia porcellus*, with an emendation of the genus. *J Protozool* 18:243–247, 1971.
149. Tzipori S: Cryptosporidiosis in animals and humans. *Microbiol Rev* 47:84–96, 1983.
150. Current WL, Upton SJ, Haynes TB: The life cycle of *Cryptosporidium baileyn* sp. infecting chickens. *J Protozool* 33:289–296, 1986.
151. Kirkpatrick CE: *Cryptosporidium* infection as a cause of calf diarrhea. *Vet Clin North Am [Food Anim Pract]* 1:515–528, 1985.
152. Anderson BC: Quick and easy diagnosis of cryptosporidiosis and Johne's disease. *Vet Med* 80:87–89, 1985.
153. Campbell I, Tzipori S, Hutchinson G, Augus KW: Effect of disinfectants on survival of *Cryptosporidium* oocysts. *Vet Rec* 111:414–415, 1982.
154. Pohjola S: Negative staining method with nigrosin for the detection of cryptosporidial oocysts: A comparative study. *Res Vet Sci* 36:217–219, 1984.

KEY FACTS

- Avian practitioners should be aware of potential zoonoses.
- Most avian zoonotic diseases are easy to prevent.
- Birds may be involved with transmission of influenza, Newcastle disease, viral encephalitis, histoplasmosis, cryptococcosis, and dermatophytosis.

Avian Zoonoses: Proven and Potential Diseases. Part II. Viral, Fungal, and Miscellaneous Diseases

Branson W. Ritchie, DVM
Department of Small
Animal Medicine

David W. Dreesen, DVM, MPVM
Department of Medical
Microbiology

College of Veterinary Medicine
University of Georgia
Athens, Georgia

Veterinary practitioners dealing with avian patients should be aware of the potential zoonotic diseases involved with commonly maintained captive birds. Under the proper conditions, over 200 diseases are transmissible from animals to humans. Birds are known to be directly involved with the transmission of a few of these disease syndromes and may be implicated with others as our knowledge of avian medicine increases. Fortunately, the majority of avian zoonoses are relatively easy to prevent through appropriate sanitation, hygiene, and veterinary care.

Influenza A

Numerous strains of orthomyxovirus cause influenza in humans and animals. Hundreds of strains of influenza have been isolated from wild and domestic birds; however, only influenza A has been definitively associated with natural infections in animals other than humans.[1]

Poultry, turkeys, ducks, terns, finches, parakeets, mynahs, weavers, owlets, bluebirds, orioles, Amazon parrots, pittas, peckers, thrush, tanager, hoopee, and cockatoos have all been shown to be naturally infected with a large variety of influenza A strains and may provide an immense reservoir for viral activity.[1-13] Influenza A was isolated from eight psittacine bird consignments and one finch consignment in 109 groups of birds at a Canadian quarantine station.[2] Virus isolation studies in asymptomatic migratory ducks reported infectivity of 3% to 30%.[3,9] Investigations into the occurrence of influenza in captive birds are limited; however, the potential is great for all avian species to provide a steady flow of viral shifts and to disseminate these new viruses worldwide.[11,14]

Morbidity and mortality associated with influenza infection vary with the species affected. Most avian viral isolates are from asymptomatic birds or those with other disease entities producing clinical signs. A South African episode of substantial tern mortality linked to avian influenza provided a sharp contrast to the usual asymptomatic nature of the disease.[10] Strains of

Originally published in Volume 10, Number 6, June 1988

the virus have been recovered from both the respiratory and gastrointestinal tracts of numerous avian species. Some investigators report viral isolation primarily from the respiratory tract, while others report isolation more commonly from the gastrointestinal tract.[3,9,12] Influenza A is considered stable in the environment and has been shown to persist in duck ponds at 22° C for 4 days and at 0° C for 30 days.[15]

Direct animal-to-human transmission of influenza has been shown to occur but is rare.[16,17] Evidence suggests that birds and swine may provide a reservoir for influenza strains that, either by themselves or following recombination with human strains, may produce influenza pandemics in humans.[3,11,14] Isolates from a 1979 epizootic of influenza in Belgium swine were antigenically related to strains isolated from ducks in North America and Germany.[3] In this outbreak, researchers were unable to determine whether avian influenza was the actual cause of disease or whether the virus isolated was merely a passenger in the infectious process.[11] Before this documentation, it was assumed that a species barrier existed, thus preventing the intraspecies transmission of influenza A.[3] Further studies have indicated that strains of influenza isolated from ducks can infect pigs, and human strains can produce disease in chickens.[11,18] Two avian influenza strains, one from a seal and one from an unknown source, have been isolated from humans.[4] People working with an avian influenza outbreak in seals contracted conjunctivitis and upper respiratory disease.[16] More studies are needed to determine the degree of influenza infectivity in captive birds and the role they may play in human disease.

Diagnosis of influenza in the avian patient is best accomplished by isolation of the virus from tracheal or fecal samples. Testing for antibody formation may be indicated if a bird is known to have been exposed. A group-specific antigen is used in the immunodiffusion test and can be employed for diagnosing avian infections.

Newcastle Disease

Newcastle disease is caused by several pathotypes of paramyxovirus that are worldwide in distribution and that cause disease syndromes in birds that vary from asymptomatic carriers to fulminating fatal septicemias. Manifestations of Newcastle disease depend on host susceptibility, general health of the host, the strain of virus, and the degree of viral exposure.[19,20] The four pathotypes of paramyxovirus responsible for Newcastle disease are lentogenic, mesogenic, neurotropic velogenic, and viscerotropic velogenic.[21] For the purpose of this article, viscerotropic velogenic Newcastle disease will be referred to as *VVND* and all other strains will be referred to as *NDV*. Clinical presentation varies with the infecting pathotype but may include depression, diarrhea, anorexia, ruffled feathers, ocular and nasal discharges, conjunctivitis, dyspnea, ataxia, wing tremors, torticollis, paralysis, muscle tremors, and sudden death.[19]

Newcastle disease is considered to affect primarily gallinaceous species; however, numerous other birds, including pheasants, partridges, quail, owls, pigeons, finches, sparrows, starlings, canaries,[19] pittas, flowerpeckers,[22] toucans, ducks, crows,[23] parakeets, Amazon parrots, half-moon conures, lesser hill mynahs, and black-headed nuns,[24] have exhibited various clinical syndromes caused by the virus. Virtually all families and subfamilies of psittaciformes have been shown to be naturally infected.[25-29] Epidemics of Newcastle disease have been responsible for devastating losses in African parrot populations.[19] In a California study of wild birds, VVND was isolated from 0.04% of free-flying birds, 0.76% of semidomesticated birds, and 1.01% of exotics. NDV was isolated in 0.29% of free-flying birds, 1.65% of semidomesticated birds, and 0.19% of exotic species. Ducks, quail, chukars, pheasant, peafowl, pigeons, and doves were considered to be semidomesticated species.[23]

In pet bird species, NDV or VVND infections typically develop before exportation as a result of association with diseased poultry or asymptomatic carriers of an avirulent pathotype.[19] Controlled studies involving VVND exposure in representative species of several pet bird groups indicated a wide range of susceptibility and virus transmission. Mortality was found to be most severe in conures, while canaries were found to be relatively resistant to disease. Infected canaries, although asymptomatic, did shed virus. Mynahs and black-headed nuns had low morbidity, but mortality in infected birds was high—19% in mynahs, 15% in nuns, and 7% in canaries.[24] Of the species studied, double yellow-headed Amazon parrots, mynahs, and budgerigars were considered to have the greatest ability to transmit disease.[24]

Transmission of Newcastle disease occurs from direct contact with viral particles in aerosolized respiratory exudates or from fecal contamination of food, water, or litter.[19,25] Recovered birds and immune carriers are believed to shed infective virus indefinitely.[25]

Newcastle disease has been isolated from numerous pet bird species, but no reports of transmission to people could be found. In a 1980 outbreak of Newcastle disease in a quarantine station, over 300 shipments of birds went to 33 states and positive avian cases were subsequently isolated in 23 states.[20] Although numerous individuals were exposed to the birds, there were no reports of human cases of Newcastle disease during this outbreak. In human infections, the clinical signs of mild acute granular conjunctivitis, general malaise, and sinusitis usually resolve in 7 to 20 days.[30] Newcastle disease in bird owners may be underreported because of clinical similarities to influenza and uneventful recoveries.

Diagnosis is based on virus isolation from tissue or feces. Demonstration of specific serum antibodies using the hemagglutination inhibition test is diagnostic. This test is also useful in detecting individuals that may be shedding the virus. It is important to note that some birds, particularly budgerigars and columbiformes, may not develop hemagglutination inhibition antibodies after infection.[30] Preventing exposure to Newcastle virus is best done by avoiding psittacines that may have entered the country illegally and obtaining birds only from reliable sources.

Viral Encephalitis

Avian species are known to be important reservoirs for several arthropod-borne viral zoonoses. Eastern equine encephalitis virus and western equine encephalitis virus are the two primary infectious agents responsible for human disease in which birds play a role in viral maintenance. Most outbreaks of both viruses occur in late summer and continue until the first mosquito-killing frost. Disease syndromes appear first in the bird population and then, depending on environmental conditions and virus prevalence, progress to involve humans.[31] People are considered to be an accidental host for both viruses and play no role in the transmission cycle.

Natural or experimental infections with eastern equine encephalitis have been described in 51 native species of birds from Canada, North America, and the Caribbean.[32] Clinical signs associated with avian infections include ataxia, trembling, weakness, paralysis, and death.[31,33] Mortality in birds is generally restricted to non-native avian species, as endemic birds are usually asymptomatic.[34] Clinical infections with this virus have been reported in Chinese ring-necked, Impeyan, Mongolian, and Tragopan pheasants[35]; English sparrows; partridges; quail; ducks[32]; blackbirds; cedar waxwings; cardinals[36]; and whooping cranes.[33] The primary mosquito species acting as the vector of either eastern or western equine encephalitis depends on the geographic location. In the United States and Canada, *Culiseta melanura, Aedes* spp., and *Coquillettidia* spp. commonly transmit the eastern variety. *Culiseta melanura* feeds primarily on birds and rarely attacks humans.[37,38] *Aedes sollicitans* and *A. vexans* may feed on birds and humans but are less readily infected with the virus.[39,40] Bird mites are known to be potential vectors of the virus and thus may provide a means other than mosquitoes for successful transmission.[34]

Western equine encephalitis is less commonly associated with avian infections than is the eastern virus. There have been sporadic reports of western equine encephalitis in partridges,[41] pheasants,[35] and ducks.[42] This disease is primarily transmitted by *Culex tarsalis* in the western United States and Canada and by *Culiseta melanura* in the eastern United States.[43,44]

The fatality rate in symptomatic humans approaches 80% for eastern equine encephalitis and 5% to 15% for western equine encephalitis.[45] For the latter, the virus was isolated in approximately 22% of wild birds examined during a 1962 human outbreak in Saskatchewan. There was a direct correlation between the number of human infections and the prevalence of virus in wild birds.[46] Although these viruses are typically transmitted by mosquitoes, eastern equine encephalitis has been transmitted in pheasants through trauma secondary to pecking.[47] The possibility of human disease resulting from trauma-related transmission of the virus has not been evaluated. Specific isolation studies of encephalomyelitis viruses from commonly maintained pet bird species could not be found.

Rabies

All warm-blooded animals are susceptible to rabies virus. The occurrence of disease, however, is extremely rare in domestic and wild birds if, in fact, it exists at all in nature.[48] In Germany, rabies was reported in 11 chickens, 2 geese, 1 duck, 1 sparrow, 1 owl, 3 hawks, 1 kite, 1 magpie, and 4 buzzards.[49] A serologic study using the passive hemagglutination test on 343 wild birds representing 22 avian species revealed that 23.1% of 65 predatory and 2.9% of 278 nonpredatory birds were seropositive for rabies.[50] A great-horned owl was experimentally infected with rabies by feeding the animal portions of an infected skunk. The bird remained clinically normal and seroconverted 27 days after oral inoculation. The virus was isolated from oral swabs, corneal smears, the brain, and the eyes.[51] Rabies has also been experimentally induced in falcons, hawks, ravens, pigeons, ducks, geese, and peafowl.[49,52-54] Chickens inoculated intracranially with rabies virus rapidly produced central nervous system–bound antibodies.[55]

Various experts state categorically that there has been no bona fide natural cases of rabies in birds—only experimentally induced cases.[a] Birds of the raptorial family may become mechanically involved in the transmission of rabies and, while there have been no documented cases of bird-to-human rabies transmission, one should handle these birds with care. Preexposure rabies prophylaxis may be warranted for individuals who routinely work with such species.

Histoplasmosis

Histoplasma capsulatum is a highly infectious imperfect dimorphous fungus that infects a wide variety of animals and humans and has worldwide distribution.[56] Histoplasmosis in humans is very common, usually benign, and self-limiting. Three typical forms are defined in human medicine: (1) primary pulmonary histoplasmosis, (2) chronic cavitary histoplasmosis, and (3) disseminated or extrapulmonary histoplasmosis. The severity of the pulmonary form depends on the infecting dose and adequacy of immune response.[56,57] All *H. capsulatum* infections can be traced to inhalation of infective spores.[56,58] The fungus proliferates in soil enriched with droppings from gregarious bird species, such as blackbirds, pigeons, and gulls.[56,57]

Contaminated roosting sites have been well documented as a source of human disease.[59,60] Following exposure to the nesting sites of a ring-billed gull colony, 138 people working in the area developed acute pulmonary disease. *Histoplasma capsulatum* was isolated from the nesting site, equipment used in the area, and the sputum of several affected workers.[57] Numerous human infections with *H. capsulatum* were reported over a 22-month period following destruction of a blackbird roost. The degree of illness in this outbreak ranged from asymptomatic to severe respiratory disease.[58] This outbreak indicated that contaminated

[a]Baer GM: Personal communication, Rabies Laboratory, Centers for Disease Control, U.S. Public Health Services, Atlanta, Georgia, 1987.

areas could remain a human health hazard for prolonged periods of time.[58] Studies on isolation of *H. capsulatum* from pet or zoologic aviaries could not be found. The potential for histoplasmosis to grow in any avian housing unit using soil as an enclosure substrate should be considered.

Diagnosis of *H. capsulatum* is best accomplished by fungal isolation from infected tissue or from soil contaminated with feces. Identification of the small yeast cells is simplified by using Giemsa and Wright's stains. Fluorescent antibody techniques may be useful for detecting yeast cells in infected tissue.[56] A positive skin reaction to injected histoplasmin is indicative of fungal sensitization.[56]

Cryptococcosis

Cryptococcus neoformans is a saprophytic yeastlike fungus associated with gelatinous or granulomatous lesions in a number of host species. In birds, *Cryptococcus* has been isolated from intraocular sites, bone marrow,[61] pectoral muscles, neck fascia, meninges,[62] hepatic veins, air sacs, trachea, pararenal areas, and lungs.[63-65] Sheets of myxomatous gelatinous material represent the most consistent type of lesion reported. The clinical presentations in birds vary widely, depending on the site of infection, but generally include depression, weakness, anorexia, weight loss, acute diarrhea, incoordination, blindness, dyspnea, nasal exudates, oral masses, and death.[63,64] Avian species reported with *Cryptococcus* infections include swallows,[64] pigeons, green-winged macaws,[63,65] canaries,[67] Becarris-crowned pigeon,[61] Bartlett's bleeding heart pigeon,[62] thick-billed parrot, African grey parrot,[65] triton cockatoo, and Moluccan cockatoo.[64]

Cryptococcosis infectivity in avian species may be low when compared with mammalian disease. In vitro tests have shown *Cryptococcus* to grow poorly at 40° C, and apparent avian resistance is believed to occur from a higher core body temperature.[63,68] It is theorized that the high percentage of avian cryptococcal infections involving the respiratory tract may be attributable to a lower mean temperature in these tissues.[64] The normal avian bacterial flora has been shown to inhibit the in vitro growth of *C. neoformans*, and a history of antibiotic therapy is often noted in avian patients with cryptococcosis.[64]

Although fulminating cryptococcosis in an otherwise healthy person is rare, human infections resulting from exposure to avian species are well documented.[66,69-73] *Cryptococcus neoformans* is a known health hazard for people exposed to pigeon droppings and has been isolated from the roosts of canaries and psittacines.[66,67,74] A person died from cryptococcal meningitis resistant to flucytosine therapy; the source of infection was traced to dust and debris associated with a swallow nest the man had handled four months previously.[66] Cryptomeningitis in another person was traced to an air conditioner laden with bird excreta.[72] Cryptomeningitis was also reported in three people exposed to the fungus in a bird sanctuary.[70] In still another instance, a primary pulmonary infection with pleural effusion resulted from human exposure to pigeon excreta.[73] In a study in a zoo, *C. neoformans* was isolated in 8 of 13 fecal samples associated with a pigeon roost, in 3 soil samples in the same area, and from the sputum of 1 of 36 employees tested. The person from whom the organism was isolated had a low-grade fever with a productive cough and recovered in approximately two months with no further complications.[69]

Antemortem diagnosis of cryptococcosis is difficult. Finding lesions consisting of typical myxomatous material in the patient is considered a presumptive diagnosis.[75] Positive identification of *C. neoformans* is usually accomplished by wet slide mounts and smears of potentially infected material along with Gram staining to demonstrate the organism. In the avian patient, laparoscopy may prove beneficial in visualizing infected areas with typical lesions. Blood parameters in avian patients are typically normal to slightly leukocytic, and reported serum chemistries have been normal.[63,64] Serum from an infected bird in a breeding aviary had a latex agglutination assay antibody titer of 1:640, while the affected bird's cage mate had no antibody response on paired samples.[64]

Amphotericin B and flucytosine in combination have been shown to be a successful treatment for mammals with cryptococcosis.[76,77] Advanced human cryptococcal infections may be difficult to treat and are often fatal. People suffering from cryptococcal meningitis have a 53% to 58% recovery rate when treated with amphotericin B alone; but when this drug is used in combination with flucytosine, the recovery rate is increased to 68%.[78-80] Successful treatment in avian species has not been described.

Dermatophytes

Pathogenic forms of dermatophytes occur worldwide, affecting a wide range of hosts. The majority of dermatophytes are in the genera *Trichophyton* and *Microsporum*.[81,82] *Trichophyton gallinae, M. gypseum,* and *T. megnini* are the primary dermatophytes that cause disease in avian species.[83,84] Dermatophytes have been isolated from European robins, dunnocks, house sparrows, bluetits, bullfinches,[85] canaries,[86,87] ducks,[81,86] chickens, quail, turkeys, pigeons,[86-89] black grouse,[90] budgerigars,[91] and parrots.[81] Clinical signs in birds include scaly encrustations; alopecia of the head, neck, and breast; hyperkeratosis; pruritus; self-mutilation; and feather plucking.[91,92]

Dermatophytes grow on and into the surface of the stratum corneum, penetrating and parasitizing the keratinous body tissues.[83,84] Lesions in the skin and feather follicles usually occur, with minimal host reaction.[91] Dermatophytosis in birds is considered sporadic and uncommon.[83] Spontaneous recovery usually occurs in the avian patient.

The dermatophytes that affect birds may be transmitted to humans and other animals.[83] A budgerigar owner suffered from swollen, erythematous, round plaques on the hands following exposure to a bird infected with *M. gypseum*.[82] *Trichophyton gallinae* was isolated from a dog and a four-year-old girl exposed to infected pet chickens. The *T. gallinae* that was isolated in these cases produced experimentally induced dermatophytosis in other chickens as well as in guinea pigs.[93]

Diagnosis of dermatophytosis is accomplished by identifying the causative organism by microscopic examination. Skin scrapings and swabs of skin or crushed feather follicles can be treated with sodium hydroxide and stained with Gram's stain or acid-fast stains to facilitate diagnosis. Dermatophytes can also be isolated by culturing infected tissue in Sabouraud's dextrose agar.[91]

Allergies

Allergies caused by exposure to a number of antigens have been documented in humans and animals. In humans, clinical signs associated with allergies to birds include malaise, chills, fever, shortness of breath, myalgia, and coughing.[94,95] These clinical signs are not caused by a bronchial obstruction; rather, they are created by a reduction of vital lung capacity with impairment of alveolar-capillary diffusion.[94,95]

Hypersensitivity pneumonitis and interstitial pneumonia in humans have been associated with exposure to feathers, aerosolized droppings, and serum from pigeons and budgerigars. Part of the allergic clinical response is believed to be caused by exposure to bacterial endotoxins in fecal extracts.[94] Many bird fanciers have been shown to have high titers of precipitating antibodies to fecal and feather extracts obtained from the birds they raise. Seven asymptomatic members of a pigeon club had high precipitating antibodies to pigeon antigens.[94] Human patients suffering from pigeon-induced allergies developed clinical signs following experimental exposure to aerosolized feces, dust, and feathers from pigeons.[94] A budgerigar owner suffered from a recurrent influenzalike illness that occurred every other week. The clinical signs were eventually linked to the biweekly cleaning of bird cages.[95] The sera and droppings of various avian species were found to contain different antigens with limited cross-reactivity between various extracts.[96] Acute clinical signs in pigeon fanciers usually develop four to eight hours after exposure to antigen and recede within 12 hours.[94,96] Sensitivities to budgerigars are usually insidious in onset.[96]

Precipitating antibodies have been shown to regress in patients in a few weeks to several months without further antigen stimulation.[95] After removal of inciting antigens, one allergic pigeon fancier remained asymptomatic for two years and was able to resume raising pigeons with no further complications.[94]

REFERENCES

1. Kaplan MM, Webster RG: The epidemiology of influenza. *Sci Am* 237:88–106, 1977.
2. Rigby CE, Pettit JR, Papp-Vid G, et al: Isolation of salmonella, Newcastle disease virus and other infectious agents from quarantined imported birds in Canada. *Can J Comp Med* 45:366–370, 1981.
3. Pensaert M, Ottis K, Vandeputte J, et al: Evidence for the natural transmission of influenza A virus from wild ducks to swine and its potential importance to man. *Bull WHO* 59:75–78, 1981.
4. Easterday BC: Animal influenza, in Kilbourne ED (ed): *The Influenza Viruses and Influenza*. London, Academic Press, 1975, pp 444–481.
5. Alexandar DJ, Allan WH, Harkness JW, Hall SA: Isolation of influenza virus from psittacines. *Res Vet Sci* 17:125–127,1974.
6. Butterfield WK, Yedloutschnig RJ, Dardiri AH: Isolation and identification of myxoviruses from domestic and exotic avian species. *Avian Dis* 17:155–159, 1973.
7. Slemons RD, Johnson DC, Malone TG: Influenza type A isolated from imported exotic birds. *Avian Dis* 17:458–459, 1973.
8. Slemons RD, Cooper RS, Orsborn JS: Isolation of type A influenza viruses from imported birds. *Avian Dis* 17:746–751, 1973.
9. Slemons RD, Easterday BC: Type A influenza viruses in the feces of migratory waterfowl. *JAVMA* 171:947–948, 1977.
10. Becker WC: Isolation and classification of tern virus: Influenza virus A/tern/South Africa/1961. *J Hyg (Camb)* 64:309–320, 1966.
11. Kaplan MM: The epidemiology of influenza as a zoonosis. *Vet Rec*:395–399, 1982.
12. Bahl AK, Pomeroy BS, Mangundimedjo S, et al: Isolation of type A influenza and Newcastle disease virus from migratory waterfowl in the Mississippi flyway. *JAVMA* 171:949–951, 1977.
13. Lalitha Rao B, Khan FU, Bhat HR, Kadam SS: Zoonotic studies on influenza in pigs and birds, India 1980–81. *Int J Zoonoses* 10:40–44, 1983.
14. Webster RG: On the origin of pandemic influenza viruses, in *Current Topics in Microbiology and Immunology*. Berlin, Springer-Verlag, 1972, pp 72–105.
15. Hinshaw VS, Webster RG, Turner B: Water-borne transmission of influenza A viruses. *Intervirology* 11:66–68, 1979.
16. Webster RG, Geraci J, Petursson G, Skirnisson K: Conjunctivitis in human beings caused by influenza A virus of seals. *N Engl J Med* 304:911, 1981.
17. Beare AS, Kendal AP, Craig JW: Further studies in man of Hsw/N1 influenza viruses. *J Med Virol* 5:33–38, 1980.
18. Ottis K, Bachmann PA: Occurrence of Hsw/N1 subtype influenza A viruses in wild ducks in Europe. *Arch Virol* 63:185–190, 1980.
19. Davis RB, Steiner CV: *Caged Bird Medicine*. Ames, IA, Iowa State University Press, 1981, pp 125–129.
20. Clubb SL, Graham DL: An outbreak of viscerotropic velogenic Newcastle disease in pet birds. *Proc 32nd W Poultry Dis Symp*:105–109, 1981.
21. Hanson RP, Spalatin J, Jacobson GS: The viscerotropic pathotype of Newcastle disease virus. *Avian Dis* 17:354–361, 1973.
22. Hanson RP: Research support for eradication of velogenic viscerotropic Newcastle disease and other diseases. *JAVMA* 163:1094–1096, 1973.
23. Pearson GL, McCann MK: The role of indigenous, wild, semidomestic, and exotic birds in the epizootiology of velogenic viscerotropic Newcastle disease in southern California 1972–1973. *JAVMA* 167:610–614, 1975.
24. Erickson GA, Mure CJ, Beran GW, Carbrey EA: Epizootiologic aspects of viscerotropic velogenic Newcastle disease in six pet bird species. *Am J Vet Res* 39:105–107, 1978.
25. Gerlach H: Viral diseases, in Harrison GJ, Harrison LR (eds): *Clinical Avian Medicine and Surgery*. Philadelphia, WB Saunders Co, 1986, pp 408–433.
26. Cavill JP: Newcastle disease in imported psittacine birds. *Vet Rec* 94:226, 1974.
27. Francis DW: Newcastle and psittacines, 1970–71. *Poult Dig* 32:16, 1973.
28. Scott GR, Winwill AJ: Newcastle disease in the grey parrot. *J Comp Path Ther* 70:115, 1960.
29. Zuydam DM: Isolation of Newcastle disease virus from the osprey and the parakeet. *JAVMA* 120:88, 1952.
30. Evans RH, Carey DP: Zoonotic diseases, in Harrison GJ, Harrison LR (eds): *Clinical Avian Medicine and Surgery*. Philadelphia, WB Saunders Co, 1986, pp 537–540.
31. Hayes RO: Eastern and western encephalitis, in Steele JH (ed): *CRC Handbook Series in Zoonoses*. Ames, IA, Iowa State University Press, 1981, pp 29–57.
32. Dardiri AH, Yates VJ, Chaug PW, et al: The isolation of eastern equine encephalomyelitis virus from brains of sparrows. *JAVMA*

1:409–410, 1957.
33. Dein JF, Carpenter JW, Clark GC, et al: Mortality of captive whooping cranes caused by eastern equine encephalitis virus. *JAVMA* 189:1006–1010, 1986.
34. Herman CM: Bird-borne diseases in man, in Petrak ML (ed): *Diseases of Cage and Aviary Birds*. Philadelphia, Lea & Febiger, 1982, pp 653–657.
35. Faddoul GP, Fellows GW: Clinical manifestations of eastern equine encephalomyelitis in pheasants. *Avian Dis* 9:530, 1965.
36. Cavill JP: Viral diseases, in Petrak ML (ed): *Diseases of Cage and Aviary Birds*. Philadelphia, Lea & Febiger, 1982, pp 515–525.
37. Edman JD, Webber LA, Kale HW: Host feeding patterns of Florida mosquitoes. II. *Culiseta. J Med Entomol* 9:942, 1972.
38. Wallis RC, Howard JJ, Main AJ, et al: An increase of *Culliseta melanura* coinciding with an epizootic of eastern equine encephalitis in Connecticut. *Mosquito News* 34:63, 1974.
39. Crans WJ: The status of *Aedes sollicitans* as an epidemic vector of eastern equine encephalitis in New Jersey. *Mosquito News* 37:85, 1977.
40. Feemster RF, Getting VA: Distribution of the vectors of equine encephalomyelitis in Massachusetts. *Am J Public Health* 31:791, 1941.
41. Ranck FJ Jr, Gainer JH, Hanley JE, Nelson SL: Natural outbreak of eastern and western encephalitis in pen-raised chukars in Florida. *Avian Dis* 9:8, 1965.
42. Burton AN, Connell R, Rempel JG, Gollop JB: Studies in WEE associated with wild ducks in Saskatchewan. *Can J Microbiol* 7:295–302, 1961.
43. Hayes RO, LaMotte LC, Holden P: Ecology of arboviruses in Hale County, Texas, during 1965. *Am J Trop Med Hyg* 16:675, 1967.
44. Chamberlain RW: Arborvirus infections of North America, in Green WH (ed): *Viruses Affecting Man and Animals*. St. Louis, WB Saunders Co, 1971, p 309.
45. Rhodes AJ, Von Rooyen CE: *Textbook of Virology*, ed 4. Baltimore, Williams & Wilkins, 1962, p 300.
46. Burton AN, McLintock JR, Spalatin J, Rempel JG: Western equine encephalitis in Saskatchewan birds and mammals 1962–1963. *Can J Microbiol* 126:133–141, 1966.
47. Herman CM: The role of birds in the epizootiology of eastern encephalitis. *Auk* 79:99–103, 1962.
48. Beran GW: Rabies and infection by rabies related viruses, in Steele JH (ed): *CRC Handbook Series in Zoonoses*. Ames, IA, Iowa State University Press, 1981, pp 75–76.
49. Paarmann E: Ein Beitrag zur lyssa der vogel. *Z Hyg Intcktionskr* 141:103, 1955.
50. Gough PM, Jorgenson RD: Rabies antibodies in sera of wild birds. *J Wildl Dis* 12:392–395, 1976.
51. Jorgenson RD, Gough PM, Graham DL: Experimental rabies in a great horned owl. *J Wildl Dis* 12:144, 1976.
52. Kraus R, Clairmont P: Ueber experimentelle lyssa bei vogein. *Z Hyg Intcktionskr* 34:1–30, 1900.
53. Remlinger P, Bailly J: La rage duc coq. *Ann Inst Pasteur* 43:153–167, 1929.
54. Von Lote J: Beitrage zue kenntnis der experimentelle en lyssa der vogel. *Zentralbl Bakteriol Parasiterık Abt I. Orig* 35:741–744, 1904.
55. Schneider LG, Burtscher H: Unterschugen uber die pathogenese der tollwut bei huhnern nach intercerebraler intektion. *Zentralbl Veterinarmed [B]* 14:598–624, 1967.
56. Ajello L, Kaplan W: Systemic mycoses, in Steele JH (ed): *CRC Handbook Series in Zoonoses*. Ames, IA, Iowa State University Press, 1981, pp 479–481.
57. Waldman RJ, England AC, Tauxe R, et al: A winter outbreak of acute histoplasmosis in northern Michigan. *Am J Epidemiol* 117:68–78, 1983.
58. Latham RH, Kaiser AB, Dupont WD, Dan BB, et al: Chronic pulmonary histoplasmosis following the excavation of a bird roost. *Am J Med* 68:504–508, 1980.
59. Dodge HJ, Ajello L, Engelke OK: The association of a bird-roosting site with infection of school children by *Histoplasma capsulatum. Am J Public Health* 55:1203–1211, 1965.
60. Emmons CW: Histoplasmosis. Animal reservoirs and other sources in nature of the pathogenic fungus *Histoplasma. Am J Public Health* 40:436–440, 1950.
61. Ensley PK, Davis CE, Anderson MP, et al: Cryptococcosis in a male Beccari's crowned pigeon. *JAVMA* 175:992–994, 1974.
62. Griner LA: *Pathology of Zoo Animals*. San Diego, Zoological Society of San Diego, 1983, pp 206–211.
63. Clipsham RC, Britt JO: Disseminated cryptococcosis in a macaw. *JAVMA* 183:1303–1305, 1983.
64. Takeshita K, Fenwick B, Wong A: Cryptococcosis in captive cockatoos. *Proc Assoc Avian Vet*:133–138, 1986.
65. Rosskopf WJ, Woerpel RW: Cryptococcosis in a thick-billed parrot. *Proc Assoc Avian Vet*:281–288, 1984.
66. Glasziou D, McAleer R: Cryptococcosis: An unusual avian source. *Med J Aust* 140:447, 1984.
67. Chute HL: Fungal infections, in Hofstad MS, et al (eds): *Diseases of Poultry*. Ames, IA, Iowa State University Press, 1972, pp 465–466.
68. Klingman AM: Effect of temperature on survival of chick embryos infected intravenously with *C. neoformans. Am J Med Sci* 221:273–278, 1951.
69. Gugnani HC, Gupta NP, Shrivastav JB: Prevalence of *Cryptococcus neoformans* in Delhi Zoological Park and its recovery from the sputum of an employee. *Indian J Med Res* 60:182–185, 1972.
70. Muchmore HC, Rhoades ER, Nix GE, et al: Occurrence of *Cryptococcus neoformans* in the environment of three geographically associated cases of cryptococcal meningitis. *N Engl J Med* 268:1112–1114, 1963.
71. Littman ML, Schneierson SS: *Cryptococcus neoformans* in pigeon excreta in New York City. *Am J Hyg* 69:49–59, 1959.
72. Littman ML: Cryptococcosis (tornlosis): Current concepts and therapy. *Am J Med* 27:976–998, 1959.
73. Procknow JJ, Benfield JR, Rippon JW, et al: Cryptococcosis hepatitis presenting as a surgical emergency. *JAMA* 191:269–274, 1965.
74. Walter J, Coffee E: Distribution and epidemiologic significance of the serotypes of *Cryptococcus neoformans. Am J Epidemiol* 97:167–172, 1968.
75. Anderson WAD: *Pathology*, ed 4. St. Louis, CV Mosby Co, 1961, pp 340–341.
76. Barrett RE, Scott DW: Treatment of feline cryptococcosis: Literature review and case report. *JAAHA* 11:511–518,1975.
77. Prevost E, McKee JM, Crawford P, et al: Successful medical management of severe feline cryptococcosis. *JAAHA* 18:111–114, 1982.
78. Bennett JE: Chemotherapy of systemic mycoses. *N Engl J Med* 290:30–32, 1974.
79. Bennett JE, Dismakes WE, Duma RJ, et al: A comparison of amphotericin B alone and in combination with flucytosine in the treatment of cryptococcal meningitis. *N Engl J Med* 301:126–131, 1979.
80. Firkia FC: Therapy of deep seated fungal infections with 5-fluorocytosine. *N Z Med J* 4:462–467, 1974.
81. Ainsworth GG, Austwick PKC: *Fungal Diseases of Animals*, ed 2, no. 6. Commonwealth Bureau of Animal Health, Farnham Royal, Commonwealth Agricultural Bureaux. Canada, 1973, p 216.
82. Alteras MD, Cojocaru MD: *Microsporum gypseum* infection in the parrot (*Melopsittacus undulatus*). *Mykosen* 13:377–379, 1970.
83. Keymer IF: Mycoses, in Petrak ML (ed): *Diseases of Cage and Aviary Birds*. Philadelphia, Lea & Febiger, 1982, pp 599–605.
84. Padhye AA: Cutaneous mycoses, in Steele JH (ed): *CRC Handbook Series in Zoonoses*. Ames, IA, Iowa State University Press, 1981, pp 441–485.
85. Blackmore DK, Keymer IF: Cutaneous diseases of wild birds in Britain. *Br Birds* 62:316–331, 1969.
86. Beneke ES: Mycotic infections, in Hitcher SB (ed): *Isolation and Identification of Avian Pathogens*. Ithaca, NY, Arnold Printing, 1975, pp 133–141.
87. Kral F: Skin diseases. *Adv Vet Sci* 7:183, 1962.
88. Gierloff BCH, Katac I: Griseofulvin treatment of ringworm in animals. *Nord Vet Med* 13:571, 1981.
89. Carnaghan RBA, et al: Falvus poultry: An outbreak of *Trichophyton gallinae* infection. *Vet Rec* 68:600, 1956.
90. Patiala R: On fungus disease in game. *Paper Game Res* 6:21–22, 1951.
91. Campbell TW: Mycotic diseases, in Harrison GJ, Harrison LR (eds): *Clinical Avian Medicine and Surgery*. Philadelphia, WB Saunders Co, 1986, pp 464–471.
92. Kabayaski GS: Fungi, in Davis BD, et al (eds): *Microbiology Including Immunology and Molecular Genetics*, ed 2. Hagerstown, MD, Harper & Row, 1973, pp 966, 1006.
93. Torres G, Georg LK: A human case of *Trichophyton gallinae* infection. *Arch Dermatol* 74:191–197, 1956.
94. Reed CE, Sosman A, Barbec RA: Pigeon-breeders lung. *JAMA* 193:81–85, 1965.
95. Warren WP: Hypersensitivity pneumonitis due to exposure to budgerigars. *Chest* 62:170–174, 1972.
96. Hargreave FE, Pepys J, Longbottom JL, Wruith DG: Bird breeders (fanciers) lung. *Lancet* 1:446, 1966.

Heavy-Metal Intoxication in Caged Birds—Part I

Richard W. Woerpel, MS, DVM
Walter J. Rosskopf, Jr., BS, DVM

Animal Medical Centre of Lawndale
Hawthorne, California

Heavy-metal intoxication, resulting primarily from the ingestion of lead substances, is surprisingly common among caged birds, but it is often misdiagnosed. This article will familiarize the veterinarian with the clinical features of plumbism and prompt the practitioner to maintain a high index of suspicion for this disease.

This article represents a compilation of 10 cases of heavy-metal intoxication in caged birds that have been diagnosed in the authors' clinic and two cases on which the authors were consulted within the last three years (1979–1982). The study includes eight Amazon parrots (*Amazona* spp.), one African grey parrot (*Psittacus erithacus erithacus*), one green-winged macaw (*Ara chloroptera*), and two cockatiels (*Nymphicus hollandicus*). During the time of this study, one case of probable inhalation lead poisoning in a blue-fronted Amazon parrot (*Amazona aestiva aestiva*) and one case of zinc toxicosis in a green-winged macaw were also treated at the authors' clinic. All except four of the patients discussed are alive and well at this time. One of the deceased parrots suffered heavy-metal toxicosis twice.

In Part I of this article, a literature summary and the results of the authors' survey are presented. This is followed by a discussion of these data. In Part II, the discussion continues, focusing on treatment and pathology, and three case reports are presented.

Literature Summary

Accidental lead poisoning has been reported in the following mammals: dogs,[1-4] cats,[5] cattle,[6,7] horses,[1,6,7] sheep,[6,8] swine,[6,7] mink,[7] primates,[9] and humans.[1,2,10] Among avian species, the most well-known lead poisoning syndrome occurs in waterfowl,[1,7,11-18] resulting from their inadvertent ingestion of spent lead shot from the bottoms of ponds and other waterways in heavily hunted areas. It has been estimated that at least 2 to 3% of the U.S. waterfowl population dies each year from this cause.[13] Consequently, a tremendous amount of research has been carried out to better understand this cause of waterfowl mortality.[11-19]

Much less research has been done on lead poisoning in nonwaterfowl avian species. Locke and Bagley reported on plumbism in mourning doves resulting from the ingestion of spent lead shot taken from the ground in areas of concentrated dove hunting.[20] Plumbism resulting from the ingestion of lead shot that was embedded in the tissues of prey (either captured by raptors in the wild,[21-23] or shot and offered for con-

Originally published in Volume 4, Number 9, September 1982

TABLE I

SOURCES OF INGESTED HEAVY METAL (14 CASES)

Leaded windows (stained glass, etc.)	4
Toy containing lead	2
Toy containing zinc/aluminum alloy	1
Costume jewelry	1
Curtain weight	1
Lead pellet from pellet gun	1
Lead fishing weight	1
Unknown	3

sumption to captive raptors[24,25]) has been documented in raptors by a number of authors.

Comparatively little has been written on the subject of heavy-metal intoxication in captive avian species from causes other than ingestion of lead ammunition. A relatively common cause of lead poisoning among poultry is the consumption of lead-based paint or orchard spray material (containing lead arsenate).[7] Janssen et al. presented a concise summary of lead poisoning in birds.[26] Kennedy et al. provided an account of plumbism in captive sandhill cranes resulting from the ingestion of lead-based paint.[27] Zook et al. reported on a similar occurrence in a zoological collection which caused the demise of 11 psittacines over a 2½-year period.[28] Comparatively few papers have been published on the subject of plumbism in caged (pet) birds.[29-33]

Clinical Cases

To simplify presentation of the information, some of the data has been summarized in tables that appear throughout the text. Results of the case studies are reported under specific headings and a discussion of each topic follows in the next section.

Source of Ingested Heavy Metal

Table I is a list of the sources of ingested heavy metal in the 14 cases (in 13 birds, one poisoned twice) studied. Lead-based paint was not implicated in this study. The lead-containing toy noted in two of the cases involving Amazon parrots was a lead-weighted plastic penguin commonly sold in pet stores.

Clinical Signs

In Table II, the relative frequency of the typical presenting signs is given for 13 heavy-metal intoxication cases studied. It should be noted that this table is based on a retrospective examination of the case records and that a minimum of four veterinarians were involved in the acquisition of the histories and recording of the physical examination findings. In some cases, thorough histories were not received or recorded. Furthermore, the thoroughness of the physical examinations of the patients and interpretation of information received undoubtedly varied between veterinarians.

TABLE II

RELATIVE FREQUENCY OF SALIENT CLINICAL SIGNS (13 CASES)

Depression/lethargy/weakness	8
Vomiting	5
Polyuria and polydipsia	5
Central nervous system signs (incoordination, head tilt, circling, seizures)	4
Hemoglobinuria	4
Diarrhea	2

Radiographic Findings

Of the 13 typical cases of heavy-metal intoxication (one parrot was poisoned twice) included in this study, five had heavy-metal–dense particles located within the ventriculus (gizzard) only at the time of first x-ray; three had similar particles within the ventriculus and intestines; two had heavy-metal–dense particles within the crop and ventriculus; two had similar particles within the ventriculus and cloaca; and one patient had heavy-metal–dense particles within the crop, ventriculus, and cloaca at the time of first x-ray. The dynamics of these particles as they resided in and passed through the gastrointestinal tract of the patients are detailed in Table III.

Clinical Pathology

Hematology and blood chemistry evaluations were conducted on all but one of the cases in this survey. In Table IV, the ranges of values from hemograms of nine Amazon parrots suffering from lead poisoning are listed. This table also provides normal ranges for each test category.

Toxicology

Only one blood lead determination was made. The patient was a yellow-naped Amazon parrot (*Amazona ochrocephala auropalliata*) and its blood lead concentration was reported to be 70 mg/dl. The source of the heavy metal ingested in this case was never determined; therefore, the significance of this value is questionable.

Pathology

Of the four cases of heavy-metal intoxication that did not survive treatment, three were confirmed to be the result of ingestion of lead. In the remaining case, the source and type of heavy metal were never positively determined, although clinical signs and radiography strongly suggested plumbism. A necropsy was performed on this bird, and the histopathological report revealed significant pathology within the spleen only.[34] Severe lymphoid follicular necrosis was noted and attributed to a probable acute viral infection rather than to heavy-

TABLE III

NUMBER OF HEAVY-METAL–DENSE PARTICLES DETECTABLE RADIOGRAPHICALLY

Case	*First X-ray*	*Second X-ray*	*Third X-ray*	*Fourth X-ray*
Amazon 1	15 particles within gizzard	1 particle within gut, 7 days after first x-ray	-	-
Amazon 2	~ 35 particles within gizzard and 5 within gut	1 particle within gut 2 days after first x-ray	-	-
Amazon 3	2 particles within gizzard and 2 within gut	No particles seen 5 days after first x-ray	-	-
Amazon 4	> 50 particles within gizzard	~ 20 particles within gizzard and gut 9 days after first x-ray	3 particles within gut 12 days after first x-ray	No particles seen 14 days after first x-ray
Amazon 5	~ 50 particles within gizzard	~ 20 particles within gizzard 3 days after first x-ray	-	-
Amazon 6	2 large particles within gizzard	Both particles present; no appreciable change in size of either 5 days after first x-ray	Both particles present; each ~ 1/3 original size 16 days after first x-ray	-
Green-winged macaw	1 177-caliber air gun pellet within gizzard	Pellet still present; ~ ½ original size 5 days after first x-ray	-	-
Cockatiel 1	Multiple particles within crop and gizzard	4 particles within gizzard 8 days after first x-ray	-	-
Cockatiel 2	4 particles within gizzard, 1 within proventriculus, and 1 within esophagus	No particles seen 7 days after first x-ray	-	-

metal intoxication. Sections of lung, liver, kidney, and intestine were found to be normal.

The only other necropsy performed, on a case of confirmed plumbism (ingestion of lead costume jewelry), revealed significant renal and hepatic pathology.[35] The kidney revealed granular hemoglobin casts within many convoluted tubules (Figure 1). Many tubular epithelial cells contained pyknotic nuclei and were sloughing into the tubular lumina. Other tubular cells exhibited vacuolar degeneration. Acid-fast stains failed to reveal inclusions within the tubular epithelial cells. The liver exhibited multiple large foci of hepatocellular dissociation and pyknosis, with dropout and necrosis of individual hepatocytes (Figure 2). The brain revealed numerous pale neurons, suggesting degenerative changes. The submitted bone marrow and ventriculus were normal.

TABLE IV

RANGE OF CLINICAL PATHOLOGY VALUES FOR NINE AMAZON PARROTS SUFFERING FROM PLUMBISM

*Test**	*Range of Values*	*Normal Values*[33,40]
WBCs ($\times 10^3/mm^3$)	10.9–30.0	6–11
PCV (%)	31–58	45–55
Total protein (g/dl)	3.0–8.7	3.0–5.0
Glucose (mg/dl)	156–298	220–350
SAST (IU/L)	151–824	130–350
Creatinine (mg/dl)	<0.2–0.8	0.1–0.4
Uric acid (mg/dl)	2.7–18.9	2.0–10.0
Polychromasia	slight to marked	slight
Hemolysis	+ or −	−
Basophilic stippling	−	−

*WBCs = white blood cells; PCV = packed-cell volume; SAST = serum aspartate aminotransferase (formerly SGOT).

Discussion

Source of Ingested Heavy Metal

Of the 13 cases of heavy-metal toxicosis studied, six were presented with the clients' knowledge of the birds' having ingested lead prior to the onset of signs. In these cases, the source of the lead could be confirmed.

Table I indicates that all the known sources of ingested heavy metal (either determined prior to presentation of the patient or subsequently) are commonly found in homes. A pet bird would have access to many of these sources if allowed unsupervised freedom outside its cage or off its perch. The avian practitioner would be well advised when taking a medical history to bear in mind that allowing caged birds such freedom is common among bird owners. Caged birds have a need to chew and an unhealthy affinity toward objects made of lead as well as curiosity about this very soft metal, and frequently lead poisoning is the result. Clients must be warned of this potential problem.

Ingestion of lead paint or lead-impregnated plaster used on cages or on walls of enclosures was not impli-

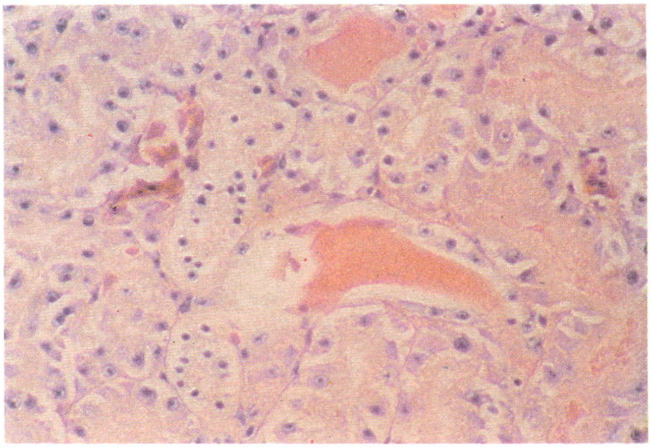

Figure 1—Histopathological appearance of kidney exhibiting granular hemoglobin casts within convoluted tubules and tubular nephrosis. No acid-fast intranuclear inclusion bodies were found within tubular epithelial cells.

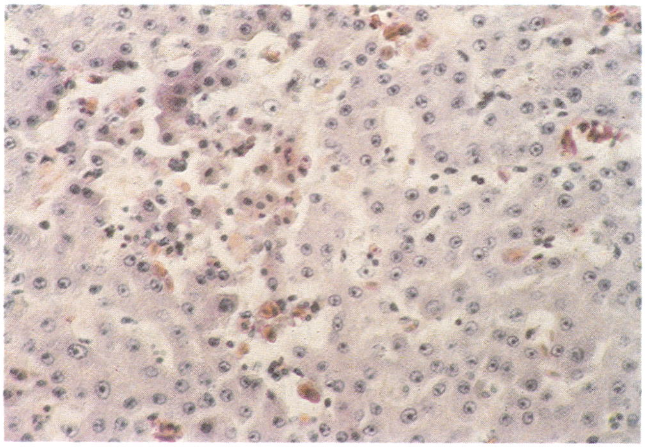

Figure 2—Histopathological appearance of liver exhibiting foci of hepatocellular dissociation and necrosis.

cated in this study, although it has been reported to be a common source of plumbism among captive birds.[27-29,36] The toy penguins implicated in the authors' study are intended for cockatiel-sized or smaller caged birds but often end up as toys for parrots. Buyers must be warned that such toys are potentially hazardous to birds larger than cockatiels, because the labels offer no warning or precautions. It is also important to note that psittacines have been known to chew on and swallow the lead clapper from bells that were suspended in their cages, and this also has resulted in clinical plumbism.[37]

Clinical Signs

The clinical signs result from the absorption of heavy-metal ions from the gastrointestinal tract and their subsequent effects on all tissues. No consistent correlation could be found between the severity of clinical signs and the number of heavy-metal–dense particles subsequently discovered within the gut. Even in cases in which the client knew of heavy-metal ingestion prior to presentation, it was not possible to accurately ascertain the

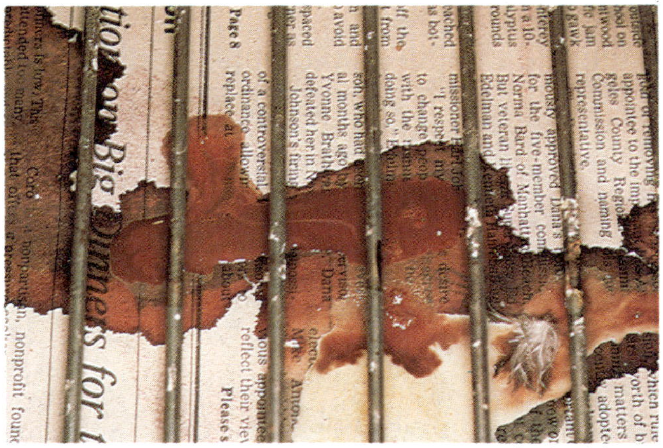

Figure 3—Hemoglobinuria in an Amazon parrot with plumbism.

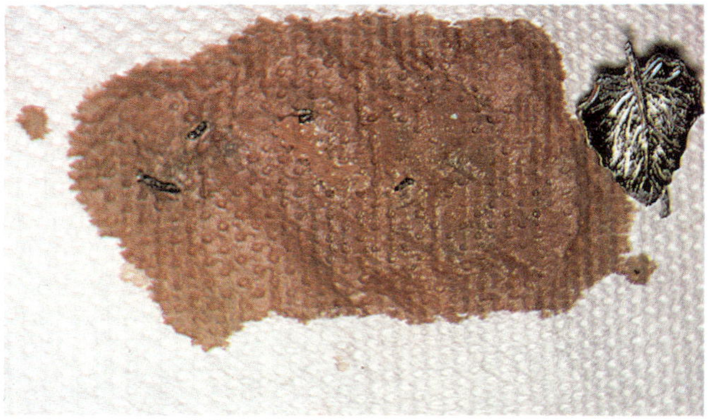

Figure 4—Hemoglobinuria often has a chocolate-milk color. Note the four small bits of relatively normal-appearing feces in the midst of the abnormal urine.

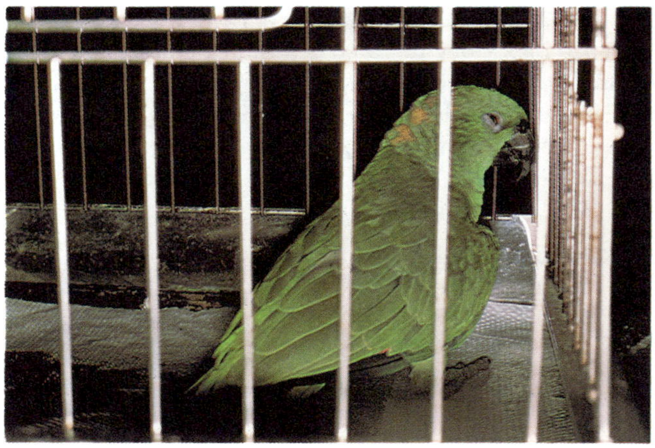

Figure 5—Yellow-naped Amazon parrot suffering from plumbism. Photo was taken within three hours of its death. Note the bird's location on cage bottom, the closed eyes, the depression, and droopy wings.

amount of time elapsed between ingestion of the heavy metal and the onset of clinical signs. In only one case (that of a green-winged macaw ingesting a single lead pellet from a pellet gun[32]) was the illness chronic. That the onset of signs in this case was relatively gradual (one week) may be because only a single lead particle was ingested; usually in cases of plumbism, many small flakes or pieces of lead are ingested. The relative surface area for loss of lead ions into the gut would be proportionately smaller in this single-particle case than that provided in the commoner situation and would result in slower absorption of the metal into systemic circulation.

No single sign or group of signs was consistently noted in this survey. The clinical signs are those suggesting gastrointestinal, renal, and/or neurologic dysfunction. Polyuria and polydipsia and vomiting were more often recorded than the central nervous system signs (incoordination, head tilt, circling, and seizures were the most frequently noted). Diarrhea was an inconsistent clinical sign. This might be due in part to the confusion that often exists in the interpretation of polyuria versus true diarrhea. The hemoglobinuria, which is perhaps the most dramatic of the presenting signs (Figures 3 and 4), was only noted in Amazon parrots. It was usually associated with hemolysis which resulted in red or pink plasma. Most patients exhibited depression, lethargy, or weakness at the time of presentation (Figure 5).

The presence of any one of these clinical signs and the order in which it was exhibited in relation to others is related no doubt to a number of factors: the type and amount of heavy metal ingested; the size of the particle(s) ingested; the length of time the heavy metal was within the gut; the coexistence of grit within the ventriculus, which would hasten the mechanical breakdown of the metal; and the preexisting health status of the animal.

Giddings reported rapid onset of anorexia, depression, incoordination (inability to perch), loose droppings ("contained small amount of blood") in a mature double yellow-headed Amazon parrot (*A. ochrocephala oratrix*) suffering from plumbism.[30] Zook et al., in a retrospective study, reported on the clinical signs of 11 psittacines that perished from lead poisoning in a large zoological park collection over a 2½-year period.[28] Six of these parrots were found dead in their cages; two exhibited seizure activity; two were unable to fly and exhibited ataxia; and one exhibited only lethargy prior to death. Janssen et al., in a concise summary of lead poisoning in captive birds, indicated that the signs were often inconclusive, including nonspecific gastrointestinal and neurological signs (seizures, incoordination, alimentary stasis, and behavioral changes).[26] They also reported other commonly noted signs: anorexia, green diarrhea, weakness, and wing droop. The latter clinical sign was noted in one sandhill crane (*Grus canadensis*) suffering from lead poisoning secondary to the ingestion of lead-based paint.[27] The wings of this bird drooped from the carpal joint because of extensor muscle paralysis. This has also been noted in poultry[7] and waterfowl[12] and is considered analogous to wrist drop in humans suffering from plumbism. Droopy wings (Figure 5) were noted in a number of patients in this study, but this sign was attributed to the stressed and debilitated condition of the patients. This posture is typical of seriously ill birds, especially just prior to death.

Watery green or lime-green feces have been reported in birds of prey,[22,23] waterfowl,[12,15,18] and poultry[7] suffering from lead poisoning. Often, green, bile staining of the vent feathers is mentioned, especially in waterfowl prior to death or at necropsy. Diarrhea was not a consistent clinical sign in the authors' study. One cockatiel exhibited chartreuse vent feathers but the diarrhea produced by this bird was light brown.

Regurgitation was mentioned only once in the literature as a specific clinical sign of plumbism in caged birds.[29] Redig et al. noted vomiting in a female prairie falcon (*Falco mexicanus*) fed shotgun-killed ducks and pheasants.[22] In the authors' survey, this clinical sign was frequently but not consistently noted.

Polydipsia was another frequently but not consistently noted clinical sign of plumbism in the authors' study. Their literature search found polydipsia associated with plumbism mentioned only in regard to poultry.[7] It is possible, however, that the watery or loose droppings so often reported as diarrhea were really a reflection of polyuria, which would most likely be accompanied by an obligatory polydipsia.

Neurologic signs were noted in many of the avian species in which plumbism has been reported. Ataxia, amaurosis, and epileptiform seizures were noted in the aforementioned female prairie falcon.[21] Petrak included the same three signs in her report of lead poisoning in caged birds.[29] Jacobson et al. noted incoordination and a head tilt in an immature bald eagle (*Haliaeetus leucocephalus*) suffering from lead poisoning which resulted from the bird's ingestion of hunter-wounded prey.[23] Decker et al. reported ataxia and apparent incoordination in an adult male king vulture (*Sarcohampus papa*) that died of plumbism.[25] It is possible that the incoordination noted in these accounts was at least in part a manifestation of weakness in the patient. Nevertheless, the authors' study and that of Zook et al.[28] clearly indicate that neurologic signs (especially central nervous system signs) are common among psittacines suffering from lead poisoning.

Nowhere in the literature was hemoglobinuria mentioned as a clinical sign of lead poisoning. It was noted in only 4 of the authors' 13 cases; all of these involved Amazon parrots, and in most cases the hemoglobinuria was associated with hemolysis. Blackwell reported hemoglobinuria in a ewe suffering from chronic lead toxicosis but indicated that it is not a commonly observed sign in this disease of sheep.[8]

In summary, the avian practitioner should include lead poisoning in the differential diagnosis when the clinical signs of the patient include one or more of the following: vomiting, diarrhea, polyuria and polydipsia, hemoglobinuria, central nervous system signs, generalized depression, and weakness.

Radiographic Findings

Of the 13 typical clinical cases of heavy-metal intoxication, only six of the patients were presented with the owner's knowing that the bird had *ingested* heavy metal. In each of these cases, the existence of heavy-metal particles within the gastrointestinal tract of the patient was subsequently confirmed radiographically. Of the other cases, the presence of heavy metal within the gut was confirmed radiographically because the history suggested the possibility of plumbism (in three cases); other diagnostic tests performed previously had not elucidated the cause of the signs and x-rays were therefore undertaken (in two cases); radiography was included as part of the routine data base on the patient upon presentation (in one case); or heavy-metal intoxication was suspected after the patient's death (in one case).

In every case, radiography was done, and this revealed a variable number of heavy-metal–dense particles within the gut. It should be emphasized that the presence of such particles confirmed on x-ray does not confirm the diagnosis of lead poisoning; it only suggests the possibility of heavy-metal intoxication. A thorough history, a determination of the concentration of lead in the blood of the patient, and the retrieval and analysis of the radiopaque material are methods that can be used to confirm the diagnosis of plumbism (or other heavy-metal poisoning).

In Table III the dynamics of these particles in and as they pass through the gastrointestinal tract of the patient are detailed. In each case, subsequent radiographs revealed a definite decrease in the number or the size of the heavy-metal–dense particles within the gut, regardless of the amount of time that had elapsed between the radiographs. No correlation could be made between these dynamic changes and the existence of grit within the ventriculus. However, the presence of grit within the ventriculus along with the heavy metal would hasten the latter's mechanical degradation and subsequent passage out of the patient. Subsequent radiographs in some of the cases revealed heavy-metal–dense particles within the intestines when prior radiographs had indicated that the particles were within the ventriculus. This suggests that the particles are passed out of the patient prior to their complete degradation and dissolution by the action of the gizzard and intestinal fluids. In none of the cases could heavy-metal fragments be found within the droppings.

The cases involving the ingestion of a few relatively large, discrete heavy-metal particles (Amazon parrot 6) and the ingestion of a single lead pellet (green-winged macaw) reveal several interesting points. These larger particles do not tend to move out of the ventriculus, as do the smaller fragments, but they do undergo a visible reduction in size (no doubt resulting from mechanical degradation and absorption) with time. This information strongly suggests that surgical intervention (ventriculotomy)[23] may be more expedient in the management of certain heavy-metal toxicosis cases than a medical approach (to be discussed in Part II of this article).

Clinical Pathology

The important features in Table IV are the leukocytosis, hemolysis, regenerative anemia, absence of basophilic stippling of erythrocytes, evidence of renal compromise (elevations of both creatinine and uric acid), and serum aspartate aminotransferase (SAST, or SGOT) elevation, suggesting hepatic toxicity. The leukocytosis and the regenerative anemia were the most consistent hematologic findings.

No basophilic stippling of erythrocytes was noted by the laboratory, even in cases where lead ingestion by the patient was known when the blood sample was submitted and examination of the blood films for this morphologic peculiarity was requested. Basophilic stippling has been noted in the blood smears of puppies and cats suffering from plumbism.[2,3,5,38] Zook et al. found this to be a nearly consistent finding in their study of plumbism in 60 puppies.[2] They concluded that the appearance of large numbers of immature (especially nucleated) RBCs and basophilic stippling of erythrocytes with a normal or slightly lowered hematocrit is nearly pathognomonic of lead poisoning in the dog. In contrast, Knecht et al., in their more recent investigation of the same subject, did not find basophilic stippling of erythrocytes and circulating nucleated RBCs to be common.[3] Janssen et al. reported that a lowered hematocrit and basophilic stippling of RBCs are indicative of lead intoxication in birds.[26] However, the authors could find only one reference to this morphologic peculiarity, and it was regarding wild ducks afflicted with lead poisoning.[11] Therefore it seems that the practitioner should not depend on this finding to aid in the diagnosis of plumbism in caged birds.

Anticoagulants such as EDTA and potassium oxalate lessen the appearance of basophilic stippling in canine erythrocytes.[4,38] All blood smears taken from the avian patients in this study were made from blood as it flowed directly from a clipped toenail.[39]

The blood of at least two of the patients in this study exhibited hemolysis. More consistent findings included a mild to moderate decrease in the hematocrit and marked polychromasia. No abnormally shaped RBCs were noted, as has been reported elsewhere.[12]

The observed elevations in the SAST and the creatinine and uric acid values (although not consistent) probably reflect toxic damage to the liver and kidneys, respectively, of the affected caged birds. These elevated values are not diagnostic of plumbism by themselves but are contributory when the history, physical examination, radiographic evidence, and the other hematologic parameters of the patient are evaluated.

Toxicology

Determination of blood lead concentration and the toxicologic analysis of tissues for lead in a caged bird at necropsy are usually economically prohibitive in clinical practice. The former determination was once more difficult because of the relatively large volume of blood needed for the assay. However, this constraint is much less of a problem now because there are laboratories (human or otherwise) that can run this assay using as little as 20 μl of plasma.

Janssen et al. indicated that lead poisoning was most reliably diagnosed by determination of blood lead concentration and noted that values ranging from 146 mg/dl to 378 mg/dl have been reported.[26,27] Zook et al. reported a whole-blood lead concentration of 40 mg/dl in an ataxic kea parrot (*Nestor notabilis*) that was suspected to have ingested lead-based paint.[28] No other hematologic abnormalities in this patient were noted.

It is the authors' opinion that if heavy-metal densities are discovered on radiographs of a patient exhibiting signs consistent with heavy-metal toxicosis and the history provided does not reveal the source or identity of the metal, the initiation of chelation therapy should have precedence over the collection of blood for blood lead concentration determination. This clinical approach is justified in situations where economics dictates a conservative workup. The treatment program will not harm the patient and will usually render it asymptomatic by the time the toxicology results are reported.

If blood is to be collected for this toxicologic test, hematology, and blood chemistry, it must be done prior to the onset of chelation therapy. However, this may not be possible because of the stress imposed on the already debilitated patient during the blood collection procedure. The empirical treatment program should therefore take precedence.

REFERENCES

1. Smith HA, Jones TC, Hunt RD: *Veterinary Pathology*. Philadelphia, Lea & Febiger, 1972, pp 956-961.
2. Zook BC, Carpenter JL, Leeds EB: Lead poisoning in dogs. *JAVMA* 155:1329-1342, 1969.
3. Knecht CD, Crabtree J, Katherman A: Clinical, clinicopathologic, and electroencephalographic features of lead poisoning in dogs. *JAVMA* 175(2):196-201, 1979.
4. Kowalcyzk DF: Lead poisoning in dogs at the University of Pennsylvania Veterinary Hospital. *JAVMA* 168:428-432, 1976.
5. Jacobs G: Lead poisoning in a cat. *JAVMA* 179(12):1396-1397, 1981.
6. Blood DC, Henderson JA: *Veterinary Medicine*, ed 4. Baltimore, The Williams & Wilkins Co, 1974, pp 784-789.
7. Siegmund OH (ed): *The Merck Veterinary Manual*, ed 4. Rahway, NJ, Merck and Co, Inc, 1973, pp 935; 1087.
8. Blackwell JG: Chronic lead poisoning (chronic plumbism) in a ewe. *VM SAC* 72(12):1879-1882, 1977.
9. Martin DP: Primates, in Fowler ME (ed): *Zoo and Wild Animal Medicine*. Philadelphia, WB Saunders Co, 1978, p 547.
10. Beyers RK: Lead poisoning. *Pediatrics* 23:585-603, 1959.
11. Johns FM: A study of punctate stippling as found in the lead poisoning of wild ducks. *J Lab Clin Med* 19:514-517, 1934.
12. Coburn DR, Metzler DW, Treichler R: A study of absorption and retention of lead in wild waterfowl in relation to clinical evidence of lead poisoning. *J Wildl Mgmt* 15:186-192, 1951.
13. Bellrose F: Lead poisoning as a mortality factor in waterfowl populations. *Bull IL Nat Hist Surv* 27:235-288, 1959.
14. Rosen MN, Bankowski RA: A diagnostic technique and treatment for lead poisoning in swans. *Cal Fish Game* 46:81-90, 1960.
15. Trainer DO, Hunt RA: Lead poisoning of whistling swans in Wisconsin. *Avian Dis* 9:252-264, 1965.
16. Locke LN, Bagley GE, Irby HD: Acid-fast intranuclear inclusion bodies in the kidneys of mallards fed lead shot. *Bull Wildl Dis Assoc* 2:127-131, 1966.
17. Bagley GE, Locke LN: Lead poisoning in Canada geese in Delaware. *Avian Dis* 11:601-608, 1967.
18. Humphreys P: Noninfectious diseases, in Fowler ME: *Zoo and Wild Animal Medicine*. Philadelphia, WB Saunders Co, 1978, p 204.
19. Grandy JW, Locke LN, Bagley GE: Relative toxicity of lead and five proposed substitute shot types to pen-reared mallards. *J Wildl Mgmt* 32:483-488, 1968.
20. Locke LN, Bagley GE: Lead poisoning in a sample of Maryland mourning doves. *J Wildl Mgmt* 31:515-518, 1967.
21. Bagley GE, Locke LN: The occurrence of lead in tissues of wild birds. *Bull Environ Contam Toxicol* 2:297-305, 1967.
22. Redig PT, Stowe CM, Barnes DM, Arent TD: Lead toxicosis in raptors. *JAVMA* 177(9):941-943, 1980.
23. Jacobson E, Carpenter JW, Meliton N: Suspected lead toxicosis in a bald eagle. *JAVMA* 171:952-954, 1977.
24. Locke LN, Bagley GE, Frickie DN, Young LT: Lead poisoning and aspergillosis in an Andean condor. *JAVMA* 155:1052-1056, 1969.
25. Decker RA, McDermid AM, Prideaux JW: Lead poisoning in two captive king vultures. *JAVMA* 175(9):1009, 1979.
26. Janssen DL, Robinson PT, Ensley PK: Lead poisoning in birds. *JAVMA* 178(2):150, 1981.
27. Kennedy S, Crisler JP, Smith E, Bush M: Lead poisoning in sandhill cranes. *JAVMA* 171(9):955-958, 1977.
28. Zook BC, Sauer RM, Garner FM: Lead poisoning in captive wild animals. *J Wildl Dis* 8(3):264-272, 1972.
29. Petrak ML: Digestive system disturbances in cage birds (lead poisoning). *Vet Clin North Am* 3(2):196-197, 1973.
30. Giddings RF: Lead poisoning in a parrot. *VM SAC* 75(6):1015-1016, 1980.
31. Rosskopf WJ Jr, Woerpel RW: Lead poisoning in a cockatiel. *Mod Vet Pract* 63(1):46-48, 1982.
32. Rosskopf WJ Jr, Woerpel RW: Removal of a lead pellet by gizzard-otomy (ventriculotomy) in a green-winged macaw. *VM SAC* 77(6):969-974, 1982.
33. Fudge AM: Clinical findings in an Amazon parrot with suspected lead toxicosis. *Calif Vet* 36(5):23-25, 1982.
34. *Case Record #96564*. Downey, CA, Section of Comparative Pathology, Los Angeles County Dept of Health Services.
35. *Case Record #91075*. Downey, CA, Section of Comparative Pathology, Los Angeles County Dept of Health Services.
36. Petrak ML (ed): *Diseases of Cage and Aviary Birds*. Philadelphia, Lea and Febiger, 1969, p 500.
37. Burke TJ: Personal communication, University of Illinois, 1977.
38. Zook BC, McConnell G, Gilmore CE: Basophilic stippling of erythrocytes in dogs with special reference to lead poisoning. *JAVMA* 157:2092-2099, 1970.
39. Woerpel RW, Rosskopf WJ Jr: Avian handling techniques: Part II. *Anim Health Tech* 3(2):81-86, 1982.
40. Rosskopf WJ Jr, Woerpel RW, Van De Water D, Rosskopf G: Normal hematologic and blood chemistry values for commonly kept pet avian species. *VM SAC*, in press.

Heavy-Metal Intoxication in Caged Birds—Part II

Richard W. Woerpel, MS, DVM
Walter J. Rosskopf, Jr., BS, DVM

Animal Medical Centre of Lawndale
Hawthorne, California

Heavy-metal intoxication is common among caged birds, but it is frequently not diagnosed. Part I of this article summarized the existing literature on the subject and presented an in-depth discussion of lead toxicosis in caged birds, focusing on the sources, clinical signs, radiographic findings, clinical pathology, and toxicology of lead poisoning. In Part II, treatment and pathology are discussed, and three case reports are presented.

Treatment

Petrak has described the use of calcium ethylenediaminetetraacetic acid (Ca EDTA) for treating plumbism in caged birds.[1] Intramuscular injections of 20 to 45 mg/kg were given two to three times daily. The drug was mixed in normal saline or 5% dextrose solution prior to administration. Giddings reported using calcium disodium edetate[a] to treat an Amazon parrot for lead poisoning at a dose of 110 mg/kg in two and later three divided doses daily for four days.[2] The drug was initially given intravenously (diluted 1:2 with 5% dextrose solution) and later intramuscularly (diluted 1:4 with 5% dextrose solution). Janssen et al. used a dose of 35 mg/kg of Ca EDTA, given intramuscularly twice daily for five days for treatment of plumbism in birds.[3] This same dosage was used by Kennedy et al. in treating sandhill cranes suffering from lead poisoning.[4]

In treating caged birds suffering from plumbism, the authors have used calcium disodium edetate[b] dosages between 35 and 50 mg/kg given by intramuscular injection three times daily for five to seven days.[5-7] They do not dilute the drug before administering it intramuscularly and have had no problems. They have found, as did the authors mentioned above, the therapeutic response to be dramatic. Often the prominent clinical signs disappear within the first 24 to 48 hours of treatment. No side effects have been seen from using this drug as often as three times daily by intramuscular injection. The authors have also sent home patients on double their injectable dose of Ca EDTA to be given directly per os three times daily (in lieu of injections). This latter therapeutic method has kept patients asymptomatic during the time that heavy metal is being cleared from their gastrointestinal tracts. In addition to

[a]Havidote®, Haver-Lockhart, Shawnee, KS 66201.
[b]Calcium Disodium Versenate®, Riker Laboratories, Inc., Northridge, CA 91324.

Originally published in Volume 4, Number 10, October 1982

Ca EDTA, the authors also routinely use parenteral ampicillin[c] prophylactically twice daily and injections every other day of stanozolol[d] to stimulate erythropoiesis, in addition to routine supportive care (e.g., force-feeding and fluids).

Some authors have used a noninvasive suction technique to aspirate heavy-metal particles from the stomach or gizzard of an afflicted bird in lieu of gastrotomy or ventriculotomy.[8,9] The authors have performed both cropotomy[10] and ventriculotomy[6] procedures in the treatment of lead-poisoned caged birds, in addition to medical therapy with Ca EDTA.

When radiography reveals heavy-metal particles within the crop of the patient, a cropotomy must be performed to prevent their inevitable movement into the ventriculus. However, the authors recommend that general anesthesia *not* be used for this procedure because of the potential risks to the patient. With the use of only physical restraint, the procedure is simple, quick, and not dependent on the total relaxation of general anesthesia for its success.[10]

One of the authors' cases involved an African grey parrot. The client knew the bird had recently ingested lead from a leaded window. Survey radiographs revealed numerous heavy-metal–dense particles within the crop and gizzard (Figure 1). Because of the large number of particles within the crop destined to become sequestered within the gizzard and result in systemic absorption of lead, and because the bird was exhibiting signs of plumbism, a cropotomy was elected. The patient was given 15 mg of intramuscular ketamine, and the surgery (Figure 2) resulted in successful removal of all the lead fragments. Unfortunately, the parrot never recovered from the anesthetic. Retrospectively, if faced with the same clinical circumstances, the authors would definitely elect to perform a cropotomy. They would, however, use only physical restraint and not take the risks of general anesthesia.

The decision to perform a cropotomy should be made as soon as possible after radiography has confirmed the presence of heavy-metal particles within the crop of a patient showing signs of intoxication. Chelation therapy may be initiated prior to the surgery, but surgery cannot

[c]Polyflex™, Bristol Laboratories, Syracuse, NY 13201.
[d]Winstrol®-V, Winthrop Laboratories, New York, NY 10016.

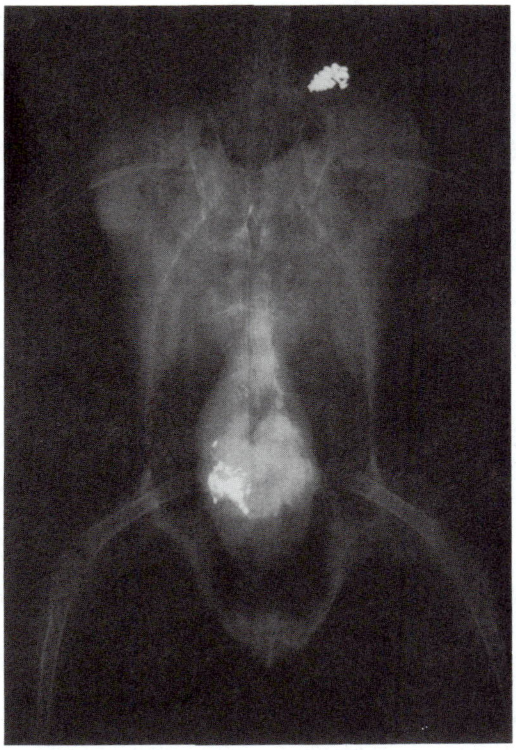

Figure 1—Radiograph of an African grey parrot suffering from clinical plumbism. Note heavy-metal–dense particles within the crop and gizzard.

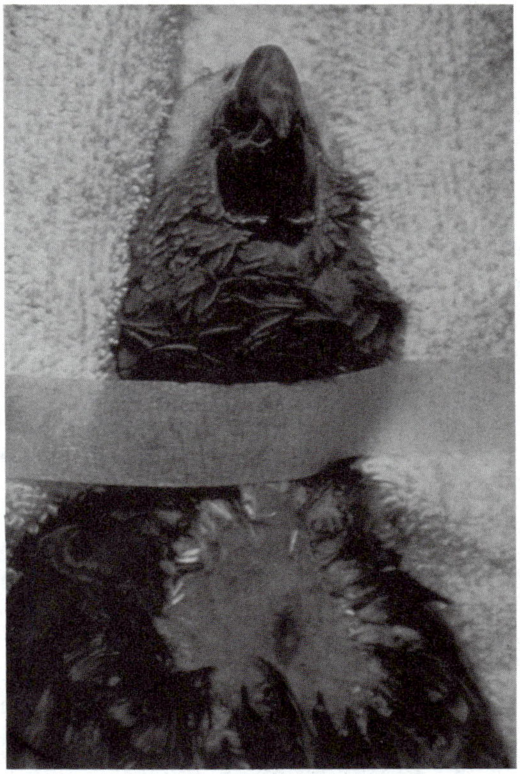

Figure 2—African grey parrot (shown in Figure 1) under ketamine anesthesia during cropotomy to retrieve lead particles.

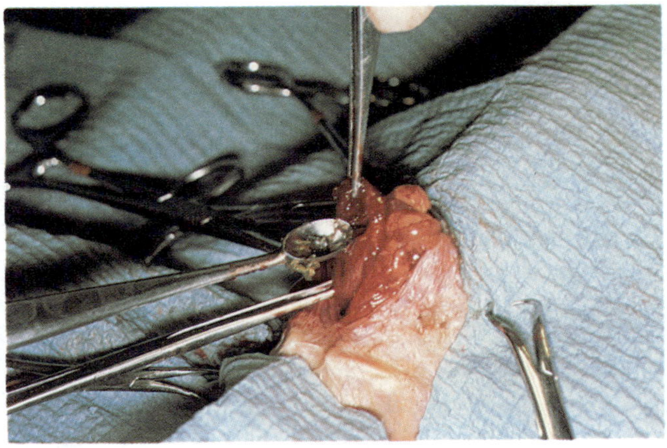

Figure 3—Ventriculotomy performed on a green-winged macaw. Note the lead pellet (from 177-caliber airgun) in the surgical spoon.

be delayed to await a clinical response. The decision to perform a ventriculotomy for retrieval of one or more heavy-metal particles (Figure 3), on the other hand, need not be as hasty. The patient probably should be receiving chelation therapy and should be asymptomatic before this procedure is attempted. The authors have performed only one ventriculotomy for this purpose, and it was successful.[6] They attribute their success to the stability of the patient, achieved by prior treatment with Ca EDTA.

Pathology

Zook et al. estimated the incidence of plumbism in psittacines necropsied at the National Zoological Park from January 1969 to May 1971 to be 50%.[11] This figure was based on the presence of multiple acid-fast, intranuclear inclusion bodies within proximal tubular epithelial cells of the kidney or within hepatocytes. These inclusion bodies within the kidney and/or the liver are specific for lead-poisoned mammals and are thought to function in the storage of lead.[12] Many other authors have reported their presence within the kidney in relation to lead-poisoned avian species.[13-19] It should be noted, however, that nearly an equal number of investigators (including the authors) have not found these inclusion bodies upon histopathologic examination of the kidney and/or liver using acid-fast stains.[4,9,20-22] Locke et al. reported that the amount of lead absorbed, the period of exposure, and the diet of the individual affected the occurrence of intranuclear inclusion bodies;[14] other unknown factors also probably influence the presence or absence of intranuclear inclusion bodies within the tissues.

Few other authors have reported the existence of hemoglobin casts within the renal tubules,[19] but a number have noted evidence within the liver of hemolysis (e.g., hemosiderin).[4,18,21,22] These same authors also noted definite evidence of hepatocellular degeneration and/or necrosis. None mentioned the existence of any pathology involving the tissues of the central nervous system.

Very little has been written regarding the pathological changes (both gross and microscopic) that accompany plumbism in psittacines. This is in part because the disease, when properly diagnosed, is treatable, and when it is not diagnosed antemortem, there are few lesions (without the use of special stains) that suggest plumbism to the pathologist.

The discovery within the gizzard or elsewhere in the gastrointestinal tract of one or more heavy-metal fragments that could be analyzed for lead content would be the most rewarding finding at necropsy on a lead-poisoned psittacine. No other gross findings should be expected. Interestingly, many investigators have noted in the tissues of lead-poisoned poultry, waterfowl, or raptors one or more of the following gross findings: gross distention of the gallbladder;[18-23] emaciation;[18-20,23] eroded mucosa of gizzard (stomach)[8,21] with bright green staining of its contents;[8,21,23] atrophy of liver and/or heart;[19,20,23] increased amount of pericardial fluid;[18,21,23] and impaction of the proventriculus.[8,21] It should be noted that a gallbladder is lacking in the budgerigar and in some species of parrots,[24] and therefore, gross distention of the gallbladder is rarely seen in caged birds. It should also be noted that in all cases the gross lesions mentioned were the result of chronic plumbism. Psittacine species, in contrast, seem to manifest clinical signs within a relatively short time following the ingestion of a critical amount of heavy metal. Therefore, these lesions would be rarely encountered during the necropsy of a parrot that succumbed to lead poisoning.

Case Report 1

A red-lored Amazon parrot (*Amazona autumnalis autumnalis*) of unknown age and sex was presented to the authors' clinic on 4/7/79 with a history of lead ingestion. The bird had apparently broken the plastic covering of a toy penguin and eaten some of its lead core. The client did not know how long the bird had been ingesting the lead.

Physical examination revealed a well-muscled bird with pronounced central nervous system signs (head tilt, torticollis, and incoordination) that was unable to perch. A blood sample was collected for hematology and chemical evaluation, and survey radiographs were obtained (Amazon 4 of Table III in Part I of this article). The latter revealed more than 50 heavy-metal–dense particles within the gizzard. The patient was immediately given 10 mg intramuscular Ca EDTA, 25 mg intramuscular ampicillin, and 0.5 mg intramuscular dexamethasone. The patient was hospitalized for the next four days, during which time it received 10 mg Ca EDTA three times daily, 30 mg ampicillin once daily, and parenteral B vitamins

The blood test results revealed only an elevated creatinine value. All other parameters were within normal limits. Throughout its stay in the hospital, the patient exhibited only slight improvement. The central nervous system signs and weakness continued. Hospitalization was terminated for financial reasons. The parrot was released on Ca EDTA to be given orally at 20 mg three times daily. On 4/13 the client indicated that the bird's general condition was not improved and that it was manifesting definite signs of blindness. The owner was instructed to continue the medication as previously directed. The patient was reexamined on 4/16. At that time the parrot was clinically normal. Radiography of the patient revealed approximately 20 particles of lead within the gizzard and gut. The owner was instructed to continue the oral Ca EDTA. The bird remained clinically normal and was reradiographed on 4/19. The x-rays revealed only three lead particles within the gut. The owner was told to stop the chelation therapy and present the parrot for final radiography on 4/21. On this date the radiographs revealed no heavy metal. The bird made a complete recovery.

This case is reported because it is typical of those seen in private practice and because it demonstrates the relative severity of the central nervous system signs sometimes seen with plumbism and the response of the patient to specific chelation therapy (even when it is administered orally).

Case Report 2

On 5/30/81, an 11-year-old blue-fronted Amazon parrot (*A. aestiva aestiva*) of unknown sex was presented with acute onset of signs that were suggestive of plumbism. The owner had noted chocolate-milk–colored droppings that morning. She indicated that the bird had suffered lead intoxication approximately 10 years previous to this visit. When questioned about the current possibility of plumbism and the availability of lead within the parrot's environment (the owner admitted that the bird was allowed substantial freedom from its cage), the owner stated that her husband frequently prepared and loaded ammunition within the house.

Physical examination of the patient revealed obvious hemoglobinuria (see Figure 3 in Part I) and a weak, stressed parrot of 375 g body weight. Survey radiographs and blood for hematology and chemical evaluation were obtained. The radiographs revealed no heavy-metal–dense fragments of any kind within the bird. Whole blood was collected in heparinized microhematocrit tubes and centrifuged, and the packed-cell volume (PCV) (23%) was recorded. It was noted that the plasma was clear and red (hemolysis). The anemia and hemolysis and presenting signs continued to suggest lead toxicosis as the likely diagnosis. The owner was again questioned regarding the possibility of the parrot's past or present exposure to heavy metal. She then mentioned that her husband had melted lead #2 alloy on the stove in the kitchen of the home on each of two days prior to 5/30 and had done so many times before. The bird had been in the living room, and her husband usually carried out this procedure with the kitchen ventilation fan on and the windows open. She was vague as to whether these two precautions had been taken this last time and mentioned the presence of smoke in the house. The tentative diagnosis was plumbism secondary to inhalation of the heavy metal.

Upon hospitalization the patient was given intramuscular injections of 30 mg ampicillin, 10 mg Ca EDTA, 12.5 mg stanozolol, 0.4 mg dexamethasone, and 1.0 mg vitamin K.[c] During its four-day stay, the parrot received 25 mg ampicillin twice daily, 20 mg Ca EDTA twice or three times daily, and every-other-day injections of 1.0 mg vitamin K and 12.5 mg stanozolol.

On the day following hospitalization, the droppings were nearly normal (Figure 4) and the bird seemed a little stronger. The blood test results were obtained on the following day and revealed no basophilic stippling, a mild leukocytosis with a heterophilia and basophilia, slight thrombocytopenia (qualitative assessment), elevated total protein, and normal values for serum aspartate aminotransferase (SAST, or SGOT) and creatinine. On each successive day of hospitalization the patient grew stronger and more aggressive. There was no hemoglobinuria noted after the day of presentation. A PCV performed on 6/2/81 (three days postpresentation) was 21% with no evidence of hemolysis. This was not considered a decrease in red cell mass because the first PCV and total protein value obtained on 5/31 were probably falsely elevated as a result of dehydration of the patient.

The patient was released on 6/3/81 and was not returned one week later as requested for a recheck. One year later it was alive and well with no repeat of similar signs. The husband continues to melt lead tape in the home, but the parrot is placed outdoors during this procedure.

This case is of particular interest because the history, physical examination, and clinical pathology results strongly suggested plumbism, but radiography could not confirm the expected presence of heavy metal within the gut of the patient. The tentative diagnosis of inhalation plumbism was never confirmed but remains the most plausible explanation for the clinical signs and dramatic response to treatment. Plumbism has been reported in horses as a result of their frequent exposure to fumes from lead smelters, and in other domestic animals as a result of exposure to fumes from burning storage batteries or from cutaneous absorption of gasoline containing tetra-ethyl lead.[12,23] Cotter reported on an inhalation lead intoxication syndrome in humans which resulted from chronic exposure of welders to fumes from the burning of lead-painted surfaces.[25]

Case Report 3

This case report involves zinc toxicosis in a seven-year-old green-winged macaw (sex unknown). This disorder resulted from the bird's ingestion of a zinc-aluminum alloy, the source of which was later determined to be a toy.

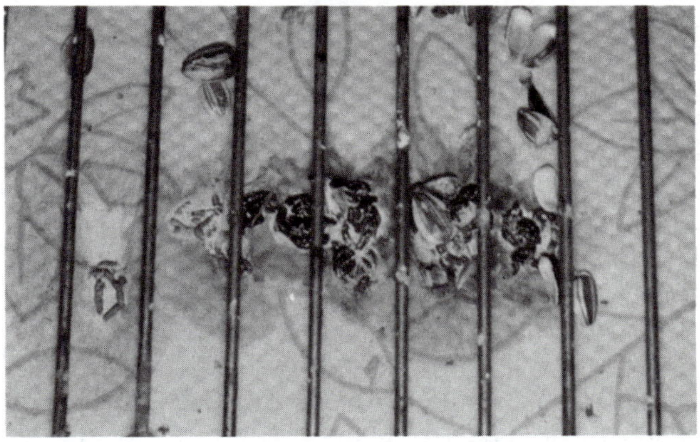

Figure 4—Droppings from a blue-fronted Amazon parrot with probable inhalation plumbism one day after presentation. The droppings from this bird on the day of presentation are shown in Figure 3 of Part I of this article.

[c] AquaMEPHYTON®, Merck Sharp & Dohme, West Point, PA 19486.

The macaw was first presented on 1/5/81 because of a relatively sudden onset of lethargy, vomiting, and diarrhea. The physical exam was unremarkable (weight—1245 g). Blood was collected for clinical pathology (hematology and chemical evaluation), and the bird was sent home on 50 mg ampicillin to be given intramuscularly once a day for seven days. The blood examination revealed only leukocytosis with heterophilia and eosinophilia. The patient was returned for a progress check on 1/12/81, at which time the owner indicated that the bird was nearly 100% normal. A blood sample collected at this time revealed that the white blood cell (WBC) count had fallen into the high normal range, with complete disappearance of monocytes and eosinophils from the differential count.

The bird was normal until 6/3/81 at which time it was presented to the authors' clinic because of anorexia, diarrhea, and a change in color of the feces. Physical examination was unremarkable (weight—1245 g). A blood sample (hematology only) was taken and the bird was sent home on parenteral ampicillin, as before, for one week. The WBC and differential counts were essentially normal. On 6/5 the bird was not doing well and had started to vomit. The macaw was reexamined on 6/10. Its weight had fallen to 1103 g and its droppings revealed green feces without form and yellow urine and urates. Another blood sample (hematology and chemical evaluation) was collected. All values were within normal limits.

The macaw continued to do poorly at home and the owner agreed to hospitalize the bird on 6/12. During its 10-day period of hospitalization the patient received parenteral antibiotics, antiemetic medication,[f] vitamins (B complex and A, D, and E[g]), and anabolic steroids (stanozolol), in addition to aggressive force-feeding. Blood examination (hematology and chemical evaluation) done on 6/16 indicated severe leukocytosis (WBC = 35,000 to 40,000/mm^3) with many toxic heterophils, with extreme elevations in both SAST (1426 IU/L) and lactate dehydrogenase (LDH) (2498 IU/L) values, suggesting severe hepatitis (probable toxic cause).

The patient continued to lose weight (on 6/19 it weighed 996 g) and exhibit intermittent vomiting and continuous diarrhea. On 6/19 the macaw was x-rayed. The radiographs revealed approximately 25 particles of heavy-metal–dense material of varying sizes, all of which appeared to be within the gizzard. The bird was started on parenteral Ca EDTA at 25 mg three times daily. A blood lead concentration determination was not done. The patient's weight and overall condition continued to decline in spite of chelation therapy and the aggressive supportive care outlined above. A blood sample (hematology and chemical evaluation) taken on 6/22 revealed a high normal WBC count with heterophilia and monocytosis and a rising SAST value (2218 IU/L).

[f]Centrine®, Bristol Laboratories, Syracuse, NY 13201.
[g]Injacom®, Roche Chemical Div., Nutley, NJ 07110.

The bird was allowed to go home on 6/22 for a short stay; the authors hoped that a more familiar environment would stimulate its appetite. No medications were sent home with the patient. On 6/24, the macaw was returned in an extremely weakened condition. Its weight had dropped to 827 g and its droppings still reflected yellow brown urates and diarrhea. Radiographs taken on this day revealed a slight decrease in the total number of particles and not all were located within the gizzard. Chelation therapy and supportive care (including force-feedings three times daily) were reinstituted and 1 mg parenteral dexamethasone was given additionally for the next three days.

On 6/26 the bird began to show mild improvement and began to gain weight. The patient was released on 6/27. No medication was sent home with the bird. It continued to exhibit gradual and steady improvement each day. The client returned the bird on 7/3, at which time it weighed 999 g. Radiography revealed no more heavy metal within the gut. Blood examination (hematology and chemical evaluation) revealed a normal WBC and differential and a nearly normal SAST (422 IU/L) value.

This green-winged macaw made a complete recovery and regained its original weight (1210 g) by 7/11/82. The owner had the toy analyzed by a private laboratory (98.8% zinc; 1.2% aluminum).

This case is noteworthy because it involves an atypical heavy-metal intoxication, where the source of the metal was zinc rather than lead. The course of the illness was chronic, which is unlike plumbism cases treated by the authors. It is impossible to ascertain just how long the zinc-aluminum particles had been in the gut. The history and clinical signs suggest that they may have been present in the bird prior to the first complaint of gastrointestinal signs on 1/5/81. They remained within the gut for a substantial period of time, probably because of their relatively large size.

The major clinical signs in this case were those of gastroenteritis. It is not known whether these signs were primary or secondary to the hepatic involvement. The salient clinical pathologic findings were leukocytosis with heterophilia and evidence of hepatic involvement (grossly elevated SAST and LDH values). The cause of the hepatitis was undoubtedly toxic.

It is interesting that this case was comparatively refractory to Ca EDTA treatment. The patient did not exhibit the rapid, dramatic improvement characteristic of lead-poisoned patients receiving chelation therapy and did not seem to benefit from it. The authors are still unsure of what caused the course of the bird's illness to reverse itself on 6/26. The mass of heavy metal within the bird had been gradually decreasing and it is possible that the amount remaining dropped below the critical level necessary to cause clinical illness.

Nevertheless, this case clearly demonstrates how aggressive supportive care and frequent monitoring of the patient (e.g., weight and hematologic parameters) can result in the successful resolution of very serious disease problems in caged birds. This bird would surely have perished without this attentive nursing care.

REFERENCES

1. Petrak ML: Digestive system disturbances in cage birds (lead poisoning). *Vet Clin North Am* 3(2):196-197, 1973.
2. Giddings RF: Lead poisoning in a parrot. *VM SAC* 75(6):1015-1016, 1980.
3. Janssen DL, Robinson PT, Ensley PK: Lead poisoning in birds. *JAVMA* 178(2):150, 1981.
4. Kennedy S, Crisler JP, Smith E, Bush M: Lead poisoning in sandhill cranes. *JAVMA* 171(9):955-958, 1977.
5. Rosskopf WJ Jr, Woerpel RW: Lead poisoning in a cockatiel. *Mod Vet Pract* 63(1):46-48, 1982.
6. Rosskopf WJ Jr, Woerpel RW: Removal of a lead pellet by gizzardotomy (ventriculotomy) in a green-winged macaw. *VM SAC* 77(6):969-974, 1982.
7. Woerpel RW, Kosskopf WJ Jr: Avian therapeutics. *Mod Vet Pract* 62(12):947-949, 1981.
8. Humphreys P: Noninfectious diseases, in Fowler ME: *Zoo and Wild Animal Medicine*. Philadelphia, WB Saunders Co, 1978, p 204.
9. Redig PT, Stowe CM, Barnes DM, Arent TD: Lead toxicosis in raptors. *JAVMA* 177(9):941-943, 1980.
10. Rosskopf WJ Jr, Woerpel RW, Pitts BJ: Cropotomy in a parrot. *Mod Vet Pract* 63(3):219-222, 1982.
11. Zook BC, Sauer RM, Garner FM: Lead poisoning in captive wild animals. *J Wildl Dis* 8(3):264-272, 1972.
12. Smith HA, Jones TC, Hunt RD: *Veterinary Pathology*. Philadelphia, Lea & Febiger, 1972, pp 956-961.
13. Bellrose F: Lead poisoning as a mortality factor in waterfowl populations. *Bull IL Nat Hist Surv* 27:235-288, 1959.
14. Locke LN, Bagley GE, Irby HD: Acid-fast intranuclear inclusion bodies in the kidneys of mallards fed lead shot. *Bull Wildl Dis Assoc* 2:127-131, 1966.
15. Bagley GE, Locke LN: Lead poisoning in Canada geese in Delaware. *Avian Dis* 11:601-608, 1967.
16. Grandy JW, Locke LN, Bagley GE: Relative toxicity of lead and five proposed substitute shot types to pen-reared mallards. *J Wildl Mgmt* 32:483-488, 1968.
17. Locke LN, Bagley GE: Lead poisoning in a sample of Maryland mourning doves. *J Wildl Mgmt* 31:515-518, 1967.
18. Locke LN, Bagley GE, Frickie DN, Young LT: Lead poisoning and aspergillosis in an Andean condor. *JAVMA* 155:1052-1056, 1969.
19. Decker RA, McDermid AM, Prideaux JW: Lead poisoning in two captive king vultures. *JAVMA* 175(9):1009, 1979.
20. Coburn DR, Metzler DW, Treichler R: A study of absorption and retention of lead in wild waterfowl in relation to clinical evidence of lead poisoning. *J Wildl Mgmt* 15:186-192, 1951.
21. Trainer DO, Hunt RA: Lead poisoning of whistling swans in Wisconsin. *Avian Dis* 9:252-264, 1965.
22. Jacobson E, Carpenter JW, Meliton N: Suspected lead toxicosis in a bald eagle. *JAVMA* 171:952-954, 1977.
23. Siegmund OH (ed): *The Merck Veterinary Manual*, ed 4. Rahway, NJ, Merck and Co, Inc, 1973, pp 935; 1087.
24. Petrak ML (ed): *Diseases of Cage and Aviary Birds*. Philadelphia, Lea & Febiger, 1969, pp 82; 115.
25. Cotter LH: Lead intoxication by inhalation. *J Ind Hyg Toxicol* 28:44-46, 1946.

Clinical Manifestations of Cervicocephalic Air Sacs of Psittacines

Michael T. Walsh, DVM
Department of Special Clinical Sciences

Maron Calderwood Mays, VMD, PhD
Department of Comparative and Experimental Pathology

College of Veterinary Medicine
University of Florida
Gainesville, Florida

An increase in ownership of psittacine birds as companion animals has led to much interest in improving their medical care. Upper respiratory tract problems, such as rhinitis, rhinorrhea, and sinusitis, are common reasons for presentation to the veterinarian. Psittacines have features of the upper respiratory system that may be overlooked. For example, the cervicocephalic air sacs of psittacines are not recognized by many veterinarians, and there are clinical problems associated with this portion of the upper respiratory system that are important in managing upper respiratory diseases.

Regional Anatomy of the Upper Respiratory System

Some terms that are used in reference to the upper respiratory system and the relationship of the nasal cavities to the sinuses are reviewed in Table I.

The two major divisions of the upper respiratory system in birds are the rhinal cavities and the infraorbital sinuses. In many species, air from the external nares first encounters the operculum protruding just inside the cere. It then travels down the rhinal cavity, which is sometimes tubular in shape, past the chonchae. The chonchae, by projecting into the passageway, give the rhinal cavity a greater surface area, which allows the cavity to act as a site for heat exchange, heat conservation, olfaction, filtration of airborne debris, and water conservation.

The right and left nasal cavities are separated by a nasal septum. They communicate at the choanae, which in turn communicate with the glottis of the trachea. The lateral walls of the rhinal cavities separate them from the sinus cavities.

The infraorbital sinus (paranasal sinus) is a fairly spacious cavity located laterally to the nasal area and rostroventrad to the eyes. The lateral borders of the sinus are the facial musculature, though there are portions caudad to the upper beak that are fairly superficial. These are the most commonly noted sites of swellings in extreme cases of sinusitis. Many diverticula of the infraorbital sinus from the main body surround the eye. Figure 1 shows the extent of this sinus in the head of a conure that has been injected with latex. Portions of the sinus may extend into the upper beak and mandible and may communicate with extensive pneumatized sections of the skull. Through small openings in its medial

Originally published in Volume 6, Number 9, September 1984

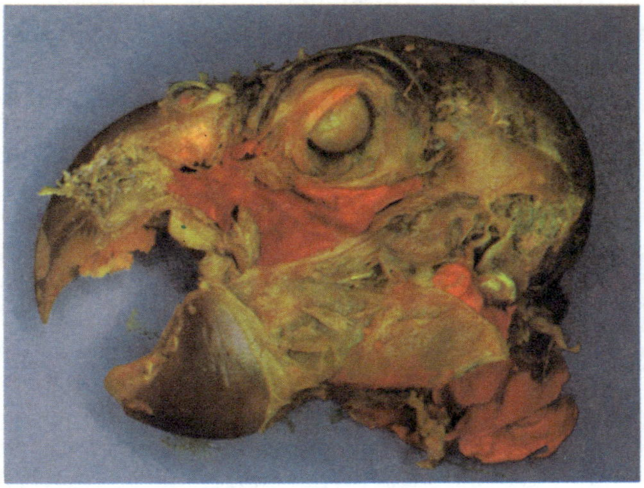

Figure 1A

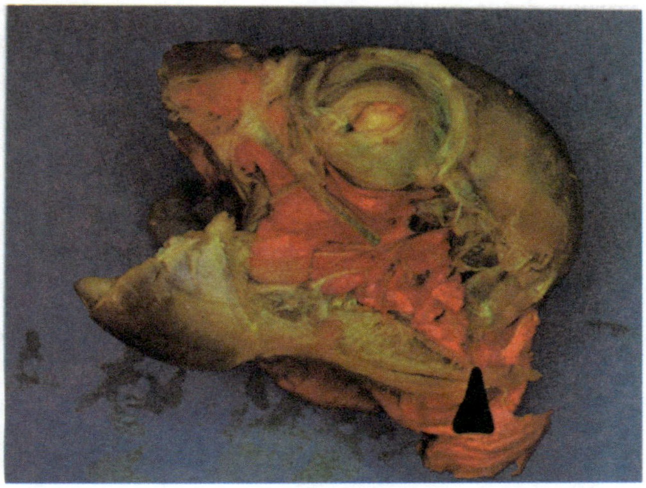

Figure 1B

Figure 1—(**A**) The skin has been removed on the head of this conure after latex injection of the infraorbital sinus. The red area at the commissure of the oral cavity is a common site of swelling associated with sinusitis. (**B**) The facial musculature and portions of the upper and lower beaks have been removed to show the extent of the infraorbital sinus cranially into the beak and caudally, exiting at the tympanic area (*arrow*) to communicate with the cervicocephalic system.

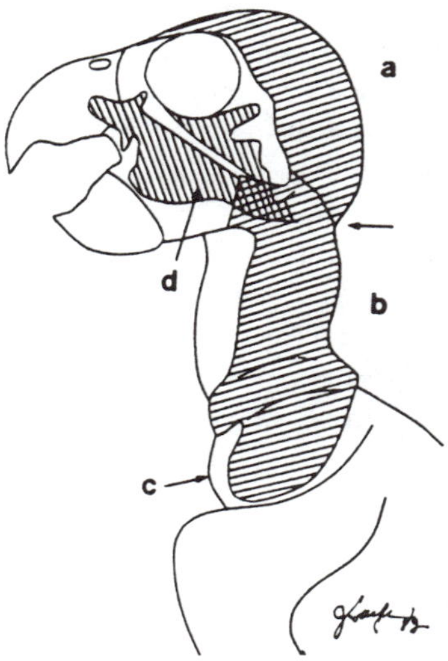

Figure 2A

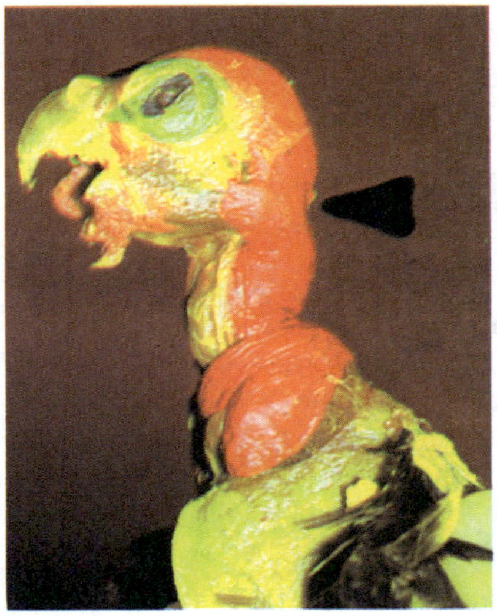

Figure 2B

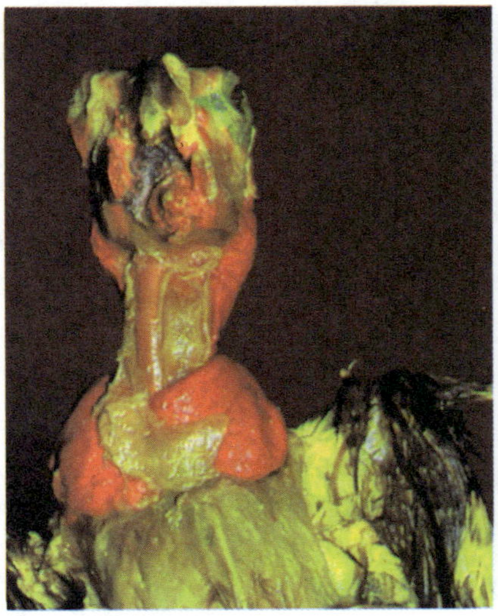

Figure 2C

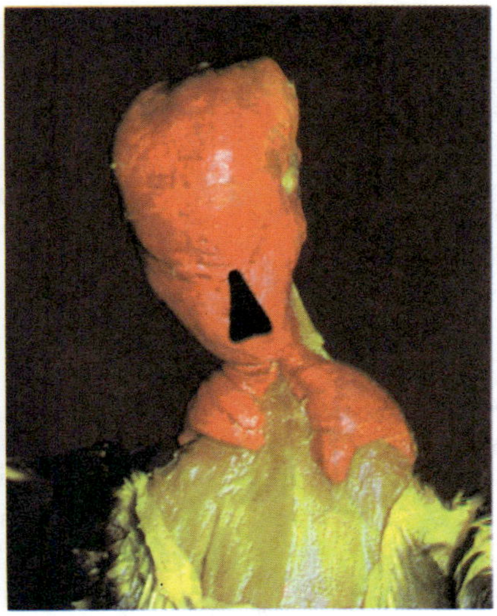

Figure 2D

Figure 2—(**A** through **D**) Illustration of the relationship of the sinus to the cerviocephalic air sacs. (**A**) *Unlettered arrow* indicates the division between the cephalic portion (*a*) and the cervical portion (*b*). *c* = crop; *d* = infraorbital sinus. The caudal aspect of the infraorbital sinus connects to the cerviocephalic air sacs. (**B**) Lateral view of a cockatiel. The cerviocephalic air sacs have been injected with red latex, and the skin is removed. Note the caplike cephalic portion over the head and the distal extent of the cervical portion to the shoulders. The *arrowhead* denotes the division between the cervical and cephalic portions. (**C**) Anterior view of the cockatiel in **B**. Note the latex filling the air sacs that surround the crop. (**D**) Posterior view of the cockatiel in **B** and **C**. *Arrowhead* indicates the point of division between the cervical and cephalic portions.

TABLE I
Some Anatomic and Pathologic Terms Relating to the Upper Respiratory System

Air sacculitis	Inflammation of the air sacs
Cere	Area surrounding the external nares; in psittacines, often ovoid and consisting of raised keratinized tissue
Choanae	Slit-like opening in the maxillary portion of the pharynx (internal nares)
Chonchae	Bony scroll-like protrusions (usually 2 to 3) into the rhinal area; consist of epithelial-lined tissue
Infundibular cleft (sphenopalatine cleft)	Small oval opening, located posterior to the choanae; connects the pharynx to the infraorbital sinus
Operculum	Flat rounded bony protrusion into the area of the external nasal opening
Rhinitis	Inflammation of the mucous membranes of the nasal passages
Rhinopathy	Any disease of the nasal passages
Rhinorrhea	Free discharge of a thin nasal mucus
Sinusitis	Inflammation of a sinus; may be acute or chronic, purulent or nonpurulent

wall, the infraorbital sinus also communicates with the corresponding nasal cavity. Ventrally, the sinus is in contact with the oral pharyngeal area through the infundibular slit. Caudally, the sinus communicates through channels in the tympanic area with the cervicocephalic air sac system, as shown by the arrow in Figure 1B.

Avian Air Sac Systems

The term *air sac* is usually used in reference to the pulmonary air sac system in birds. William Harvey gave the first detailed description of the air sacs in 1651, and it has been said that Aristotle knew of them 2000 years before. In fact there are three systems of air sacs: the pulmonary system, the pharyngeal tracheal system, and the cervicocephalic system.

The pulmonary system is the most familiar. It is widely recognized that there are nine air sacs present in the adult psittacine. The embryonic fusion of one pair forms the clavicular sac,[1] and the remainder are the cervical,[2] anterior thoracic,[2] posterior thoracic,[2] and abdominal air sacs.[2]

The pharyngeal tracheal system is used mainly in courtship in some species. This system consists of saclike diverticula that extend from the oral cavity or trachea and are inflated during display behaviors, such as those seen in the frigate bird *(Fragata magnificens)*.

The third system, the cervicocephalic air system, was first well described by Bignon in 1889. Though present in at least six avian orders, the system is absent in diving birds, such as penguins and grebes. Ratites (emu, rhea), pigeons, and chickens have only a partially developed cervicocephalic system. This system is most extensively developed in strong flyers (e.g., stork, albatross) and in birds with large heads and beaks (psittacines). Within the psittacine family there is a great deal of variability in the sacular development.

There are two main divisions of the cervicocephalic system: a cranial cephalic portion and a cervical, or neck, portion. As seen in Figure 2A (arrow), the system is connected by bilateral channels that travel below the ear to the infraorbital sinuses. The relationship is best visualized by injecting latex into the system through the infundibular cleft, to fill the sinuses and then the cervicocephalic system. The cephalic portion is extensive in some species, such as the conures and parakeets. This caplike portion (Figures 2A through C) is connected to the cervical portion by a small median communication. The cephalic portion of the system may extend from the occipital region to just caudad to the cere rostrally and dorsad to the eyes laterally. The cervical portion, which originates in the tympanic area, extends in two columns bilaterally down the neck to rest in a saddlelike fashion over the shoulders (Figure 2D). In some species, e.g., macaws, there may be discrete communications between the two columns at various intervals. The crop is flanked on each side by the distal cervical portions. When viewed externally, the inflated air cells appear nearly to encase the vertebral column. This development is extensive in parakeets, cockatiels, conures, amazons, macaws, and some members of the cockatoo family.

Histology of the Cervicocephalic Air Sac

In amazon parrots, the epithelial lining of the lateral wall of the cervical air sac is apparent histologically (Figure 3). These cervical air sacs are thin-walled extensions of the upper respiratory system and are completely lined by a single layer of very low cuboidal or flat squamous cells. Beneath the epithelial lining of the air sac is a thin layer of loosely arranged collagen and elastic fibers, which attaches the walls of the air sacs to adjacent tissues. Because the cervicocephalic air sacs are not used for oxygen exchange, the vasculature beneath the epithelial lining is not prominent.

Clinical Implications

Because of the direct connection between the cervicocephalic air sacs and the infraorbital sinuses, diseases can involve both the sinuses and the cervicocephalic air sac system. Many clinicians are not aware of the existence

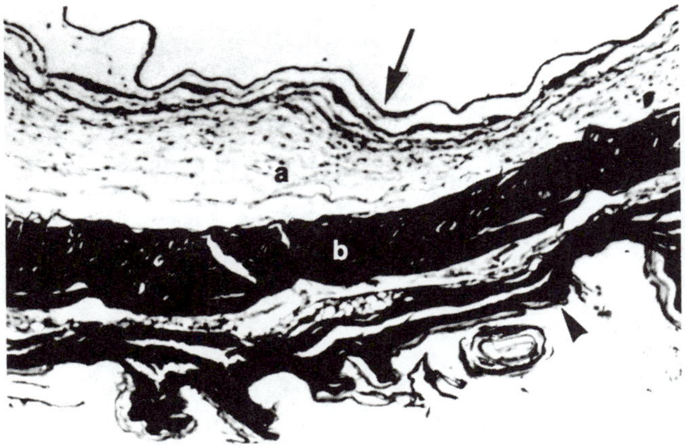

Figure 3—Histologically, the lining of a cervicocephalic air sac is a single layer of flattened cells (*arrow*). Underlying the sac are layers of loose connective tissue (*a*), skeletal muscle (*b*), and the skin of the neck (*arrowhead*). (H&E, ×56)

of the cervicocephalic air sacs, thus they may be overlooked in examination of a bird with a respiratory problem.

Three case histories are presented to illustrate problems that involve the cervicocephalic air sacs.

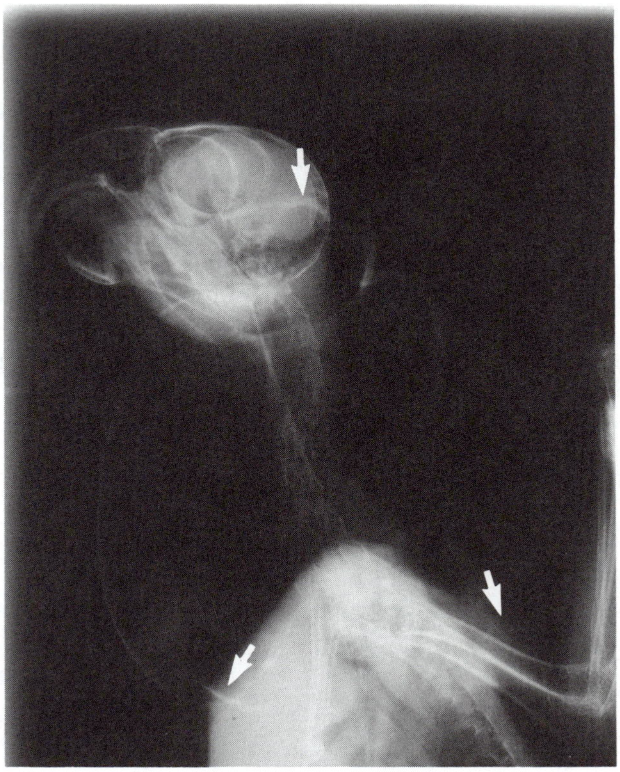

Figure 4B

Case 1

A 12-year-old amazon parrot presented with an eight-month history of having "an enlarged neck area" (Figure 4A). The problem had been previously diagnosed as a

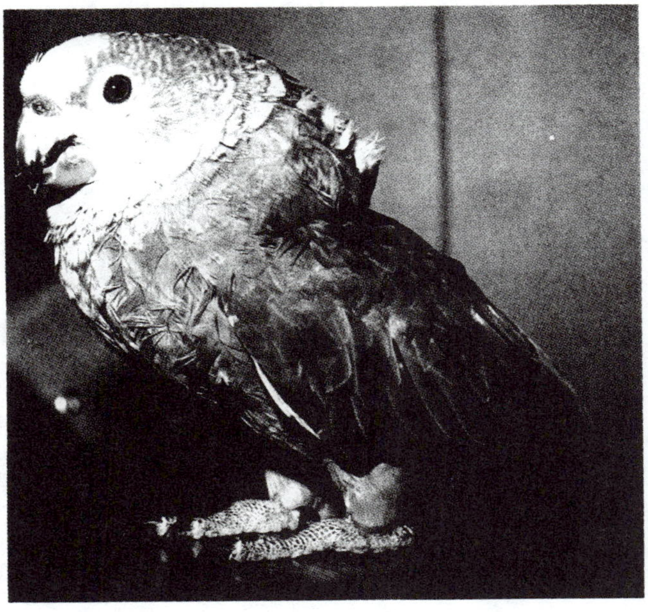

Figure 4A

Figure 4—(**A**) An amazon parrot with cervicocephalic air sac involvement showing a neck area that is distended to be two to three times normal size. (**B**) Lateral radiograph of the amazon parrot seen in **A**. The borders of the trapped air from the tympanic area to the shoulder (*arrows*) are shown. (**C**) Anterior-posterior view of the same amazon parrot. Because it can be seen that the air is limited to the cervical area, subcutaneous emphysema can be ruled out as a diagnosis. The crop and trachea are made very evident by the trapped air.

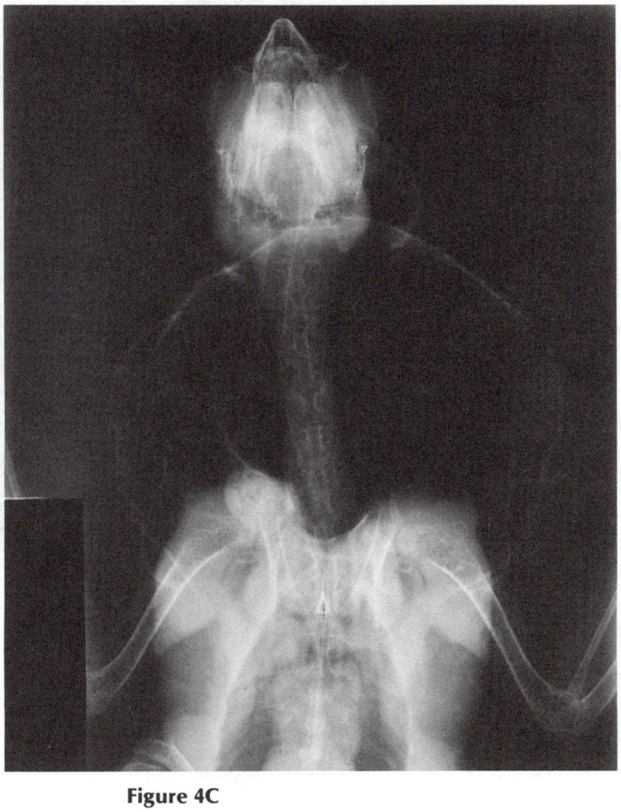

Figure 4C

ruptured pulmonary air sac. It was noted in the history that the bird was being offered a poor diet and had clinical signs of respiratory disease (sneezing, nasal discharge) before development of swelling. There was no history of trauma. Physical examination revealed air distention from the occipital area to the shoulders. After brushing away the feathers on the back of the neck with an alcohol swab, an extra layer of tissue below the skin was revealed. The orientation of the vasculature in this layer suggested that the layer was not associated with the dermis. Radiographs were taken (Figures 4B and C), which showed trapped air that had definitive borders and did not extend below the shoulder area or above the tympanic area.

Three hundred milliliters of air were aspirated from the distended air sac; the air was replaced within 12 hours. This indicated that the connection between the infundibular cleft and the tympanic area might be obstructed in such a way as to allow air to enter the air sacs and not allow it to escape.

Case 2

A mature albino cockatiel presented with a swelling of the head and neck, which had been noted when the bird was first given to the owners 15 months previously (Figure 5A). The bird did not appear to be in any discomfort and it ate well and acted normally. There

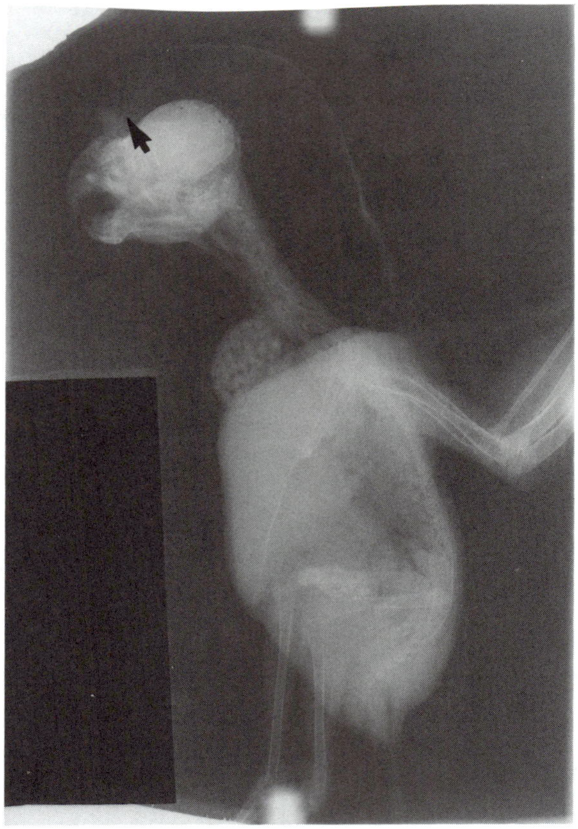

Figure 5B

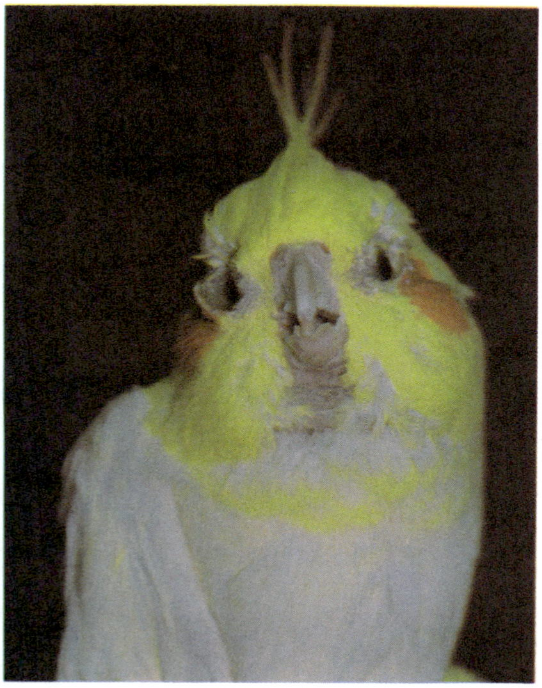

Figure 5A

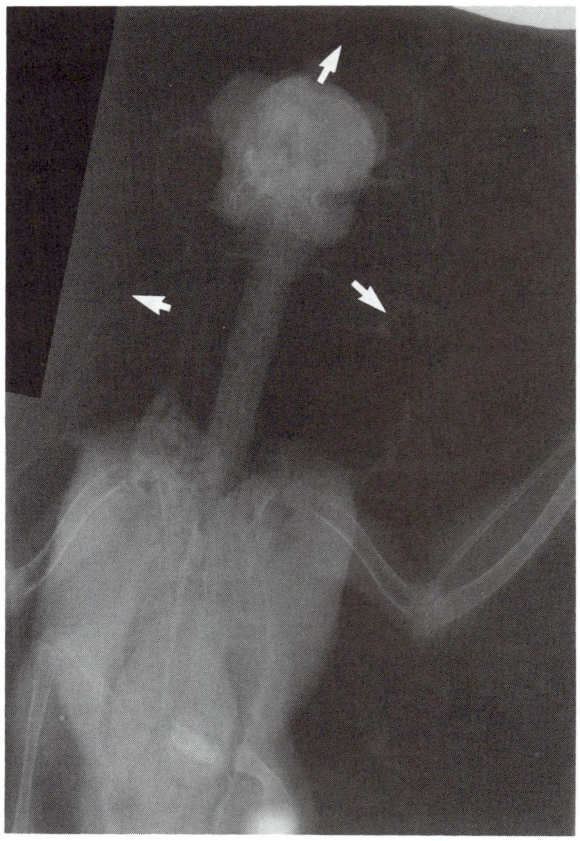

Figure 5C

Figure 5—(**A**) A cockatiel with chronic cerviocephalic air sac inflation. This case differs from the one illustrated in **4A** in that the cephalic portion is more prominent. (**B**) Lateral radiograph of the cockatiel shown in **A**. The film has been lightened to show the distention of the soft tissue. Note the cephalic involvement caudal to the cere (*arrow*). (**C**) Anterior-posterior view of the cockatiel in **A** and **B**. *Arrows* indicate distention of the air sac. The cervical portion does not extend beyond the shoulders caudally.

had been episodes of respiratory disease that had been treated with antibiotics. Physical examination revealed a very pliable air-filled swelling that extended the length of the neck and involved the head. Determination of the extent of the swelling was facilitated by clearing away feathers with an alcohol swab. As in Case 1, there was a second layer of tissue present in close proximity to the skin. No other abnormalities were detected. Radiographs were taken to verify cervicocephalic air sac involvement and as part of a routine workup (Figures 5B and C). These showed that the air did not extend beyond the shoulder and that there was more cephalic involvement than there was in Case 1.

Case 3

A three-year-old male sulfur-crested cockatoo presented with a history of collapsing in its cage. The bird had been purchased three months previously and was on an all-seed diet. Though the appetite was good, the bird had lost weight over the preceding two weeks. Antibiotics were prescribed by a veterinarian for a "lameness problem."

Physical examination revealed an emaciated bird weighing 280 g with anemia and hypoproteinemia. Supportive therapy strengthened the bird adequately for radiographic evaluation the next day. Endostosis of the left femur as well as multiple circular densities in the soft tissue of the cervical area were noted on radiographs. The significance of the neck opacities was not appreciated at that time.

After some improvement, the bird again collapsed and died on the third day of hospitalization. Lesions found at necropsy consisted of granulomas in the medullary space of the left femur, left tibia, liver, and the soft tissue of the neck. Bacteria in these lesions were determined histologically to be acid-fast and thus consistent with mycobacteria. The reason for the multiple lesions in the soft tissue at the neck was not determined. The slides were reviewed at a later date when the possibility of cervicocephalic air sac involvement was being considered. Review of the radiographs showed that the location of the granulomas was compatible with the normal anatomic location of the air sacs (Figure 6A). Subsequent examination of the histologic sections from the neck area revealed that the granuloma was within the air sac (Figure 6B).

Diagnosis

The absence of inflated air sacs does not rule out a pathologic process in the cervicocephalic air sac system. Any bird with a history of upper respiratory disease should be examined closely for cervicocephalic air sac involvement. The first step is to examine the oral cavity visually and give particular attention to the infundibular cleft and choanae. Swelling, discoloration, obstruction, and discharge should be noted, and bacterial and fungal cultures should be taken when indicated. Visual and otoscopic examination of the ears should be routinely performed to detect signs of otitis, which may interfere with the passage of air through the tympanic area. Palpation of the cervical region from the tympanic area to the shoulders to detect focal granulomas or debris lying within the air sac should also be performed as part of a complete examination. The feathers behind the ears, along the right and left jugular area, and over the shoulders can be brushed away with an alcohol swab to aid in visualization. The skin is best seen when feathers are parted over the apterylae, the tracts of skin relatively devoid of feather follicles. These featherless tracts are the tracts used when attempting to locate the jugular vein for obtaining a blood sample.

Whole-body radiographs can help confirm a diagnosis of cervicocephalic air sac distention and detect granulomas. The most common differential diagnosis of subcutaneous emphysema can usually be ruled out on the basis of the location of the distention and a history of

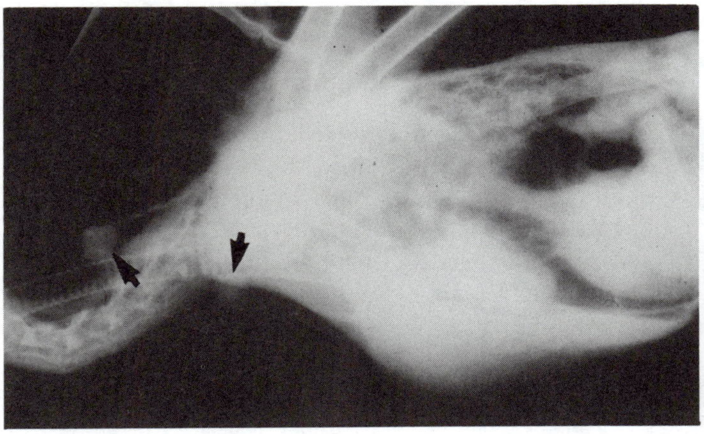

Figure 6A

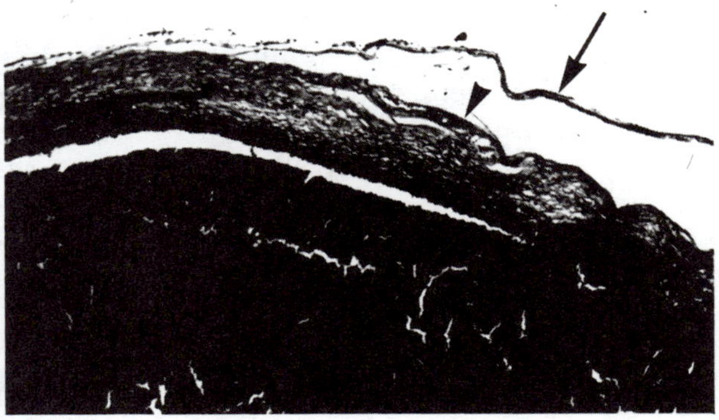

Figure 6B

Figure 6—(**A**) Lateral radiograph of a three-year-old cockatoo. The *arrows* show the positions of the granulomas in the region of the cervical air sacs of the neck. (**B**) Histologic appearance of a granuloma within a cerviocephalic air sac. The granuloma has been "peeled out." Surrounding it is a thin membrane of flattened cells, which are remnants of the air sac lining (*arrow*). Within this membrane is a band of fibrous connective tissue (*arrowhead*) and a central mass of epithelioid macrophages and necrotic debris. (H&E, ×56) trauma. Subcutaneous emphysema, as a result of tracheal trauma or air sac rupture, results in air dissecting in a diffuse irregular pattern that commonly spreads to other portions of the body.

The air sacs can be filled voluntarily on expiration. Bacteria, fungi, and other airborne pathogens may thereby be deposited in these air cells. As a result, air sacculitis and granuloma formation are probably fairly common problems but may not be easily detected. The presence of lesions, such as the granuloma detected in the neck area of the bird in Case 3, necessitates aspiration or surgical removal. Culture, cytology, and histopathology help to pinpoint the cause and aid in determining therapy.

To determine the frequency of cervicocephalic disease in birds accurately, necropsy techniques should be adapted to include a close examination of the cervicocephalic area following removal of the skin.

Therapy

Because pathology involving the cervicocephalic air sacs is not well documented or understood, definitive therapeutic principles have not been formulated. The most common problems that have been noted by the authors are granulomatous air sacculitis[2] and chronically distended air sacs.[3]

Treatment for chronically distended air sacs is mainly symptomatic. Simply aspirating the trapped air may only give short-term relief. Chronic deflation is more successful, but there is no information that can be used to compare results with known causes or to determine the recurrence rate. Basically, the treatment technique for chronic deflation involves creating a *sacculostomy*, or stoma of the air sac. The stoma is created and the skin and air sac are sutured together or are sutured to an O-ring made of silicone or Teflon® (DuPont) to maintain the opening. It appears that one opening is sufficient to relieve the distention in many species. The site for placement of the stoma can be verified by first aspirating the air to determine if bilateral drainage is achieved.

More consideration should be given to determining the initial cause of chronically distended air sacs; the cause may be related to concurrent or previous upper respiratory disease, such as chronic sinusitus. It is probable that inflammation and debris between the infundibular cleft and the tympanic area may be creating a one-way valve effect so that air is pumped in with pressure but cannot escape. The chronic release of this pressure with the air sacculostomy may be providing symptomatic relief or simply giving the involved area adequate time to heal.

Antibiotic therapy based on culture and sensitivity testing may be helpful in treatment of air sacculitis, granulomas, and the early stages of the distended air sac.

Discussion

Bignon believed that the air sacs have three functions.[1] The first is heat retention, which is important during cold periods. Birds inflate the sacs to produce an insulating layer of air to aid in heat conservation. In high-flying birds, the sacs may be inflated to decrease heat loss during flight. The second function is buoyancy control, a function exemplified in such birds as the pelican and albatross that spend long periods in the water. The third function of the air sacs is supporting the head during sleep. Other possible functions include inflation during flight for head support and reducing the force of impact during free-fall fishing (another function of the pelican).

For the most part, the results of the authors' study agreed with those of Bignon's. Bignon found that of the species she investigated, the Carolina parakeet and Ledbetters cockatoo had the most extensive development of both portions of the cervicocephalic air sac system. It is also evident that cockatiels and small conures have well-developed cervical and cephalic portions. Amazon parrots have a well-developed cervical portion and a reduced cranial portion. The macaw also has a well-defined cervical portion but no cephalic portion. It appears that both portions of the cervicocephalic system are well developed in smaller species. Development of the cervical portions of the system seems generally more advanced than that of the cephalic portion in larger birds. No direct connection has yet been found between the cervicocephalic air sac system and the pulmonary air sac system.

The veterinarian should be aware of certain problems associated with the cervicocephalic air sac system. As previously noted, this system has differences in form, function, and distribution between the species. Keeping the variations in mind will help to explain some of the subtle differences in presentation and lesion location. Although pathology of the cervicocephalic system seems rare when compared with that of other upper respiratory conditions, such as sinusitis, it is also likely that pathology in this area is overlooked by the clinicians and pathologists. It would be interesting to examine every necropsied bird for cervicocephalic air sac involvement because pathologic processes in this system may play a role in the development of other airway diseases.

Acknowledgments

The authors thank Marisa Mitchell for her translation of Bignon's article; Dr. Claus Buergelt for his translation of the Groebbels article; Jody Sayle for her artwork; Mark Hoffenberg for the photographs; and Dr. George Kollias and Lisa Biles for their help with the manuscript.

REFERENCES

1. Bignon, F: Contribution to the study of pneumacity of birds—The cervicocephalic air cells of the birds and their relation with the bones of the head. *Mem Soc Zool Franc* 2:260-318, 1889.
2. Groebbels F: *Der Vogel*, vol 1. Berlin, Borntrager, 1932.
3. King AS: Structural and functional aspects of the avian lungs and air sacs. *Int Rev Gen Exp Zool*:171-267. 1966.
4. Coe MJ: Letter. *Nature* 188:598, 1960.

Disorders of the Avian Crop

Terry W. Campbell, DVM, PhD
Colorado State University
Fort Collins, Colorado

The crop (ingluvies) is a dilatation or diverticulum of the esophagus in birds. It is subject to several medical disorders, and the knowledge of these conditions is important to the avian practitioner. Common noninfectious surgical disorders include fistulas, lacerations, and obstructions. Common infectious crop disorders are candidiasis, trichomoniasis, and sour crop. This article provides a basic understanding of crop anatomy and physiology and describes the various crop disorders and current treatments.

Anatomy

The crop is a specialized, permanent diverticulum or expansion of the esophagus. The esophagus is divided into two sections in relation to the crop, the pars cervicalis (the area between the pharynx and crop) and the pars thoracica (the area between the crop and proventriculus). The esophagus and crop generally lie to the right of the midline and in the subcutaneous space bound by delicate fascia and adipose tissue. Gallinaceous, psittacine, and columbiform birds have a muscular sling that surrounds the crop and inserts into the skin.[1,2] This sling aids in emptying of the crop. Depending upon age, species, and size of the bird, the crop usually lies near the thoracic inlet. A full crop in hawks extends ventrally. It also extends ventrally in parrots, whereas in some psittacines it protrudes laterally and dorsally. Not all crops are identical, nor do all birds have crops. The crop may be a spindle-shaped enlargement of the esophagus, a unilateral enlargement or evagination, a unilateral sac, or a bilateral double sac.[3] The parakeet crop is a fusiform widening of the esophagus that narrows at the pectoral end.[4] Some birds (e.g., canaries, owls, and gulls) do not have crops but can store food by temporary expansion of the esophagus.[3,5]

Avian esophageal and crop tissues have the same general organization as the mammalian esophagus. The musculature of the crop, the tunica muscularis, is in three layers in the chicken and two layers in psittacines and birds of prey.[2] The external longitudinal muscle is usually thin, while the circular and interlongitudinal muscle layers are well developed.[3] The epithelium (lamina epithelialis mucosae) varies in thickness with species, and the outer layer may be cornified into a stratum corneum. In some passerines the epithelium is thickest in the crop with the greatest cornification in the pars cervicalis. The tunica mucosa of the crop contains mucous glands, which vary in location among species.[2] The

Updated from Volume 5, Number 10, October 1983 for publication in
Exotic Animal Medicine in Practice, Volume 1, VLS Books, Trenton, NJ, 1991

glands are tubular to alveolar and have merocrine secretion.

The crop is innervated by esophageal branches of the glossopharyngeal nerve anastomosing with recurrent branches of the vagus.[6] Normal peristalsis is maintained by the vagal efferent input and the myenteric nervous system. The vagus also controls the crop sphincter.[3] The crop of pigeons and chickens has stronger rhythmic contractions when empty than when full. Feeding or cerebral inhibition causes a temporary cessation of these movements. Birds that swallow large food particles (i.e., raptors) temporarily store the food in the crop before peristaltic contractions move it into the proventriculus.

The crop is supplied by the left ascending esophageal artery, which is a branch from the common carotid artery. The venous return is through the esophageal veins draining into the left and right caudal veins of the crop. These veins enter the jugular directly.

Crop Function

The crop functions as a food storage chamber where ingesta undergoes softening, moistening, and swelling.[7] The crop supplies ingesta to the proventriculus at an appropriate rate for digestion. Food initially consumed may be delivered directly to the proventriculus without entering the crop. Later, the crop sphincter relaxes allowing food to enter the crop. Ingesta leaves the crop at irregular intervals reflexively controlled by the degree of fullness of the gastrointestinal tract.[3] The crop allows the bird to consume large quantities of small food rapidly, thus minimizing exposure time to predation.[7] Food to feed the young is stored in the crop from which it is regurgitated by reverse peristalsis in such birds as hawks, parrots, and pigeons. Maximum storage capacity is obtained by the saclike diverticula-style crops.

The role of the crop in chemical digestion is controversial. Some authors feel that starch digestion within the crop is due to amylase activity derived from saliva and crop secretions.[8] Others believe carbohydrate digestion is primarily microbial in origin.[9] Lactic acid can be found in significant concentration within the crop lumen, indicating carbohydrate hydrolysis. Protein digestion probably occurs from proventricular proteinases regurgitated into the crop. Any chemical digestion within the crop is of minor importance since it precedes the physical digestion by the gizzard.

Some birds produce a milklike secretion (crop milk) that is formed in the crop and regurgitated to feed nestlings. In pigeons and doves, this fluid is produced by the desquamation of fat-laden cells of the crop. In both sexes prior to hatching, this superficial nutritive cell layer begins to proliferate under the stimulation of oxytocin and prolactin.[7,10,11] The liquid produced is rich in fat and protein but low in carbohydrates and is fed to the young during the first two weeks of life.[3] Crop milk production allows parents to feed at irregular intervals while providing nestlings with a stable and constant food supply.[12]

The crop functions in courtship behavior in some birds. Males of certain species (i.e., grouse and pigeons) have inflatable esophageal diverticula, which act as resonating chambers or display devices.[3]

Examination of the Crop

Examination of the crop should be included in the physical examination of the avian patient. The crop is palpated to determine the degree of fill and consistency of its contents. Presence (or absence) of contents, dilatation, loss of tone, and masses inside the crop wall should be noted. An impacted crop may be enlarged, doughy, or firm upon palpation. An extremely dilated, atonic, fluid-filled crop can result from obstruction distal to the crop (i.e., in the proventriculus or gizzard). Crop atony can result from bacterial, protozoal, or mycotic infections. Parrots with access to food should have food in the crop;[13] thus, an empty crop is abnormal. In some birds the crop can be visualized through the skin by wetting the feathers. Better visualization is achieved by transillumination of the skin and crop wall with a bright light, such as that of an otoscope.

Contrast radiology is useful in the diagnosis of certain crop disorders. A 10 to 25% solution of barium sulfate is introduced into the crop using an infant feeding tube. The barium dosage for birds the size of a parakeet (30 gm) is 0.5 to 2.0 ml and for parrots is 5.0 to 10.0 ml.[14,15] Survey radiographs are taken before the barium is given. Second radiographs are taken immediately after barium administration. Subsequent radiographs are taken at 10- to 30-minute intervals. Barium should be in the proventriculus within 15 minutes and the small intestine within 30 minutes. The usual transit time of barium through the gastrointestinal tract is less than three hours.[11] Air can be used as the contrast medium for contrast radiology of the crop.[16,17]

Aspiration and evaluation of the crop contents is valuable in the diagnosis of crop disease. Whenever a crop disorder is suspected, aspiration of the crop contents should be considered. Sterile disposable feeding tubes are used (Figure 1). Tube sizes include No. 5 French for birds the size of a parakeet or smaller, No. 8 to No. 10 French for birds the size of cockatiels and medium-sized parrots (i.e., conures), and No. 14 to No. 18 French for larger birds (i.e., Amazon parrots, macaws, and raptors). A speculum will aid passage of the tube through the mouth. In parakeets or smaller birds, a small paper clip or thumb forceps can be used for this purpose; a larger paper clip or laboratory animal speculum can be used in a cockatiel or medium-sized parrot. An open-handle–style hoof pick or laboratory animal speculum can be used for aid in passing a feeding tube into the mouth of large parrots.

The head and neck should be extended to straighten the esophagus when inserting a tube into the crop. The tube is inserted into the mouth and passed over the tongue into the esophagus. The tube should pass easily into the crop and can be palpated through the skin. If

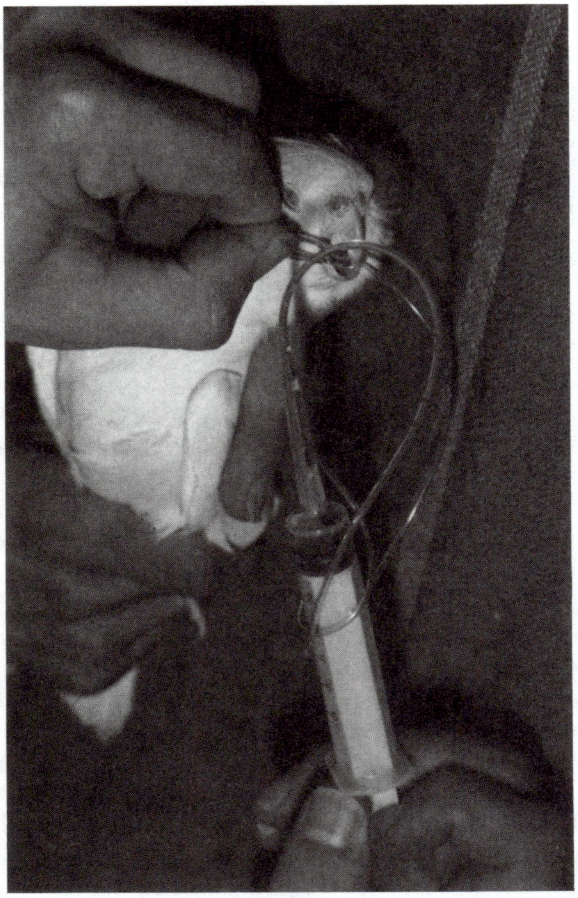

Figure 1—Crop aspiration technique using a sterile feeding tube.

any resistance occurs during the passage of the tube, the process should be stopped and repeated. The wall of the esophagus and crop is easily punctured, and excessive force should be avoided. In larger birds the mouth can be examined to insure the tube is in the esophagus and not in the trachea. When the end of the tube is within the crop, contents of the crop can be aspirated with a sterile syringe attached to the external end of the tube. Aspirated crop material should be submitted for mycotic and bacterial culture, antibiotic sensitivity, and cytologic examination. A wet mount is examined for trichomonads or other protozoa. An air-dried smear can be stained with Diff Quik®,[a] Wright's stain, or other suitable cytologic stain. The stained smear is examined for the presence of inflammatory cells, *Candida*, or any other abnormal content.

Ingluvotomy

Crop disorders that require surgery include lacerations, foreign bodies, calculi, fistulas, punctures, impactions, obstructions, and chronic dilatation. An ingluvotomy is indicated for removal of foreign bodies or obstructing material and repair of chronic dilatation. General anesthesia is usually required, although the procedure may be done without anesthesia in young birds.[17] Since the crop is relatively avascular and subcutaneous in location, surgery is relatively easy. However, the crop wall is thin and easily torn and care should be taken when handling the tissue. The crop should be emptied of excess gas and liquid prior to surgery using the crop aspiration technique described above. Patency of the esophagus and crop is maintained before and after surgery with a soft feeding tube or catheter placed in the esophagus and crop. The bird is placed in dorsal recumbency with proper consideration for preservation of body temperature. Feathers are removed from the incision site. The skin is prepared with a gentle surgical scrub and swabbed with tincture of iodine. A skin incision is made using a scalpel blade. The crop is bluntly dissected from surrounding tissue, and an incision is made into the crop for the removal of foreign bodies or obstructing material. The skin and crop should be sutured separately when closing.[10,18-20] The crop wall is closed using an inverting pattern (i.e., continuous Lembert suture) using 3-0 to 5-0 surgical gut or 4-0 absorbable suture on an atraumatic needle. The skin is closed with a simple interrupted or continuous pattern using 2-0 to 4-0 surgical gut. Optimum healing is obtained if suture lines of the crop and skin are offset.

Food and water should be withheld as long as possible following surgery, but no longer than 18 hours depending upon the size and condition of the bird.[21] Generally, food and water are withheld for three to four hours postoperatively and small amounts of soft foods are offered for 12 to 24 hours. Normal feeding is resumed after 24 hours. A common complication of ingluvotomy is a fistula, which requires resuturing. An Elizabethan collar may be required to prevent the bird from removing the sutures.

Crop Fistula

Crop fistulas result from postoperative ingluvotomy complications, lacerations, penetration of foreign bodies, and trauma or necrosis of the crop lining. A puncture of the crop occurs frequently in birds being force-fed using feeding tubes. Baby birds often develop marked edema and bruising in the area where the crop was punctured by a feeding tube and die quickly. Necrosis of the crop mucosa also may result from trauma induced by a tube or hot foods. The subcutaneous location of the crop predisposes it to punctures and lacerations (a common occurrence from encounters with cats). Raptors may suffer from punctures of the esophagus or crop as a result of bones ingested with their prey.[22,23] Crop fistulas can be difficult to treat and require immediate attention. Examination of the bird may reveal only a small opening and a few feathers matted with crop content. In acute cases the bird appears healthy, but a ravenous appetite and marked weight loss may be associated with a more chronic disorder. After feeding, the food may be deposited externally or subcutaneously; the latter is usually fatal.[24]

Repair of a fistulated crop requires debridement and separation of the crop wall from the skin. The freshened

[a]Harleco, Gibbstown, NJ 08027.

edges of the opened crop and skin are closed independently as in an ingluvotomy. Altman[25] suggests using 4-0 nylon to repair the crop because of the rapid absorption of 4-0 surgical gut. If more than eight hours have elapsed, the crop tissue becomes difficult to dissect from the surrounding tissue.[25] If the fistula repair is delayed longer than 24 hours, the prognosis is guarded.[10] A soft, seedless diet should be fed for the first 24 to 48 hours following fistula repair. Soaked and softened seed and soft foods should be continued for one week postoperatively.[11] A broad-spectrum oral antibiotic for one week is recommended.

Crop Impaction

Impaction of the crop is uncommon in caged birds. When it occurs, the impaction usually is due to a dry food mass resulting from obstructive foreign bodies, greedy feeding, inflammation lower in the gastrointestinal tract, or neuromuscular stasis of the crop.[26] Chickens, quail, and pheasants deprived of greens often gorge themselves when given access to long grass and this may result in crop impactions.[11,27] Ingestion of certain types of foods (e.g., oatmeal) or seeds (e.g., soybeans) frequently results in crop impactions.[11,28,29] If a large amount of these foods is ingested, crop impaction can result when the food rapidly swells within the crop. Grit impactions frequently occur when a bird denied access to grit suddenly is given grit free choice.

Raptors ingest large chunks of food or the entire carcass of small prey. The undigested parts are regurgitated as a pellet or casting, which involves gastric and esophageal antiperistalsis. Crop impactions in captive birds of prey often occur when a diet containing no castings (or roughage) is suddenly changed to one with castings.[30] Calculi causing crop impaction (crop lithiasis) are rare but have been reported.[11,31]

Clinical signs of crop impaction include repeated nonproductive regurgitation attempts, an interest in food but reluctance to eat, and picking at the base of the neck in the area of the crop. The crop is usually enlarged, has a doughlike consistency, and fails to empty. Acute impactions lead to crop rupture, toxicity due to absorbed toxins, or compression of the trachea. Chronic impactions result in emaciation and death due to starvation.[11]

Nonsurgical attempts to relieve the impaction should be attempted. In small birds a few drops of mineral or vegetable oil are given by crop gavage followed by gentle manual massage to break up the mass.[26] In raptors and gallinaceous birds 20 to 30 ml of vegetable oil can be given to soften the mass. Flushing or purging of the mass with warm isotonic saline may be attempted, but care must be taken to prevent respiratory aspiration of the fluid. If nonsurgical attempts fail, then an ingluvotomy to remove the impacted material is indicated.

Young hand-fed psittacines frequently develop crop impactions. Predisposing conditions include feeding foods that are cold, low in fiber, or spoiled; introducing air into the crop during feeding; and overfeeding the bird.[32] These conditions result in delayed emptying or impaction of the crop. Treatment should be prompt and requires evacuation of the crop by turning the chick upside down and milking out the contents. The bird is then fed small amounts of food at frequent intervals. If the retained food has fermented, then treatment may require administering a sodium bicarbonate solution (1 tsp/pt of water).

Chronic Dilatation of the Crop (Pendulous Crop)

The crop may become extremely dilated as a result of chronic obstruction distal to the crop, excessive food intake, atony from crop infections (bacterial, protozoal, or fungal), or unknown causes. This disorder frequently leads to ingluvitis, frequent regurgitation, and malnutrition. Birds with chronic dilatation of the crop lose body weight, as most of the ingested food is unable to pass out of the enlarged crop. Physical examination reveals an extremely enlarged and flaccid, fluid-filled crop that lies over the cranial aspect of the thorax. This condition is seen in older parakeets with a history of excessive food intake or hand-fed young psittacines that have been overfed. It can also be secondary to gastrointestinal tract obstruction (i.e., impaction of the proventriculus or gizzard) or pressure due to lesions at the thoracic inlet (i.e., abscess, neoplasia, fat deposits, or thyroid dysplasia). (See Figure 2.) Once the crop has been distended, it rarely corrects itself.

Diagnosis of the primary lesion may require crop aspiration for cytologic evaluation, culture of the crop contents, and contrast radiology to reveal obstructive lesions distal to the crop. Treatment of the primary lesion should be the first consideration. Excess crop fluid can be removed by turning the bird upside down and quickly milking the fluid out. The crop may require emptying two to three times a day. Force-feeding small amounts of a liquid diet at frequent intervals may be required, especially in obstructive cases. Oral antibiotics, as indicated from bacterial culture and sensitivity tests, should be given. Chloramphenicol palmitate[b] (0.05 to 0.01 ml/50 gm body weight) is a good broad-spectrum antibiotic to use while waiting for antibiotic sensitivity test results. Nystatin[c] (given at 0.05 to 0.01 ml/50 gm body weight) is indicated for candidiasis. Obese birds with fat deposits at the thoracic inlet should be fed reducing diets. Thyroid dysplasia should be treated by adding 10% sodium iodide to the drinking water (1 drop/30 ml). The distended crop is often refractory to medical treatment and usually requires a partial ingluvectomy. Using the technique described for an ingluvotomy, 40 to 60% of the distended crop wall can be removed with a fair to good prognosis.[21] Distention may recur, especially if the primary lesion is uncorrected.[20]

---

[b]Chloromycetin® Palmitate, Parke-Davis, Morris Plains, NJ 07950.
[c]Mycostatin®, E.R. Squibb & Sons, Inc., Princeton, NJ 08540.

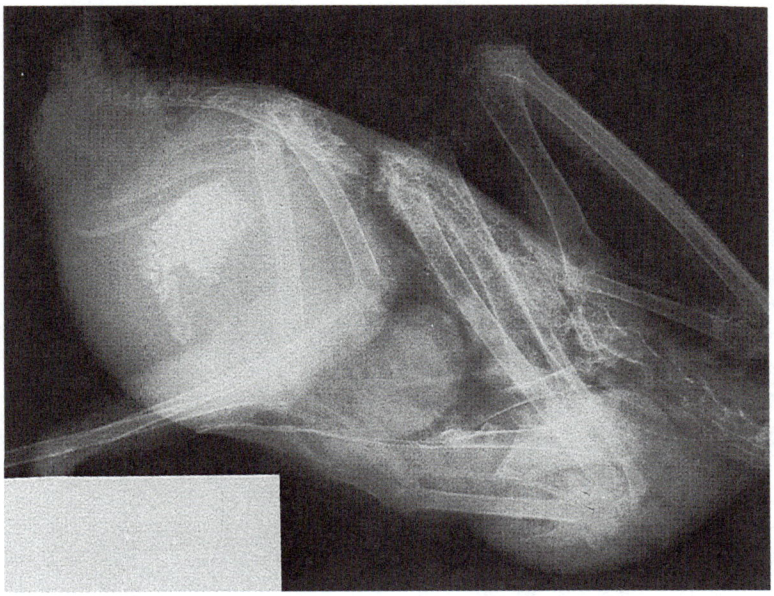

Figure 2—Lateral radiograph showing dilatation of the crop resulting from an obstruction of the proventriculus.

Ingluvitis (Inflammation of the Crop)

Ingluvitis can be caused by infectious agents such as bacteria, protozoa, and fungi; by chemical irritants, including such toxic plants as ivies, lilies, and oleander; by nutritional imbalances or deficiencies; and by unknown etiologies. Regurgitation is a common clinical sign. The crop becomes flaccid and filled with mucoid fluid, which is frequently regurgitated and flipped on the bird's head and objects in its cage. This material will paste head feathers together. Polydipsia is common.[33] The diagnosis is based upon clinical signs of regurgitation, the presence of an enlarged atonic crop, and cytologic evidence of inflammation on examination of the crop contents.

Cytologically, a normal crop aspirate from seed-eating birds has moderate numbers of cornified squamous epithelial cells and extracellular bacteria with a variety of morphologic types (Figure 3). An occasional *Candida*-like yeast can be seen, and there is a moderate amount of debris and plant fibers depending upon the sample. A Gram's stain reveals primarily gram-positive cocci and small to medium rods. Presence of many inflammatory cells (i.e., heterophils and macrophages) and an increased number of bacteria (especially intracellular), protozoa, or yeasts is indicative of ingluvitis (Figure 4). A smear with a large number of bacteria predominantly of one morphologic type or many gram-negative bacteria (in seed-eating birds) is abnormal.

Treatment requires emptying the crop two to three times a day and using oral antibiotics based upon the culture and sensitivity tests. Liquid vitamins are recommended. Supplemental digestive enzymes, lactobacillus, and nutritional yeasts may aid in restoration of normal crop flora. Ingluvitis has an inconsistent prognosis and can become a chronic or recurrent condition.

Sour Crop

Sour crop is an inflammation or ulceration of the crop associated with a foul-smelling, fermenting crop

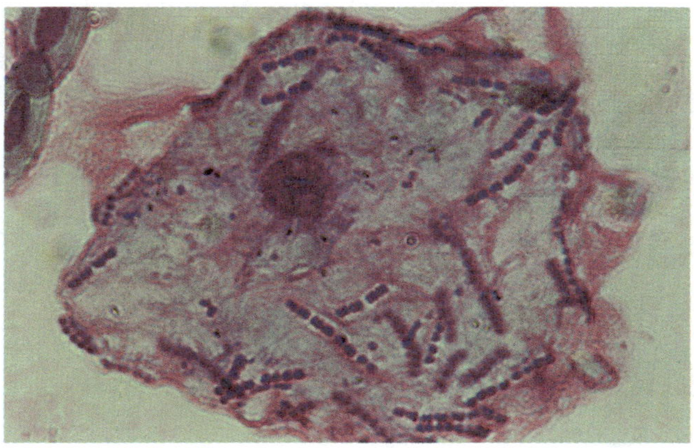

Figure 3—Crop aspirate from a scarlet macaw showing *Alysiella filiformis*, a normal bacterial inhabitant of the avian crop frequently seen on the surface of squamous epithelial cells. (Diff Quik, 100×)

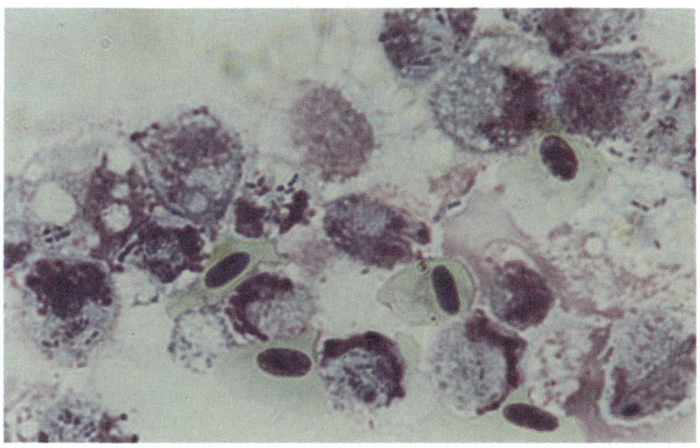

Figure 4—Septic ingluvitis in a cockatiel. Cytology of the crop aspirate shows a marked number of heterophils and macrophages with phagocytosis of bacteria. (Diff Quik, 100×)

fluid. Crop content is often acidic, which is presumably due to excessive lactate production (normal crop pH of seed-eating birds is between 4.5 and 6.7).[3] Predisposing factors include ingestion of spoiled food, irregular feeding, chilling, lower digestive tract disorders, vitamin deficiencies, protein deficiencies, regurgitation of the proventriculus content into the crop, and such infectious agents as *Candida* and *Trichomonas*.[11] Disorders causing delayed emptying of the crop predispose to this condition. Death results from malnutrition and dehydration due to vomiting and diarrhea.[11] Treatment requires emptying the crop several times a day. A broad-spectrum antibiotic (e.g., chloramphenicol palmitate), an antacid (e.g., sodium bicarbonate), and a digestive tract protectant (i.e., Kaopectate®[d]) should be given. A liquid diet given every two hours for one to three days is followed by a semisolid diet and finally a normal diet after three to five days.[11] Specific treatment for any infectious agent should be provided.

Candidiasis of the Crop

Candidiasis is caused by a fungus in the genus *Candida. Candida albicans* is the most common species isolated. The organism is part of the normal intestinal flora and is frequently isolated from droppings of healthy birds.[34-36] *Candida* is usually found in low numbers but will cause disease if allowed to overgrow. Predisposing factors to candidiasis include prolonged antibiotic treatment, avitaminosis (especially in avitaminosis A), nutritional disorders, bacterial or viral infections, feeding damp spoiled foods, and poor sanitation.[36,37] Jungerman and Schwartzman[36] list possible reasons for antibiotic enhancement of candidiasis: (1) direct stimulation of mycotic growth, (2) removal of bacteria competing for nutrients, (3) removal of organisms producing antifungal substances, (4) direct tissue damage allowing local invasion by *Candida*, (5) conversion of *Candida* to a more invasive form, (6) toxic products produced by *Candida*, (7) depression of the host immune response, (8) destruction of the normal flora resulting in avitaminosis that leads to lower tissue resistance to *Candida* invasion, and (9) use of certain antibiotics (especially tetracyclines) by *Candida* as a nitrogen source.

Young birds are more susceptible to candidiasis. *Candida* and bacterial infections of the crop are common causes of crop impaction and death in baby psittacines.[37] The organism is usually confined to the crop, causing delayed emptying of the crop and malnutrition. Cytologic evaluation of the crop contents shows an absence of inflammation (i.e., no heterophil or macrophage infiltration). The organism can invade the mouth, infraorbital sinuses, esophagus, proventriculus, gizzard, and intestinal tract.[36,38] Systemic infections can occur, especially in young birds. Venereal candidiasis has been reported in geese.[39]

[d]The Upjohn Co., Kalamazoo, MI 49001.

A normal healthy crop has a white to pale pink mucosal lining with many smooth convoluted folds. Candidiasis causes crop mucosa to become rough and thickened. The crop surface may be coated with a catarrhal to mucoid tenacious exudate.[36] Infected crops show mild white streaking, erosions, pseudomembranous white areas, or diphtheritic membrane formation.[40] Oral lesions are not always present with crop lesions.

Clinical signs are variable. They include general malaise, loss of body weight (often with an increased appetite), delayed emptying of the crop, frequent regurgitation, and a thickened or dilated crop. Crop candidiasis in raptors is characterized by pseudomembranous patches of epithelium, foul-smelling crop contents, and impairment of ingestion.[30] Frequently, the only sign is of general malaise.

Suspicion of candidiasis of the crop is based on clinical signs, a history with predisposing factors, and demonstration of crop lesions. A presumptive diagnosis is based on the identification of the organism either by microscopic examination or mycotic culture of the crop contents. If blastospores and pseudohyphae (or true mycelia) are present, a presumptive diagnosis of candidiasis can be made, since these forms indicate tissue invasion (Figure 5).[36] Aspiration of the crop contents will usually reveal oval, thin-walled budding yeasts measuring 3 to 6 μ in diameter. Dry smears stained with Diff Quik®,[a] Gram's stain, or new methylene blue or a wet mount stained with lactophenol cotton blue will aid in identifying the yeasts (Figure 6). Selective media are required to culture *Candida*. The organism grows on blood or Sabouraud's agar producing soft, white, smooth colonies with a characteristic yeast odor. Older colonies will show feathery margins due to mycelial growth. Cornmeal agar is used to identify *Candida albicans*, which produces characteristic chlamydospores.[36,41] Differential diagnosis for avian candidiasis includes pox, trichomoniasis, histomoniasis, and avitaminosis A lesions.

Treatment of crop candidiasis involves correcting the predisposing factors. Specific medications include nystatin,[c] chlorhexidine,[e] ketaconizol,[f] amphotericin B,[g] and iodine.[37] Supplemental A and B-complex vitamins are indicated. Nystatin[c] is commonly used to treat *Candida* at a dose of 100,000 units/300 gm body weight once or twice a day for seven days.[37,42] Other antifungal drugs, amphotericin B[g] and flucytosine,[h] are used in cases refractory to nystatin.[37] A 2% chlorhexidine solution[e] in the water or 15% formic acid solution sprayed on the food can be used to treat flocks.[37,43]

Trichomoniasis

Trichomoniasis is a common disease affecting the crop in pigeons, doves, and raptors. It has been reported

[e]Nolvasan®, Fort Dodge Laboratories, Fort Dodge, IA 50501.
[f]Nizoral®, Janssen Pharmaceutica, Inc., New Brunswick, NJ 08903.
[g]Fungizone®, E.R. Squibb & Sons, Inc., Princeton, NJ 08540.
[h]Ancobon®, Roche Products, Inc., Manati, PR 00701.

in chickens, turkeys, finches, canaries, and rarely in psittacines.[44-46] Trichomoniasis is called "canker" by pigeon fanciers and "frounce" by falconers. The disease is caused by *Trichomonas gallinae*, an ellipsoid or piriform flagellate protozoan. The organism measures 5 to 19 μ by 2 to 9 μ and has four anterior flagella, a narrow axostyle that protrudes 2 to 8 μ from the body, an undulating membrane, and no posterior flagellum.[45,47,48] The disease primarily affects young birds. Adult pigeons and doves may be healthy carriers and transmit the organism through the crop milk to their young. Trichomonads are sensitive to drying and do not form cysts, therefore direct transmission or contamination of food and water by material from the mouth (but not the feces) is necessary.[45,49] Raptors become infected by eating feral pigeons and doves. The susceptibility of pigeons and doves varies among breeds and the pathogenicity varies among strains of *T. gallinae*. Stress due to concurrent illness or environmental changes may predispose the bird to infection. Young pigeons appear to be most susceptible during weaning or molting.[45] Chemical irritants affecting the mucosa of the upper digestive tract will allow the normal protozoan population to become pathogenic.[50]

Trichomonas infections have an affinity for the esophagus and crop. Early lesions are small, white or yellow caseous nodules on the mucosa that may develop into large necrotic masses, which can occlude the lumen.[45] These firm masses may extend between folds in the mucosa and are often palpated as hard masses in the esophagus and crop. Soft, moist lesions occur with acute forms whereas dry, firm, cheesy lesions are seen in chronic forms.[11] Lesions may involve the oral cavity and upper respiratory tract. Highly pathogenic strains are invasive with lesions extending into the head and neck musculature or causing systemic infection.[51,52]

Clinical signs of trichomoniasis are more severe in young birds. Initially, regurgitation may occur due to invasion of the esophagus or crop mucosa. Sudden death without signs of illness occurs in some acute cases. Clinical signs of the chronic forms depend upon the severity and location of the lesions. Common signs include anorexia, weight loss, dyspnea, general malaise, and depression. The bird with occlusion of the esophagus or crop may die from starvation. A large amount of foul-smelling fluid may accumulate in the crop and may exude from the mouth.

The lesions caused by trichomoniasis must be differentiated from those of candidiasis, avitaminosis A, pox, and bacterial abscess. The diagnosis is based on history, clinical signs, and demonstration of the organisms from lesions or crop contents. A sample is collected by swabbing the crop with a moist cotton swab or aspirating the contents. A wet mount is prepared and the organisms can be seen microscopically. Trichomonads move through the fluid, and a wavy motion of the flagella and undulating membrane can be seen. The organisms can also be cultured in the laboratory (Figure 7).

Treatment for trichomoniasis involves use of antiprotozoal drugs. Dimetridazole[i] has been used successfully at a dose of 50 mg/kg body weight orally for two to seven days or 0.6 mg/L drinking water (2.27 g/gal) for six to seven days.[27,37,44,48,52] A single oral dose of 500 mg dimetridazole[i]/kg body weight has also been recommended.[42] Metronidazole[j] can be used orally at a dose of 50 to 60 mg/kg body weight or 66 mg/L (250 mg/gal) of drinking water for five to seven days.[42,52] The drug, 2-amino-5-nitrothiazole[k] can be used orally at a dose of 30 to 45 mg/kg body weight or 1 to 2 g/L of drinking water for seven days.[27,42,45,48] Ipronidazole[l] at a dose of 132 mg/L (500 mg/gal) of drinking water for seven days has also been used.[37] Broad-spectrum antibiotics and vitamin supplementation by crop gavage may aid in preventing secondary bacterial infections and vitamin deficiencies.

Recovery from infection or previous exposure to trichomonads will lead to immunity. Infection with an avirulent strain produces immunity against virulent strains, and passive immunity using serum from an infected bird provides protective immunity.[45] Trichomoniasis is controlled by eliminating carrier birds with treatment, preventing feral birds from contaminating food and water, and regular cleaning of food and water containers.

Neoplasia of the Crop

Neoplasms affecting the crop are rare. Petrak[53] describes a leiomyosarcoma of the crop in a budgerigar. The tumor measured 5 cm in diameter and was attached to the crop wall. A green-wing macaw with multiple papillomas affecting the esophagus, crop, and cranial proventriculus was referred to the author's clinic.[54] The bird was extremely emaciated, weak, and had inspiratory wheezing. Physical examination revealed marked weight loss, marked stress barring of the feathers, and a small papilloma in the glottis. Radiographs, hemogram, and blood chemistry results were within normal limits except for a slight elevation of aspartate aminotransferase. The bird continued to eat but was supplemented by tube feeding. Necropsy revealed multiple papillomatous growths partially occluding the lumen of the esophagus, crop, and proventriculus (Figure 8).

[i]Emtryl®, Salsbury Labs, Charles City, IA 50616.
[j]Flagyl®, Searle & Co., San Juan, PR 00936.
[k]Enheptin®, American Cyanamid Co., Princeton, NJ 08540.
[l]Ipropran®, Roche Chemical Div., Nutley, NJ 07110.

REFERENCES

1. Vanden Berge JC: Aves myology, in Getty R (ed): *Sisson and Grossman's The Anatomy of the Domestic Animals.* Philadelphia, WB Saunders Co, 1975, p 1803.
2. Koch T: *Anatomy of the Chicken and Domestic Birds.* Ames, IA, The Iowa State University Press, 1973, pp 70-71.
3. Ziswiler V, Farner DS: Digestion and the digestive system, in Farner DS, King JR (eds): *Avian Biology*, vol 2. New York, Academic Press, 1972, pp 343-430.
4. Stone RM: Clinical examination and methods of treatment, in

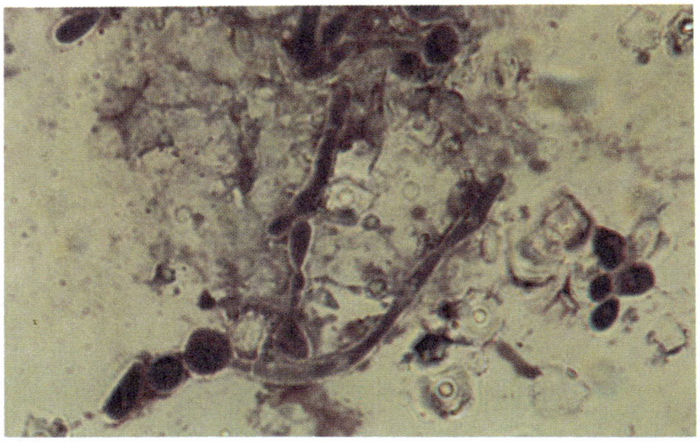

Figure 5—Candidiasis in a young cockatiel. The crop aspirate shows budding yeasts, pseudohyphae, and chlamydospores of *C. albicans*. (Diff Quik, 100×)

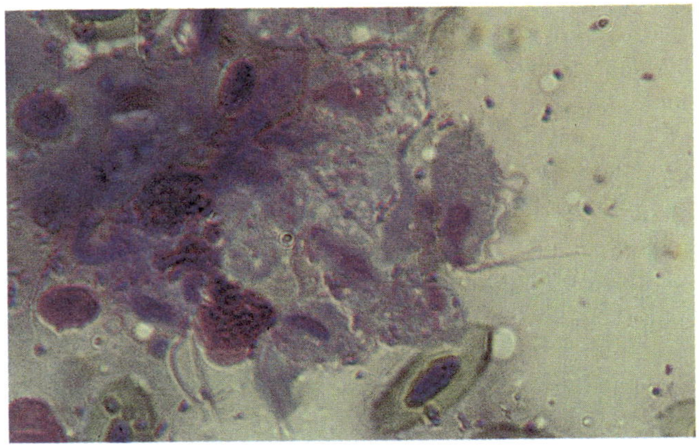

Figure 7—Crop aspirate from a pigeon with trichomoniasis. Note the piriform flagellate protozoa with anterior flagella and the undulating membrane. (Diff Quik, 100×)

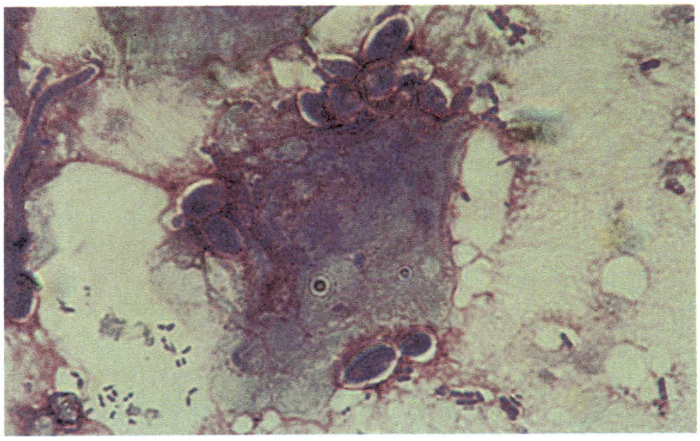

Figure 6—Candidiasis in a yellow-naped Amazon parrot. Note the thin-walled budding yeasts. (Diff Quik, 100×)

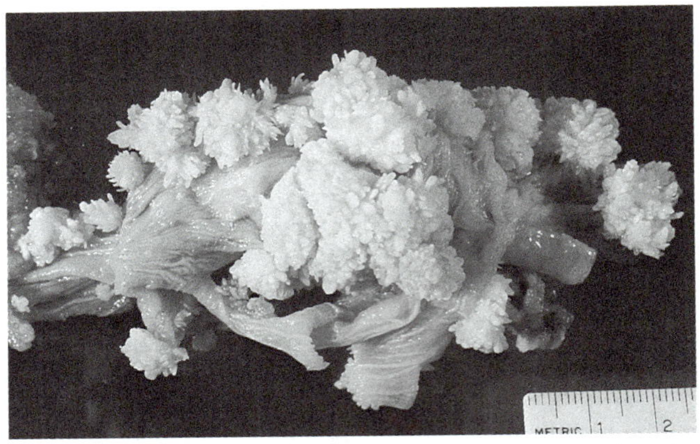

Figure 8—Multiple papillomatous growths partially occluding the esophagus and crop in a green-wing macaw.

Petrak ML (ed): *Diseases of Cage and Aviary Birds*. Philadelphia, Lea & Febiger, 1982, p 261.
5. Duke GE: Raptor physiology, in Fowler ME (ed): *Zoo and Wild Animal Medicine*. Philadelphia, WB Saunders Co, 1978, p 225.
6. McLelland J: Aves digestive system, in Getty R (ed): *Sisson and Grossman's The Anatomy of the Domestic Animals*. Philadelphia, WB Saunders Co, 1975, p 1867.
7. McCauley WJ: *Vertebrate Physiology*. Philadelphia, WB Saunders Co, 1971, p 200.
8. Prosser CL: Nutrition, in Prosser CL (ed): *Comparative Animal Physiology*. Philadelphia, WB Saunders Co, 1973, p 134.
9. Ivorec-Szylit O, Mercier C, Raibaud P, Calet C: Contribution a l'e'tude de la de'gradation des glucides dans le jabot du Coq. Influence du taux de glucose du re'gime sur l'utilisation de l'amidon. C.R. *Acad Sci* 261:3201-3203, 1965.
10. Stunkard JA: *A Guide to Diagnosis, Treatment and Husbandry of Caged Birds*. Bonner Springs, KS, Veterinary Medicine Publishing Co, 1980.
11. Arnall L, Keymer IF: *Bird Diseases*. Neptune City, NJ, TFH Publications, Inc, 1975.
12. Schmidt-Nielsen K: *Animal Physiology*. Cambridge, Cambridge University Press, 1979, p 128.
13. Spira A: Practice tips from an avian practice. *Proc AAHA 47th Annual Meeting*:56, 1980.
14. Galvin C: Laboratory diagnostic aids in pet bird practice. *Proc AAHA 47th Annual Meeting*:50, 1980.
15. Altman R: Radiology, in Fowler ME (ed): *Zoo and Wild Animal Medicine*. Philadelphia, WB Saunders Co, 1978, pp 364-367.
16. Evans SM: Avian radiographic diagnosis. *Compend Contin Educ Pract Vet* 3(7):660-666, 1981.
17. Rosskopf WJ, Woerpel RW, Pitts BJ: Cropotomy in a parrot. *Mod Vet Pract* 63(3):219-222, 1982.
18. Redig P: Orthopedic and soft tissue surgery in raptorial birds, in Fowler ME (ed): *Zoo and Wild Animal Medicine*. Philadelphia, WB Saunders Co, 1978, pp 246-253.
19. Madill DN: Avian Surgery, in Hungerford TG (ed): *Proceedings No. 55 Refresher Course on Aviary and Caged Birds*. Sydney, Australia, The Post-graduate Committee in Veterinary Science, 1981, pp 208-209.
20. Amand WB: General techniques for avian surgery, in Kirk RW (ed): *Current Veterinary Therapy VI*. Philadelphia, WB Saunders Co, 1977, p 713.
21. Gandal CP: Anesthetic and surgical techniques, in Petrak ML (ed): *Diseases of Cage and Aviary Birds*. Philadelphia, Lea & Febiger, 1982, p 316.
22. Brooks NG: Crop wall necrosis in a sparrowhawk. *Vet Rec* 111(22):513, 1982.
23. Pepper WJ: Crop wall necrosis. *Vet Rec* 111(25/26):591, 1982.
24. Lafeber TJ: Respiratory diseases. *Vet Clin North Am* 3(2):218, 1973.
25. Altman RB: Conditions involving the integumentary system, in Petrak ML (ed): *Diseases of Cage and Aviary Birds*. Philadelphia, Lea & Febiger, 1982, pp 368-381.
26. Minsky L, Petrak ML: Diseases of the digestive system, in Petrak ML (ed): *Diseases of Cage and Aviary Birds*. Philadelphia, Lea & Febiger, 1982, pp 432-448.
27. Schultz DJ: Alimentary tract disease, in Hungerford TG (ed):

Proceedings No. 55 Refresher Course on Aviary and Caged Birds. Sydney, Australia, The Post-graduate Committee in Veterinary Science, 1981, pp 535-562.
28. Hurst GA: Crop impactions in bobwhite quail in Louisiana. *J Wildl Dis* 14:355-357, 1978.
29. Jarvis RL: Soybean impaction of waterfowl, in Hoff GL, Davis JW (eds): *Noninfectious Diseases of Wildlife*. Ames, IA, The Iowa State University Press, 1982, pp 109-112.
30. Halliwell WH: Diseases of birds of prey. *Vet Clin North Am* 9(3):541-568, 1979.
31. Batwell R: Crop lithiasis in a budgerigar. *Aust Vet J* 54:452-453, 1978.
32. Eamens GJ: Zoonoses and other human diseases associated with aviary and cage birds, in Hungerford TG (ed): *Proceedings No. 55 Refresher Course on Aviary and Caged Birds*. Sydney, Australia, The Post-graduate Committee in Veterinary Science, 1981, p 546.
33. Perry RA: Aspects of examination, diseases and therapy of caged birds, in Hungerford TG (ed): *Proceedings No. 55 Refresher Course on Aviary and Caged Birds*. Sydney, Australia, The Post-graduate Committee in Veterinary Science, 1981, p 118.
34. Kocan RM, Hasenclever HF: Normal yeast flora of the upper digestive tract of some wild columbids. *J Wildl Dis* 8:365-368, 1972.
35. Kocan RM, Hasenclever HF: Seasonal variation of the upper digestive tract yeast flora of feral pigeons. *J Wildl Dis* 10:263-266, 1974.
36. Jungerman PF, Schwartzman RM: *Veterinary Medical Mycology*. Philadelphia, Lea & Febiger, 1972.
37. Clubb SL: Infectious diseases. *Proc 1982 Annual Meeting of the AAV*:91-119, 1982.
38. Humphreys PN: Debilitating syndrome in budgerigars. *Vet Rec* 101:248-249, 1977.
39. Beemer AM, Kuttin ES, Katz Z: Epidemic venereal disease due to *Candida albicans* in geese in Israel. *Avian Dis* 17:639-649, 1973.
40. Chute HL: Fungal infections, in Hofstad MS (ed): *Diseases of Poultry*. Ames, IA, The Iowa State University Press, 1972, pp 458-463.
41. Carter GR: *Essentials of Veterinary Bacteriology and Mycology*. East Lansing, MI, Michigan State University Press, 1976.
42. Woerpel RW, Rosskopf WJ: Avian therapeutics. *Mod Vet Pract* 62:947-949, 1981.
43. Wood NA: Treatment of established infections of candidiasis in partridges with formic acid. *Vet Rec* 87:656-658, 1970.
44. Keymer IF: Parasitic diseases, in Petrak ML (ed): *Diseases of Cage and Aviary Birds*, Philadelphia, Lea & Febiger, 1982, pp 538-539.
45. Levine ND: *Protozoan Parasites of Domestic Animals and of Man*. Minneapolis, Burgess Publishing Co, 1973, pp 102-104.
46. Ahmed A, Pandurang A, Acharya RS, Ali G: Some observations on trichomoniasis of the upper digestive tract of love birds (budgerigars) in Hyderabad, Andhra Pradesh. *Indian Vet J* 47:210-212, 1970.
47. Griffiths HJ: *A Handbook of Veterinary Parasitology*. Minneapolis, University of Minnesota Press, 1978.
48. Soulsby EJL: *Helminths, Arthropods and Protozoa of Domesticated Animals*. Philadelphia, Lea & Febiger, 1982, pp 562-564.
49. Greve JH: Parasitic diseases, in Fowler ME (ed): *Zoo and Wild Animal Medicine*. Philadelphia, WB Saunders Co, 1978, p 380.
50. Conrad R: Pigeons-hygromycin-trichomoniasis. *Proc 19th Western Poultry Disease Conference, 4th Poultry Health Symposia*:15, 1970.
51. Kocan RM, Banko W: Trichomoniasis in the Hawaiian barred dove. *J Wildl Dis* 10:359-360, 1974.
52. Fowler ME: Doves, hornbills, toucans, and tinamous, in Fowler ME (ed): *Zoo and Wild Animal Medicine*. Philadelphia, WB Saunders Co, 1978, p 330.
53. Petrak ML, Gilmore CE: Neoplasms, in Petrak ML (ed): *Diseases of Cage and Aviary Birds*. Philadelphia, Lea & Febiger, 1982, pp 623-624.
54. Campbell TW: Unpublished case report, Kansas State University, 1981.

UPDATE

Capillariasis can occasionally affect the oral cavity, esophagus, and crop of birds. *Capillaria* spp. cause thickening of the crop mucosa and can be identified by the presence of the characteristic double operculated oval ova in crop aspirate or swab samples. Anthelmintics such as fenbendazole (Panacur®—American Hoechst Corporation), 10 to 50 mg/kg body weight given orally once a day for five days, or mebendazole (Telmintic™—Pitman-Moore), 25 mg/kg body weight given orally twice a day for five days, can be used for the treatment of capillariasis.

During the physical examination, the esophageal and crop mucosa can be inspected by direct endoscopy.

General Principles of Avian Surgery

Veterinary Surgical Associates, Inc.
Coral Springs, Florida
Douglas M. MacCoy, DVM

KEY FACTS

- **Before starting a procedure, the practitioner should have all materials ready; significant time can be spent retrieving instruments.**
- **Drapes should allow the anesthetist to monitor the patient visually for general depth of anesthesia and should provide a sterile barrier for the surgical field.**
- **Because of small patient size, rapid heat loss, and the lack of easily recognized indicators of anesthetic depth, general anesthesia in birds is more risky than in mammals.**
- **With some modifications, Kirschner-Ehmer external fixators are useful in birds.**
- **Visualization is crucial; a good light source and meticulous hemostasis are necessary for success.**

Before beginning a procedure, it is important to have all materials ready. A significant amount of time can be lost gathering instruments. Preparation for surgery in birds is different from that in mammals. Feather plucking should be done during anesthesia; preparation time thus markedly increases total anesthesia time. Because avian skin is delicate compared with mammalian skin, care must be taken to avoid skin tears during removal of feathers.[1,2]

PREPARATIONS FOR SURGERY

Even though preparation is difficult, a wide area must be cleared to allow truly aseptic surgery. Feather loss can be minimized if a featherless (apteric) area can be used for the center of the incision site or if sterile, water-soluble lubricating jelly can be applied to surrounding feathers.

Care must be taken in scrubbing the site. Gentle cleansing using cotton balls instead of gauze sponges minimizes skin trauma. If an adhesive drape is used during the procedure, the site must be dried with sterile cotton. If towel clamps are used, the site may be sprayed with antiseptic solution and left to dry. To protect personnel from injury, the feet and talons of birds of prey should be wrapped around a ball of gauze and covered with bandage material.

Acceptable cleansing agents include chlorhexidine diacetate 0.05%, povidone-iodine 1%, or chlorhexidine gluconate 4%. Chlorhexidine diacetate seems to be the least irritating and has broad antimicrobial activity and long residual activity.

DRAPES

Drapes should allow the anesthetist to monitor the patient visually for general depth of anesthesia and should provide a sterile barrier for the surgical field. A transparent drape (Avian drape sheet, fenestrated, #8263V-ST—General Econopak, Philadelphia, PA) is ideal for the anesthetist and helps the surgeon by allowing good visualization of surrounding structures for orientation. A secondary benefit is the heat-retaining characteristics of plastic film.[3]

Although the transparent drape may be large enough for simple procedures or small birds, it is usually inadequate for large species or involved procedures. In such cases, the plastic drape must be covered with an impermeable, lightweight overdrape, such as a disposable paper drape (Drape sheet 60 × 80-inch [8206V] or 40 × 40-inch [8203V]—General Econopak).

Updated from original publication in Volume 13, Number 6, June 1991

In draping wings, just the incision site should be covered with plastic drapes. If both sides of the wing must be accessible, complete feather removal is performed and the entire area is prepared. Areas outside the surgical field may be wrapped in a sterile towel or sterile adhesive strips (Econo-Tape® [8138V-STV]—General Econopak) or covered with sterilized manila envelopes. Where possible, towel clamps should be placed around the feather shafts rather than through the easily torn skin.

Heating pads should be used for all avian patients except arctic birds, in which ice packs are substituted. The safest pads are circulating water pads (Hamilton Aquamatic®—Hamilton Industries, Cincinnati, OH), which provide even, nonburning heat. Hot-water bottles (which can be made from surgical gloves or ziplock bags) serve for short periods but drain heat from the patient as they cool.

Clear drapes also are available from Veterinary Specialty Products (Boca Raton, FL), Incise (Johnson & Johnson), and Iodophor (3M).

INSTRUMENTS

Small, delicate instruments allow the surgeon to manipulate small organs and see the tissue past the tip of the instrument.[4] Curved-tip instruments with thin tips enhance visualization. Mosquito forceps (Halsted curved mosquito forceps, 5-inch, 18-2310—Pilling Co, Fort Washington, PA) are good hemostatic forceps for general use. Tiny serrefine clamps (Serrefine, 1.5-inch, 18-2210—Pilling Co) may be needed for budgerigars and canaries.

Bipolar cautery (Surgitron™—Ellman International Manufacturing, Hewlett, NY) is an excellent way to achieve hemostasis for small vessels. Carefully controlled use of cutting currents can decrease bleeding and surgical time. Stainless steel hemostatic clips (Hemoclip®—Edward Weck & Co, Research Triangle Park, NC) are a good alternative to hand ligation of vessels that cannot be cauterized.

Magnification of the surgical site is strongly suggested. This can be accomplished by the use of surgical loops of 1.5 to 3 times magnification or by surgical or dissecting microscopes (Prescott's, Inc., Monument, CO). Microsurgical instrumentation also is very beneficial for manipulation of delicate avian tissues and is available from a variety of sources. Suture material in the 6-0 to 9-0 range may be needed for vascular work, with larger sizes for more general suturing.

For cutting and dissecting, fine Metzenbaum or Lahey scissors (curved Lahey scissors, 5.75-inch, 14-1452—Pilling Co) or tenotomy scissors (Curved Stevens tenotomy scissors, OP5690-V. Mueller) are good choices. Retraction of tissue can be done with thumb forceps (Adson thumb forceps #18-1223—Pilling Co), self-retaining ophthalmic retractors (Alm retractor SU 3147—V. Mueller), or handheld retractors (Senn retractor #16-4752—Pilling Co). Care must be taken to avoid hanging instruments from the patient; the weight may cause damage.

ANESTHESIA

Because of small patient size, rapid heat loss, and lack of easily recognized indicators of anesthetic depth, general anesthesia holds greater risks for birds than for mammals. Preanesthetic agents are not normally needed unless there are problems with copious oral secretions or bradycardia. Atropine tends to thicken tracheal secretions; such thickening might lead to endotracheal tube obstruction. Atropine can be given intramuscularly at a dose of 0.04 mg/kg.

Diazepam (0.1 mg/kg) can be used to reduce excitement or in combination with an injectable induction agent. Ketamine hydrochloride can be given intravenously (beginning at 5 mg/kg) for rapid induction of a hypnotic state, which allows intubation or minor procedures.[5] This dose combined with intravenous diazepam (0.1 mg/kg) provides light general anesthesia.[6]

With the advent of isoflurane and the availability of precision vaporizers for use with the agent, there is little reason to use anything else.[7] Isoflurane is a safe anesthetic with the advantage of rapid induction and rapid recovery. Induction may be performed via face mask at 4% to 5% concentrations; maintenance is usually at 2% to 3%. High flow rates (two to three liters per minute) are usually used for induction; rates of 0.5 to 1.0 liters per minute are used for maintenance.

Minimal cardiac arrhythmias occur with this agent; profound respiratory depression is possible with high concentrations. If a concentration above 3% is necessary, the setup should be reviewed to be sure that no tubes are kinked or occluded with mucus and that the respirations are deep enough to ensure gas exchange. The practitioner should be prepared for a rapid recovery and should plan to support the patient until it is ready to perch (in 5 to 15 minutes).

Trachea intubation is possible in large birds; in small species, mask inhalation must be used. The practitioner should be prepared for breath holding in aquatic species and should not hesitate to assist respiration. A nonrebreathing system should be used in all cases.

Complete control of ventilation is possible via reverse-flow, positive-pressure ventilation administered through the interclavicular or caudal thoracic air sac with a suitable catheter.[8,9] Gas flow through the air sacs is slowly increased until respirations cease. During recovery, spontaneous respirations should begin 60 to 90 seconds after gas flow through the air sac cannula is discontinued.

Immediately after surgery, an ambient temperature of

85°F to 90°F should be provided until the patient has completely recovered. A darkened recovery box minimizes struggling. Patients that are excitable, have very fragile limbs, or exhibit violent recovery should be wrapped in towels and held by hand until danger subsides. Corticosteroids and fluids are administered as required for shock or blood loss.

Respiratory and apnea monitors (Medical Engineering, Jackson, MI) have been adapted for use in small birds. Normal respiratory rates are reported as 55 to 75 minutes for budgies, 10 to 20 for larger parrots, and 2 to 20 for ostriches. It has been determined that a 10°F drop in body temperature can predispose birds to arrhythmia and prolong recovery times. As body temperature drops, anesthetic gas levels should be decreased.[9a]

Normal reflexes checked to evaluate anesthetic depth (e.g., palpebral response and response to toe pinching) are not as reliable in birds as in mammals. Other signs must also be observed. The respiratory rate should not be allowed to decrease below six breaths/min in any size bird. It is generally advisable to decrease anesthetic depth or support respirations if the rate drops more than one third of the initial rate during the procedure. The same is true of the heart rate. An electrocardiography unit that is equipped with an oscilloscope display should be used to monitor the heart rate.

Special caution must be exercised with supported respirations; the air sacs and lungs of birds are not as elastic as the lungs of mammals. The practitioner should observe expansion of the keel when the bird is awake and should not exceed that degree of movement with supported breathing. Properly performed assisted respiration provides a steady anesthetic depth while ensuring proper oxygenation.

It is necessary to be alert for decreased tidal volume or slowed expiratory flow caused by accumulation of mucus in the endotracheal tube or trachea. Suction (by machine or syringe and urinary catheter) should be available to clear secretions.

As the anesthetic period increases, body temperature decreases markedly (heat loss from warming the inspired gas and humidifying it at one liter of flow is approximately 37 cal/min).[10] Hypothermia allows reduced dosages of anesthetic agents.

FRACTURE REPAIR

The goals of fracture repair in birds are identical to those in mammals. Of first importance is accurate alignment of the fragments to maintain the normal biomechanics of the part. Second is the need to achieve rigid stabilization of the fracture fragments. This stabilization promotes rapid, firm callus formation; allows rapid growth of blood vessels; and minimizes the damage to adjacent structures and the risk of trapping nerves, vessels, or muscles between fragments.

When fractures occur near joints, the prognosis for function is worse because of the potential damage to articular cartilage and periarticular support structures. Proximal limb fractures often have less effect on limb function, perhaps because of a decreased need for delicate movement of the large bones and muscle masses. The further distal a fracture is located, the poorer the prognosis.

Massive soft tissue damage and direct tissue loss limit blood supply to the fracture. This limitation may result in delayed union or nonunion of the fracture. The increased adhesions associated with scar tissue may directly limit muscle and joint movement. It is important but difficult to evaluate nerve function in the injured limb. Damage to motor nerves may preclude normal function of the limb regardless of what happens to the fracture.

Easily overlooked is the damage surgical intervention may add to the existing injury. Vessels, nerves, and muscles are manipulated during surgical repair; iatrogenic injury is a risk. The surgeon must determine what structures will be affected by the surgical approach and fixation devices and must consider the sequelae of surgical and conservative therapy. If the sequelae of conservative therapy are no worse than those of surgery and if equal function will be gained, then the risks of surgery and general anesthesia are not justified.

External stabilization by bandaging can be an excellent way to manage fractures temporarily or, in some cases, as primary treatment. Because of the streamlined curves of the avian body, simply holding the humerus or femur against the body can produce reasonable reduction. Standard adhesive tape, or sticking plaster, is not appropriate for use in birds; glue may remain on the feathers after tape removal, attracting dirt and preventing proper preening. Appropriate materials are masking tape, draftsman tape, wound tape, or self-adhesive materials. Commonly used splint materials are wooden applicator sticks, wooden tongue depressors, soda straws, and lightweight plastic or fiberglass cast materials. With some modifications, Kirschner-Ehmer external fixators are useful in birds. The weight of the device must be reduced as much as possible by the use of small pins (not more than 20% of the diameter of the bone) and lightweight connecting bars (e.g., of cast epoxy).[11]

The device should be as small as possible. The device should be positioned as close to the skin as is consistent with good medical practice. This position decreases the risk of damage to the fixator by catching on cage bars or perches. The device must also be protected from the powerful beak of a large psittacine bird.

There are several configurations of Kirschner-Ehmer splints: type Ia double clamp, type Ia single bar, type Ia double bar, type Ib, type II, and type III. Type Ia single bar and type II splints are usually used because of their simplicity.

Intramedullary pins in avian fracture fixation provide the same advantages as in mammals. In birds, however, placing pins without damaging surrounding structures is difficult because of the pneumatized bones with scant cancellous metaphyseal bone for pin engagement, the thin cortices, and the shape of the wings.[12]

Compared with steel pins, plastic rods have several advantages. They are light; do not require surgical manipulation of tissue away from the fracture site; provide accurate axial alignment of fracture fragments, good rotational stability (even with transverse fractures), and adequate stability for bone healing; are readily available and easily sterilized; and are easily cut with hand tools. The application technique involves shuttling the pin into position.[13]

SOFT TISSUE INJURY

Management of skin injury in birds is complicated by poor skin blood supply, inadequate knowledge of collateral circulation, and the potential for self-mutilation exhibited by some birds. Birds have scant extra skin or skin elasticity to help in the closure of large defects; large wounds usually must be managed open (with supportive medical care) while contracture and epithelialization occur. Large wounds on the extremities may lead to loss of the part as a result of complications of wound care. If degloving occurs, amputation should be strongly considered.

Muscle lacerations usually heal with minimal complications if blood and nerve supplies survive. Simple suturing after cleansing is usually sufficient. Closing muscles that have been divided is difficult because of the tension on the tissue and the damage to the blood supply. Mattress pattern or locking-loop sutures are best in such situations.

Crop lacerations are simple to manage and respond well to cleaning, debridement, and watertight closure. Various suture materials have been used; medium chromic catgut in a simple continuous pattern usually works well if the site is not grossly infected.

Advances have been made in the management of large wounds, with some skin grafting being done.[13a]

ABDOMINAL SURGERY

Abdominal surgery in birds presents special hazards.[14] Because of the lack of a diaphragm, some respiratory compromise and a change in the delivery of anesthetic gases occur when the abdomen and abdominal air sacs are opened. There is a minimum of stretch to the musculature of the abdomen; approaches usually must be centered over the area of interest, and the surgeon must be prepared for limited exposure.

The intestinal vessels are delicate and short; retraction of bowel is thus limited. Care must be taken to avoid tearing vessels free from the bowel. Because visualization is very important, a good light source and meticulous hemostasis are necessary for success. Bipolar cautery should be available during all procedures. Closure of abdominal wounds usually requires only abdominal wall closure and skin sutures.

About the Author

Dr. MacCoy, who is a Diplomate of the American College of Veterinary Surgeons, is affiliated with Veterinary Surgical Associates, Inc., Coral Springs, Florida.

REFERENCES

1. Altman RB: Disorders of the skeletal system, in *Diseases of Cage and Aviary Birds*, ed 2. Philadelphia, Lea & Febiger, 1982, pp 382–394.
2. MacCoy DM: Orthopedic surgery, in *Diseases of Cage and Aviary Birds*, ed 3. Philadelphia, Lea & Febiger, 1991, pp 312–313.
3. MacCoy DM: I.M.E. #589: Commercially available, clear, adhesive drape designed specifically for bird surgery. *Newsletter Assoc Avian Vet* 6(2):57, 1985.
4. MacCoy DM: Avian fracture management. *Proc Avian/Exotic Anim Med Symp*:63–74, 1990.
5. Boever WJ, Wright W: Use of ketamine for restraint and anesthesia of birds. *VM SAC* 70:86–88, 1975.
6. Redig PT, Duke GE: Intravenously administered ketamine HCl and diazepam for anesthesia of raptors. *JAVMA* 169(9): 886–888, 1976.
7. Harrison GJ: Anesthesiology, in *Clinical Avian Medicine and Surgery*. Philadelphia, WB Saunders Co, 1986, pp 549–559.
8. Whittow GC, Ossorio N: A new technic for anesthetizing birds. *Lab Anim Care* 20(4):651–656, 1970.
9. Burger RE, Lorenz FW: Artificial respiration in birds by unidirectional air flow. *Poult Sci* 39:236–237, 1960.

9a. La Bonde J, Michel C: Anesthesia monitoring and intraoperative support of the avian patient. *Proc Annu Conf AAV*: 271–274, 1995.

10. Stewart BJ, MacCoy DM: Evaluation of reverse flow anesthesia in birds. Unpublished data, New York State College of Veterinary Medicine, Cornell University, Ithaca, NY, 1979.
11. MacCoy DM: Modified Kirschner splints for application to small birds. *VM SAC* 76:853, 1981.
12. MacCoy DM: Techniques of fracture treatment in birds and their indications: External and internal fixation. *Proc ACVS Forum*:114–118, 1986.
13. MacCoy DM, Sykes G: Evaluation of high density polymers as intramedullary fixation devices in birds. *JAAHA* 19:767, 1983.

13a. Hannon DE, McGehee NW, Weber TD: Use of a single pedicle advancement flap for wound repair in a great horned owl (*Bubo virginianus*). *Proc Annu Conf AAV*:285–289, 1995.

14. Harrison GJ: Intra-abdominal procedures, in *Clinical Avian Medicine and Surgery*. Philadelphia, WB Saunders Co, 1986, pp 585–593.

Avian Anesthesia

Florida Atlantic University
Robert B. Altman, DVM

KEY FACTS

- Careful assessment of an avian patient's cardiopulmonary system is essential before a physical examination is performed.
- The minimal data base for pathologic evaluation should include a packed cell volume, total solids, and serum glucose.
- Radiographs are a valuable adjunct in evaluating the status of avian patients undergoing surgery.
- Neonatal and pediatric patients require more rigorous attention than do their adult counterparts.
- Local anesthesia is infrequently used on birds, while parenteral anesthesia is reserved for use in large species. Isoflurane is the anesthetic of choice for all species of birds.

Before gas anesthesia was used for avian surgery, high mortality and a low success rate discouraged most practitioners from performing surgery on birds. Methoxyflurane and eventually halothane reversed the poor odds, and the introduction of isoflurane[1] significantly improved the statistics by allowing surgeons to perform longer procedures with much higher safety and recovery rates. Today even high-risk complicated procedures have become a daily occurrence for avian clinicians.

Administration of anesthesia for the more complex and lengthier procedures requires a high level of skill and a thorough understanding of patient support. The veterinary anesthetist must not only understand anesthetic regimens but have comprehensive knowledge of physiology, anatomy, critical care techniques, anesthetic monitoring, intraoperative methods of support for stabilizing a patient, and postoperative care and support.

PREANESTHETIC EVALUATION

Any bird undergoing a surgical procedure should have a complete history taken, with as much biologic data accumulated as is practical and affordable. Assessment of the bird's cardiopulmonary system by evaluating stress tolerance is essential. With careful observation of the patient at rest, signs of respiratory distress characterized by increased respiratory rate and effort, increased thoracic excursions, tail bobbing, open-mouthed breathing, or tachypnea (rapid, shallow respirations) should be noted. When possible, correction or alteration of these clinical signs must occur before induction of anesthesia.

After the cardiopulmonary system has been evaluated, the bird should undergo a thorough physical examination. Auscultation is important to assess any areas of air sac involvement as characterized by dull or absent inspiratory and expiratory sounds. If the patient's nares are obstructed with dried exudate, they should be cleared to permit unobstructed nasal breathing.

When the physical examination has been completed, the bird should be returned to its cage and respiratory patterns observed and evaluated again. Any open-mouthed breathing, panting, or increased thoracic excursions that may occur after a bird has been subjected to the stress of handling should return to normal within five minutes. Abnormal breathing patterns persisting beyond five minutes can be indicative of cardiopulmonary abnormalities. If recovery exceeds 10 minutes, cardiopulmonary compromise must be suspected.

An alternate method of evaluating stress is to permit the bird free flight in an enclosed room for three or more minutes, capture the bird and place it in a cage, and observe recovery time. This technique, however, can be awkward if the client is present and the bird resists capture.

First-time publication

TABLE I
Doses for Chemical Anesthetic Agents[12]

Agent	*Patient*	*Dose*
Tiletamine–zolazepam	Most species	10–30 mg/kg IM
Tiletamine–zolazepam	Ratites	2–8 mg/kg IV, 4–12 mg/kg IM
Ketamine	Raptors	15–20 mg/kg IM, IV
	Pigeons, ratites	25–50 mg/kg IM

TABLE II
Doses for Combined Anesthetic Agents[12]

Patient	*Combination Agents*	*Amount*
Psittacines	Diazepam }	10–50 mg/kg IM
	Ketamine }	0.5–2.0 mg/kg IM
	Diazepam }	0.5–2.0 mg/kg IV
	Ketamine }	5–25 mg/kg IV
	Ketamine }	10–30 mg/kg IM
	Xylazine }	2–6 mg/kg IM
Pigeons	Diazepam }	0.5–1.0 mg/kg IM or IV
	Ketamine }	10–25 mg/kg IM or IV
Ratites	Diazepam }	0.1–2.0 mg/kg IV
	Ketamine }	5–10 mg/kg IV
	Ketamine }	10 mg/kg IM
	Xylazine }	0.5–1.0 mg/kg IM

The minimal data base for pathologic evaluation should include a packed cell volume (PCV), total solids, and serum glucose.[1,2] Packed cell volume can determine whether dehydration or anemia is present. A volume exceeding 55% requires administration of 2.5% dextrose in half-strength saline before and during the surgical episode. For low normal or mildly decreased glucose levels, subcutaneous fluids usually suffice. For very low glucose levels, intravenous or intraosseous administration is necessary.

Anemic birds (PCV < 20%) should not undergo surgery until the anemia has been treated. If surgery is essential, a blood transfusion could be lifesaving; however, the safety and efficacy of blood transfusions are controversial. Some authors[3] believe that the half-life survival time of red blood cells is too short to be of value. Others authors[4,5] (including me) believe that blood transfusions can be lifesaving. Homologous transfusions are certainly of greater benefit; however, in critical emergency situations, heterologous transfusions have apparently been beneficial. Crossmatching is essential to avoid fatal transfusion reactions. A simple crossmatch can be performed by mixing red blood cells from the donor with serum from the recipient. If immediate agglutination occurs, the blood is incompatible.

Total solids can be determined by placing a drop of serum on a refractometer to assess total protein levels.

Serum glucose levels should be evaluated before administration of anesthesia. Reestablishing glucose levels in hypoglycemic patients or patients in the low normal range is critical.

A complete chemistry panel, including aspartate aminotransferase (AST), uric acid, and calcium, can be beneficial in evaluating the patient. Time, affordability, or the size or physical condition of the patient may, however, preclude completing a chemistry panel.

Radiographs are a valuable adjunct in evaluating the status of surgical patients. Assessing the skeletal structures and the respiratory system is of particular benefit. Birds demonstrating respiratory abnormalities, egg-bound birds, and orthopedic cases require radiographs. Many birds with respiratory conditions (e.g., aspergillosis) or with bacterial infection can be asymptomatic on presentation but are poor anesthetic risks. Birds with poorly calcified bones must be handled with care to avoid iatrogenic fracture.

Although not essential, performing a cloacal Gram's stain can alert the clinician to the presence of heavy gram-negative bacterial flora that require antibiotics before and after surgery. Proliferation of bacterial organisms can cause immunosuppression enhanced by surgical stress. Antibiotic therapy, however, should not be a routine regimen after surgery.

Developing a comprehensive data base is essential for determining pre- and intraanesthetic surgical support and stabilization of the patient. Correction of all abnormal physiologic findings should be attempted and the patient stabilized before anesthetic induction.

ANESTHETIC CONSIDERATIONS IN NEONATAL AND PEDIATRIC PATIENTS

Neonatal and pediatric patients require more scrutiny and attention than adults do. Organ development is immature in younger birds, and renal and hepatic function have not fully developed. Anesthetic detoxification in many instances can be prolonged. Because the rate of oxygen consumption is two to three times greater than that of adults, the respiratory rate must be two to three

TABLE III
Anesthetic Induction and Maintenance

	Methoxyflurane	*Halothane*	*Isoflurane*
Induction			
Time	4–8 min	1–5 min	1–4 min
Concentration	3% to 4%	2% to 3%	3% to 4%
Oxygen flow rate	0.5–2.0 L/min	0.5–2.0 L/min	1–2 L/min
Maintenance			
Recovery time	10–20 min	3–8 min	2–5 min
Concentration	0.25% to 0.5%	0.5% to 1.5%	1.5% to 2.5%
Oxygen flow rate	0.5–1.0 L/min	0.5–1.0 L/min	0.5–1.5 L/min

times greater to meet the oxygen demand. The high respiratory rate must be maintained to avoid excessive carbon dioxide buildup and resultant hypoxemia.

Baby birds have a large body surface-to-volume ratio and an immature, poorly developed thermoregulatory system. Because many birds are hatched featherless, hypothermia becomes a major problem. Body temperature therefore must be monitored and supplemental heat provided throughout surgery and the recovery period. The heart rate also must be monitored to detect bradyarrhythmia. Hypoglycemia can occur because of rapid depletion of glycogen reserves. Dehydration is also a major risk because baby birds have a high fluid requirement and rapid fluid loss, particularly during prolonged surgical procedures. Meticulous hemostasis is essential because neonates are particularly susceptible to blood loss, which can result in hypovolemic shock.

ANESTHETIC AGENTS

Local Anesthesia

Local anesthesia is infrequently used because the stress of restraint is not eliminated, the margin of safety (which is dose related) is narrow, and the requirement for local anesthesia is minimal. Lidocaine toxicity is characterized by excitement, depression, seizures, cardiovascular collapse, and respiratory arrest.[6]

Topical anesthesia using anesthetic ointments to relieve discomfort of the skin or cloacal mucosa and ophthalmic anesthetic drops are beneficial but should be used sparingly.

Parenteral Anesthesia

Parenteral anesthesia is reserved for use in large species, primarily as a preanesthetic for restraint and for short surgical procedures. The benzodiazepines (diazepam, zolazepam, midazolam) produce a sedative effect with muscle relaxation and anticonvulsant effects. Benzodiazepines cause ataxia and incoordination, have poor analgesic properties,[7] and are unpredictable in their effect. Diazepam, when given rapidly in an intravenous route to hypovolemic birds, can cause hypotension and cardiac arrest. Benzodiazepines are used most effectively when combined with dissociative anesthetics.

The combination of zolazepam and tiletamine is used effectively for restraint during radiologic procedures, as a preanesthetic for large birds, and during ultrashort surgical procedures. There is considerable dose variation in the different avian species (Table I) and poor analgesic effect.

Ketamine has been used in avian anesthesia for many years. This dissociative anesthetic does not inhibit ocular reflexes, produces inadequate muscle relaxation, has a wide dose variation, and often causes excitatory activity characterized by fluttering and seizures during induction. Diazepam must be administered to control the seizures. Prolonged recovery with excitatory activity can also occur. Ketamine depresses cardiac contractility, which can cause cardiac arrest, particularly in birds with marginal cardiovascular reserves.[6] Another major disadvantage of ketamine is its inability to offer adequate analgesic effect. Because of its disadvantages, it is infrequently used alone. It is used most often in conjunction with other anesthetic agents, such as diazepam or xylazine. Table I lists doses for ketamine.

A diazepam–ketamine combination can increase the duration of anesthesia, can improve muscle relaxation, has a longer recovery period, and is safer than a xylazine–ketamine combination because diazepam–ketamine does not produce as much cardiopulmonary depression. Table II lists doses for psittacines, pigeons, and ratites. In raptors, slow intravenous administration or divided doses were used successfully[8] at a dose of 1 to 1.5 mg/kg diazepam and 30 to 40 mg/kg ketamine. Xylazine–ketamine is used by mixing equal parts of xylazine (20 mg/ml) with ketamine (100 mg/ml) for psittacines. The mixture should be administered intramuscularly. Table II lists doses. With xylazine–ketamine, improved muscle relaxation and analgesia occur and a shorter recovery period is required; however, the potential for cardiac complications is increased compared with the use of a diazepam–ketamine combination.

Medetomidine in combination with ketamine has

been used in Europe. Medetomidine is not available in the United States.

Inhalation Anesthesia

The four inhalation anesthetic agents currently being used are nitrous oxide, methoxyflurane, halothane, and isoflurane.

Nitrous oxide is used infrequently for avian anesthesia. Although it has rapid uptake and excretion, provides good analgesic action, and enhances the effect of other anesthetic gases being used concurrently, nitrous oxide can cause cardiovascular depression.[6] It has been used to some degree in ratites but has very little application for general avian anesthesia.

Methoxyflurane was the first inhalation anesthetic with a relatively wide margin of safety that permitted longer surgical procedures with lower anesthetic mortality. With the introduction of halothane and particularly isoflurane, however, methoxyflurane should no longer be a choice of anesthetic agent. Table III lists induction and maintenance times and concentrations for methoxyflurane.

Halothane was considered an effective and relatively safe anesthetic agent until the introduction of isoflurane. Because halothane causes myocardial sensitization to catecholamine-induced arrhythmia and has been incriminated in causing hepatotoxicity to both the patient and operating room personnel,[9] isoflurane is currently the anesthetic of choice. In addition, unless a very effective waste-gas evacuation system is used, halothane levels can quickly rise above OSHA–accepted levels, placing operating room personnel at risk and exposing the hospital owner to possible fines and litigation. Because halothane vaporizers can easily be converted for use with isoflurane, there is little reason not to convert to isoflurane. Table III lists induction and maintenance levels for halothane.

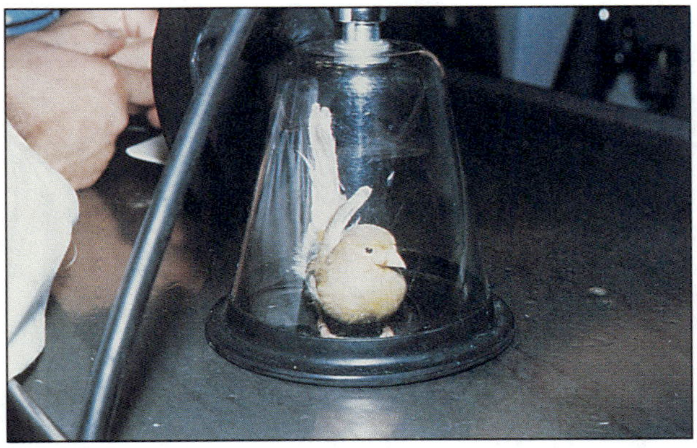

Figure 1A

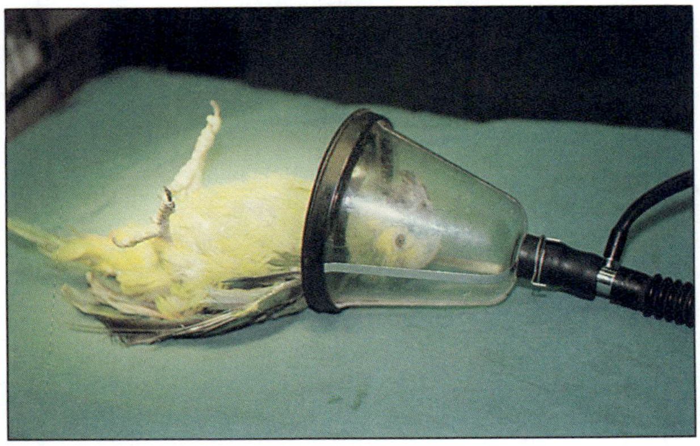

Figure 1B

Figure 1—(**A**) A canary is placed into a facemask and observed during induction of anesthesia. (**B**) The parrot's head is carefully inserted into the facemask. As soon as induction has been accomplished, the bird should be intubated.

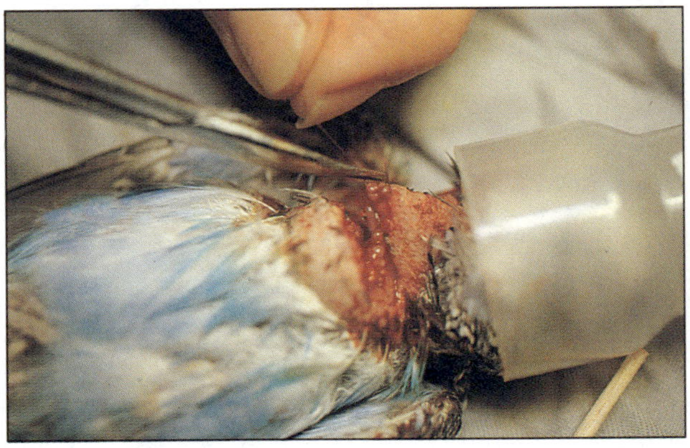

Figure 2—To maintain anesthesia, a budgerigar's head is inserted into a modified 30-cc syringe case. This method, however, allows leakage of waste gas into the operating room.

Isoflurane is unquestionably the anesthetic of choice for all species of birds. It has the most rapid induction and recovery. Because isoflurane is insoluble in blood, birds can recover sufficiently to perch and fly in as few as three to five minutes after cessation of the gas. With isoflurane, there is less depression of cardiac output than occurs with other volatile anesthetic agents and apparently no associated hepatotoxicity. Some dose-dependent cardiopulmonary depression and decreases in blood pressure can, however, occur. Table III lists induction and maintenance levels.

During long surgical procedures (in excess of 10 minutes), the bird should be ventilated three times per minute throughout the anesthetic period. Gentle pressure on the nonrebreathing bag can avoid damaging the air sacs. Just enough pressure should be placed on the bag to accomplish a slight thoracic rise.

ADMINISTRATION OF ANESTHESIA

For birds weighing less than 10 to 11 kg, a nonrebreathing system, such as the Ayre's T-piece, should be used to minimize dead space and resistance. An accurately calibrated vaporizer must be used. Every bird large enough to be intubated should have an endotracheal tube gently placed into the trachea to deliver the anesthetic, secure a means of ventilation, and minimize the escape of waste gas into the operating room.

For induction, the patient can be placed in an anesthetic chamber and monitored until there is enough relaxation to allow intubation. A standard small animal facemask can be used. Small birds can be placed directly into the mask (Figure 1A) and the mask placed on the table with the opening against the table to minimize leakage. For larger birds (weighing more than 100 grams), the bird's head can be placed into the mask and a hand towel used to close the opening (Figure 1B). When inserting the bird's head, care should be taken to avoid having the bird bite the rubber dam covering the opening of the mask. As soon as the bird is relaxed and can be intubated, the head should be removed from the mask.

Large birds, such as ratites, must be given a preanesthetic agent and then intubated. Once anesthetized, small birds that cannot be intubated can have the gas delivered by way of a facemask made from a 30-ml syringe casing (Figure 2).

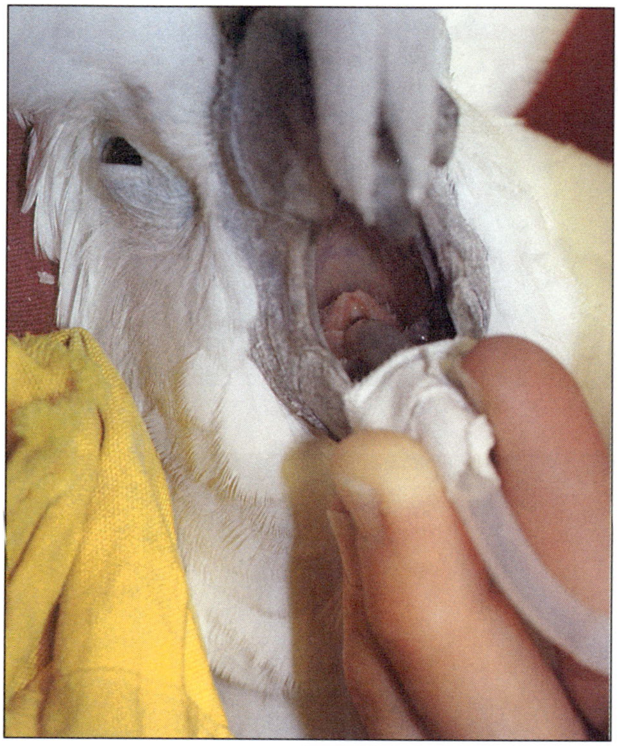

Figure 3—The endotracheal tube is gently passed into the trachea through the glottis and secured to the beak. (Courtesy of Dr. Michael Doolen, Oakhurst Veterinary Hospital, Oakhurst, New Jersey)

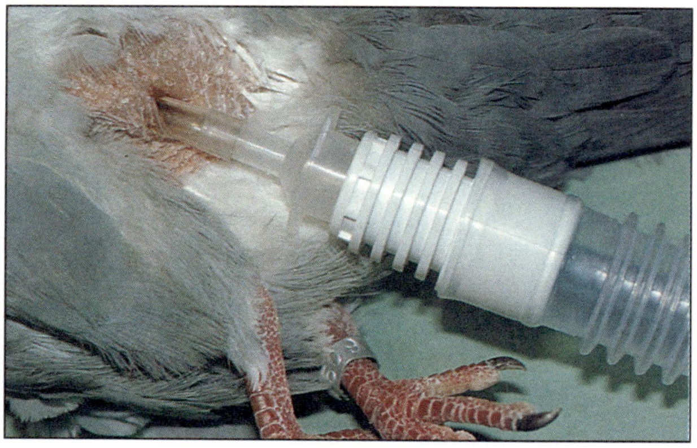

Figure 4—Placement of an air sac tube in a pigeon caudal to the left thigh. (Courtesy of Dr. Michael Doolen, Oakhurst Veterinary Hospital, Oakhurst, New Jersey)

Intubation

Endotracheal intubation must be done carefully to avoid injuring the trachea. Birds have complete tracheal rings and therefore no elasticity of the trachea. Tracheal tubes must first be tested for patency and then slightly lubricated with water and passed into the glottis on inspiration or expiration (Figure 3). If a cuffed tube is being used, the cuff should be placed just beyond the glottis. In psittacines, placing digital pressure at the base of the tongue under the mandible can elevate the glottis and facilitate passage of the tube.

All endotracheal tubes should be cut down to reduce dead space. When inflating the balloon, enough air should be used to move the walls of the balloon slightly. Excessive pressure can rupture the tracheal rings or compress the tracheal mucosa and cause ischemia and sloughing. In neonatal and pediatric patients, extreme care must be taken during intubation because of the small size and friability of the glottis and trachea.

In psittacines, the endotracheal tube should be secured by taping the tube to the maxilla, unless the area within the mouth or the maxilla itself is the area to be worked on. A flap should always be placed on the end of the tape to permit rapid removal in the event of an emergency.

For small birds, noncuffed or Cole tubes can be used. The smallest cuffed tube available is 2.5 mm in diameter. For surgery of the mouth or trachea or in emergency situations in which there is occlusion of the airways, placement of an air sac tube allows the bird to breathe in the event of airway obstruction and permits uninterrupted administration of anesthesia[10] (Figure 4).

Anesthetic Monitoring

The anesthetist's singular responsibility is to monitor the patient constantly while administering the anesthesia. The surgeon's job is to perform the surgical procedure as quickly and efficiently as possible and get the patient to recovery. The surgeon must therefore have no responsibilities for anesthesia. A third person can act as circulating nurse and supply any necessary assistance.

Although many reflexes (e.g., corneal, palpebral, cere, and pedal) can be evaluated, they are difficult to ascertain and interpret. The only accurate means of monitoring anesthesia is to visualize thoracic movement. Transparent surgical drapes are therefore necessary. It is important that no pressure be placed on the drape or on the bird's thorax.

The ideal plane of surgical anesthesia is characterized by slow, regular, and deep respirations, with slight corneal and pedal reflexes. If respirations are shallow or all reflexes are absent, the patient is anesthetized too deeply; apnea can result.

For surgical procedures in excess of 10 minutes, body temperature and heart rate must be monitored. Electronic thermometers are available for measuring body temperature. The bird should be placed on a heating platform or circulating hot water jacket throughout the procedure to combat heat loss and hypothermia associated with inhalation anesthesia.

The heart rate should be followed throughout the procedure; however, small changes in rate are difficult to evaluate and arrhythmia usually cannot be detected. An electrocardiograph or cardiac monitor is an effective means of monitoring the heart rate. An ultrasonographic Doppler flow apparatus can be used to monitor arterial flow.

At termination of the procedure, the anesthetic gas should be discontinued and the bird maintained on 100% oxygen until reflexes have returned and the bird starts to chew on the endotracheal tube. The bird should then be carefully extubated and, to decrease the potential for orthostatic hypotension, kept from making rapid changes in body position. The bird should be placed in an unobstructed holding area until it is stable and ready to perch. Supplemental heat should be supplied until the bird has completely recovered from anesthesia. Food and water should be offered as soon as the bird is able to perch.

Analgesia

In birds, postoperative discomfort is infrequent. Pain can be associated with such sensitive surgical areas as the feet and the area around the cere. Butorphanol at 0.5 to 2.0 mg/kg intramuscularly and flunixin meglumine at 1 to 10 mg/kg intramuscularly[11] have been used successfully.

About the Author

Dr. Altman has been involved with the practice of small animal, avian, and exotics specialties for almost 40 years. At present, he is Professor of Research at the Florida Atlantic University in Boca Raton, Florida. Dr. Altman is an honorary member of the American Board of Veterinary Practitioners and lectures and writes extensively on avian medicine and surgery.

REFERENCES

1. Altman RB: Avian anesthesia. *Compend Contin Educ Pract Vet* 2(1):38–42, 1980.
2. Sinn LC: Anesthesiology, in Ritchie B, Harrison GJ, Harrison LR (eds): *Avian Medicine: Principles and Applications.* Lake Worth, FL, Wingers Publishing, 1994, pp 1067–1080.
3. Stauber E, Washizuka A, Wilson E, Waredrop J: Cross-matching reactions of blood from various avian species. *Proc 3rd Conf Euro Comm Assoc Avian Vet*:142–144, 1995.
4. Quesenberry KE, Hillyer EV: Supportive care and emergency therapy, in Ritchie B, Harrison GJ, Harrison LR (eds): *Avian Medicine: Principles and Applications.* Lake Worth, FL, Wingers Publishing, 1994, pp 400–401.
5. Bos JH, et al: Treatment of anemic birds with iron dextran therapy: Homologous and heterologous blood transfusions. *Proceed Assoc Avian Vet*:221–225, 1990.
6. Stoelting RK: *Pharmacology and Physiology in Anesthetic Practice.* Philadelphia, JB Lippincott, 1987.
7. Harvey SC: Hypnotics and sedatives, in Gilman AG, Goodman LS, Rall TW, et al (eds): *The Pharmacological Basis of Therapeutics.* New York, MacMillan, 1985, pp 339–371.
8. Redig PT, Duke GE: Intravenously administered ketamine HCl and diazepam for anesthesia of raptors. *JAVMA* 169(9): 886–888, 1976.
9. Altman RB: A method for reducing exposure of operating room personnel to anesthetic gas. *J Assoc Avian Vet* 6(2): 99–101, 1992.
10. Korbel R, et al: Aerosacular perfusion with isoflurane, an anesthetic procedure for head surgery in birds. *Proceed Eur Assoc Avian Vet*:9–37, 1993.
11. Carpenter JW, Mashima TY, Rupiper DJ: *Exotic Animal Formulary.* Manhattan, KS, Greystone Publications, 1996, pp 125–134.

Surgical Correction of Impaction of the Proventriculus in Ostriches

Dallas Zoo and Aquarium
Dallas, Texas
Kathryn C. Gamble, DVM

Texas A&M University
Clifford M. Honnas, DVM

KEY FACTS

- **Impaction of the proventriculus is a common cause of vague, chronic unproductivity and results from consumption of indigestible foreign objects.**
- **Prevention is the most appropriate method of minimizing proventricular impaction.**
- **Typical clinical signs of an impacted proventriculus include anorexia, scant defecation, dehydration, and weight loss.**
- **The condition usually develops over a period of time; affected birds are thus often severely debilitated by the time of diagnosis.**
- **Specific techniques for diagnosis of proventricular impaction include abdominal palpation, radiography, and endoscopy.**

Ostriches (*Struthio camelus*) have become popular ranch exotics for breeding stock and as sources of hide, feathers, and meat. Zoos often display these birds for their unusually large size and inability to fly. In either situation, they are exposed to stresses associated with captivity that can result in medically significant behavioral patterns. Foraging behaviors of these captive birds are most commonly affected.[1–3] In the wild, ostriches must forage daily to supply their nutritional needs. This instinctive behavior is unnecessary in captive ostriches because their diet is supplied in the form of a pelleted ration. As a result, these naturally curious birds are instead afforded the opportunity to forage for inedible objects.

Not discriminating in their tastes, ostriches are attracted to foreign objects, which they readily consume. Bright objects (such as nails) or moving objects (such as paper blowing in a breeze) are accepted as suitable types of food by the bird. By instinct, they peck off the ground, and stones (which compose many impactions) often are ingested. Most captive birds eagerly consume pelleted rations but fail to differentiate between these rations and substrates of pea gravel or sand in their environment. These abnormal consumption habits can be enhanced in periods of stress, such as transport to a new location or introduction of additional birds to the farm.[3] The occurrence of impaction of the proventriculus can be minimized by instituting management techniques that limit the opportunities to ingest foreign bodies and by modifying the ostriches' behavior.[3]

Minimizing ingestion of foreign objects can be accomplished by removal of debris from the pens. Substrate of the pens should preferably be pasture, which is digestible if consumed, as opposed to stone or sand. Feeding from pans or other containers prevents inadvertent consumption of foreign bodies, which can occur when ostriches eat off the ground.

To modify the behavior of an ostrich, the best approach is to diminish stress. Slow introductions to new areas or birds are beneficial for many reasons and are very beneficial for decreasing incidence of impaction.

Updated from original publication in Volume 15, Number 2, February 1993

PATHOPHYSIOLOGY OF IMPACTION

Ostriches are classified in a group of flightless birds known as ratites. Ratites lack the traditional avian crop and instead have a well-developed proventriculus.[4] This organ is located within the abdominal cavity and has both secretory and storage functions. In ratites, ingested foreign objects initially lodge in the proventriculus.

Ingested foreign objects produce mechanical obstruction to the flow of ingesta[2] or act as valves by blocking outflow into the ventriculus.[a] In addition, they can perpetuate the obstruction by entangling dietary roughage. With prolonged impaction, foreign material can progress into the ventriculus and initiate impaction of the organ. Impaction of the ventriculus minimizes ingesta flow further and damages the ventricular mucosa during the grinding motions of digestion.

With a full proventriculus, affected birds are satiated and exhibit anorexia with resultant weight loss, dehydration, and scant defecation.[2,3] As a result of inappetence, they lose body condition and become less able to compete with penmates, resulting in decreased growth and breeding efficiency. Impaction of the proventriculus therefore represents a problem of serious economic importance to the ratite producer and usually prompts veterinary intervention.

MEDICAL OR SURGICAL THERAPY?

The value of ostriches is such that economics are not usually the limiting factor determining selection of treatment; rather, duration of the problem and health status of the bird are important in deciding whether medical or surgical therapy is indicated. For sand impaction, birds can be administered psyllium laxatives to promote passage of ingesta[2,3]; however, the bird must be willing to eat or be able to accept the laxative through a stomach tube. The most important consideration is that for medical therapy to be undertaken, the bird must be healthy enough so that enough time can be devoted to impaction relief without the bird becoming critically ill. Many impactions are already chronic by the time of diagnosis, and surgical removal of the impacting material often is indicated.[3]

Before the technique for proventriculotomy was developed,[2] a procedure of ventriculostomy had been attempted to treat ventricular impaction in several avian species.[1,5] This procedure, however, was fraught with complications. Even in cases for which surgical intervention was necessary, hesitation would occur. It was difficult to suture the strong muscular walls together adequately enough to withstand the grinding motions of the ventriculus,[5] and accessibility to the proventricular material could not readily be made. Anesthetic and postsurgical requirements also tended to be demanding. By contrast, the proventriculus, although it is muscular, acts as an organ for storage and not one for grinding. Suturing is thus much more secure with less possibility of dehiscence. The proventriculus is also readily accessible in most impacted ostriches through a simple skin incision followed by blunt dissection of the air sac surrounding the proventriculus.[2] Using this approach, abdominal air sac integrity is maintained and there is less chance of generalized peritonitis in the event of dehiscence of the suture line. In addition, the lumen of the ventriculus can be accessed, thereby allowing removal of foreign objects from the proventriculus as well as the ventriculus.[3,4] Over a period of 27 months, 25 ostriches with impaction of the proventriculus were treated surgically at the Texas Veterinary Medical Center.[2,3]

[a]Honnas CM: Personal observation, Texas A&M University, 1991.

DIAGNOSTIC TECHNIQUES

Most birds are presented with an ambiguous history of lack of productivity for a period ranging from several days to weeks. Physical examination usually reveals decreased body condition and generalized weakness. In many cases of impaction of the proventriculus, palpation in the region caudal to the sternum often reveals an enlarged visceral organ.[2,3] Standard hematology (with samples submitted in heparinized tubes as standard for avian profiles) and serum chemistry profiles are nonspecific in supporting the diagnosis of impaction. Routine blood work is important, however, in alerting the clinician to concurrent problems (e.g., transport stress, dehydration, or infection) and in assessing the patient's ability to withstand sedation or surgery.[6-9] Radiographs are used to confirm an impacted proventriculus. Dorsoventral and lateral oblique radiographs of the abdomen are sufficient to document impaction resulting from ingestion of radiodense materials.[1–3] For impactions that are less discernible on survey radiographs, such as sand or roughage, endoscopic examination of the proventriculus can be of diagnostic use. Before endoscopic examination, sedation or immobilization usually is necessary because even weakened ostriches may resist handling and present significant danger to the clinician and themselves.

SEDATION AND ANESTHESIA

Because ostriches are large and potentially dangerous, sedation and anesthesia are challenging to the practitioner attempting to diagnose and treat impaction of the proventriculus.[8] Before administration of pharmacologic agents is considered, a planned approach should include placing the bird in a small enclosure at presentation. Patients debilitated by impaction can sometimes be approached and restrained for intravenous catheterization without premedication. Restraint for most mature birds, however, takes several people[9,10]; and the bird may still effectively resist intravenous injections. Administering drugs by intramuscular routes can provide an alternative for initial sedation of intractable animals.

Many drugs, alone or combined, have been used with varied success for sedation and induction; however, none has been reported as superior.[2,11–13] Agents to consider include xylazine,[2] ketamine hydrochloride,[2,11] telazol,[2] carfentanil,[2] and diazepam.[2] The benzodiazepines (diazepam and midazolam) have been empirically observed to give reliable sedation and smoother inductions than do other agents. Specifically, midazolam has demonstrated excellent sedation 15 minutes after a split intramuscular and intravenous dose, with sedation lasting approximately 30 minutes. A combination of ketamine hydrochloride (1 to 1.5 mg/kg intravenously) and diazepam (0.1 mg/kg intravenously) has shown the most promise for inducing anesthesia.[b] Birds that have been sedated but not anesthetized can be transported to surgery on a cart or walked with an escort from the stall. Sedated or lightly anesthetized birds should be handled with caution to avoid their powerful forward kicks.[9,10] A person on either side of the bird to hold the wings where they join the body and the tailhead controls the bird's direction while keeping the handlers in a safe position. A hood made from an orthopedic stockinette that is rolled over the eyes and cranial neck[2,10] is effective in calming the bird during transport. Manual restraint remains necessary until gas anesthesia has eliminated purposeful movement.

Inhalant anesthesia is initiated with a mask using isoflurane and oxygen before intubation. Endotracheal intubation is simple to accomplish because the glottis is visible immediately on opening the mouth.[4] The cuff requires minimal inflation to allow secure placement of the tube but prevents injury to the complete tracheal rings.[4] Tape can then be used to secure the tube to the bill and cover the nares. Oxygen (20 ml/kg/min) and isoflurane, often required at concentrations of 4% to 5% throughout surgery, are delivered in a semiclosed system.[2] Cloacal temperature, heart rate, respiratory rate, electrocardiography, and direct arterial pressures are monitored during surgery.[2,8,12]

Recovery from anesthesia presents a second period of danger to the handlers and the bird. Benzodiazepines are excellent for induction and allow for smooth recovery if given immediately before transport to the recovery area. During this period, ostriches can thrash severely and a padded stall is recommended to minimize injury to the waking bird.[3] The optimum sequence of recovery begins with the bird in lateral recumbency; then sternal recumbency with the head held normally; followed by sitting on the hocks; and finally, sedate standing. The last stage allows safe return of the bird to its enclosure.

[b]Matthews NS: Personal communication, Texas A&M University, 1991.

PROVENTRICULOTOMY

Once the decision for surgery is made and anesthesia is induced, the bird is positioned in right lateral recumbency with the left leg restrained in abduction and pulled caudally[2,3] (Figure 1). A left paramedian approach is required for access to the proventriculus. The surgical site is delineated by several landmarks. A quilled band of feathers on either side of midline coincides with the ventrolateral surface of the proventriculus to the left of midline. This quilled band is plucked free of feathers[14] from the caudal sternum to 20 centimeters behind the thigh. The cranial aspect of the incision is in line with the cranial aspect of the thigh (approximately 15 cm caudal to the xiphoid) and centered in the quilled band[2,4] (Figure 1). The proventriculus position also can be palpated transabdominally and then used to approximate the area of incision. The surgical site is aseptically prepared and draped routinely.[14]

The skin, subcutaneous tissue, and rectus abdominus muscle are incised with a scalpel. The abdominal air sac is encountered once the rectus abdominus muscle is incised. The abdominal air sac covers the abaxial surface of the proventriculus and is bluntly separated from it by the surgeon's fingers. The thick wall of the proventriculus is grasped with Allis tissue forceps and stabilized by an assistant. The site of the proposed proventriculotomy is isolated by saline-moistened sponges before incision.

The lumen of the proventriculus is stabbed, and a suction tip is introduced to evacuate liquid surrounding the impaction. The suction and sponge packing minimize contamination of the surrounding tissue during relief of impaction. The incision is extended cranially and caudally with Metzenbaum scissors in an avascular region of the proventriculus (Figure 2). The edges of the proventriculotomy incision are stabilized with Allis tissue forceps. A long-handled spoon, introduced concave side down, is then scooped through the proventricular lumen and withdrawn (Figure 3). This procedure is repeated until the lumen is free of impacting material.[2,3] By advancing the spoon cranially and ventrally, the ventriculus also can be emptied. Sponge forceps are useful for effective removal of roughage impactions from the proventriculus and ventriculus.[3] In larger birds, the inside of both organs can be swept by the surgeon's

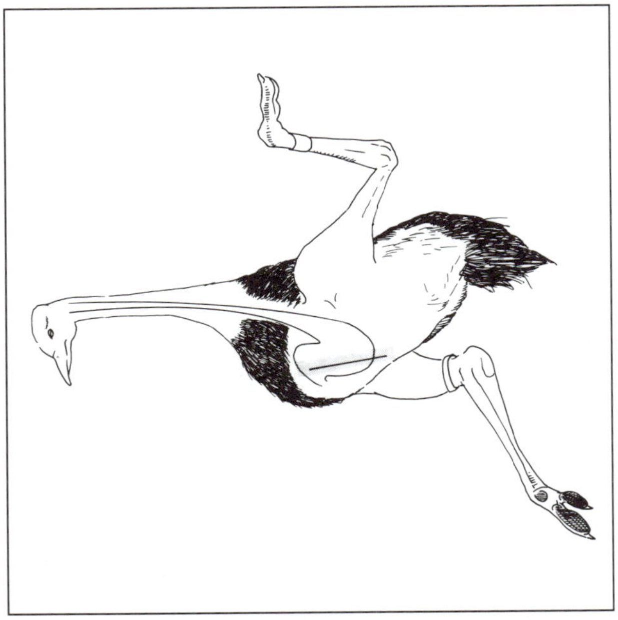

Figure 1—Ostrich in right lateral recumbency for proventriculotomy. The left hindlimb is pulled caudally and abducted. Note the incision (—) centered in the plucked quilled band and the position of the ventriculus cranial to the proventriculus.

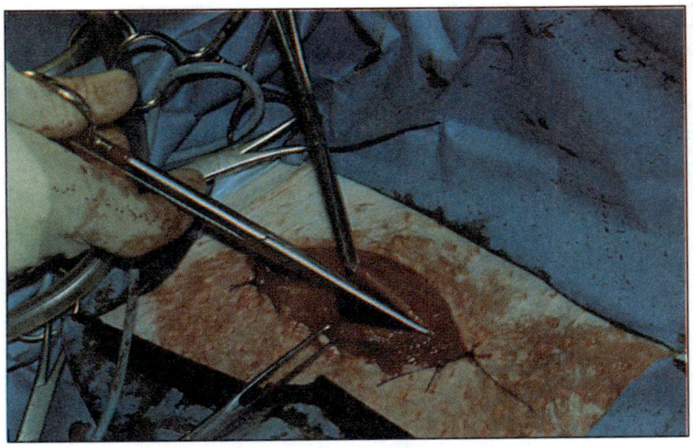

Figure 2—After evacuation of the fluid contents of the proventriculus, Metzenbaum scissors are used to lengthen the incision.

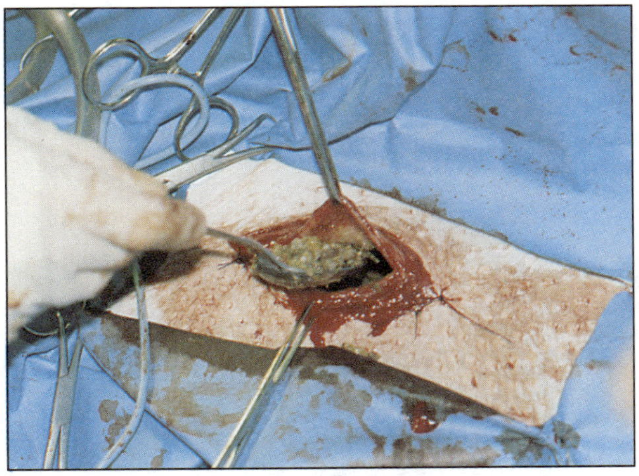

Figure 3—The spoon used to remove the impaction is introduced concave side down and rotated within the proventriculus to maximize recovery of foreign objects.

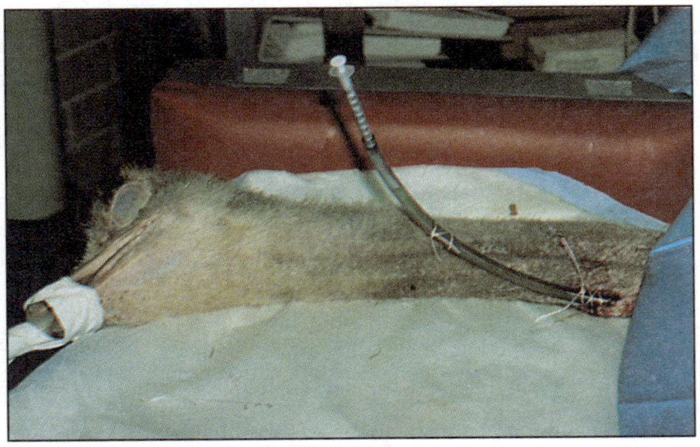

Figure 4—The neck of an ostrich after placement of an esophagotomy tube for postsurgical supplementation. Note the exit of the tube in the caudal third of the neck and the sutures that secure it. The syringe is placed in the open end to prevent bloating of the gastrointestinal tract with outside air.

hand to confirm complete removal of impacting material.[2,3] Before closure of the proventriculotomy, the incision is copiously lavaged with sterile saline and suctioned free of contaminating debris.

Absorbable sutures are used for closure. We prefer polydioxanone suture. The proventricular incision is first apposed with No. 0 polydioxanone suture in a simple continuous pattern. The surface is thoroughly lavaged, and the incision is oversewn with a simple continuous Cushing's pattern using the same material. The paramedian muscular incision is closed with No. 1 polydioxanone suture in a simple continuous pattern. The subcutaneous tissue is sparse and does not require closure. The skin is closed with No. 0 polydioxanone suture in a simple continuous pattern. Absorbable suture material is recommended in the skin to avoid having to remove sutures in aggressive birds after surgery.

POSTSURGICAL CARE

For a patient that is debilitated on presentation, an esophagotomy tube is placed before surgical recovery to reduce postsurgical care.[3] An equine stomach tube of appropriate size is passed orally to the site of the esophagotomy in the caudal third of the neck. An incision is made over the end of the tube through the skin and esophagus. The tube is then withdrawn from the mouth and inserted through the esophagot-

TABLE I
Hematology Profiles of Case Presentations and Normal Values

Parameters	*Bird A*	*Bird B*	*Normal*[a]
Red blood cells (×10^6/µl)	—[b]	—[b]	1.3–1.7 1.48–3.02
Hemoglobin (g/dl)	13.5	12.1	10.8–16.8 12.5–16.5
Packed cell volume (%)	55	48	40 40–61
White blood cell count (×10^3/µl)	22.8	31.3	3.6–6.8 9.2–18.3
Differential[c]			
Heterophils	86 19,608	96 30,048	58.3–68.3 5359–15,704
Lymphocytes	8 1824	1 313	22.4–31.8 1153–3788
Monocytes	2 456	3 939	1–2.8 0–527
Eosinophils	4 912	—[d]	0–0.5 0–612
Basophils	—[d]	—[d]	0–0.4 0–153
Platelets (/hpf)	0–3	1–4	—[d]
Protein (g/dl)	7.1	7.2	—[d]
Fibrinogen (mg/dl)	100	300	—[d]

[a]Normal values are taken from Levy, Perelman, Waner, et al[6] and Stoskopf, Beall, Ensley, et al[9] and are tabled in that order except in the white blood cell differential (see footnote *c*).
[b]These values were unavailable because of sample submission in EDTA.
[c]The white blood cell differential is reported as percentage of white blood cells (top line)[6] and absolute number (bottom line).[9]
[d]There are no reportable values for this category.

omy incision. The proximal end of the tube is sutured to the skin (Figure 4).

A pelleted ration or grain is typically offered within six to eight hours of anesthetic recovery. Ostriches with an esophagotomy tube can be supplemented until a normal appetite returns. The supplement diet is an adult canine maintenance kibble (five to six cups) blended with warm water (one gallon) to a slurry consistency.[3] The mixture is pumped into the proventriculus three times daily. Because the tube does not interfere with normal alimentation, feeding by means of the esophagotomy tube is continued until the bird is passing adequate food boluses. Once normal alimentation returns, the tube can be removed and the wound is allowed to heal by second intention. In patients that seem to require nutritional support, an equine stomach tube can be passed orally intermittently to allow supplemental feedings. Supplemental feedings require additional personnel for restraint of the bird and are time-consuming when compared with an esophagotomy tube placed during surgery.

With the potential mucosal irritation from the foreign objects and clean–contaminated status of the proventricular and esophageal surgical procedures, perisurgical antibiotics are warranted and are continued for five to seven days after surgery.[3] A regimen of 48% trimethoprim-sulfadiazine injected intramuscularly twice daily is preferred at the Texas Veterinary Medical Center; the dose is calculated by metabolic energy scaling for individual birds from the dose given to dogs.[15] Oral enrofloxacin also can be prescribed for postsurgical care after the bird is discharged from the clinic. With a long-standing impaction, postsurgical care can be a significant commitment and may ultimately determine the success of surgery.

CLINICAL CASES OF PROVENTRICULAR IMPACTION

Presentation and Diagnostics

Two mature ostriches were presented to the Texas Veterinary Medical Center for evaluation. Bird A, presented in May 1991, was a four-year-old breeding

Table II
Preoperative Hematology and Clinical Pathology of Bird A (Day 5 of Hospitalization)

Parameters	*Value*
Red blood cells (×10^6/μl)	—[a]
Hemoglobin (g/dl)	12.9
Packed cell volume (%)	52
Platelets (/hpf)	0–2
Protein (g/dl)	7.1
Fibrinogen (mg/dl)	100
Glucose (mg/dl)	219
Uric acid (mg/dl)	3.9
Blood urea nitrogen (mg/dl)	2.0
Creatinine (mg/dl)	0.1
Ca^{2+} (mg/dl)	9.6
PO_4 (mg/dl)	3.1
Na^+ (mMol/L)	148
K^+ (mMol/L)	3.8
Cl^- (mMol/L)	110
White blood cells (×10^3/μl)	20
Differential (%)/absolute	
Heterophils	(78)/15,600
Lymphocytes	(11)/2200
Monocytes	(11)/2200
Eosinophils	—[b]
Basophils	—[b]
Total carbon dioxide (mMol/L)	31
Total protein (g/dl)	4.8
Albumin (g/dl)	2.3
Aspartate transaminase (U/L)	531
Creatinine kinase (U/L)	15,818
Alkaline phosphatase (U/L)	22
Gamma glutamyl transferase (U/L)	10
Total bilirubin (mg/dl)	0.1

[a]This value is unavailable because of sample submission in EDTA.
[b]There are no reportable values for this category.

male that exhibited anorexia and weight loss. In this bird, the vigorous attitude and vibrant skin coloration exhibited for three weeks of the breeding season had diminished in conjuction with the bird's appetite during the previous 7 to 10 days. Two juvenile male and three mature female penmates chased the bird from the pasture as its strength declined.

Bird B, presented in August 1991, was a 12-year-old female with a past history of high egg production. During the current breeding season, a male became aggressive after mating and kicked the patient's right stifle. The lameness affected the bird's ability to compete with the other adult birds in the pen for food, and the bird presented in a severely cachectic state.

Both birds were housed in pastures but had access to foreign objects. A pelleted ratite diet and water were offered free choice to both patients. Although the animals presented with totally different complaints and not specifically for gastrointestinal dysfunction, proventricular impaction remained high on the differential list because of the clinical appearance of the birds.[3] Diagnostic workup began with nonspecific hematology and serum chemistries.

A hematology profile (Table I) confirmed that both birds were dehydrated with an elevated packed cell volume and total protein. Both birds exhibited profound leukocytosis with significant heterophilia. Because the elevation in the heterophil count of Bird A could not be attributed to anything other than mucosal irritation, an aerobic and anaerobic blood culture was done and empirical trimethoprim-sulfadiazine therapy was begun (1560 mg or 12 mg/kg intramuscularly twice daily for 10 days). Results (at 72 hours) indicated an *Acinetobacter* species bacteremia that was sensitive to trimethoprim-sulfadiazine. When the hematology profile was repeated five days after the initial blood work (Table II), the heterophils and the total white blood cell count had decreased. The eosinophilia noted in Bird A was likely the result of undiagnosed parasitism.

The profile of Bird B exhibited a severe stress and inflammatory leukogram with monocytosis and lymphopenia in addition to the heterophilia; the antibiotics trimethoprim-sulfadiazine (1920 mg or 19.2 mg/kg subcutaneously twice daily for five days) and ceftiofur (650 mg or 6.5 mg/kg intramuscularly twice daily for five days) were given before hematology or serum chemistry profiles had returned from the laboratory.

Serum chemistry profiles (Table III) provided confirmation of the stress, dehydration, anorexia, and transport bruising for both birds. Stress was evident from the elevation in glucose and dehydration interpreted from elevations in creatinine, sodium (Bird A), total protein, and albumin. The electrolyte abnormalities could be attributed to prolonged anorexia. Liver enzymes also were affected by the inappetence and injured muscles. The creatinine kinase of Bird B was elevated, which was diagnostic of muscular damage from transport or previous injury, and remained so from the intramuscular administration of antibiotics. The second profile of Bird A (Table II), which was done immediately before surgery, revealed similar abnormalities from hospitalization stress and contin-

TABLE III
Clinical Pathology of Case Presentations and Normal Values

Parameters	*Bird A*	*Bird B*	*Normal*[a]
Glucose (mg/dl)	278	207	160
			150–200
Uric acid (mg/dl)	5.9	7.3	4–15[10]
Blood urea nitrogen (mg/dl)	2.0	< 2.0	1–2[7]
Creatinine (mg/dl)	0.1	< 0.1	0.4–0.8[10]
Ca^{2+} (mg/dl)	10.0	9.5	9.6–10.4
			10–14
PO_4 (mg/dl)	2.6	4.3	12.5–14.4[7]
Na^+ (mMol/L)	150	—[b]	118–184
			130–145
K^+ (mMol/L)	3.4	—[b]	2.3–3.3
			3.5–4.5
Cl^- (mMol/L)	112	—[b]	94–118[7]
Total carbon dioxide (mMol/L)	31	—[b]	—[b]
Total protein (g/dl)	5.1	5.3	3.8–5.2
			3.6–4.6
Albumin (g/dl)	2.3	2.0	25% total protein[10]
Aspartate transaminase (U/L)	411	719	105–129
			90–150
Creatinine kinase (U/L)	6591	16,000+	457–749[7]
Alkaline phosphatase (U/L)	25	76	212–448[7]
Gamma glutamyl transferase (U/L)	10	10	0.6–2.2[7]
Total bilirubin (mg/dl)	0.1	0.2	0.1–0.3[10]

[a]Normal values are taken from Levy, Perelman, Waner, et al[6] and Bruning and Dolensek[10] and are tabled in that order except as individually referenced. The values from the former article are for the adult animals reported.
[b]There are no reportable values for this category.

ued lack of consumption of food and water. Confirmation of proventricular impaction was made by palpation; radiography; and, for Bird B, endoscopy.

Palpation of the proventriculus of Bird A was unremarkable and thus not diagnostic. The proventriculus of Bird B was palpated and found to be a greatly enlarged, gritty viscus caudal to the sternum. Radiographs verified impaction of the proventriculus in both animals. Bird A (Figure 5) had a minor impaction of the proventriculus with radiodense objects and significant fluid in the gastrointestinal tract. Bird B (Figure 6) had a more tightly packed proventriculus with the ventriculus also containing numerous radiodense foreign objects. Endoscopy of the proventriculus of Bird B showed minor amounts of greenish ingesta and an occasional rock. The proventricular mucosa exhibited some small areas of ulceration that were suspected to have resulted from damage cause by foreign bodies. Neither bird could survive with the impaction and relief could not occur naturally; therefore, the owners elected proventriculotomy for their animals.

Surgical Anesthesia and Procedure

The previously outlined anesthetic and surgical procedures were used for both birds; therefore, only significant deviations from the prescribed protocol are noted here. Diazepam and isoflurane were used for both birds. Ketamine hydrochloride was added to the induction of Bird A, and Bird B was masked with isoflurane to effect. Bird A experienced an extended, difficult induction from premature transport attempts to the surgery suite; however, recovery was difficult for only a brief period, and (with additional diazepam) the bird attained sternal posture in minutes. Because of the extremely weakened state of Bird B, induction proceeded quickly and without incident. Recovery was quiet but prolonged. Intraarterial catheterization for blood pressure; electrocardiography; and measurement of blood gas, heart rate, and respiratory rate were used to monitor anesthetic induction.

During surgery, eight pounds of small pebbles and coastal Bermuda grass hay were removed from Bird A. This was consistent with the previous radiographic view of fluid and minimal radiopacity. As anticipated from presurgical radiographs, the proventriculus of Bird B was impacted with five pounds of rocks (some of which were quite large) and a small amount of grass. Bird A, a mature male that was in relatively

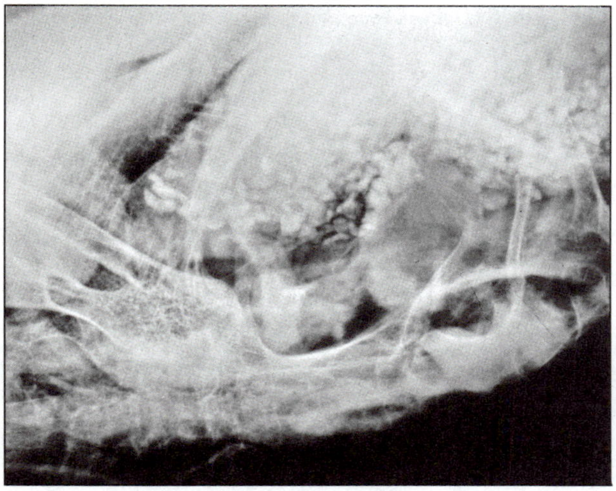

Figure 5—Lateral oblique radiographic view of the abdominal region of Bird A reveals numerous radiodense foreign bodies lodged primarily in the proventriculus. The right side of the radiograph is the cranial aspect of the ostrich.

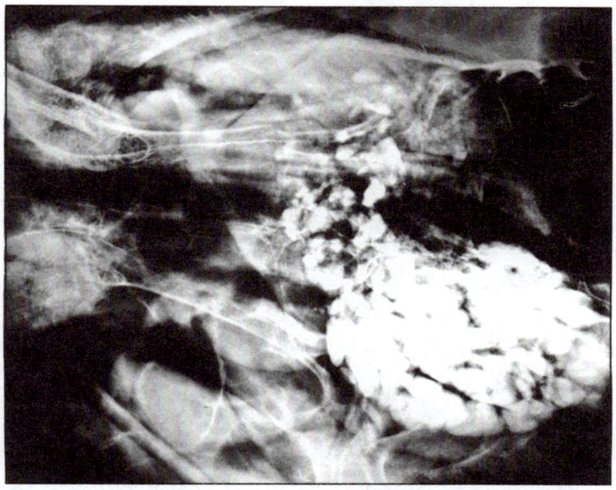

Figure 6—Dorsoventral radiographic view of the abdominal region of Bird B reveals proventricular impaction of radiodense foreign objects as well as the beginning of a ventricular impaction. Note the position of the proventriculus on the left side of the abdominal cavity.

good health before surgery, was not considered a candidate for intensive postsurgical handling; an esophagotomy tube was therefore not placed. Bird B, which was debilitated and severely cachectic before surgery, had an esophagotomy tube placed at surgery. After the proventriculotomy, the proventriculus and rectus abdominus muscle of Bird A were sutured with No. 1 polyglactin 910 and the skin was sutured with No. 1 polydioxanone. Bird B had No. 0 polydioxanone used consistently throughout closure. Minimal differences in healing between birds were noted after surgery; however, Bird A had slight incisional swelling for 24 hours.

Postsurgical Care

The birds had differing postsurgical needs. Bird A was offered grain approximately five hours after surgery and showed active interest by midmorning of the next day. Food passage was confirmed three days after surgery by food boluses passing down the esophagus. Minimal fecal material was passed during hospitalization, but the bird remained alert and ate well. The bird was discharged six days after surgery with enrofloxacin (28.5 mg or 0.22 mg/kg orally once daily for five days), and the owners were instructed to keep it physically separated but visible to its former penmates. Five weeks after surgery, follow-up revealed that the bird had regained much of its coloration, interest in breeding, and weight (approximately 50% of weight loss regained) with no complications noted as a result of surgery.

In contrast to the usual recovery from proventriculotomy, the eating habits of Bird B did not improve until nearly five days after surgery. The bird was supplemented with dog food slurries three times daily through the esophagotomy tube until the tube dislodged two days after surgery. To continue supplementation, an equine stomach tube was passed orally once a day and a dog food slurry was given for four additional days. Because there was still no significant increase in appetite, the esophagotomy tube was again placed. Before marked improvement in the condition of the bird was noted, it fell as a result of instability of the injured stifle. Three days later, it was euthanatized for reasons unrelated to the proventricular impaction.[3]

SUMMARY

These cases depict the common presentation of a proventricular impaction in ostriches. Clinical signs are manifested as vague, chronic unproductivity that complicates or is complicated by other medical problems. History reveals availability of foreign objects or recent stresses in the environment that may induce indiscriminate eating of foreign material. Affected birds present with anorexia, weight loss, and dehydration. Many of these birds require surgical intervention to survive. The method of proventriculotomy discussed in this article has advantages of procedural consistency between patients and excellent access to the gastrointestinal tract for relief of impaction.

Ratites (and ostriches in particular) are increasing in popularity in exotic animal collections, and the incidence of proventricular impaction has developed concurrent with the increasing captive maintenance of these birds. Prevention is the best means to minimize this problem in a ratite operation, but the inquisitive nature of an ostrich often results in proventricular impaction even with the best management. Proventriculotomy, as done at the Texas Veterinary Medical Center and discussed in this article, can provide a novel approach to this aspect of exotic animal practice, which before proved difficult if not impossible to manage successfully.

About the Authors

Dr. Gamble is associate veterinarian at the Dallas Zoo and Aquarium, Dallas, Texas. Dr. Honnas is affiliated with the Texas Veterinary Medical Center, Large Animal Clinic, College of Veterinary Medicine, Texas A&M University, College Station, Texas. Dr. Honnas is a Diplomate of the American College of Veterinary Surgeons.

REFERENCES

1. Jacobsen ER, Ellison GW, McMurphy R, et al: Ventriculostomy for removal of multiple foreign bodies in an ostrich. *JAVMA* 189(9):117–119, 1986.
2. Honnas CM, Jensen J, Cornick JL, et al: Proventriculotomy to relieve foreign body impactions in ostriches. *JAVMA* 199(4):461–465, 1991.
3. Honnas CM, Blue-McLendon A, Zamos DT, et al: Proventriculotomy in ostriches: 25 cases (1989–1992). *JAVMA*, in press.
4. Fowler ME: Comparative clinical anatomy of ratites. *J Zoo Wild Anim Med* 22(2):204–227, 1991.
5. Bush M, Kennedy S: Ventriculostomy for removal of foreign bodies from Sarus cranes. *JAVMA* 173(4):1107–1110, 1978.
6. Levy A, Perelman B, Waner T, et al: Haematological parameters of the ostrich (*Struthio camelus*). *Avian Pathol* 18(2): 321–327, 1989.
7. Levy A, Perelman B, Waner T, et al: Reference blood chemical values in ostriches (*Struthio camelus*). *Am J Vet Res* 50(9):1548–1550, 1989.
8. Matthews NS, Burba DJ, Cornick JL: Premature ventricular contractions and apparent hypertension during anesthesia in an ostrich. *JAVMA* 198(11):1959–1961, 1991.
9. Stoskopf MJ, Beall FB, Ensley PK, et al: Immobilization of large ratites: Blue necked ostrich (*Struthio camelus austrealis*) and double wattled cassowary (*Casuarius casuarius*) with hematologic and serum chemistry data. *J Zoo Anim Med* 13(4):160–168, 1982.
10. Bruning DF, Dolensek EP: Ratites, in Fowler ME (ed): *Zoo and Wild Animal Medicine*, ed 2. Philadelphia, WB Saunders Co, 1986, pp 277–291.
11. Ensley PK, Launer DP, Blasingame JP: General anesthesia and surgical removal of a tumor-like growth from the foot of the double-wattled cassowary. *J Zoo Anim Med* 15(1):35–37, 1984.
12. Gandini GCM, Keffen RH, Burroghs REJ, et al: An anesthetic combination of ketamine, xylazine and alphaxalone-alphadolone in ostriches (*Struthio camelus*). *Vet Rec* 118(26): 729–730, 1986.
13. Grubb B: Use of ketamine to restrain and anesthetize emus. *VM SAC* 78(2):247–248, 1983.
14. Bush M: Laparoscopy and surgery, in Fowler ME (ed): *Zoo and Wild Animal Medicine*, ed 2. Philadelphia, WB Saunders Co, 1986, pp 254–261.
15. Sedgwick C, Pokras M, Kaufman G: Metabolic scaling: Using estimated energy costs to extrapolate drug doses between different species and different individuals of diverse body size. *Proc Am Assoc Zoo Vet*:249–254, 1990.

UPDATE

Since publication of this article, the value of ratites in private practice has declined in many areas. Economic considerations now dictate choice and administration of treatment options. One of the authors (KCG), however, has been able to apply this surgical approach in additional clinical situations. In other long-legged (even flighted) birds, the procedure has proven helpful in retrieval of ingested foreign objects. Although the surgical procedure remains unchanged, more timely comments on anesthetic management of ratites are needed.

Induction remains the most variable aspect of anesthesia; therefore several suggestions have been made. Telazol (2 to 8 mg/kg intravenously) has been reported to induce anesthesia within 15 seconds and maintain it for 20 to 40 minutes,[1] which would provide ample time for intubation. Telazol has been associated with particularly rough recoveries; however, as mentioned in the original article, they can be managed by administering benzodiazepines after surgery.[2] Benzodiazepines also are being used more often during the induction phase. Diazepam (0.4 to 1.0 mg/kg intramuscularly) and midazolam (0.4 mg/kg intramuscularly) in combination with ketamine have produced smoother overall anesthesia.[2] As presented in the original article, inhalant anesthesia remains the primary means of maintenance.

Juvenile ratites still benefit from both induction and maintenance with isoflurane. Adult birds (even young adults), however, should be induced using parenteral regimens and then transferred to isoflurane. The prolonged induction times required for even elevated isoflurane levels introduce a protracted period of danger for both the bird and the handlers. Further investigation since original publication has determined that 8 to 16 minutes of intermittent positive-pressure ventilation (IPPV) is important during anesthetic maintenance.[2] Depressed ventilation is typical, and IPPV not only improves oxygenation but apparently counteracts the potential shunting of anesthetic gases that can occur with a ratite surgical patient.[2]

Using these current anesthetic guidelines, surgical correction of impaction of the proventriculus in ostriches remains useful. In addition, the surgical procedure has garnered successful application beyond the original context of the article.

REFERENCES

1. Stewart J: Ratites, in Branson BW, Harrison GJ, Harrison LR (eds): *Avian Medicine: Principles and Application*, ed 2. Lake Worth, FL, Wingers Publishing, 1994, pp 1284–1326.
2. Ludders JW, Matthew N: Birds, in Thurmon JC, Tranquilli WJ, Benson GJ (eds): *Lumb & Jones' Veterinary Anesthesia*, ed 3. Baltimore, Williams & Wilkins, 1996, pp 645–669.

Surgical Correction of Maxillofacial Defects in Pet Birds

KEY FACTS

❑ **Accurate repair requires a thorough understanding of the embryologic development of the beak and its mechanical use.**

❑ **The axioms for avian beak repair are both returning the bird to a level of acceptable function and reestablishing a protective barrier against infectious agents.**

❑ **Beak repair becomes necessary with malocclusions, scissors beak, mandibular prognathism, acquired disorders, epidermal wounds, and fractures of the beak tip and skeleton.**

Thousand Oaks, California
Robert Clipsham, DVM

Beak repair has traditionally been one of the most frequent reasons birds are presented for physical correction. From the viewpoint of structure and function, however, beak repair is perhaps one of the least understood aspects of avian clinical care.

Newly developed synthetic adhesives and dental bonding agents have allowed improved protocols for beak reconstruction and correction. The greatest demand for such protocols involves owners of pet birds (particularly psittacine owners), despite the fact that these surgical protocols are equally necessary for wild and zoologic avian species and equally justifiable in terms of ecology.

Such factors as species-specific jaw kinetics and marked variability in structure can make both beak reconstruction and correction of congenital defects seem incomprehensible. Serious attempts to identify jaw biomechanics, tissue-healing strategies, and materials application have only been made during the past 25 years. Fortunately, significant progress has been made. With emphasis on psittacines, these insights are presented in this article to promote further investigation and participation in the field. Accurate repair requires firm comprehension of embryologic development at both gross[1–3] and molecular[4–7] levels as well as an understanding of mechanical use, which is a direct result of evolutionary adaptation.[8]

BEAK ANATOMY

The bones of the avian face are derived from the first two pharyngeal arches, and the structures of the mouth are largely deviations of the first arch.[9] The beak is barely visible in the chicken embryo at 5½ days and becomes a recognizable structure by day 7. Beak cornification begins by day 10, and a hard surface structure is present by day 13.[2,3,10]

The skull of birds is composed of a greater number of bones than that of mammals; but the sutures, including those of the beak, fuse early in life to give the appearance of a single bone.[11] While many species (e.g., Amazon parrots, owls, and rhamphastidae) have extensively pneumatized skulls to lighten the skeleton for flight, species that need to sustain force to the skull (e.g., woodpeckers and diving birds) lack such structure.[11–13] Pneumatization may take up to two years for completion in some species and includes extensive diverticula

First-time publication

of the beak and periorbital region, which are especially evident in psittacines.[11,12,14–17]

Jaw articulation is achieved through direct craniomaxillary contact as well as through contact with the bilaterally paired quadrate bones. Rostrally, the quadrate bones articulate with the quadratojugal bones, which in turn articulate rostrally with the jugal bones and collectively form the quadrate mechanism. Each quadrate bone acts as a pivotal point for the kinetic upper beak joint as well as being a suspensory structure for lower beak articulation.[17] A kinetic nasofrontal hinge is present in all birds but is most highly developed in psittacines, where it also serves as a synovial joint. Some species (e.g., eagles) sustain fusion of the joint.[11]

The bones of the beak are covered by multiple keratin plates that vary in number and shape.[15,18] The suture lines are no longer visible in most modern birds, but a few species show vestiges (e.g., ostriches, skuas) or obvious plate anatomy (e.g., shearwaters, petrals). According to the literature, Coures in 1903 identified seven names for the various plates and gave locations for each in the Procellariiformes (e.g., albatrosses, petrals, shearwaters, fulmars); in puffins, Bureau described nine plates that are shed every fall in an annual postbreeding moult.[15,18] These plates have been incorrectly identified in previous publications as being derived from growth centers.[19–22] The theory that the plates remain as separate entities has been contested by most modern investigators, as a majority of birds have no persistent identifiable landmarks. Fossil bird remains, however, clearly show the evolutionary origins; various modern species provide supporting evidence.

Histologically, the rhamphotheca can be divided into two general categories of beak keratin: a very thick weight-bearing horn (also referred to as a working horn) and a thinner covering horn.[15,23,24] The cornified keratin migrates externally to the surface from all areas of the beak, where the germinal layer exists.[15,20,25] In addition, the cornified layers are tilted toward the tip of the beak in columns, with variances in degree of angle (from approximately 45° ventrolateral at the level of the nares to nearly vertical at the beak tip), depending on the original location on the beak. Transitional cell columns from the edges of the upper beak also migrate toward the tomium (cutting edges of the beak), where excess keratin is worn away during use.[15]

Many species have a thickened bone at the tip of the premaxilla (e.g., parrots) and the mandible (e.g., anseriformes), where bony canals carry nerves into the dermis and form bill-tip organs[26] that act as highly complex sensory receptors and assist in prehension.

PRINCIPLES OF REPAIR

Axioms for avian beak repair include (1) return to a level of acceptable function whereby the patient can become capable of self-feeding and (2) reestablishment of the protective barrier against subdermal infectious agents.[21] Preening and speech mimicry are less crucial. For zoologic species on public display, cosmetic appearance and reproductive capability, especially for feeding altricial chicks, must be given higher priority during the restorative process.

Prosthetic devices and appliances should be designed and fitted for simplicity and smoothness. They should have no moving parts, must be easy to disinfect, and should be permanent during the entire healing process. Minimizing anesthesia time, invasive penetration of beak tissue, and human handling after surgery promote success.[19–21,27]

DEVELOPMENTAL BEAK DISORDERS

Many beak disorders are malocclusions with moderate regularity in avicultural and pet practice. The specific cause of each disorder remains unknown, although widely diverse factors are known to be associated with congenital beak deformities in poultry, cormorants, and a few psittacine species. Causative factors include gene disorders,[10,28–33,a] malnutrition,[10,29,34,35] malpositioning within the egg,[16,29–31,34,35] improper incubation,[16,29–31,36] fungal toxins,[10,29–31,36] and chemical toxins.[10,37,38]

The true cause of craniofacial deformities probably lies in the complex relationship of individual genetic codes and their specific susceptibility to environmental factors that trigger developmental abnormalities. Early efforts to explore the molecular biology of chick development has brought some significant revelations that match similar findings in other experimental species. The entire field of molecular and genetic embryology is exceedingly complex. The pursuit of this specialty may reveal the early answers in diagnosing conditions and may eventually force practitioners to address very fundamental breeding practices that prevent perpetuation of deformities in closed aviaries. In keeping with this tenant, husbandry and consanguinity apparently play significant roles in the appearance of congenital beak defects.[21,29–31,35,36,39] A review of management practices in one large commercial psittacine aviary reduced the incidence of beak deformities in weaned chicks from 8% severely defected to 4% slightly to imperceptibly deviated during a three-year period by improving egg and chick care despite a 250% increase in total chick production.[35]

SCISSORS BEAK

Scissors beak results in lateral deviation of the rhinotheca, thereby reducing proper occlusion and effective use of the internal rhinothecal keratin ridge. De-

[a]Cunningham M: Personal communication. Los Angeles, CA, Los Angeles Zoo, 1993.

viation may be to the left or right side but has been statistically noted by me to be predominantly right sided. The incidence was found to be nearly equal by another independent survey.[35] The defect is found predominantly, but not exclusively, in psittacines.

The deformity may affect only the keratin of the rhinothecal tip (a majority of cases), the premaxilla, or the entire rostrum maxillaris and nasofrontal hinge (a small minority of cases). Detailed radiology is highly recommended as a prognostic tool before corrective attempts are made. In all cases, placement of the upper beak off the sagittal plane leads to excessive wear on the ipsilateral aspect and proliferation of uninhibited keratin on the contralateral corner of the gnathotheca (Figure 1). Cockatoos and macaws are the most commonly affected species, but a variety of large and small psittacines have been documented with scissors beak.[16,21,22,35,40]

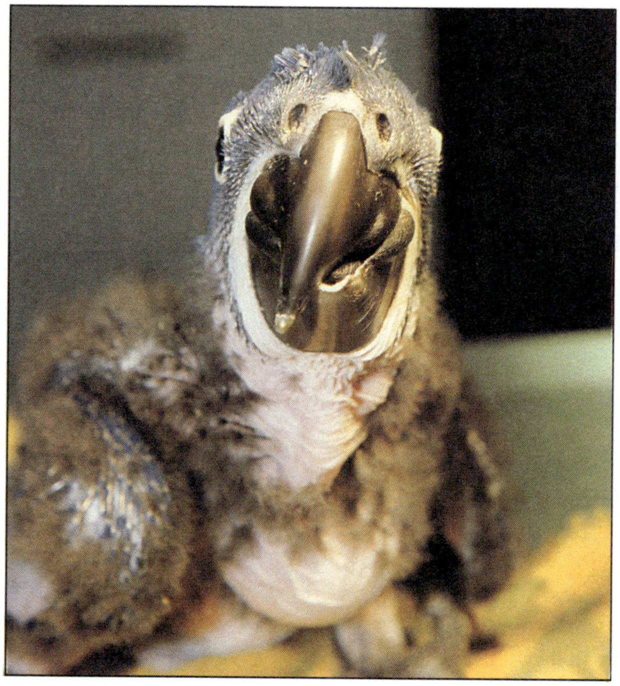

Figure 1—Scissors beak in a nyacinth macaw.

In very young chicks, correction may be as simple as giving frequent digital pressure each day. Self-corrections have been noted in rare cases. A majority of self-corrections necessarily require surgical intervention to realize permanent correction.

Use of a rhamphorthotic appliance promotes redirection of the premaxilla through keratin and/or bony remodeling. Construction of a sharply sloped ramp applies increasing resistance to the rhinotheca (as the beaks are apposed) and has been the most efficient procedure to date. This device is similar to the inclined plane devices used in human and small mammal orthodontics for repositioning teeth through bite pressures.[41] Attempts to use beak stalls, halo devices, dental brackets, or buttons with masal (rubber) chains have all been unsuccessful because of the reduced anchorage achieved at the attachment sites and unacceptable levels of intense labor, patient handling, and patient noncompliance.[12–22,36]

Before administering anesthesia or performing surgery, patients should be given a full diagnostic workup to identify any ongoing disease process. General anesthesia is fundamental for patient cooperation. Isoflurane remains the agent of choice, but a ketamine-diazepam combination has been used on occasion. While an endotracheal tube traditionally has been used for gas delivery, abdominal air sac intubation can eliminate problems in cases of unpredictable apnea, mucus obstruction in the trachea, and operating field interference. At isoflurane concentrations of 2½% to 3%, respiratory arrest during surgery is common when using air sac tubes because of the continuous cranial flow of oxygen through the parabronchi and air capillaries. Electrocardiographic hookup is a sensitive method for monitoring anesthetic status when coupled with perfusion and pulse observation.

The rostral aspects of the beak are brought into normal shape with a grinding tool, and the contralateral corner is reduced to below the occlusal plane to enhance the bite correction at approximately a 30° angle. Frontal and lateral aspects of the mandibular keratin are scored in a grid-like fashion to increase the cement interface with the appliance. The grid pattern should extend down into the intermandibular keratin and the inner aspects of the rostral gnathotheca. Any loose keratin should be removed and the area flushed with disinfectant. It is critical that the subdermis is not penetrated. Experience and a light touch can assist practitioners in recognizing the different tissue densities while working in this area. If any hemorrhaging occurs because of overgrinding, the area should be disinfected and sealed with a tissue glue.

The entire work area should be coated with a light layer of thin methyl or methoxy cyanoacrylate to create an intimately adhered lamina over the keratin grid. A strip of stainless steel mesh should be molded to the frontal facet of the rostral gnathotheca in a vertical fashion so that the mesh rests between the midline of the beak and the ipsilateral corner on the affected side of the face. The mesh strip becomes the framework for the inclined ramp that forces the upper beak medially back to the midline (Figure 2). Some discretion in placement usually is required in small species.

The upright mesh should be cemented to the foundation layer with more of the liquid cyanoacrylate, and the dorsal mesh should be cut at a 45° angle toward the midline. The entire mesh should then be infiltrated with cyanoacrylate and allowed to cure. Additional coats of acrylic should envelope the framework and beak, including the lingual aspects. The top of the structure should be even with the medial canthus of the affected side.

A thin drill can be used to create guide holes through the mandible along both lateral edges of the mesh strip. Three sets of perforations placed equally between the occlusal surface and the lingual membranes of the oral cavity are desirable, but four pairs of holes provide greater strength in large parrots. Only two sets of holes may be possible in small patients. Sterile stainless steel wire should be threaded through the mandible and around the vertical mesh and tightened carefully to avoid breakage. The wires must be secure to prevent the device from being dislodged if subjected to heavy jaw pressure. A hypodermic needle can serve as an excellent wire guide, if required, in tight work areas.

Any hemorrhaging must be controlled and the wire holes flushed, disinfected, and dried. A topcoat of acrylic or composite resin should be placed over all wires to create a confluent surface. The mesh, cyanoacrylate foundation, and cranial gnathotheca are incorporated into a uniform structure by layering these surfaces with a visible light-curing acrylic (paste or sheet). The acrylic can be layered in sectional sheets or as balls of provisional material and then smoothed into place by digital manipulation to create the final appliance form. Each area should be hardened with the aid of a special ultraviolet light designed to polymerize plastic dental materials.

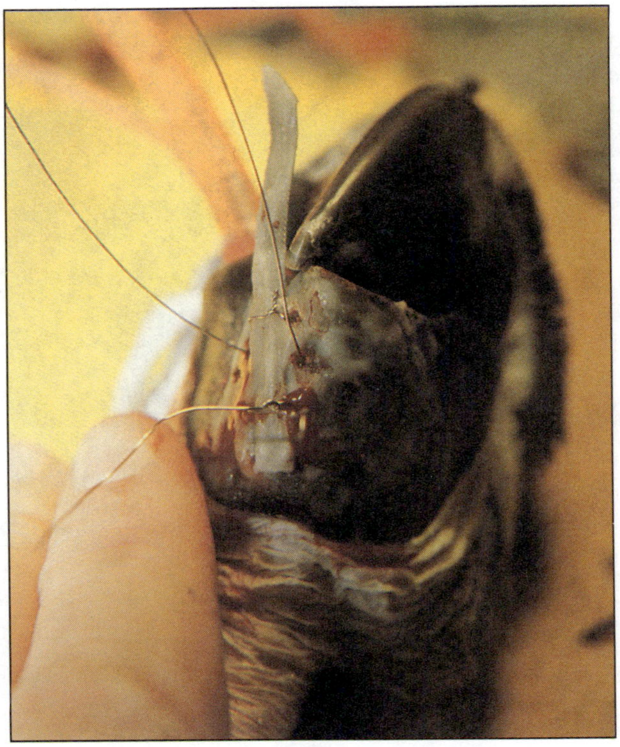

Figure 2—Cyanoacrylate-impregnated stainless steel mesh wired to the gnathotheca.

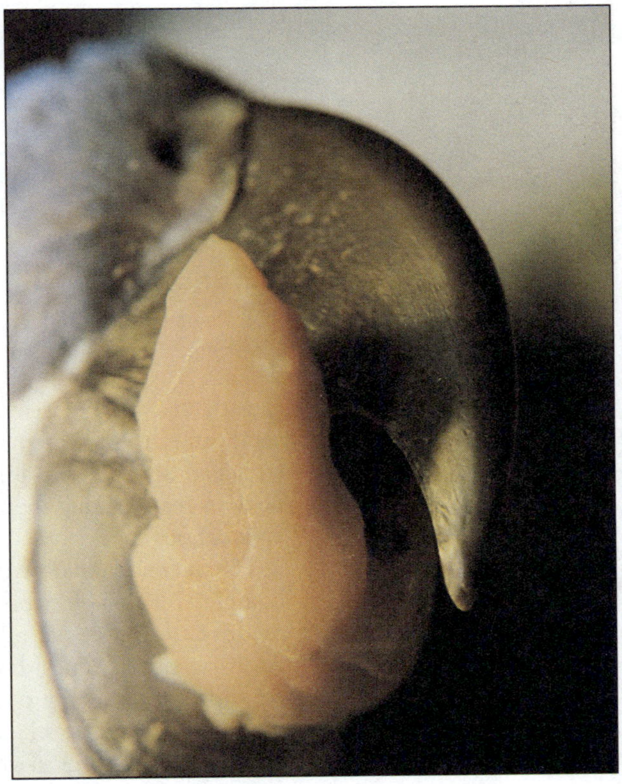

Figure 3—A corrective appliance for scissors beak.

Extra sections should be added to achieve adequate acrylic at the frontal aspects. The appearance should be a slope that has a sharp vertical curve and is continuous from the lateral occlusal edge of the unused side of the gnathotheca to the highest point of the appliance. The back half of the device should have a 45° angle formed by a moderately thin wall of acrylic from the dorsal point of the mesh to the angle of the gape. Failure to achieve sufficient height for the appliance or adequate bulk caudal to it on the affected side allows the patient to slip the abnormal beak over the top point and aggravate the condition by catching the premaxilla behind the device. The ventral aspects should envelop the whole front of the gnathotheca, inside and out, to prevent jaw pressure from cracking the base. The lateral aspects should wrap distally enough to provide resistance to forward motion when the bird grips stationary objects during climbing or attempts to remove the device (Figure 3).

After the procedure has been completed, the surgeon should evaluate the device for smoothness (to prevent accumulation of debris), total mass, functional compatibility, occlusion, and directional medial pressure on the rhinotheca. If these criteria are met, the entry site of the air sac tube can be sealed (using tissue glue). Analgesics and antiinflammatory agents should be administered to reduce discomfort from surgery. Systemic antibiotics are not needed if proper surgical technique has been followed.

The device should be cleaned several times by the owner and rechecked by the practitioner at least weekly for slippage and sanitation. Thirty days' duration apparently is the average for correction; but a few young macaws have been corrected in five days, while some adult cockatoos have required up to 90 days. A juvenile hyacinth macaw required three months because of the slower growth rate in these species.[36] The acrylic usually becomes loose about every two to three weeks because of exfoliation of natural keratin and constant work pressures. Application of a thin layer of cyanoacrylate over and beneath the device recements the new keratin and the device.

Final removal of the appliance requires isoflurane anesthesia. A cutting burr should be used along the sagittal mandibular midline, inside and out, until the keratin and wires are moderately exposed. A line along the occlusal surface should also be cut and the appliance slowly dislodged in pieces. The excess keratin under the device should be removed, the surface cleansed, and the wire holes disinfected. The wire holes should be covered, not filled, with cyanoacrylate and the bird allowed to recover. Relapses have not been documented to date if the final visual appearance and beak manipulations have been returned to normal (Figure 4).

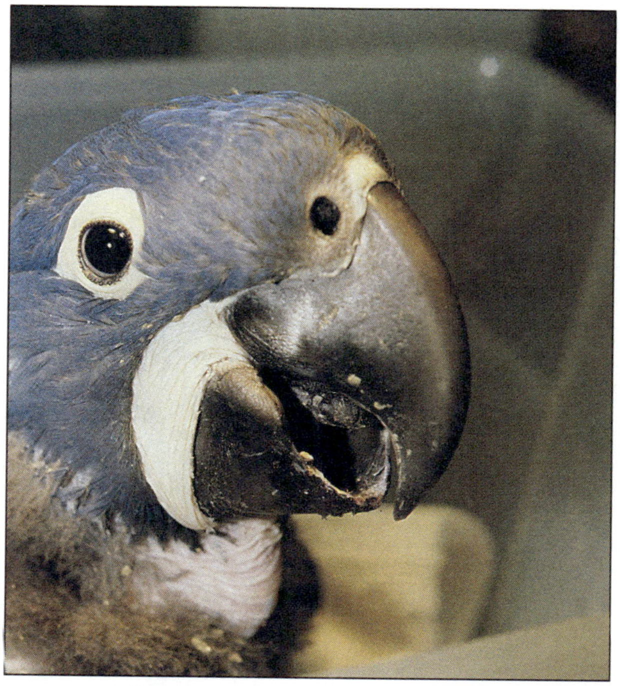

Figure 4—Full correction after 30 days.

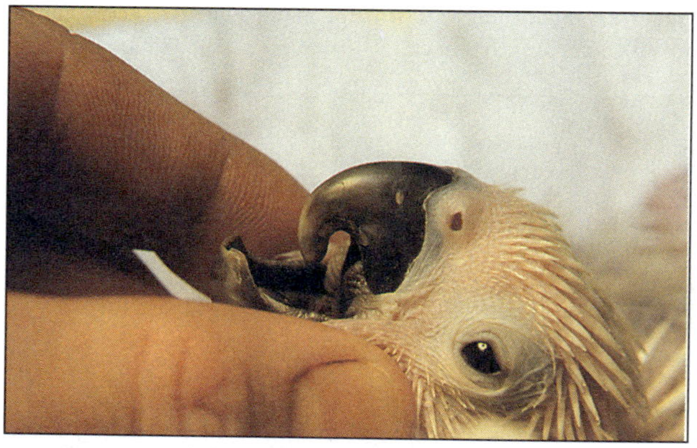

Figure 5—Severe mandibular prognathism.

MANDIBULAR PROGNATHISM

Mandibular prognathism, which is referred to as parrot beak, can be a debilitating deviation of the upper beak. The condition can range from a slightly lazy beak with the tip of the rhinotheca resting on the gnathotheca to an extreme deviation whereby the upper beak is curled under at 180° or more, sometimes with penetration of the tongue (Figure 5).

Correction by use of a premaxillary appliance is highly preferable over the cumbersome alternative that consists of constant cutting, grinding, and trauma to the sensitive bill-tip organ and beak surfaces.

Species susceptibility is wide; but mandibular prognathism is most commonly noted in cockatoos,[20,21,35] where the result in very mild cases may appear the equivalent of that observed with behavioral thumbsucking in children.

An anatomic review of cases of mandibular prognathism reveals a shortened premaxilla and/or nasal and frontal bones. Practitioners should be aware that the mandible of the normal psittacine hatchling is longer than the premaxilla and that growth of both jaws occurs in stages.[9,36,42] This temporary imbalance of length may be beneficial for parents feeding altricial chicks, and studies suggest that parents may promote beak development by pulling on the rhinotheca.[35] Very rarely has this condition ever been documented in wild hatched or parent-fed chicks.

A synthetic apparatus has been designed to accomplish the equivalent effect that the parents are believed to provide. The artificial rostral extension of the rhinotheca over the gnathotheca correctly forces its direction of growth in chicks or remodeling in older birds. At the same time, the ligaments of the nasofrontal hinge are stretched and prevent abnormal joint contracture. For obvious reasons, this approach works most effectively in epignathous species.

The patient should be induced with isoflurane after a complete diagnostic workup for occult disease. Placement of the anesthetic tube in the abdominal air sac is advantageous at times; but the inconvenience associated with upper airway delivery when repairing scissors beak is not as great when repairing mandibular prognathism, as less surgical time is required.

Any hyperplasia of the rhamphotheca should be removed but only to a state of normal shape; otherwise any leverage advantage may be lost and final recovery time prolonged. A full circumferential groove should be cut around the keratin of the rhinotheca halfway between the rostral tip and the inner keratin ridge. The chick must be old enough to have developed sufficient hard keratin so that injury is not sustained by the younger membranous keratin. Second and third circular grooves should be incised dorsal to the initial groove, as allowed by the beak size. The notches accommodate sustained gripping by the acrylic. The grooves should be cleansed and disinfected and any evidence of dermal invasion sealed with tissue glue. The external surface of the keratin should be scarified over the entire surface of the rhinotheca on at least 50% and up to 75% of the upper beak. The area should be sealed with a low-viscosity cyanoacrylate and allowed to dry.[19,40]

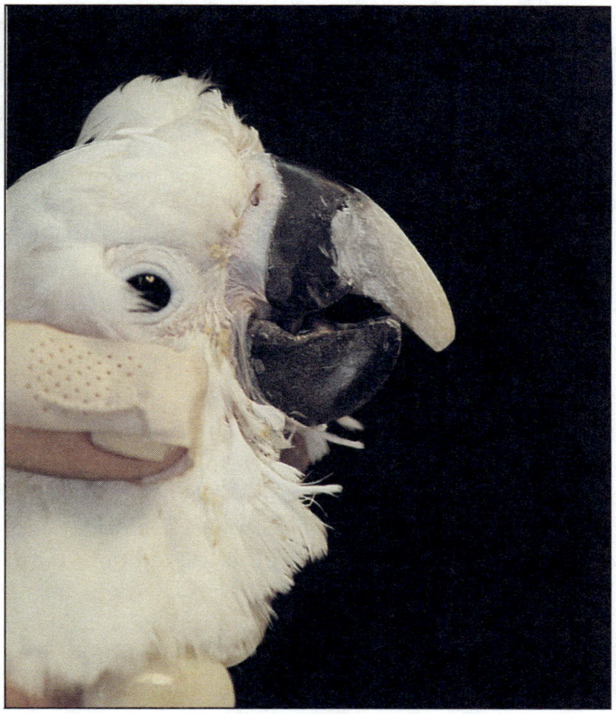

Figure 6—Finished corrective appliance.

Visible light–curing acrylics should be rolled into a conical form and the tip of the rhinotheca inserted evenly into the soft base. Latex gloves can minimize the handling problems associated with tackiness. In addition, chilling the acrylic (sheet, tube, or provisional) material in a cup of cold water can minimize any time that is loss because of prolonged handling, which can cause tackiness and poor retention of shape. The softened acrylic should be worked in an upward direction and back along all three facets of the rhinotheca in a uniform layer, spreading the acrylic until more is required. Additional aliquots of hand-warmed material can be added into the leading edge until a uniform, tightly adhered cast is formed. The acrylic can be light cured in sections while it is being added or as one final product when all acrylic has been applied, depending on surgeon preference. Electing to cure the cast in small portions to prevent movement of earlier sections is usually easiest. The rostral cast also should be extended forward at a 60° to 90° angle in a concave curve with the angle, depending on species anatomy and degree of corrective pressure required. The tapered end of the device should be smoothly pointed and sufficiently extended to prevent replacement into the oral cavity.

The final thickness of the appliance should be great enough to prevent fracture with use but thin enough to eliminate excess weight. The surface should be smooth and the edges confluent with the natural beak to prevent food retention. A grinding wheel can be used to smooth any rough spots. The critical contact areas to check are the inner rhinothecal keratin ridge (where the greatest pressures develop) and at the occlusal edge. The higher up the beak body the device is applied, the more widely distributed the forces that promote the risk of losing the device. One final check involves attempting to place the appliance tip digitally into the gnathotheca while the bird remains under anesthesia. If this check is not possible or very difficult, the patient should be allowed to recover (Figure 6).

Normal activity should be expected with temporary discomfort during the first few hours to days, as the nasofrontal joint is now forcibly extended. Hand-fed or recently weaned chicks may refuse to eat for a few meals and should be hand- or force-fed. Adults may persist in trying to dislodge the appliance because of discomfort and/or frustration. Light sedation should be considered if these efforts become too vigorous. Especially resistant patients may require a smooth sidebox or plexiglass cage to prevent violent detachment before the appliance has been accepted.

Aftercare involves routine sanitation, especially for hand-fed juveniles, and checking the periphery for movement. Scheduled rechecks each week to evaluate patient progress and to cement loose edges with a low-viscosity cyanoacrylate for 14 to 30 days after surgery are usually sufficient for most patients, particularly unweaned birds.

Excision for removal of the device is usually accomplished by digital manipulation, especially in juveniles, and by detaching the hardened acrylic cone through the exfoliated keratin layer. For patients with minimal growth or with deep notches that continue to interdigitate with the acrylic, cutting the cast along lines that are 180° from one another allows the device to separate in halves. Surgeons should be cautious when using a cutting burr, as the beak is much less dense than the acrylic.

ACQUIRED BEAK DISORDERS

Traditionally, acquired disorders of the beak are the result of trauma. The nature of the trauma in decreasing incidence involves wounds inflicted by parents or cage mates; self-induced fractures; owner-induced trauma; facial concussion; subluxation; and thermal, electrical, or chemical burns.

Beak malocclusion, defects, and overgrowth also can be generated by chronic liver disease, infection, hormonal disorders, malnutrition, and inappropriate hand-feeding techniques.[12,17,18,29,36,43–52] In addition to surgical correction, significant effort should be devoted to diagnostic studies, medical care, and improved husbandry that can correct the cause of the trauma and prevent recurrence.

EPIDERMAL WOUNDS WITHOUT FRACTURE

Punctures, lacerations, and tears are most often acquired through bites delivered by parents, siblings, or cage mates.[19,20,22,29,31,53] A fundamental concept that must be grasped is that beak wounds are soft tissue wounds involving thin, delicate tissue layers with a blood supply that is interfaced between two harder tissue layers (cortical bone and keratin). The injuries are often complicated by orthopedic lesions. Such wounds must be assessed on the basis of size, duration, contamination level, position relevant to impact on functional use, degree of damage (especially with crush injuries) sustained to the region, and any sign of subkeratin hematoma.

Beak-tip tears and minor lacerations to the keratin and dermal layers, especially in patients presented within the golden period, are good candidates for immediate closure. The wounds should be copiously flushed with chlorhexidine solution or tamed iodophor to remove foreign debris, tissue fragments, and opportunistic bacteria. Surgical scrub should be used to remove any oily contaminants. Practitioners should be certain to avoid introduction of detergents or significant volumes of fluids into the sinus cavity. Sedatives and positioning the patient with the wound in a ventrally dependent manner can prevent flush inhalation.

The wound edges should be brought into apposition by using blunt instruments, such as sterilized flat plastic toothpicks or dental hand instruments, especially picks or probes that have had their tips modified into blunt hooks for manipulation of thin tissue. Delicate handling is necessary to avoid causing further loss of capillary vitality in the wound area.[21] Fresh wounds with an intact vascular supply should undergo first-intention healing in the same manner as occurs with other epithelial lesions. Exposed tissue must be protected from further contamination by normal beak use during the healing period.

A variety of adhesives can be used to cover the area until healing is achieved. The intent of adhesive application is to create a topical bandage that allows epithelization or fibrosis under sterile conditions. The extent of healing that may occur for part or all of the wound during the initial repair process is often difficult to predict. Because neovascularization and cellular reorganization depend on a fragile dermal layer, it is critical that further disruption to the wound site be avoided during the entire healing process. The integrity and biocompatability of synthetic adhesives act as ideal topical shields. Good results have been achieved with multiple thin layers of N-butyl cyanoacrylates.[21,22,36,54] Additional adhesives include ethyl cyanoacrylates with or without methyl methacrylate powder thickeners and methoxycyanoacrylate. Compared with ethyl cyanoacrylate products, the methoxycyanoacrylate has the lowest potential to produce fumes and irritate tissue and has little exothermic activity when not used with an accelerator.[b] Patch design and coverage need to be adapted to the size, conformation, and location of the individual beak. In addition, the type of keratin involved (covering versus weight bearing) depends on lesion location and must be considered, as the stratum corneum requires more time for regeneration in weight-bearing (work contact) areas. Patch reapplication depends on the healing time required and persistence of the patch. Most acrylics and composites are lost through normal desquamation of keratin in about two or three weeks. Overlay integrity may be compromised more quickly if oral pressures are being transmitted directly or by keratin flexing into the site.

Larger wounds that require second-intention healing must be protected for a longer duration. The fundamental goal for all beak wounds is to achieve any format for tissue healing possible, regardless of whether by first or second intention. Because of the variations in anatomy and limited understanding of beak biomechanics among species, the type of healing that may occur at different beak locations with different wound patterns is impossible to predict. The primary focus should always be to minimize the likelihood of tissue loss and subsequent establishment of a permanent defect. Aggressive initial care can minimize the need for second-intention healing after necrosis or exuberant granulation occurs at the wound site. Such cases are especially noted when wounds are not treated immediately, are inadequately cleansed, or are partially protected from external invasion. It is also important not to fill the wound defect with adhesives that can interfere with capillary invasion and bridging. Many wounds heal through fibrosis with a lack of reepithelization at the defect site, and pink granulation tissue often persists with a lack of keratin for years after certain injuries. These options are perfectly acceptable for pet birds, and no techniques for implementing sliding flaps or grafts are known at present (Figure 7).

[b]Lyon A: Personal communication. Elgin, IL, Henkel Adhesive Company, Technical Department, 1992.

Antimicrobial therapy should be broad spectrum, systemic, and routine, even in cases of acute wounds, as fecal and environmental contamination are common sources for fungal and bacterial infection. Fluconazole and itraconazole have proven to be excellent antimycotic choices. Nystatin is not systemically absorbed and should not be used except for initial topical treatment. Antimycotic therapy is recommended for five to seven days in patients with acute wounds, and antibacterial therapy is recommended for 10 to 14 days. Broad-spectrum antibiotics are recommended, especially such β-lactams as piperacillin and cefotaxime. In cases of deep wounds with gram-negative contamination suspected or confirmed by culture results, broad-spectrum antibiotics also can be combined with such aminoglycosides as amikacin or netilmicin for added efficacy. Birds with more chronically exposed wounds should receive antimycotics for 10 to 14 days and antibiotics for two to eight weeks to prevent osteomyelitis. Even wounds of apparently little significance, such as macaw baby acne (seen as a result of sibling nail punctures), can result in an insidious case of osteomyelitis months after an injury if not treated properly in the initial stages.[53]

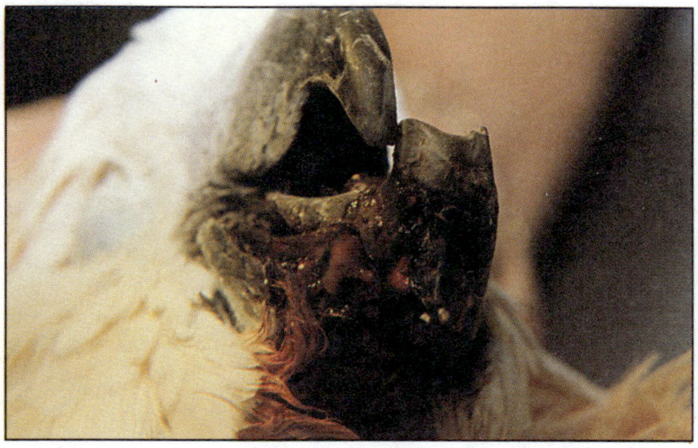

Figure 7—Mate trauma with degloving of mandible.

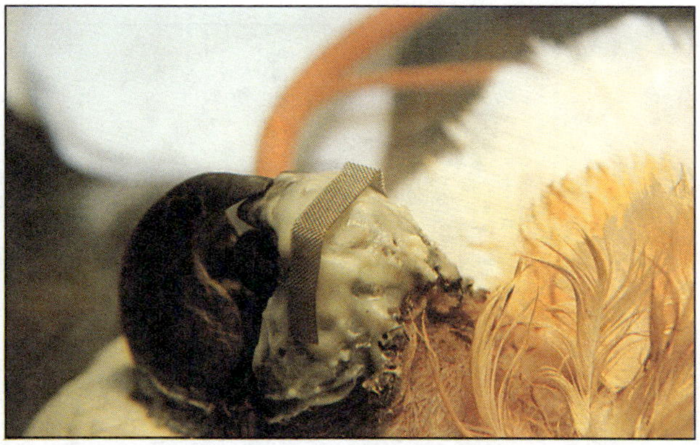

Figure 8—Wired fracture covered in cast material before support mesh has been incorporated.

FRACTURES OF THE BEAK TIP

Fractures of the tip of the rhinotheca are common in pet birds, especially African grey parrots and cockatoos.[20,21,55] Patients usually present with the premaxillary beak tip intact and a fracture line 3 to 5 mm above the point. The wound can be glued with a cyanoacrylate and allowed to heal through internal replacement.[25] Injuries in which the tip of the beak has been lost or has been significantly displaced respond well to amputation, hemostasis, and disinfection. Research in poultry has shown that traumatic beak amputation can result in full regeneration of bone, cartilage, and keratin but not nerve fibers,[56] indicating a good prognosis.

The same guidelines for treatment and antimicrobial therapy of punctures apply for fracture wounds. In addition to the pain patients sustain from the immediate impact and tip fracture, many undergo subkeratic hemorrhage and experience a condition similar to a hoof bruise. The use of nonsteroidal antiinflammatory drugs (NSAIDs), especially flunixine and analgesics, can have a positive effect and assist the patient in returning to normal self-feeding. Cases in which clinical signs support or are suspicious for central nervous system trauma from forces transmitted through the beak should receive corticosteroids instead of NSAIDs.

FRACTURE REPAIR

Fractures of the beak skeleton are significant, as they tend to be extremely painful, rapidly lead to debilitation through anorexia, and are highly prone to nonunion without surgical stabilization. In psittacines, fractures of the mandible and zygomatic arch tend to be more challenging than those of the premaxilla.

The principles of fracture repair of beaks are the same as those for other bone fractures in that stabilization against external (biting) and intrinsic (muscular) forces must be sustained. Such stability may be obtained easily when heavy cortical bone is involved but can be more difficult when the bones are small (e.g., passerines) or density low (i.e., a high degree of cancellous bone, as with anseriformes) or when pneumatization is present.[15]

Presurgical considerations should include standard assessment through routine examination and radiology. Any devitalization of the dermis, loss of vascular supply to affected bones, and potential for reapposition of the fracture site and soft tissue are major prognostic factors.

Simple unilateral fractures of the mandibular ramus can compress with jaw closure; such fractures lend themselves to synthetic casts that envelop the damaged area on at least three facets. The approach is similar to the use of dental splinting in dogs or cats by using an acrylic pour to stabilize the teeth in a fractured mandible.[41,42] In birds, intact keratin is used as a base point to mold the cyanoacrylate around any closure with an open defect. It is important to enclose a minimum of three facets of the beak adjacent to the fracture site to prevent premature cast movement but is more effective to use five or six surfaces of the gnathotheca (medial/lateral side walls and dorsal/lateral surfaces of the dentary portion) in most cases. Premaxillary fractures of the same type also respond well to cyanoacrylate-type casts or splints (Figure 8). One key to success is to envelop the damaged beak so that the splint absorbs and distributes working forces across undamaged beak sections.

Jaw fractures subjected to distractive forces, distal fractures of the mandibular ramus, and especially bilateral mandibular fractures require use of cerclage wire or internal rigid fixation. Cruciate and hemicerclage patterns placed to nullify the forces of distraction can provide stability and protect new capillary bed growth without strangulation (Figure 9).

Persistence is a mandate for success when approaching open or comminuted jaw fractures. Initially, any wound should be flushed, scrubbed, and sealed with a biocompatible cyanoacrylate that is strengthened by a light-sensitive acrylic. Medical support should include hospitalization and administration of NSAIDs, analgesics, and antimicrobials. Tube-feeding aided by administration of mild sedatives to help prevent the patient from chewing on the tube is critical during the initial postoperative period and may be required for the follow-up period as well. Diazepam is the sedative of choice. Flunixine and butorphanol are excellent for inflammation and pain control, respectively.[20–22,39,53]

Follow-up evaluations should be done every few days initially and then weekly after day 10. The area should be radiographed three to four weeks later. With the patient under gas anesthesia, the synthetic cast should be removed very cautiously for debridement and reevaluation of the healing process every 30 days (Figure 10A). Food and/or debris are commonly found around the edges of the cast during follow-up checks. Because fractures may require several months to heal, replacement of oral splints or casts one or two times after initial surgery is common (Figure 10B).

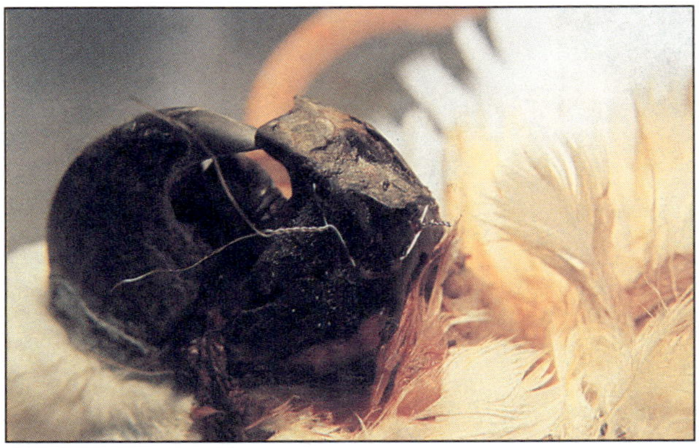

Figure 9—Cerclage wires in place.

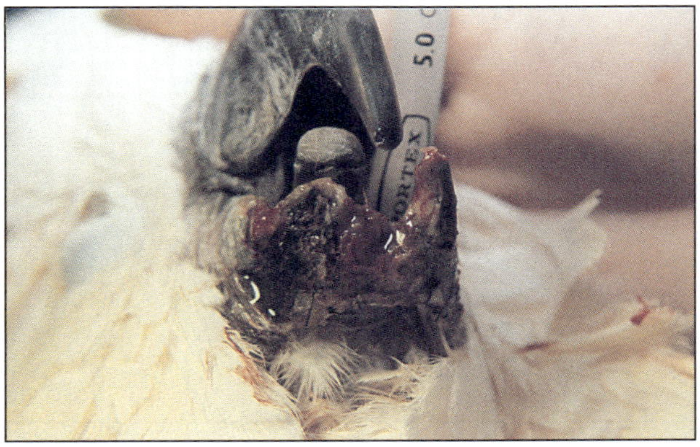

Figure 10A

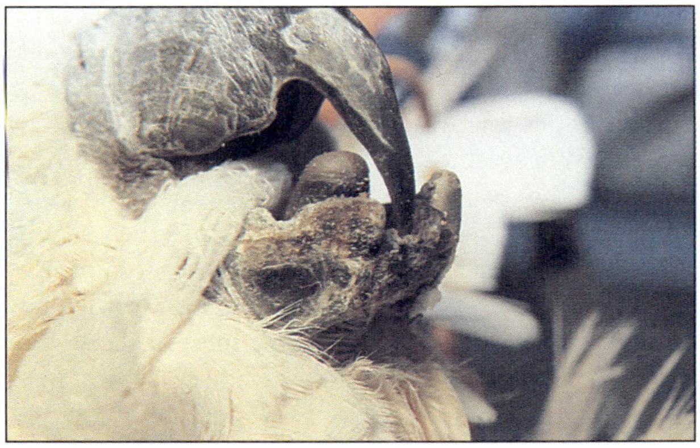

Figure 10B

Figure 10—(A) Reevaluation eight weeks (60 days) after surgery. **(B)** Reevaluation 11 weeks after surgery.

Of equal importance as the surgeon's skills is postoperative management. Smooth-sided cages large enough for feed dishes, a low perch (requiring no climbing), and ample exercise room are fundamental. Finding a suitable soft and nutritionally balanced diet also is crucial. Successful healing depends on a high-quality diet. Often these patients have been lifelong seed eaters with mineral, protein, and vitamin deficiencies. Self-feeding the new diet would be preferable, but usually these birds must be force-fed for the first several days to weeks until the new diet has been accepted. Sedation should prevent the bird from rubbing its jaw against feeding equipment.

Bilateral mandibular and to a lesser extent premaxillary fractures carry a poor prognosis. Acutely traumatized patients may be salvaged with rapid reapposition of the fragments by using a combination of internal and external fixation once the patient has been stabilized and any soft tissue wounds treated. The premaxilla may be repaired with an encompassing acrylic cast. Plastic and/or steel cast implants, such as wire mesh strips or bars, can be used to minimize the risk of fracture movement during healing. Internal fixation, in all except the largest of birds, is generally unsuccessful because of radical tissue displacement within the intercortical space, distraction of the fracture site despite the presence of pins, and thin jaw cortices that do not retain orthopedic screws or plates.

Mandibular midline fractures are seen with regularity in cases of blunt facial trauma (e.g., contact with a wall). These fractures are extremely frustrating to treat, especially in small species; nonunion apparently is the rule.[18,28] As in cases of bilateral jaw fractures, wound duration is apparently a pivotal factor. The more acute the wound, the greater the potential for persistence of the blood supply and less contamination of deep tissue. Wounds older than several hours seem to respond poorly despite extensive efforts using adhesives, wires, and pins. Smaller species apparently do not respond as well as birds weighing more than 150 to 200 grams; the relatively large amount of pressure created by wire insertion may compromise the vascular dermis. In addition, leakage of any thermoplastic adhesive from the wound edge can obstruct capillary and epithelial cell migration, thereby leading to surgical failure.[b]

CONCLUSION

The techniques and observations offered in this article are the distillation of several thousand patients. The suggestions are the most practical ones for use by moderately experienced to advanced avian practitioners. Novices are strongly advised to review the literature covering species-specific feeding habits, anatomy, histology, and beak surgery for both adults and neonates, as the impact of ignoring these vital foundations is irreparable for avian patients.

A definitive treatise addressing all corrections for beak disorders remains elusive. The burgeoning field of molecular biology holds phenomenal promise in the benefits gained from using new tools[57] and the discoveries they elicit. Eventually, innovative tools may aid in an understanding of how a complex organ that has sustained damage could be rectified with little question of success.

About the Author

Dr. Clipsham owned and operated an exclusive avian and exotic animal clinical practice and continues to consult avicultural clients. Beak repair and correction of congenital beak malformation have been leading interests of Dr. Clipsham since 1980. He has lectured and published extensively on both subjects.

REFERENCES

1. McKibben JS, Harrison G: Clinical anatomy, in *Clinical Avian Medicine and Surgery.* Philadelphia, WB Saunders Co, 1986, pp 31–66.
2. Romanoff AL: *The Avian Embryo: Structural and Functional Development.* New York, MacMillan Co, 1960.
3. Yasui K, Hayashi Y: Morphogenesis of the beak of the chick embryo: Histological, histochemical and autoradiographic studies. *Embryologia* 10:42–74, 1967.
4. Rowe A, Richman J, Brickell P: Development of the spacial pattern of retinoic acid receptor-beta transcripts in the embryonic chick primordia. *Development* 114(3):805–813, 1992.
5. Richman J, Tickle C: Epithelial-mesenchymal interactions in the outgrowth of limb buds and facial primordia in chick embryos. *Devel Biol* 154(2):299–308, 1992.
6. Francis-West PH, Tatal T, Brickell PM: Expression patterns of the bone morphogenetic protein genes. BMP-4 and BMP-2 in the developing chick face suggest a role in outgrowth of the primordia. *Devel Dynam* 201(2):168–178, 1994.
7. Shames RB, et al: Region-specific expression of scutate scale type beta keratins in the developing chick beak. *J Exp Zool:* 258–266, 1994.
8. Hertel F: Ecomorphological indicators of feeding behavior in recent and fossil raptors. *Auk* 112(4):890–903, 1995.
9. Langman J: *Medical Embryology,* ed 3. Baltimore, Williams & Wilkins, 1975.
10. Calnek BW, et al: *Diseases of Poultry,* ed 9. Ames, IA, Iowa State University Press, 1991.
11. Smith S, Smith B: *Atlas of Avian Radiographic Anatomy.* Philadelphia, WB Saunders Co, 1992.
12. Harrison G, Harrison L: *Clinical Avian Medicine and Surgery.* Philadelphia, WB Saunders Co, 1986.
13. King AS: Aves respiratory system, in Getty R (ed): *The Anatomy of Domestic Animals,* vol II, ed 5. Philadelphia, WB Saunders Co, 1975.
14. Petrak ML: *Diseases of Cage and Aviary Birds,* ed 2. Philadelphia, Lea & Febiger, 1982.
15. Lucas AM, Stettenheim PR: *Avian Anatomy: Integument Agriculture Handbook 362.* Washington, DC, Agriculture Research Service, U.S. Department of Agriculture, 1972.
16. Rubel GA, Isenbugel E, Wolvekamp P (eds): *Atlas of Diagnostic Radiology of Exotic Pets.* Philadelphia, WB Saunders Co, 1991.
17. Feduccia A: Aves ostelogy, in Getty R (ed): *The Anatomy of Domestic Animals,* vol II, ed 5. Philadelphia, WB Saunders Co, 1975.
18. Freethy R: *Secrets of Bird Life.* New York, Blandford Press, Sterling Publishing Co, 1990, pp 1–23.
19. Clipsham R: Surgical beak correction. *J Assoc Avian Vet* 3(4):188–189, 1989.
20. Clipsham R: Surgical beak restoration and correction. *Proc Assoc Avian Vet*:164–176, 1989.
21. Clipsham R: Surgical correction of beaks. *Proc Assoc Avian Vet*:325–333, 1990.
22. Clipsham R: Surgical beak restoration and correction. *Proc Am Fed Avicul*:81–98, 1991.
23. Lucas AM: Integument, in Getty R (ed): *The Anatomy of Domestic Animals,* vol II, ed 5. Philadelphia, WB Saunders Co, 1975.
24. Graham D: The avian integument—Its structure and selected diseases. *Proc Assoc Avian Vet*:33–51, 1985.
25. McDonald S: Anatomical and physiological characteristics of birds and how they differ from mammals. *Proc Assoc Avian Vet*:372–389, 1990.
26. McLelland J: *A Color Atlas of Avian Anatomy.* Philadelphia, WB Saunders Co, 1991.
27. Morris P, Weigel J: Methacrylate beak prosthesis in a Maribou stork (*Leptoptilos crumeniferus*). *J Assoc Avian Vet* 4(2): 103–107, 1990.
28. Welty JC: *Life of Birds,* ed 2. Eastbourne, WB Saunders Co, 1975.

29. Clipsham R: Prenatal medical management. Part I. *Am Fed Avicul Watchbird* XVIII(5):20–23, 1992.
30. Clipsham R: Prenatal medical management. Part II. *Am Fed Avicul Watchbird* XIX(6):14–20, 1993.
31. Clipsham R: Prenatal medical management. Part III. *Am Fed Avicul Watchbird* XX(7):44–46, 1993.
32. Vellman SG, Clark SH: The cartilage proteoglycan deficient mutation, nanomelia, contains a DNA polymorphism in the proteoglycan core protein gene that is genetically linked to the nanomelia phenotype. *Matrix* 12(1):66–72, 1992.
33. Vellman SG, et al: Screening for carriers of the avian cartilage proteoglycan core protein defect nanomelia by denaturing gradient gel electrophoresis. *J Hered* 84(2):147–149, 1993.
34. Perry R, Gill J: Disorders of the avian integument. *Vet Clin North Am Small Anim Pract* 21(6):1307–1325, 1992.
35. Schubot R, Clubb K, Clubb S: *Psittacine Aviculture.* Loxahatchee, FL, Avicult Breeding and Research Center, 1992.
36. Clipsham R: Noninfectious diseases of pediatric psittacines. *Semin Avian Exotic Pet Med* 1(1):22–33, 1992.
37. Coniff R: Why catfish farmers want to throttle the crow of the sea. *Smithsonian* 22(2):44–55, 1991.
38. Burgaz S, et al: Effect of hydroquinolone (HQ) on the development of chick embryos. *Drug Chem Toxicol* 17(2):163–174, 1995.
39. Clipsham R: Beak repair: Orthodontics, in Altman R, Clubb S, Dorrestein J, et al (eds): *Avian Medicine and Surgery.* Philadelphia, WB Saunders Co, in press.
40. Clipsham R: Surgical correction of beaks: Wet lab protocol. *AAV Lab Manual.* Chicago, Association of Avian Veterinarians, 1991.
41. Holmstrom S: *Veterinary Dental Techniques for the Small Animal Practitioner.* Philadelphia, WB Saunders Co, 1992.
42. Harvey C, Emily P: *Small Animal Dentistry.* St. Louis, MO, Mosby-Yearbook, 1993.
43. Gerlach H: Viruses, in Ritchie B, Harrison G, Harrison L (eds): *Avian Medicine: Principles and Application.* Lakeworth, FL, Wingers Publishing, 1994, pp 862–948.
44. Greiner EC, Ritchie B: Parasites, in Ritchie B, Harrison G, Harrison L (eds): *Avian Medicine: Principles and Application.* Lakeworth, FL, Wingers Publishing, 1994, pp 1007–1129.
45. Bauck L: Mycosis, in Ritchie B, Harrison G, Harrison L (eds): *Avian Medicine: Principles and Application.* Lakeworth, FL, Wingers Publishing, 1994, pp 997–1006.
46. Lumeij JT: Endocrinology, in Ritchie B, Harrison G, Harrison L (eds): *Avian Medicine: Principles and Application.* Lakeworth, FL, Wingers Publishing, 1994, pp 582–697.
47. Flammer K, Clubb S: Neonatology, in Ritchie B, Harrison G, Harrison L (eds): *Avian Medicine: Principles and Application.* Lakeworth, FL, Wingers Publishing, 1994, pp 805–841.
48. Lumeij JT: Hepatology, in Ritchie B, Harrison G, Harrison L (eds): *Avian Medicine: Principles and Application.* Lakeworth, FL, Wingers Publishing, 1994, pp 522–537.
49. Cooper JE, Harrison G: Dermatology, in Ritchie B, Harrison G, Harrison L (eds): *Avian Medicine: Principles and Application.* Lakeworth, FL, Wingers Publishing, 1994, pp 608–639.
50. Bengoa A, et al: Beak infection by penicillium cyclopium in a macaw (*Ara ararauna*). *Avian Dis* 38:922–927, 1994.
51. Latimer KS: Oncology, in Ritchie B, Harrison G, Harrison L (eds): *Avian Medicine: Principles and Application.* Lakeworth, FL, Wingers Publishing, 1994, pp 640–672.
52. Kufuor-Mensah E, Watson GL: Malignant melanomas in a penguin (*E. chrysolophus*) and a red-tailed hawk (*B. jamaicensis*). *Vet Pathol* 29:54–356, 1992.
53. Clipsham R: Introduction to psittacine pediatrics. *Vet Clin North Am Small Anim Pract* 21(6):1361–1392, 1993.
54. Harrison G: IME 211: Some suggested uses for surgical glue. *Assoc Avian Vet Newsletter* 3(2):34, 1982.
55. Rich G: Fractures of the tip of the maxillary beak. *J Assoc Avian Vet* 5(3):129, 1991.
56. Gentle MJ, Thorp BH, Hughes BO: Anatomical consequences of partial beak amputation in turkeys. *Res Vet Sci* 58(2):158–162, 1995.
57. Bartels T, Flachsbarth MF: Scanning electron microscopic investigations on the development of the avian beak. *Zool Anzeiger* 232(3–4):97–110, 1994.

Avian Orthopedics

KEY FACTS

- **Presurgical evaluation should include measurements of serum glucose, packed cell volume, serum uric acid, and total protein; although normal values vary depending on the species, general guidelines apply to most birds.**
- **Stable fractures with minimal displacement can usually be treated adequately by external splinting or casting.**
- **Fractures involving the humerus and the femur are hard to treat by splinting alone.**
- **Internal fixation by intramedullary pinning is the most common means of fracture repair in avian orthopedics.**

Pacific Spirit Veterinary Surgery
Richmond, British Columbia, Canada
Lyndell Levitt, BSc, DVM, MVSc

AVIAN ORTHOPEDICS is uniquely challenging to veterinary surgeons. Many methods and devices, developed to manage fractures in mammals, have been adapted for the repair of avian fractures. There have been numerous articles describing the use of intramedullary pins and variations of the Kirschner-Ehmer device in avian fractures.[1-10] In some instances, bone plating has been advocated[11]; this method is not widely used. A recent study detailed success rates and the rate of return to normal function after fracture repair.[12]

ANATOMIC AND PHYSIOLOGIC FACTORS

Various avian anatomic and physiologic factors affect the outcome of surgery to correct fractures. These factors include bone strength, joint involvement, rotational deformity, synostosis, fracture type, soft tissue injury, and infection.

Bone Strength

Avian bones are designed for lightweight, aerodynamic strength and have thin, brittle cortices. These cortices provide scant stability or purchase for such implants as screws or half-pin Kirschner-Ehmer devices.[13]

Joint Involvement

Fractures that involve a wing frequently occur near or through a joint. Although such fractures often can be repaired, permanent joint dysfunction is a common sequela. Serious restriction of joint mobility can result from impingement of the fracture callus on the joint or from adhesions involving adjacent ligaments and tendons. Even mild joint impingement can lead to severe loss of function and inability to fly. Prolonged immobilization of the wing with external coaptation can also lead to joint stiffness and dysfunction.

Rotational Deformity

The strong rotational forces exerted by the flight muscles and tendons can cause considerable torsional deformity. In humeral fracture repair, any degree of rotation can magnify the deformity at the wing tip and can interfere with flying ability.[10] Even if axial alignment of humeral fractures is excellent, a few degrees of rotation can mean the difference between functional and nonfunctional healing.[14]

Synostosis

The longitudinal sliding motion between the radius and the ulna is important for normal wing function. If a synostosis develops between these bones during fracture healing, the pronation–supination activity of the distal wing will be seriously limited. Wing extension and precision flying ability will be affected. This limitation is particularly important in raptors.

Fracture Type

Many avian fractures present as comminuted, open fractures with significant soft tissue damage. Such fractures are often difficult to reduce and stabilize; healing can be

Updated from original publication in Volume 11, Number 8, August 1989 prolonged. The sparseness of tissue in the area often precludes coverage of the fracture site with soft tissue. This lack of coverage can result in vascular compromise of the bone or exposure of the bone to the environment and can lead to delayed healing and increased risk of infection.

Soft Tissue Injury

In wild birds, severe trauma (e.g., injuries from gunshots, traps, or car collisions) can result in significant soft tissue injury as well as orthopedic problems. In addition to evaluating the fractured bone, the surgeon must systematically evaluate the injured soft tissues. Specific attention should be devoted to blood vessels, nerves, and musculotendinous units within the zone of trauma. Fascial and muscular planes as well as the accompanying vessels and nerves must be identified.[15] Abnormal repositioning of tendons and muscles during fracture repair will compromise the normal function of the wing or limb. Severe vascular disruption can compromise fracture healing and can increase the risk of infection.

Infection

Many avian fractures are presented as open, contaminated wounds. The general principles of wound treatment and debridement must be followed in the initial management of such fractures. Antibiotic therapy, initiated before surgery, is based on culture and sensitivity results or on knowledge of the probable contaminant. Cephalosporin antibiotics are generally useful in treating open fractures in birds.

PRESURGICAL EVALUATION AND PRESENTATION

Minimizing stress is essential when handling injured birds. The stress of handling and examination can be reduced by covering the patient's head with a towel or a falconry hood. Sedation is rarely required for initial examination. The factors evaluated during this examination include the nutritional status, the nature of the injury, and the degree of associated contamination.

MANY PATIENTS are severely to moderately debilitated on presentation. Enteral alimentation and fluid therapy are necessary presurgical procedures. Definitive fracture repair should be delayed until the patient is adequately stabilized. Temporary immobilization of the fracture should be maintained by the judicious use of external splints or slings. Such immobilization limits further damage during stabilization.

Presurgical evaluation should include measurements of serum glucose, packed cell volume, serum uric acid, and total protein. Although normal values vary depending on the species, general guidelines apply to most birds.[14,15] Birds with serum glucose levels less than 200 mg/100 ml should receive dextrose supplementation before and after surgery.[16] If the packed cell volume is less than 30%, surgery is postponed or a blood transfusion is given during surgery.

Birds with uric acid levels greater than 30 mg/100 ml might have renal failure or dehydration and prerenal azotemia. Concurrent evaluation of serum protein and packed cell volume differentiates increased uric acid levels caused by dehydration from those caused by renal failure. The source of the elevated uric acid level should be determined before therapy is instituted. Such patients should receive fluid therapy, and surgery should be postponed until the uric acid level is reduced.[16] A serum protein level less than 2 mg/100 ml indicates severe debilitation; the prognosis for patient survival after successful anesthetic and surgical outcome is guarded.

ALTERNATIVES FOR FRACTURE REPAIR

Most fractures of the pelvis and the pectoral girdle (the scapula, the clavicle, and the coronoid process) can be left without support. Strict cage rest for two to three weeks is usually the only required treatment for such fractures. Minimally displaced fractures and greenstick fractures also can heal without support if the patient's exercise is restricted. In such cases, early return to function and rehabilitation should be stressed.

External Immobilization—Splints

Stable fractures with minimal displacement can usually be treated adequately by external splinting or casting. As in mammalian orthopedics, immobilization of one joint above and one joint below the fracture is advised.

Minimally displaced radial fractures rarely require surgical intervention if the ulna is intact. Such fractures are successfully managed by external immobilization and appropriate wound therapy. Immobilization of radial fractures and nondisplaced radioulnar fractures can be achieved by folding the wing in flexion with a braile or figure-of-eight bandage or by taping the injured wing to the body.

I prefer the use of the braile sling because it is usually well-tolerated by patients and does not interfere with respiratory excursions. The sling consists of a long, narrow strip of cloth or soft leather with a longitudinal slit cut near the middle. This slit is slipped over the folded carpal joint; the two loose ends are wrapped around the folded wing and tied behind the humerus to prevent the slit from slipping off the folded carpus. The ends are then wrapped around the flight feathers and tied so that the feathers are bound compactly[11] (Figures 1 and 2).

Fractured metacarpal bones are amenable to treatment with external immobilization via the braile sling. The sling can also be used to maintain alignment after closed reduction of elbow luxations.

SIMPLE FRACTURES of the leg often heal with minimal fixation. Various splints and casts of fiberglass or plaster have been used with satisfactory results.[11,17,18] In simple tarsometatarsal or phalangeal fractures, plastic con-

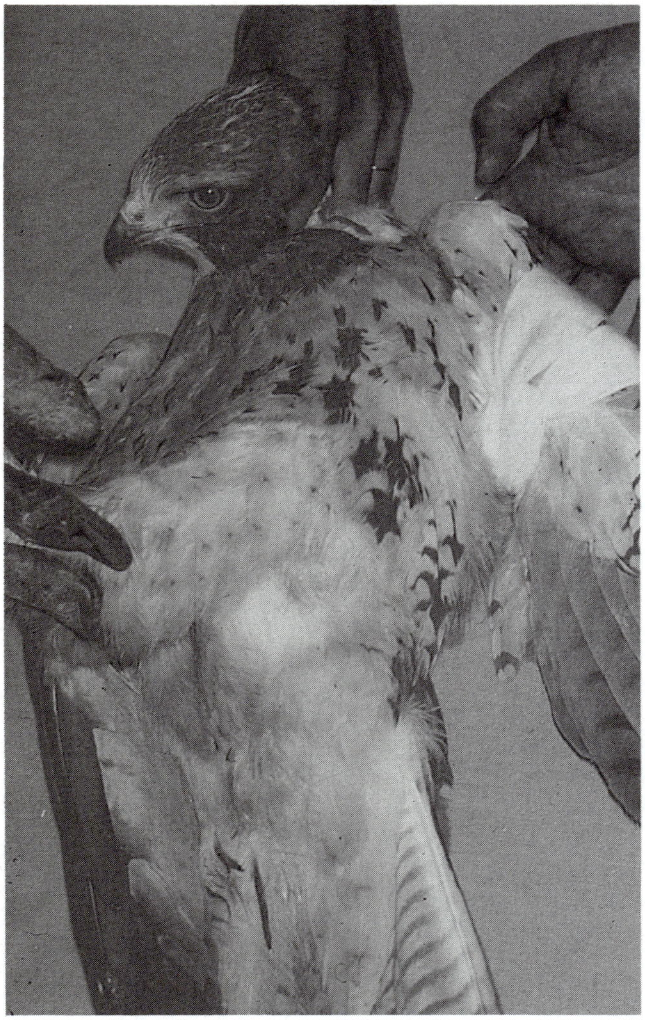

Figure 1A

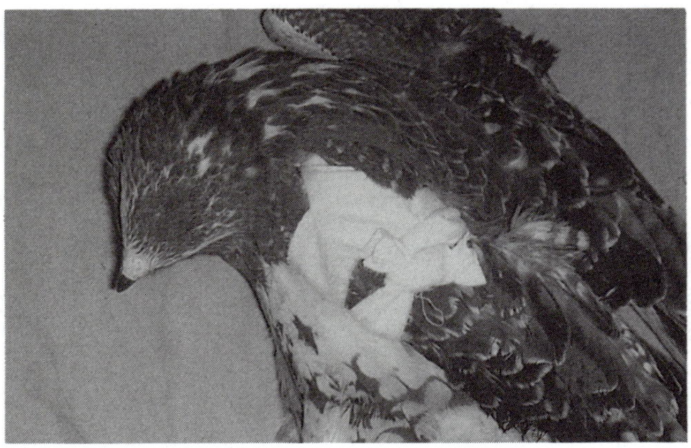

Figure 1B

Figure 1—(**A** and **B**) A rough-legged hawk (*Buteo logopus*) with a fractured radius. External immobilization was achieved by means of a braile sling.

duits (e.g., syringe cases) can be halved, padded, and applied as Mason's metasplints. Phalangeal fractures can also be treated successfully by bandaging the digits to an appropriately shaped object (e.g., a padded dowel or a tennis ball), with the talons maintained in an extended position.

Ehmer slings are designed to stabilize metatarsal and nondisplaced tibiotarsal fractures.[11] These slings are economical and easy to apply; the tarsometatarsus and the tibiotarsus are bound together in a flexed position with gauze. If necessary, the bound leg can be folded against the body with an encircling piece of tape. Alternatively, a modified spica splint provides limited immobilization of the stifle and hip joints while the limb is maintained in an extended position (Figure 3). Spica splints are inadequate for most femoral fractures but provide stability for tibiotarsal and metatarsal fractures.

Fractures involving the humerus and the femur are hard to treat by splinting alone because of the difficulty of completely immobilizing the shoulder joint and the hip joint, respectively. Such fractures often present with moderate to severe displacement and overriding caused by strong muscular contractions. External splinting techniques usually cannot maintain alignment of the fracture fragments.

In order to minimize the possibility of joint ankylosis, external immobilization should be discontinued when radiographic signs of fracture healing are evident. In most uncomplicated cases, immobilization is required for two to three weeks (adolescents) or for three to six weeks (adults).

External Fixation—Kirschner-Ehmer Splints

Variations of the Kirschner-Ehmer splint provide excellent means of fixation for many avian fractures. Modifications of the pin, clamp, and bar device described by Bush in 1981[5] include the use of lightweight casting materials (e.g., Hexcelite®—Hexcel Medical),[8] epoxy resins,[6] and methylmethacrylate. These materials bind the pins together after they are implanted in the bone. The devices provide rigid fixation, do not interfere with joint function, and are easy to apply. A Kirschner-Ehmer device permits relatively normal use of the injured wing or limb during the convalescent period; such movement minimizes disuse atrophy and allows rapid return to normal function.

A properly applied through-and-through external pin splint (i.e., full-pin splintage) is usually ideal for radioulnar or tibiotarsal fractures (Figure 4). Because of the thin cortices of avian bones, half-pin splintage tends to be inadequate; there is premature loosening of the pins and the fixation device. Although half-pin splintage techniques might not be suitable for primary fixation, such techniques can help counteract rotational forces in fractures treated concurrently with intramedullary pins (Figure 5).

Internal Fixation

Intramedullary Pins

Intramedullary pinning is a very common means of fracture repair in avian orthopedics. Pinning is simple, available, and economical; it also facilitates implant removal. The major disadvantage of pinning is the lack of rotational stability it affords. This lack is particularly evident in the humerus, a pneumatic bone with a large medullary cavity

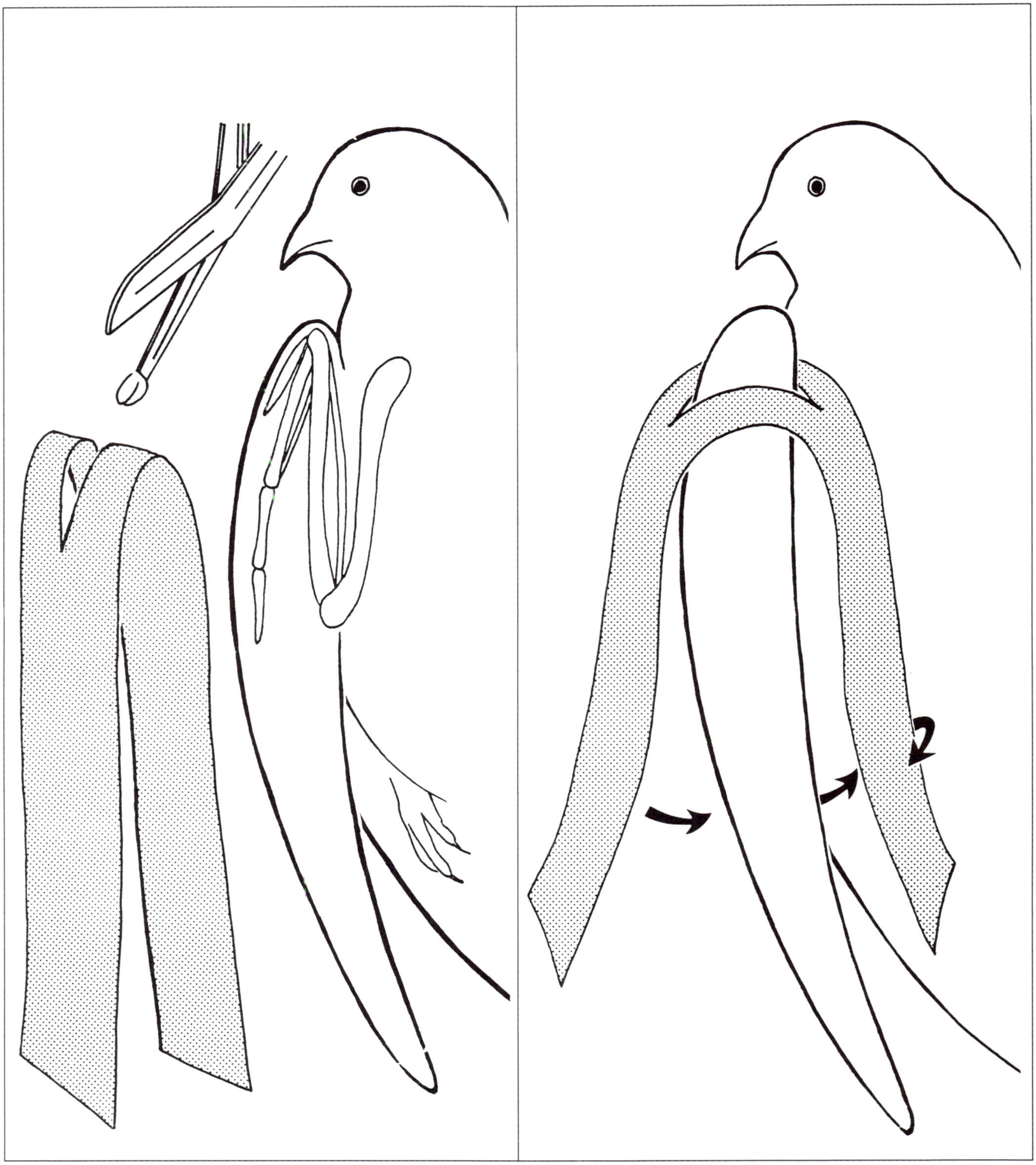

Figure 2A

Figure 2B

and scant cancellous metaphyseal bone for pin engagement. Hemicerclage wires, full-cerclage wires, or external-pin splintage can be used to maintain rotational stability while intramedullary pins maintain axial alignment.

THE VARIOUS SURGICAL APPROACHES and methods of pin placement are well-documented.[10-11] In femoral, humeral, and ulnar fractures, intramedullary pins are usually placed in a retrograde direction; in tibiotarsal fractures, the pins are placed in a normograde direction. Closed reduction and normograde placement can be used in humeral fractures involving the proximal diaphysis and in ulnar fractures involving the distal two-thirds of the diaphysis.[19] Rush pin techniques involving Kirschner wires

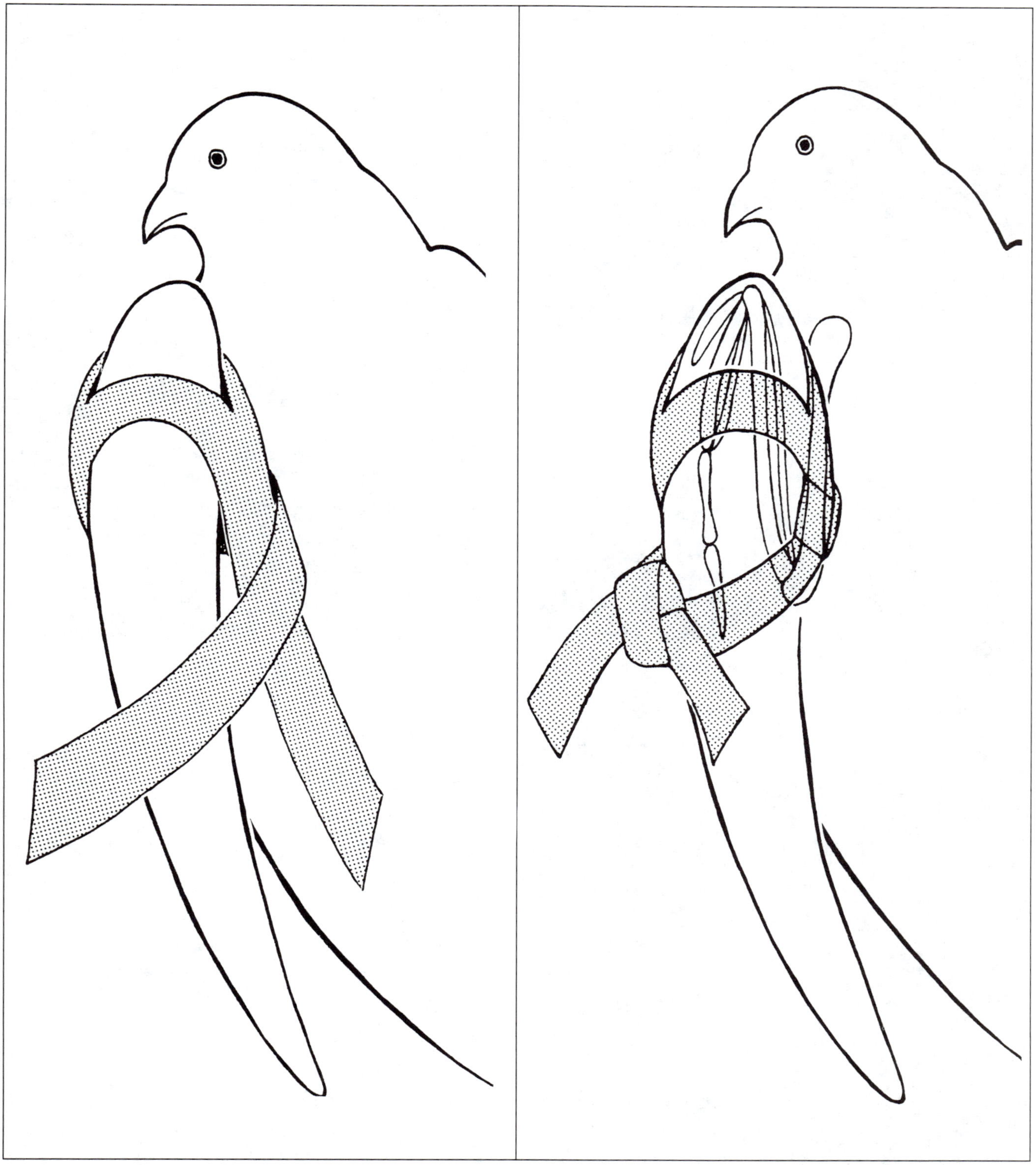

Figure 2C **Figure 2D**

Figure 2—(A) The braile sling consists of a strip of cloth or leather with a longitudinal slit cut in the middle. (**B**) The slit is placed over the folded carpus (*arrows* indicate how straps will be wrapped). (**C**) The straps are wrapped firmly behind the humerus. (**D**) The straps are then wrapped around the flight feathers and are tied.

or small Steinmann's pins are particularly well-suited to distal femoral fractures, tarsometatarsal fractures, and radial fractures.

The surgeon must ensure that the pins do not interfere with normal joint mobility. Intramedullary pins can cause significant postoperative joint problems, particularly in cases involving ulnar fractures. Intramedullary pins must be placed accurately in order to avoid interfering with

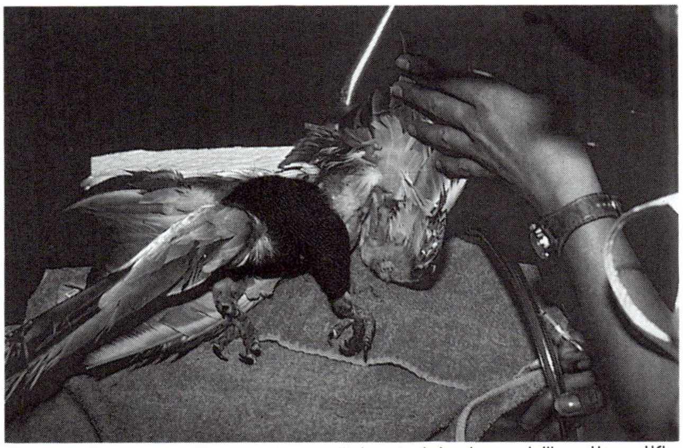

Figure 3—A modified spica splint used to immobilize the stifle and the hip of a macaw (*Ara ararauna*).

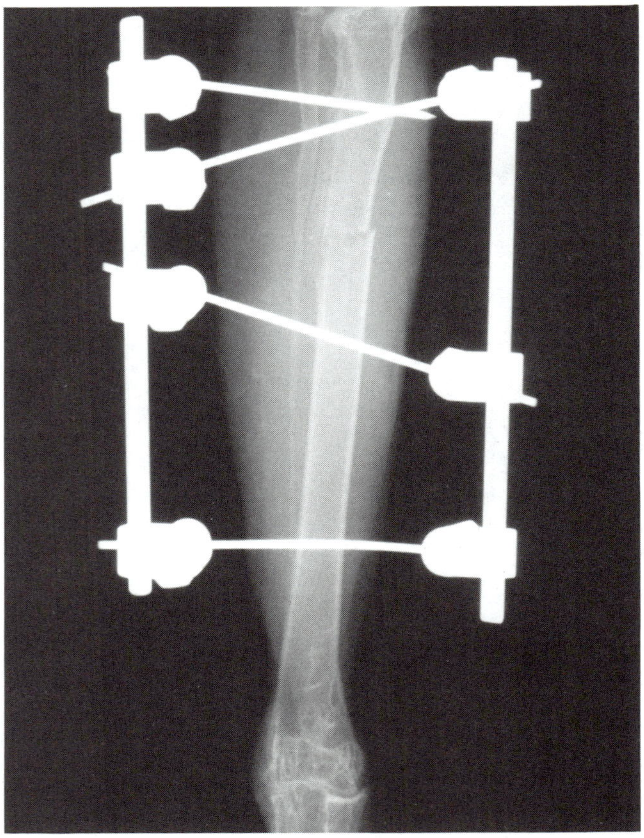

Figure 4B

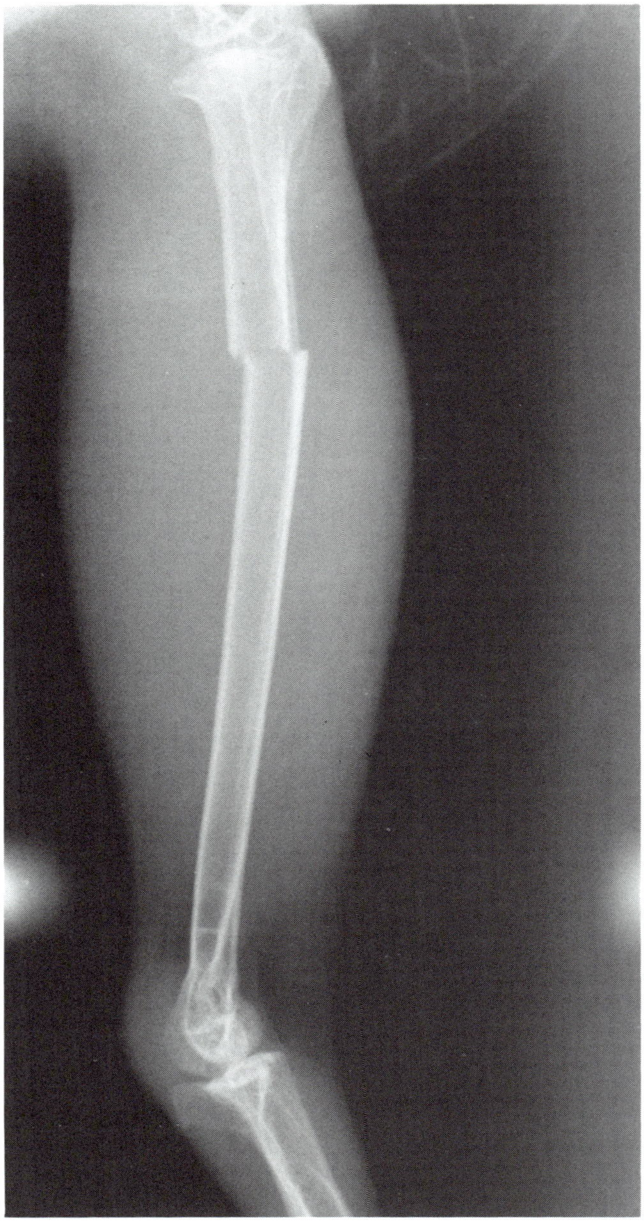

Figure 4A

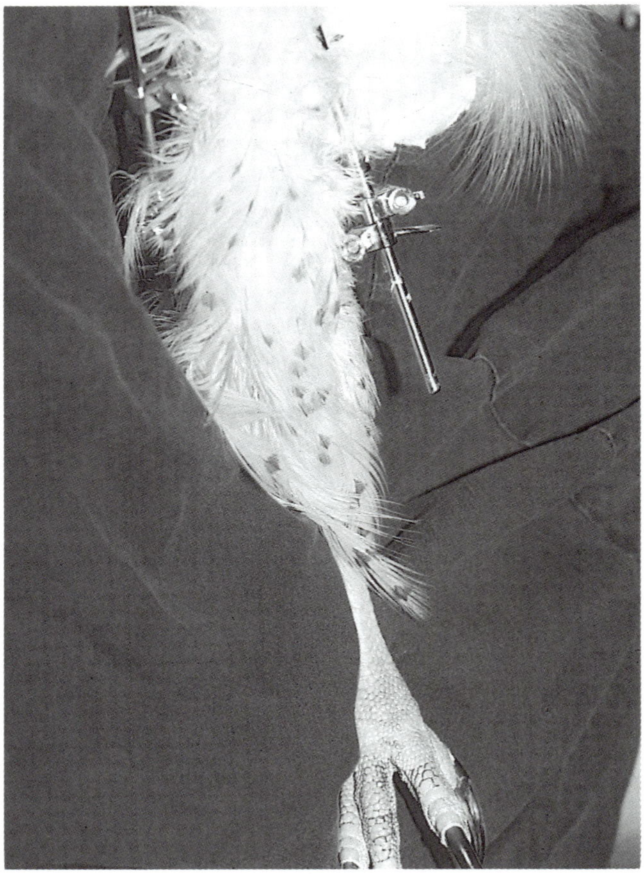

Figure 4C

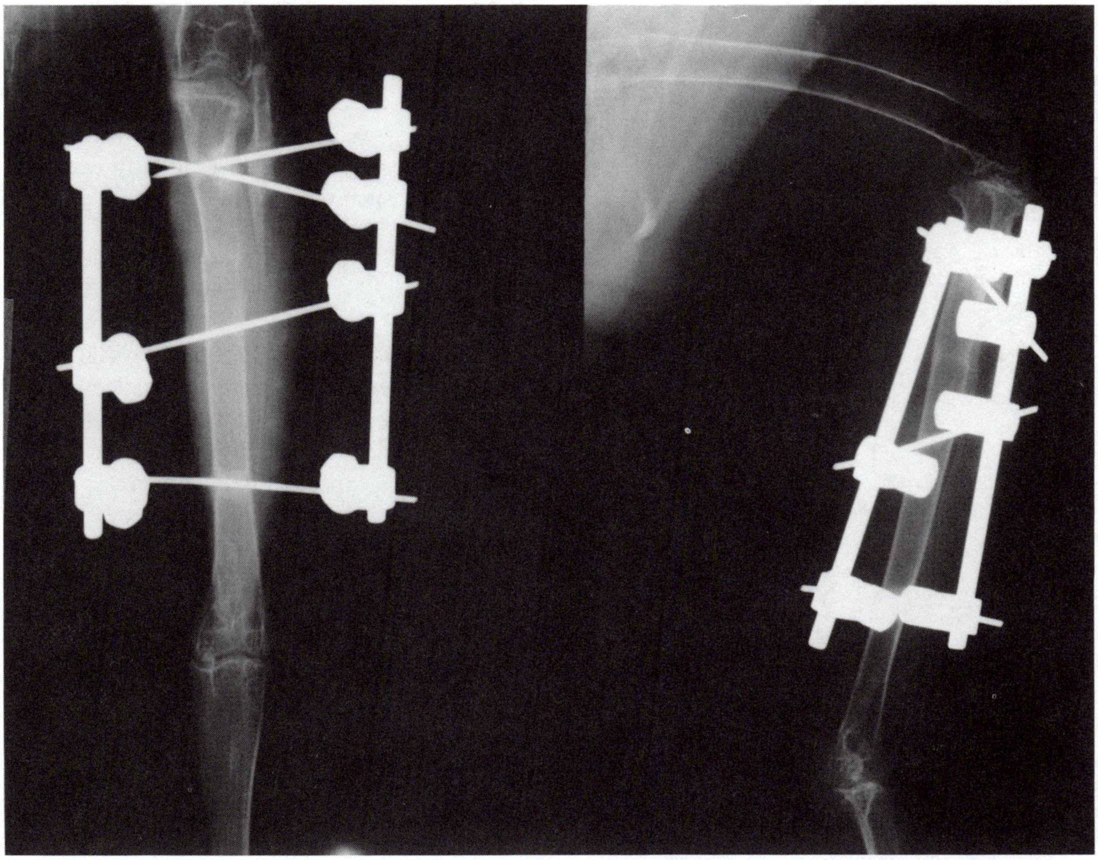

Figure 4D

Figure 4—(A) A radiograph of a simple transverse fracture of the tibia (tibiotarsus) in a red-tailed hawk (*Buteo jamaicens*). **(B)** A through-and-through external pin splint used to achieve satisfactory reduction and alignment. **(C)** A postoperative photograph of the splinted leg. **(D)** Radiographic evidence of the healed fracture six weeks after surgery.

adjacent joints. In ulnar fractures, a straight pin can be drilled in a retrograde direction through the caudal cortex of the proximal segment to exit just behind the elbow joint; this placement will prevent interference with the elbow joint. Intramedullary pins should be removed when complete healing is radiographically evident.

HIGH-DENSITY POLYMER RODS (Kyner Natural Rod®—Penwalt Chemical) used as intramedullary fixation devices have been researched.[20] The lightweight plastic rod can be inserted in a shuttle-pin maneuver; rotational stability is permitted by transverse insertion of Kirschner wires through each fracture fragment and through the intramedullary rod.[20,21] The rod enhances the rigidity and strength of the fixation and prevents rotation without adding excessive weight. Because the material is inert, the rod can be left in place.

ADVANTAGES of high-density polymer rods over Steinmann's pins include (1) lighter weight, (2) the prevention of periarticular and soft tissue damage because the rods do not exit from the bone, and (3) the avoidance of an additional anesthetic and surgical procedure for pin removal. Disadvantages of the rods include (1) a lack of absolute rigidity because of the short usable length of the rod and (2) the concentration of stress at the pin holes, which is caused by the transfixation of the rod with Kirschner wires (this concentration increases the risk that cortical fissures will be distracted to the point of fracture). Tissue reaction to implanted rods apparently is low; long-term complications from rod use have not been reported.[20,21]

Plates

Plating techniques are rarely warranted in avian orthopedics. The poor screw-holding power of thin avian cortical bones makes plating difficult.[10] Bone plating has been used in some large birds, primarily in leg fractures and corrective osteotomies.[13,22–24]

Plating has the advantages of rigid immobilization and rotational stability. Because joint interference is avoided, the bird can maintain normal joint function as the fracture

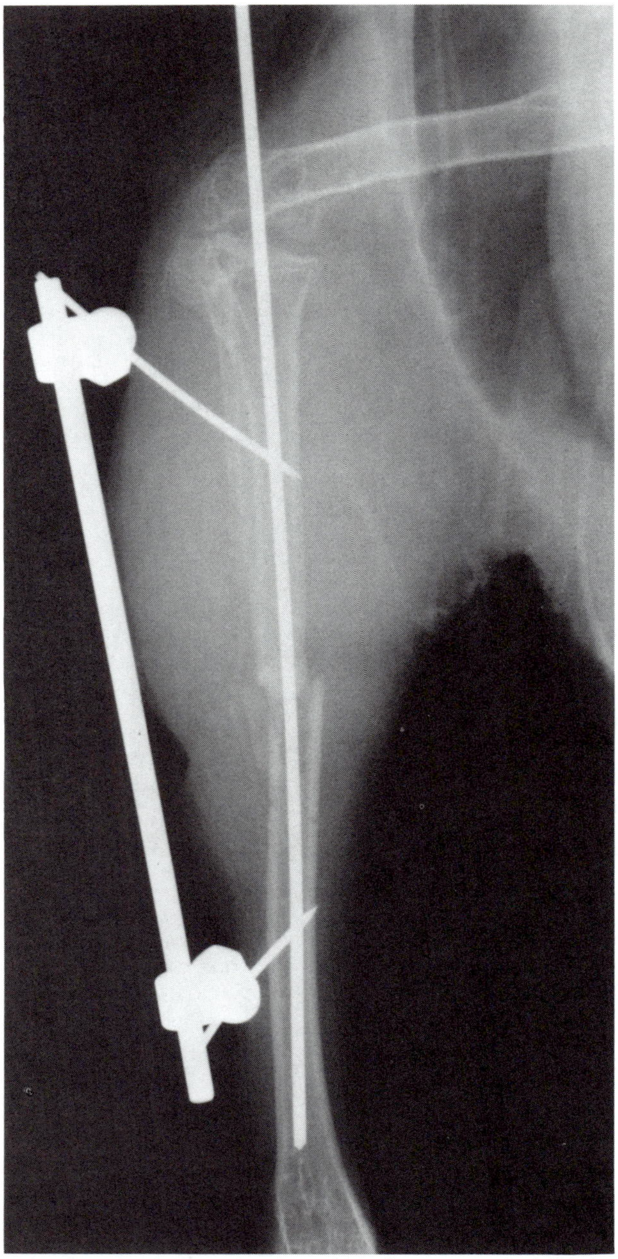

Figure 5—A radiograph of a midshaft, comminuted tibiotarsal fracture in a lesser snow goose (*Chen cacrulescens*). Fixation was achieved with a single intramedullary pin combined with a ½ Kirschner-Ehmer device for rotational stability. Alignment was not perfect, but the 75% cortical contact was acceptable.

heals. Large surgical exposure and long surgical time are disadvantages of plating techniques in birds. The size and weight of the plates might prohibit their use in small patients.

POSTOPERATIVE CONSIDERATIONS

The quality of postoperative care has a significant effect on the case's outcome. Surgical wounds are covered with sterile, nonadhering dressings and are bandaged as needed. Kirschner-Ehmer devices or external splinting devices are well-padded. Elizabethan collars are used as needed to prevent self-mutilation or destruction of bandages or splints; such destruction is common with psittacines.

Postoperative antibiotics are routinely given. Evaluation of healing is accomplished by palpation of the sedated patient at two-week intervals and by periodic radiographic evaluation. Clinical union is usually achieved in three to six weeks; such union is verified radiographically.

POSTOPERATIVE REHABILITATION is vital to the total management of orthopedic patients. Passive and active use of the limb is encouraged when fibrocallus formation is sufficient to partially stabilize the fracture. If return to the wild is expected, gradual increase in exercise and in range of motion must be encouraged.

Proper nutrition and conditioning of raptors are essential to promote healing and to maximize physical condition before release. Flight and food-gathering capabilities must be restored. The assistance of an experienced falconer or a wildlife rehabilitation center can be indispensable in preparing raptors for return to nature.

CONCLUSION

The specialized, aerodynamic bones of birds present unique challenges in veterinary orthopedics. The thin, brittle cortices tend to shatter when stressed and do not react well to conventional means of fixation. The body size of an injured bird often prohibits the application of procedures or appliances proven successful in larger species.

Various means of fixation have been used in avian fracture repair. Simple leg fractures and minimally displaced wing fractures distal to the humerus often heal with external immobilization alone. Techniques to immobilize fractured bone via external fixation include the use of simple splints or slings as well as the use of half-pin and full-pin splinting with variants of the Kirschner-Ehmer apparatus.

The variations of the Kirschner-Ehmer device have provided inexpensive, lightweight, and flexible means of stabilizing many avian fractures. Because the device does not interfere with joint mobility, return to function of the fractured wing or limb can be encouraged early in the healing process.

Internal fixation of fractures with intramedullary pins is a very common method of repair in avian orthopedics. Such fixation is the preferred method for treating most humeral and femoral fractures, in which external fixation is inadequate. With intramedullary pinning, pin placement must be accurate to prevent interference with adjacent joints. High-density polymer rods and intramedullary fixation devices are useful alternatives to steel pins in repairing certain long-bone fractures.

Many treatments are available for managing avian fractures. The preferred method in a specific case depends on the nature of the fracture, the intended use of the bird (i.e., rehabilitation and eventual release or confinement in a zoo or aviary), and the surgeon's judgment and experience.

ACKNOWLEDGMENTS

The author thanks Peter H. Cribb, DVM, and Sharon Prus, DVM, of the University of Saskatchewan, for their advice in preparing this article.

About the Author

Dr. Levitt, who is a Diplomate of the American College of Veterinary Surgeons, is affiliated with Pacific Spirit Veterinary Surgery, a surgical specialty practice located in Richmond, British Columbia, Canada.

REFERENCES

1. Bush M, James AE: Some considerations of practice of orthopedics in exotic animals. *JAAHA* 11(4):587–594, 1975.
2. Cooper JE: *Veterinary Aspects of Captive Birds of Prey*. Gloucestershire, England, Standfast Press, 1978.
3. Spink RR: Fracture repair in rehabilitation of raptors. *VM SAC* 73(11):1451–1455, 1978.
4. Westfall ML, Egger EL: The management of long bone fractures in birds. *Iowa State Vet* 2:81–87, 1979.
5. Bush M: Avian fracture repair using external fixation, in Cooper JE, Greenwood AG (eds): *Recent Advances in the Study of Raptor Disease*. Keighley, England, Chiron Publications, 1981, pp 176–185.
6. MacCoy DM: Modified Kirschner splints for application to small birds. *VM SAC* 76(6):953–955, 1981.
7. Rowley J, Psyhy BW: Repair of a fractured humerus in a red-tailed hawk (*Buteo jamaicens*). *VM SAC* 76(8):1180–1181, 1981.
8. Satterfield W, O'Rourke KI: External skeletal fixation in avian orthopedics using a modified through-and-through Kirschner-Ehmer splint technique (the Boston technique). *JAAHA* 17:635–637, 1981.
9. Elkins AD, Blass CE: Management of avian fractures—Pins and wires. *VM SAC* 77(5):825–828, 1982.
10. Withrow SJ: General principles of fracture repair in raptors. *Compend Contin Educ Pract Vet* 4(2):116–122, 1982.
11. Rousch JC: Avian orthopedics, in Kirk RW (ed): *Current Veterinary Therapy. VII*. Philadelphia, WB Saunders Co, 1980, pp 663–673.
12. Redig PT: A clinical review of the orthopedic techniques used in the rehabilitation of raptors, in Fowler ME (ed): *Zoo and Wild Animal Medicine*, ed 2. Philadelphia, WB Saunders Co, 1986.
13. Bush M, Hughes JL, Ensley PK, James AE: Fracture repair in exotics using internal fixation. *JAAHA* 12(6):746–753, 1976.
14. Fowler ME: *Zoo and Wild Animal Medicine*, ed 2. Philadelphia, WB Saunders Co, 1986, pp 388–401.
15. Harrison GJ, Harrison LR: *Clinical Avian Medicine and Surgery*. Philadelphia, WB Saunders Co, 1986, pp 543–548, 596–598.
16. Altman RB: General principles of avian surgery. *Compend Contin Educ Pract Vet* 3(2):177–183, 1981.
17. Altman RB: Fractures of the extremities of birds, in Kirk RW (ed): *Current Veterinary Therapy. IV*. Philadelphia, WB Saunders Co, 1975, pp 400–403.
18. Gandal CP: Long bone fractures in larger birds, in Kirk RW (ed): *Current Veterinary Therapy. IV*. Philadelphia, WB Saunders Co, 1975, p 403.
19. MacCoy DM, Redig PT: Surgical approaches to and repair of wing fractures. *Proc First Int Conf Zool Avian Med*:360–367, 1987.
20. MacCoy DM: High-density polymer rods as an intramedullary fixation device in birds. *JAAHA* 19(5):767–772, 1983.
21. MacCoy DM: Techniques of fracture treatment in birds and their indications: External and internal fixation. *Proc First Int Conf Zool Avian Med*:367–376, 1987.
22. Wingfield WE, Young DW: Anesthetic and surgical management of eagles with orthopedic difficulties. *VM SAC* 67(9):991–993, 1972.
23. Leeds EB: Tibial fracture repair in a double-wattled cassowary. *J Vet Orthop* 1(1):21–27, 1979.
24. Bauck L, Fowler JD, Cribb P: Tibial osteotomy in an emu. *Compan Anim Pract*:26–30, 1987.

UPDATE

When selecting a treatment for avian fractures, veterinarians must make decisions that depend on the degree of function the bird needs to have after treatment. The goal for treating fractures of captive birds (companion, aviary, and breeding stock) differs from that for wild birds. For wild birds, the goal is to return the bird to full functional capabilities and subsequent return to the wild. With captive birds, client expectations are important to define before deciding on an appropriate treatment for fracture repair. The result of the repair should be one that the client considers acceptable.

Birds presented to a veterinary practice for fracture treatment may range in size from small canaries and finches to psittacines to wild raptors. Thus, avian surgeons must be prepared to treat a variety of fractures effectively. The techniques described in the original article can all be modified for use in psittacines and smaller birds.

Pelvic limb injuries occur more frequently in pet birds than in wild birds.[1] The application of splints and bandages is a common practice in pet bird medicine. Materials commonly used for external coaptation include porous bandage tape, elastic bandaging tape, wire clips and paper clips, wooden dowels, plastic dowels, acrylics, and fiberglass casting materials.[2] Tape splints[3] work well for fractures of the tibiotarsus and tarsometatarsus in birds weighing less than 100 grams. Incorporating a cotton swab's wooden dowel into the splint gives additional support for birds weighing between 100 and 150 grams.[2] A modification of the Altman[3] tape splint with tissue glue has been described as useful in birds weighing up to 500 grams.[1] The Redig modification of the Schroedar-Thomas splint provides good support for tibiotarsal and tarsometatarsal fractures in birds weighing more than 150 grams. Paper clips work well in smaller birds, while clothes hangers or equivalent-sized wire supports are appropriate for larger birds (e.g., macaws).[4]

Acrylics and visible-light–curing composites (VLCCs) can be used to splint tibiotarsal fractures in canaries, finches, and small psittacines. Internal fixation of pelvic limb fractures is less often required in pet birds, as conservative management with external coaptation often yields acceptable functional results; however, internal fixation techniques used in pet birds may include intramedullary pinning, polymethylmethacrylate bone cement (PMMBC), and various modified external fixators.

Fractures of the pectoral limb in pet birds that do not require a return to full flight may be managed through external splinting with a body bandage. If full flight is required, humeral fractures can be treated with the use of shuttle pins embedded in polymethylmethacrylate bone cement, intramedullary pins, Rush pins, or modified Kirschner-Ehmer devices.[6] Fractures of either the radius or ulna heal well with splinting because the intact bone provides an internal splint. If a return to full flight is required, fractures of both the radius and ulna are best managed with Kirschner-Ehmer devices applied to the ulna. Carpal and metacarpal fractures are best treated with external bandaging.[6]

REFERENCES

1. Hess RE: Management of orthopedic problems of the avian pelvic limb. *Semin Avian Exotic Pet Med* 3(2):63–72, 1994.
2. McCluggage DM: Application of splints, bandages and collars. *Proc Assoc Avian Vet*:287–290, 1988.
3. Altman RB: Fractures of the extremities of birds, in Kirk RW (ed): *Current Veterinary Therapy. VI.* Philadelphia, WB Saunders Co, 1977, pp 400–403.
4. Redig PT: Evaluation and nonsurgical management of fractures, in Harrison GJ, Harrison LR (eds): *Clinical Avian Medicine and Surgery.* Philadelphia, WB Saunders Co, 1986, pp 382–383.
5. Rupiper DJ: Application of visible light curing composite splints to fractured avian legs. *JAAV* 7(3):147–149, 1993.
6. Howard DJ, Redig PT: Orthopedics of the wing. *Semin Avian Exotic Pet Med* 3(2):51–62, 1994.

Avian Beak Prosthesis

KEY FACTS

- **The success and longevity of the prosthesis are determined by the type of beak; the amount of normal, functional beak; and the use of sound orthopedic principles in anchoring the prosthesis.**
- **Diving birds and seed-cracking psittacines have limited success with prosthetic beaks.**
- **Anchorage of the prosthesis must oppose bending, shearing, and rotational forces.**
- **Dental acrylics and methyl methacrylate can be used to build prosthetic beaks.**
- **Flexible isobutyl acrylic and silicone sealer can be used to fill cracks in prosthetic beaks.**

Dunn Road Animal Hospital
Florissant, Missouri
Martin Greenwell, DVM

Veterinary Surgical Referrals
Citrus Heights, California
John J. Robertson, DVM

University of Missouri-Columbia
Gheorghe M. Constantinescu, DVM, PhD

DENTAL ACRYLICS can be used to create oral prostheses for birds with amputated, unstable, and nonfunctional beaks. Instability of beaks may result from nutritional deficiencies or from infections, neoplasia, congenital defects, or trauma.

PRELIMINARY ASSESSMENT

Before a patient is fitted with a beak prosthesis, many factors must be evaluated. The overall health of the bird; the species; and the nature, location, and extent of the oral injury should be considered. The characteristics of the materials used in the prosthetic device, the biomechanics of the avian skull, and the application of proper orthopedic principles determine the long-term success of the device.

Avian patients presented for acute, severe oral trauma may be in shock or hemorrhaging and may have dyspnea. These birds must be stabilized before anesthesia and surgical repair are attempted. Beak trauma is often associated with accidental injury, attack by another animal, or even mutilation by humans; any organ system may be compromised.

Avian patients presented for chronic beak injury may be weak or debilitated because of inanition. The reason for presentation of such birds is often difficulty in prehension or mastication of food. These patients require hand- or crop-feeding with a high-energy, low-protein, vitamin-rich, mash gruel. Once the bird has regained strength and has an acceptable weight (as assessed by daily weight monitoring), it can be evaluated for a possible beak prosthesis.

Oral prostheses with wire implants have reportedly been successful in psittacines,[1,2] a duck,[3] a goose,[4] a black eagle,[5] and a white stork.[6] Factors contributing to a successful prosthesis in these cases were individual beak morphology and function and periodic reassessment and revision of the device.

Large birds with a light, pneumatic maxilla and mandible (e.g., pelicans) have difficulty in supporting a prosthesis.[3] Birds that exert enormous forces on their beaks (such as diving birds and seed-cracking psittacines) have limited success with prosthetic beaks.[1,2] Psittacines that can adapt to pelletized food and are subjected to daily observation have a better prognosis for a successful prosthesis. Early reassessment and revision in a controlled environment reduce the incidence of prosthesis failure.

Assessing the nature, location, and extent of beak injury is important in determining the approach to application of a prosthesis. Radiographs of the skull reveal the extent of any fractures and the involvement of growth centers. A case involving a blue crowned pigeon revealed injury to the physis of the left mandibular ramus.[7] On radiographs, the mandible appeared atrophic and deviated to the left. As the mandible grew, the midline moved to the left. No surgical correction was attempted, and the patient adapted well to the malformed lower jaw.

Longitudinal beak fractures beyond the layer of germinal epithelium meet with limited success on reconstruction because the defect remains as the new beak grows. In these cases, artificial beaks serve only as temporary splints that

Originally published in Volume 11, Number 11, November 1989

allow the patient to adapt to the handicap. Such fractures are analogous to hoof cracks involving the coronary band in ungulates.

ANATOMY AND SKULL BIOMECHANICS

Most avian species have prokinetic, streptostylic skulls.[9] The prokinetic skull is characterized by a hinge or region of bending at the junction of the nasal and frontal bones. Unlike that in mammals, the entire maxilla moves as a unit. *Streptostylic* refers to the quadrate bone, which moves on the braincase relative to the surrounding bones.[9] The quadrate bone is connected to the maxilla by the quadratojugal, jugal, pterygoid, and palatine bones (Figure 1). These structures constitute a single movable unit.

Most birds also possess a postorbital ligament (the lacrimomandibular ligament in anserines) extending from the postorbital process of the braincase to the external process of the mandible slightly rostral to the jaw articulation (Figure 2A). This ligament allows the mandible and maxilla to move interdependently. Such movement is called coupled kinesis.[9]

The nature and magnitude of the forces exerted on the beak determine the success or failure of the prosthesis. When the bird bites an object, three external forces act on the upper jaw. The pterygoideus muscle applies a force in the caudal to rostral direction; this force is transferred to the maxilla by the palatines. The pterygoideus muscle originates from the pterygoid and palatine bones and inserts on the medial surface of the mandibular ramus (Figure 2B). The second force is perpendicular to the beak and results from the object being bitten. The third force is an angular force at the nasofrontal hinge.

For the maxilla to maintain its structural stability, the sum of these forces must equal zero.[10] Vector analysis confirms that a greater force is exerted on the bitten object either by increasing the force of the pterygoideus muscle or by decreasing the distance from the object to the base of the bill.

WHEN A BIRD PECKS, compressive force applied to the bill tends to compress and depress the maxilla. Protraction of the maxilla is provided by the protractor quadrati et pterygoidei muscle and counteracts this depression. The protractor quadrati et pterygoidei muscle originates from the rostral wall of the braincase below the optic foramen and inserts on the dorsal surface of the pterygoid–quadrate articulation and the medial surface of the quadrate bone (Figure 2B).

Internal stresses also act on the avian bill, and most of these forces are asymmetrical. Maximum stress from asymmetrical loading depends on the bending moment provided by the forces and the distance between the material and the center of bending. These internal stresses are offset by the trabecular pattern of the bone, bone diameter, muscular and ligamentous counterbalances, and redistribution of the force to other bones.

When a bird bites, a compressive force is applied to the maxilla and resisted by an opposite tensile force from the pterygoideus and other muscles (Figure 2). In addition, this force is redistributed to the thick braincase by the arrangement of the palatine, jugal, and quadrate bones. This configuration explains why birds can survive despite thin cortical bone on the skull roof and lateral walls. The decreased skull weight enhances the efficiency of flight.

The sum of the external and internal forces is applied at the nasofrontal hinge, which acts as a fulcrum when compressive and depressive forces are applied. A fulcrum also exists at the junction of the beak and prosthesis. The forces applied at this point are only opposed by the tensile strength of the materials used and by the method of anchorage. The longer the beak remnant is, the shorter is the lever arm of the prosthesis. The shorter the lever arm is, the smaller are the applied stresses and the better the prognosis is.

MEDICAL ASSESSMENT

A thorough physical examination to evaluate neurologic, cardiopulmonary, renal, and gastrointestinal function is recommended. Survey radiographs are indicated in most cases.

When a bird with an oral injury is presented, hemostasis, debridement, flushing, and subsequent drying of the traumatized tissues are indicated. Broad-spectrum antibiotics are administered if contamination or infection is present. When viable beak epithelium is exposed, the tissue should be protected with an ointment, such as zinc oxide.[1]

In hard-billed birds, exposure of germinal epithelium stimulates regeneration of the horny bill and results in beak malformation.[5,6] Any prosthetic repair in these cases should be designed to protect the beak during its regenerative period; frequent reassessment and multiple revisions over a lengthy time period should be planned.

SURGICAL MANAGEMENT

An understanding of the biomechanics of the avian beak is essential for fashioning the prosthesis; and if anchorage to the skull is not secure, the prosthetic device will fail. The guidelines for successful fracture fixation of mammalian bones apply. Longitudinal pins resist angular bending and are anchored securely in the beak remnant and into the prosthesis.

To counteract shearing forces, wires of the largest feasible diameter should be used. The wires should be inserted in pairs to counteract rotational forces. A second pair of wires is inserted in the transverse plane to further counteract rotational forces resulting from asymmetrical dorsoventral and lateral displacement (Figure 3). Good pin anchorage to the beak remnant helps to negate the forces of distraction. In hard-billed species, drilling wedge-shaped holes in the beak with a dental drill results in a dovetail pattern that increases the area of contact between the acrylic and beak.

In addition to the mentioned orthopedic principles, the anatomy of the maxilla should be considered. The light pneumatic bones of the avian skull are weaker than those

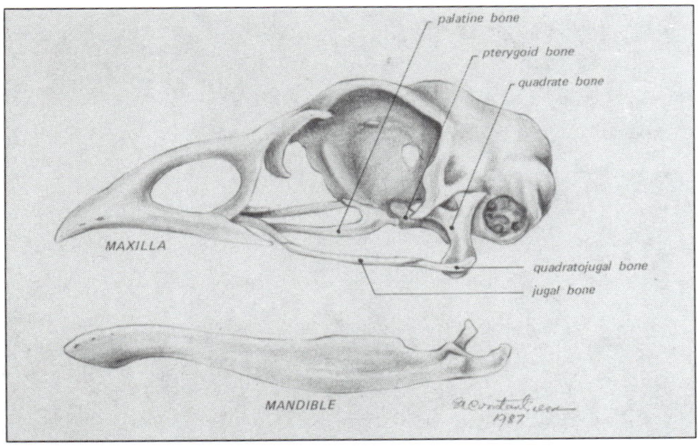

Figure 1A

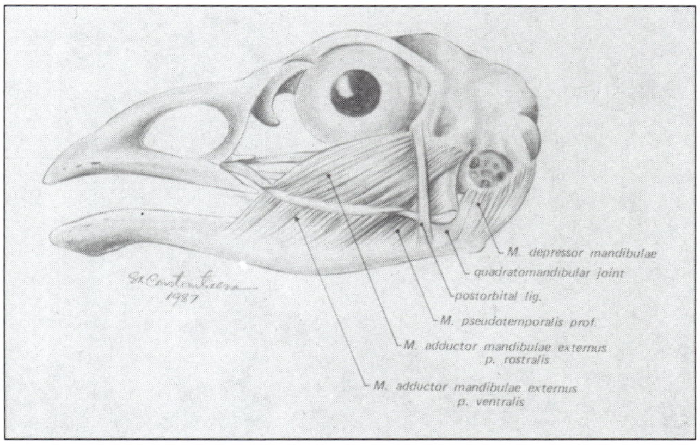

Figure 2A

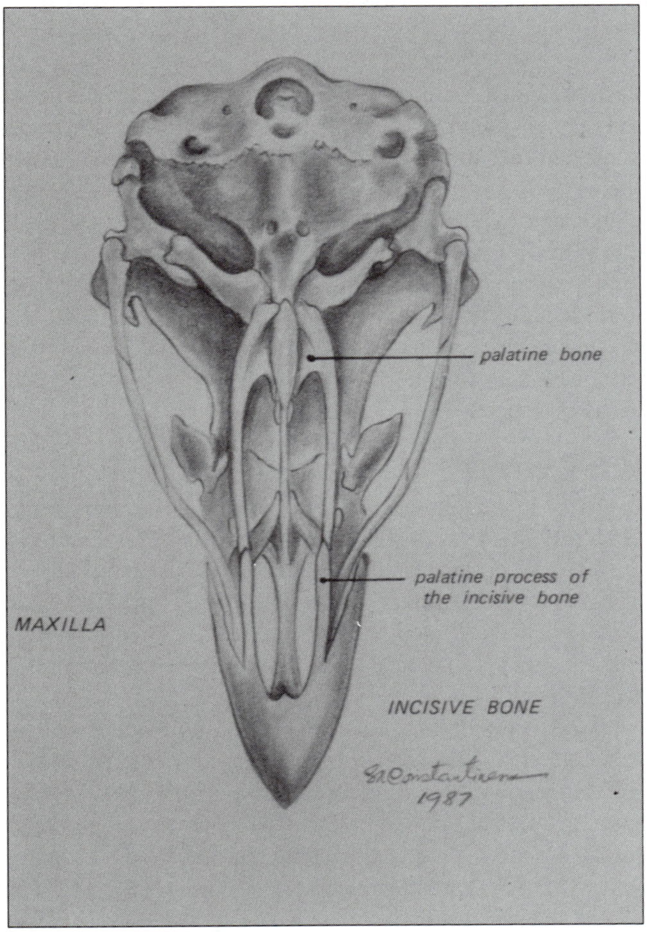

Figure 1B

Figure 1—(**A**) Lateral and (**B**) dorsoventral views of an avian (Galliformes) skull.

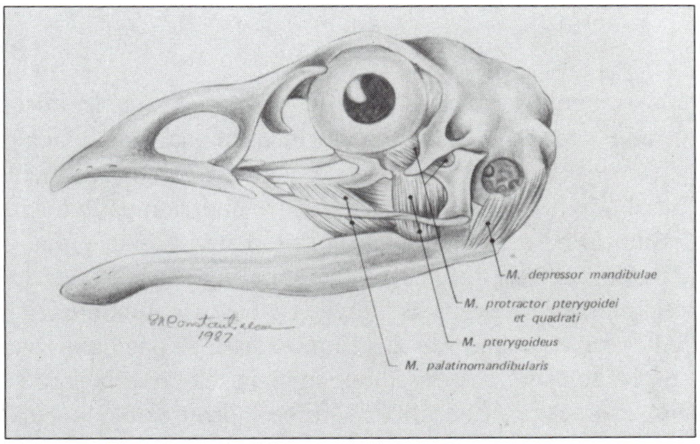

Figure 2B

Figure 2—Important (**A**) superficial muscles and (**B**) ligaments of an avian (Galliformes) skull with underlying deeper muscles.

of mammals. As discussed, birds have adapted to this weakness with anatomic specializations. The muscular forces that result in normal resistance to stress on the maxilla act through the palatine bone.

SCREWS OR PINS implanted in the maxilla should ideally be seated in the palatine process of the incisive bone to gain optimal mechanical advantage. In most avian species, the incisive bone and maxilla are fused and the palatine process connects to the palatine bone (Figure 1). Pin placement is confirmed by postoperative radiographs (Figure 3). Prosthetic devices anchored in the palatine process carry a more favorable prognosis for long-term success.

In anserines (ducks, geese, and swans), the maxillary bone, the incisive bone, and the palatine process of the incisive bone are all fused into a single, sturdy ossicle. Good anchorage and a successful long-term prosthesis are therefore more easily achieved in these species.

Prosthetic Materials

Various materials are available for building prosthetic beaks. The setting times, physical properties (such as thin versus thick flow), strength, and particle size of the various materials differ. When planning the prosthetic device, the veterinarian should attempt to select materials that are lightweight and resistant to temperature extremes, have high tensile strength and fast setting times, and bond well to different surfaces.

Such dental acrylics as ethyl acrylic,[2] methyl acrylic,[2]

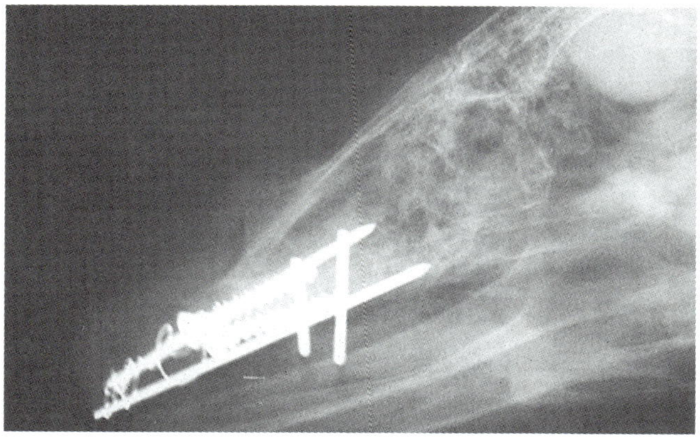

Figure 3A

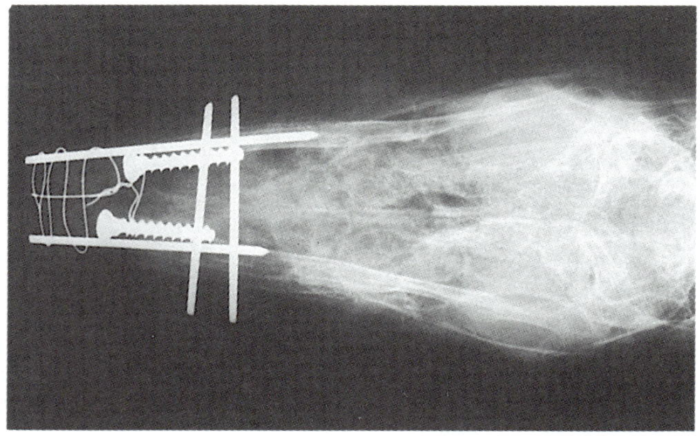

Figure 3B

Figure 3—(A) Lateral and **(B)** dorsoventral postoperative radiographs of a dewlap Toulouse goose with an upper beak amputation 1.5 cm rostral to the nares. Note the placement of two longitudinal Kirschner wires in the maxillary bone (palatine process in other species), the transverse Kirschner wires, two 3.5-mm cortical bone screws, and the 22-gauge orthopedic wire used to anchor the prosthesis.

and isobutyl acrylic (these materials are available in the Cyano-Veneer Kit™—Ellman International Manufacturing)[2] work well in combination with wire reinforcement. Ethyl acrylic and isobutyl acrylic are both compatible with tissue. Ethyl acrylic cures to form a hard substance that is durable and suitable for use in splinting, bone repair, or beak reconstruction.[8] Isobutyl acrylics are flexible after polymerization and can therefore be used as bandages over surgical closures. A prosthetic implant that gradually loosens or cracks can be filled with the more flexible isobutyl acrylic.

CARE SHOULD BE TAKEN when using acrylics near highly vascular surfaces while the patient is anesthetized. A synergistic effect between acrylics and halogenated gases deepens the anesthetic plane.[8]

A syringe case filled with clear silicone rubber cement[3] served as a prosthetic bill for a duck. The bill was contoured and fixed to the beak remnants with orthopedic wire.[3] Like isobutyl acrylic, silicone rubber cement is flexible and is useful in filling defects at the prosthesis–bill interface.

Methyl methacrylate[4] (Technovit™—Jorgensen Laboratories) is an acrylic resin that is somewhat toxic to tissue but is relatively inert when applied to keratinous beak material.[2] This resin expands and contracts in alternate periods of wetting and drying and reaches a high temperature during polymerization. Distortion of the material does not seem to be a clinical problem, and immersion in cold water reduces tissue damage resulting from heat of polymerization. A cold-cured methyl methacrylate[5] (Jet Repair Acrylic™—Lang Dental) does not reach the high temperature during polymerization.

Postoperative Care

Atraumatic surgical technique prevents iatrogenic fracturing of the delicate pneumatic skull bones, and aseptic technique and the use of prophylactic antibiotics minimize secondary infection. If the patient is of a seed-eating species, the diet must be altered to a pelletized food or soft items (e.g., oatmeal or other cooked cereal or strained fruits and vegetables). Daily weight monitoring using a gram scale is advised to assess compliance with the new diet.[11] If prehension is difficult after surgery, hand- or crop-feeding three to four times daily may be necessary. Such sequelae as acute or chronic sinusitis, beak deformities secondary to abnormal regrowth, and soft tissue infections may occur.

CASE REPORT

An adult female dewlap Toulouse goose, *Anser anser*, was presented to the University of Missouri Veterinary Teaching Hospital for evaluation of an upper bill injury. The cause of the injury was unknown. Physical examination revealed a transverse amputation of the rostral half of the maxilla approximately 1.5 cm cranial to the nares (Figure 4A).

There was minimal hemorrhage and no evidence of tissue infection. The mandible and tongue were intact. The bird appeared to have appropriate weight and was well hydrated. There was no evidence of involvement of any other organ systems. The goose could not eat, and the owner opted for a bill prosthesis.

Anesthesia was induced with methoxyflurane by face mask followed by intubation and maintenance anesthesia. The upper bill was debrided and scrubbed with povidone-iodine. Radiology confirmed that sufficient bone and soft tissue remained to support a prosthesis.

Two 3.5-mm bone screws were anchored rostrocaudally in the maxilla. Lateral to each screw, one 0.0625-inch Kirschner wire was driven rostrocaudally into the maxillary process; 22-gauge orthopedic wire was secured to the heads of the screws and wrapped spirally around the two longitudinal Kirschner wires (Figure 3). This device served as scaffolding for a methyl methacrylate prosthesis.

Two additional 0.0625-inch Kirschner wires were driven

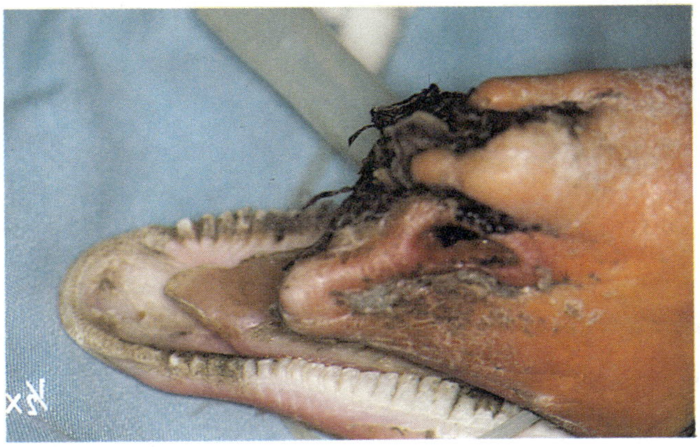

Figure 4A

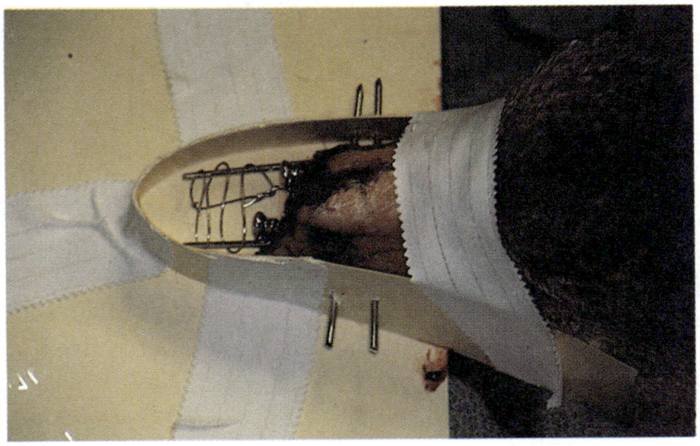

Figure 4B

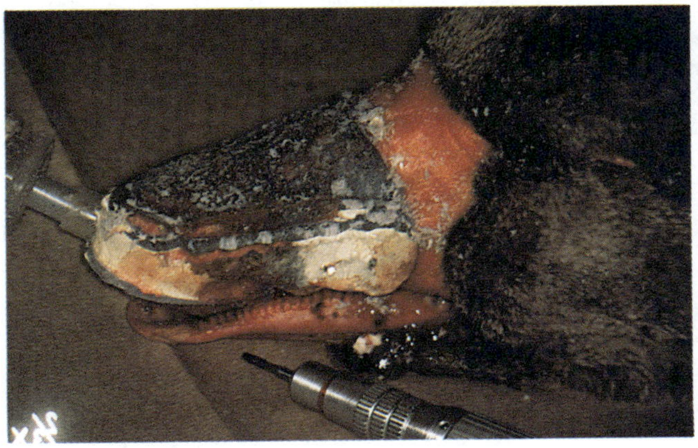

Figure 4C

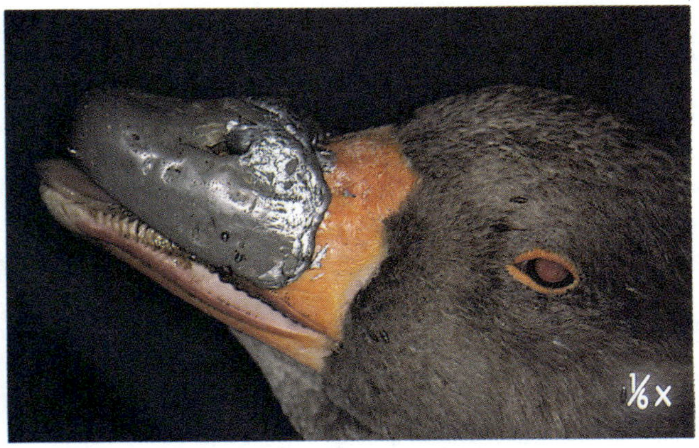

Figure 4D

Figure 4—(A) Preoperative photograph of the patient in Figure 3. **(B)** A cardboard mold is built around the scaffolding to approximate the size and shape of the upper bill. The floor of the mold shapes the roof of the mouth. **(C)** A high-speed dental drill is used to sculpt the prosthesis to make it resemble a true beak. **(D)** Silicone rubber cement was used to fill defects at the bill–prosthesis interface 15 months after discharge. The migrating Kirschner wire has been cut at the rostral edge of the prosthesis.

transversely through the beak just rostral to the junction of the maxilla and germinal epithelium. The wires were approximately one centimeter apart and served as an anchor to be incorporated into the prosthesis and to reduce torque at the bone–prosthesis interface (Figure 3).

To form a mold, a cardboard strip was folded around the metal scaffold to approximate the size and shape of the bird's upper bill. The floor of the mold (which shaped the roof of the mouth) was constructed by taping a sheet of cardboard to the strip with one-inch adhesive tape (Figure 4B). Sticks from cotton swabs were inserted into the nasal openings to simulate nares and preserve the openings. Methyl methacrylate was mixed in a ratio of two parts powder to one part liquid and poured into the cardboard mold. The methyl methacrylate was continuously cooled as it hardened by irrigation with ice water.

The sticks were removed from the nares, and the crude prosthesis was shaped with a high-speed dental drill to approximate the dimensions of the natural beak[6] (Figure 4C). The goose was discharged the same day, was returned to its normal surroundings, and was fed a mash diet for ducks.

After 15 months, the goose was presented for revision of the prosthesis. The client reported that the methyl methacrylate seemed to be loosening. The goose was able to secure and masticate food easily.

The left longitudinal Kirschner wire had migrated 1 cm rostrally. The goose was sedated with ketamine hydrochloride (10 mg/kg) for close examination, manipulation, and revision of the prosthesis. Slight movement existed at the prosthesis–beak junction; and there were a few small, irregularly shaped areas where the material was chipped around the artificial external nares. No tissue irritation was apparent.

The protruding Kirschner wire was cut flush with the rostral aspect of the prosthesis, and the perinasal defects were filled with silicone rubber cement (Figure 4D). The patient recovered from the anesthesia uneventfully and was discharged on the same day. The prosthesis has remained functional, and the owner has reported no problems.

DISCUSSION

The goals of beak reconstruction are to create a durable,

functional, and aesthetically pleasing artificial bill. Long-term maintenance of function is difficult if high stresses are applied to the prosthesis. Psittacines use their beaks for climbing as well as mastication of hard seeds and nuts. In these species, prostheses have a less favorable long-term prognosis unless the bird can be fed a pelletized diet. Beak prostheses in which the beak is wired to the lateral prominences of the frontal bone have been successful in psittacines.[1,2] In diving birds, high stress is applied to bills as birds enter the water and the prognosis is therefore guarded.

The maxillary bone, the incisive bone, and the palatine process of the incisive bone in anserines (i.e., ducks, geese, and swans) are fused into a single, sturdy ossicle. In these species, there is little movement of the maxilla during opening and closing of the mouth. It may be easier to achieve good anchorage of the metal implants in the maxilla in this group of birds, thereby achieving a more successful long-term outcome.

The prosthesis in the dewlap Toulouse goose was successful. The patient was healthy, had no complications, and was a good candidate for anesthesia and surgery. The germinal epithelium of the bill was not involved, and secondary growth deformities posed no problem. The amputation occurred within the rostral portion of the beak. The length of remaining normal bill decreased the lever arm of the prosthesis, and the resultant angular forces exerted on the artificial bill were reduced. Longitudinally directed Kirschner wires were placed in the maxillary process, and bone screws were used to increase stability at the beak–prosthesis interface. Transversely placed Kirschner wires provided additional stability and countered natural dorsoventral and torsional forces.

Methyl methacrylate provided a sturdy, durable, and functional prosthesis. The goose was a farmyard pet, and regular observation was routine. The prosthesis showed few signs of loosening for 15 months, and no toxic or abrasive effects were noted at the prosthesis–beak interface. Eventual loosening of the prosthesis is certain but can be minimized by application of sound orthopedic principles.

In this case, a silicone bathtub sealer that is pliable on curing was used at the interface of the prosthesis to seal the gap while allowing for movement of the soft tissues. The migration of the Kirschner wire might have been prevented by the use of threaded pins.

About the Authors

When this article was submitted for publication, Dr. Greenwell was affiliated with the Dunn Road Animal Hospital in Florissant, Missouri. He is currently in private practice in St. Louis, Missouri. Dr. Robertson was affiliated with the Department of Medicine and Surgery of the College of Veterinary Medicine, University of Missouri, Columbia, Missouri, when this article was submitted for publication. Dr. Robertson is a Diplomate of the American College of Veterinary Surgeons and is currently affiliated with Veterinary Surgical Referrals, Citrus Heights, California. He specializes in small animal, avian, and exotics surgery. When this article was submitted for publication, Dr. Constantinescu was affiliated with the Department of Physiological Sciences of the College of Veterinary Medicine, University of Missouri, Columbia, Missouri. Dr. Constantinescu is currently Professor of the Department of Veterinary Anatomy at the University of Missouri, Columbia, Missouri.

REFERENCES

1. Sleamaker TF: Prosthetic beak for a salmon-crested cockatoo. *JAVMA* 183(11):1300–1301, 1983.
2. Vollmar VA: Behandlung eines Unterschnabelabrisses bei einem Graupapagei durch Anbringen einer Kunstharprosthese. *Kleintier Praxis* 30:165–168, 1965.
3. Frye FL: Prostheses enhance quality of life. *Vet Med* 79(7):931–935, 1984.
4. Wolf L: Prosthetic bill technique for a Canada goose. *Proc Assoc Avian Vet*:177–180, 1985.
5. Fagan D: Beak repair in a South American black eagle. *Assoc Avian Vet Newsl* 3:2(41):225, 1982.
6. Murata K: Preparation and attachment of a prosthetic bill in a white stork. *J Jpn Vet Med Assoc* 37(12):805–808, 1984.
7. Fagan D: Oral diseases in avian species. *Annu Proc Am Assoc Zoo Vet*:30–32, 1981.
8. Harrison GJ: Surgical instrumentation and special techniques, in Harrison GJ, Harrison LR (eds): *Clinical Avian Medicine and Surgery*, ed 2. Philadelphia, WB Saunders Co, 1986, pp 563–565.
9. Bock WJ: Kinetics of the avian skull. *J Morphol* 114:1–42, 1964.
10. Bock WJ: An approach to the functional analysis of bill shape. *Auk* 83:10–51, 1966.
11. Woerpel RW, Rosskopf WJ, Holechek JD: Surgical repair of beak trauma in caged birds. *Vet Med Small Anim Clin* 77(7):1068–1072, 1982.

Avian Radiosurgery in Practice

Florida Atlantic University
Robert B. Altman, DVM

KEY FACTS

- With radiosurgery, pressure is contraindicated because the radio wave being emitted from the electrode tip incises the tissue quickly and smoothly.
- Because hemostasis is total, the surgeon has a continuous, clear view of the incision site.
- The accessories available for radiosurgical equipment can help the surgeon work more efficiently and effectively.
- When choosing radiosurgical equipment, one of the most important criteria is that the unit operates at a frequency of 3.8 to 4 MHz.
- The length of time the electrode is in contact with tissue is directly proportional to the amount of tissue alteration; electrode-to-tissue contact should be restricted to two to three seconds.

Since its introduction to avian surgery in the early 1980s, radiosurgery (also called electrosurgery) has become an integral part of general veterinary practice, particularly small animal dentistry, ophthalmology, and dermatology. Radiosurgery is very well-suited for avian surgery because the procedure fulfills requirements stipulated by avian surgeons. For example, total hemostasis is essential to minimize the potential of developing hypovolemia and hypotension. Another essential requirement is conservation of time, as speed is directly related to survival. Survival is affected by the length of the anesthetic period, and anesthetic time declines when surgical speed is increased. The faster the patient leaves the operating table, the shorter the anesthetic period.

Radiosurgical skills can be acquired easily in a relatively short time with minimal instruction and practice. To comprehend radiosurgical principles and techniques, the surgeon must understand the physical properties and principles of the equipment.

The radiosurgical unit is a radio-frequency generator that converts alternating current (AC) to direct current (DC) by a power supply within the electrosurgical unit and passes the DC current into a tuned coil capacitor that generates radio-frequency waves. Radio waves are then passed through a high-frequency waveform adapter that alters the shape and magnitude of the wave to create different waveforms.[1] The waveforms are passed through a high-frequency amplifier that increases their power levels. The amplified radio waves are then passed through a series of coupling circuits to connect them to the electrode. When the electrode is applied to body tissue, the electromagnetic field that was created heats up the intracellular fluid and volatilizes the cell.

ADVANTAGES OF RADIOSURGERY

Radiosurgery is preferred to a scalpel when incising avian tissue because the former provides total hemostasis and allows rapid, simple contouring of the incision.[2] When a scalpel is used, pressure must be applied to the blade in order to make the incision. Pressure can compress the epithelium and disrupt cells along the incision line (Figure 1). With radiosurgery, pressure is contraindicated because the radio wave emitting from the electrode tip incises the tissue quickly and smoothly and can be controlled to affect only one to two cell layers. Because the electrodes can be bent for a customized fit, the time saved also is a major advantage (Figure 2). Shaping and contouring incisions even in small difficult-to-reach areas require no effort.

As soon as the radio-frequency current passes through the electrode, all bac-

First-time publication

teria on the electrode are destroyed. The exposed metal tip of the electrode is self-sterilizing, and bacteria on contaminated tissue cannot seed into the incision site. Because hemostasis is total, the surgeon has a continuous clear view of the incision site. Surgical efficiency coupled with conservation of time and decreased anesthetic time can improve the survival rate.

HAZARDS OF RADIOSURGERY

Because inflammable or explosive products can be ignited during radiosurgical incision, such products as ether and ethyl chloride should not be used. If alcohol is used for skin preparation and sterilization, enough time for total evaporation should elapse before an incision is made.

Channeling is a condition in which radio-frequency waves travel along a blood vessel or nerve and destroy tissue at a point away from the surgical site. Channeling does not occur with radio frequencies below 4 MHz. If noninsulated or poorly insulated ground plates (passive electrodes) are used, burns can occur at the point of contact with skin.[3,4] In addition, if poorly insulated ground plates come into contact with a stainless-steel tabletop, the tabletop can act as a passive electrode and cause burns on the assistant who is holding the bird. Because the current tends to travel toward the point of least resistance, holding the bird securely may avert the problem.

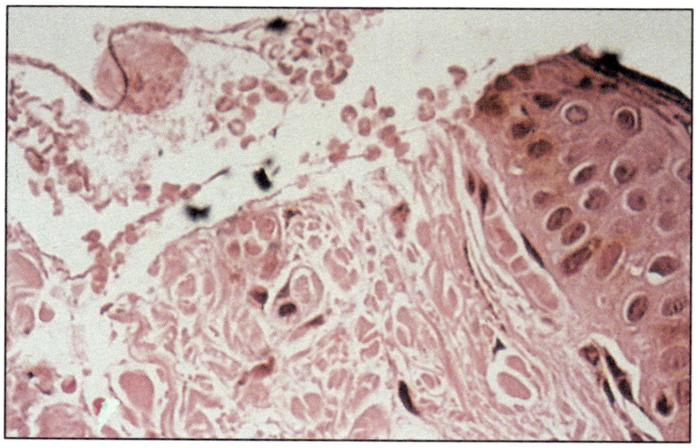

Figure 1A

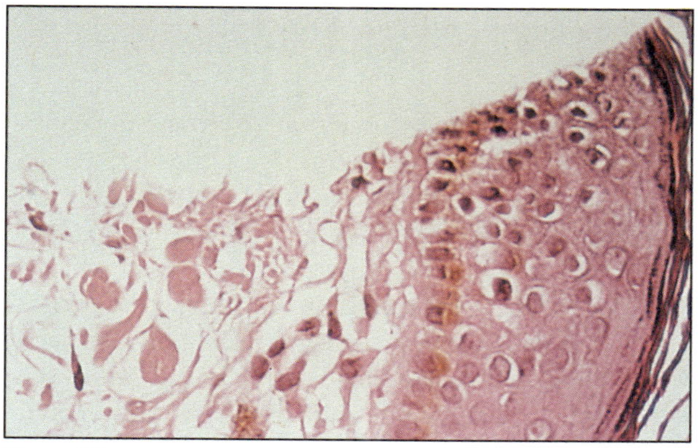

Figure 1B

Figure 1—(A) A human eyelid incised using a scalpel blade. **(B)** A human eyelid incised by radiosurgical section. Note how clean the incision line is compared with the disruption of cells along the scalpel incision and the lack of compression of the epithelium on the radiosurgical incision.

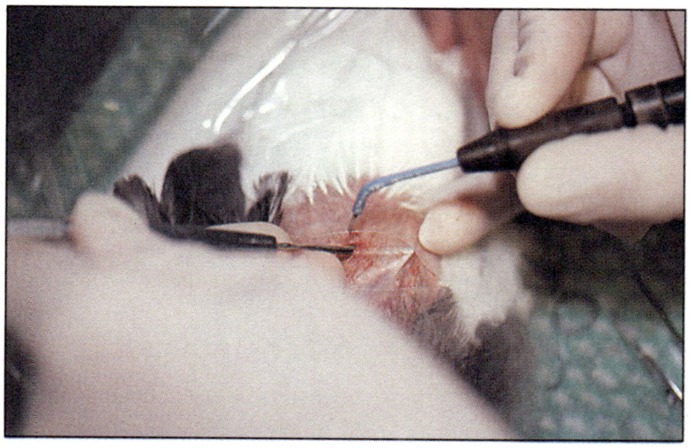

Figure 2—Skin incision on a bird. Note how the electrode is bent to permit comfortable grasping and holding of the electrode handle. It is comparable to holding a pen when signing your name, which requires no pressure.

Because avian tissue is thin, the surgeon must be careful to incise only the desired layer and avoid lacerating underlying muscle or viscera. Poor technique or inferior radiosurgical equipment can cause excessive lateral heat, which can result in poor tissue healing. Kalkwarf et al[5] showed that radiosurgical incisions in gingiva produced wound-healing characteristics similar to those that occurred with scalpel incisions.

RADIOSURGICAL EQUIPMENT

A number of radiosurgical units are available, although they vary in waveforms, radio-frequency output, and power output. Four waveforms are offered: fully filtered, fully rectified, partially rectified, and fulgurating. Not all manufacturers supply all four waveforms. Units are manufactured with a radio-frequency output ranging from 1 to 4 MHz, although 3.8 to 4 MHz is recommended. Maness et al[6] proved that 3.8 MHz was the optimum frequency for incising epithelial tissue, connective tissue, and muscle.

Unit power varies from 25 to 140 watts, with 90 to 140 watts being the most functional. Some radiosurgical units have a vaccum tube, while others have solid-state circuitry. Units with a vacuum tube–transistor combination are less prone to overheating and burnout and minimize variations in the power and frequency of the radio signal.[1] UL approval or similar standards of acceptance should be verified before a unit is purchased.

Other important features to consider include a steam autoclaving function for hand pieces and accessories. Insulated ground plates and flexible electrodes also are advantageous. Accessories can help the surgeon work more efficiently and effectively. Common accessories include bipolar forceps, bipolar converters, finger-switch adapters, suction electrodes, and an assortment of monopolar electrodes.

Bipolar forceps provide precise, pinpoint coagulation and thus can increase the surgeon's speed and efficiency. Pinpoint coagulation is achieved when one jaw of the forceps becomes the active electrode while the other jaw becomes the passive electrode. Some surgeons[7,8] use bipolar forceps to incise tissue by grasping the skin and pulling the forceps along the incision line. Although this technique conserves time because the surgeon does not have to change electrode handles, it violates a surgical principle that the smallest electrode possible should be used to prevent a buildup of lateral heat. Therefore, I do not use the technique. Instead, I recommend bipolar converters that include a convenient toggle switch that allows the surgeon to use either the bipolar or monopolar mode. Finger-switch adapters allow concurrent use of two hand pieces: one with the standard foot switch and the other with a finger-switch hand piece. By using two hand pieces, the surgeon can incise and coagulate tissue without changing the electrode.

When choosing radiosurgical equipment, one of the most important criteria is that the unit operates at a frequency of 3.8 to 4 MHz. A power output of between 90 and 140 watts is also optimum for avian procedures. In addition, the unit should be equipped with three of the four available waveforms. Although helpful, fulguration is not essential.

RADIO-FREQUENCY WAVEFORMS

As already mentioned, four waveforms (i.e., types of current) are available: fully filtered, fully rectified, partially rectified, and fulgurating.

Fully filtered current creates a continuous nonpulsating flow of current that produces the least amount of tissue alteration and lateral heat and allows microsmooth cutting.[1] This mode is used for cutting tissue and has very little coagulatory effect. A fine-wire or loop electrode should be used if the surgeon is taking biopsy samples. In general, a fully filtered current causes the least amount of scarring of the skin.

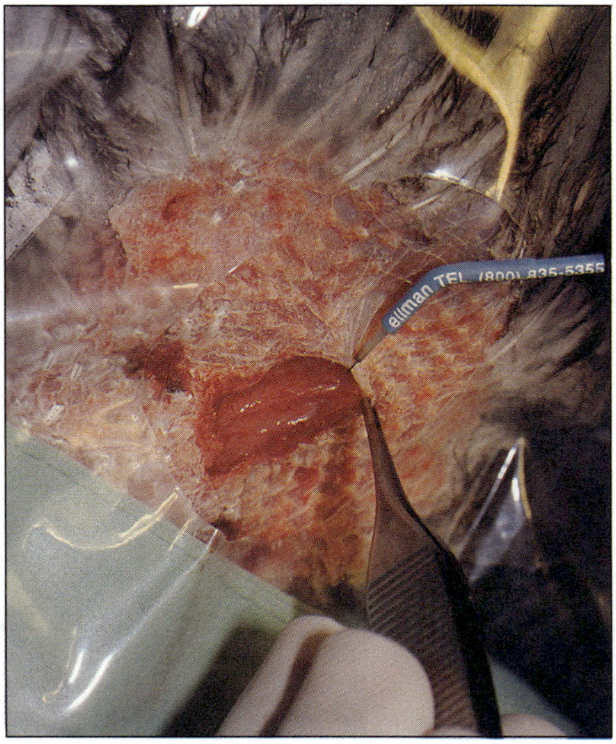

Figure 3—The skin is incised while it is being grasped with thumb forceps and lifted off the muscles. (Courtesy of Dr. Michael Doolen, Oakhurst Veterinary Hospital, Oakhurst, New Jersey)

Fully rectified current is the ideal current to use for all incisions on birds. Skin and muscle can be cut with minimal bleeding because this mode allows equal cutting as well as coagulation. Hemostasis is excellent, and cutting results in little tissue alteration. A fine-wire electrode should be used for incisions and cutting. Debulking, which is a technique used to reduce large tissue masses quickly and bloodlessly, also can be done by using this current.

Partially rectified current has the least number of pulsations per minute and is primarily used for coagulation. The mode has very little cutting quality and therefore should be used exclusively for coagulation and desiccation. Small ball and bipolar forceps are the electrodes used with this current.

Fulgurating current superficially chars and cauterizes tissue and has little use in avian surgery. A spark is emitted from the tip of the electrode to the tissue. The electrode never touches the tissue. The greatest amount of lateral heat is generated in this mode. A heavy straight-wire electrode should be used for fulguration.

PRINCIPLES OF RADIOSURGICAL TECHNIQUE

The primary objective of radiosurgical technique is to minimize the amount of lateral heat.[9] The resistance of tissue to radio-frequency waves can cause heat buildup in tissue. Destructive lateral heat can build up rapidly. A simple mistake may have minimal effect on healing; however, multiple errors in technique could have major consequences.

The length of time the electrode is in contact with tissue is directly proportional to the amount of tissue alteration. Electrode-to-tissue contact should be restricted to two to three seconds. To make an incision, the surgeon should move the electrode across the tissue as rapidly as possible at a minimal speed of 7 mm per second.[9] The surgeon should initiate the current before the electrode comes into contact with the tissue and remove the electrode as soon as the incision has been completed. Doing so prevents excessive heat buildup (which can result from the initial surge of current) and excessive contact time between the electrode and skin. If an incision needs to be longer or deeper, the surgeon should wait at least eight seconds if using a straight-wire electrode or 15 seconds if using a loop electrode to allow the tissue to cool from the initial incision.

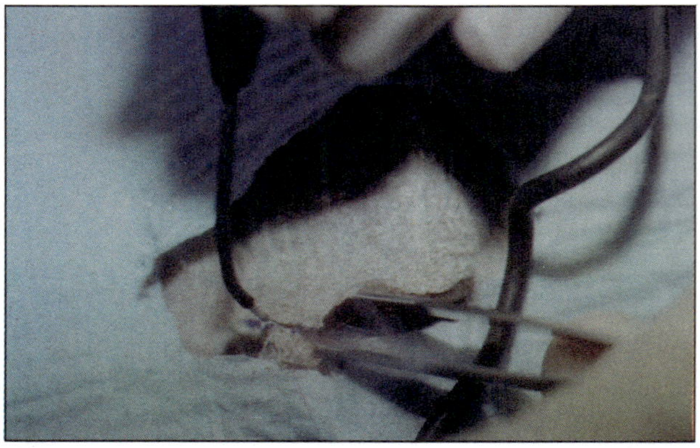

Figure 4—During transabdominal laparotomy, thumb forceps are used to elevate the abdominal muscles and peritoneum away from the abdominal viscera.

The larger the electrode (thickness and length of noninsulated metal), the more lateral heat generated. Using the smallest electrode that can accomplish the required task is therefore essential. Likewise, the intensity of power (watts) should be as low as possible because the more power used, the greater the lateral heat. In addition, the lower the frequency (below 3.8 MHz), the greater the tissue alteration. Therefore, the surgeon should operate as close as possible to the optimum frequency. The proper waveform is necessary to accomplish the task correctly. For example, taking a biopsy using an unfiltered current would create excessive lateral heat and render the biopsy sample useless.

When the surgeon makes an incision, the electrode should be held at a right angle (perpendicular) to the tissue to minimize the amount of current coming from the sides of the electrode. The more acute the electrode-to-tissue angle, the more lateral heat that is directed onto the tissue.

If a passive electrode is not used, the heat buildup in tissue increases. Although the ground plate does not have to be in direct contact with the bird's body, the plate should be as close as possible to the surgical site. All electrode-to-tissue contact (regardless of the electrode being used) should be light, with no pressure applied. When using a ball electrode for coagulation, applying pressure can decrease efficiency and increase the amount of lateral heat.

If problems occur during radiosurgery, the surgeon must be able to correct them quickly and efficiently. Rarely is the problem associated with equipment failure but is more likely procedural in nature. The surgeon should be able to rely on a systematic protocol to solve the problem and continue with surgery. Some manufacturers offer a troubleshooting chart for this purpose.

SPECIFIC SURGICAL TECHNIQUES

When making a skin incision, the skin should be tented from the surface of underlying tissue to avoid lacerating subcutaneous structures (Figure 3). To avoid damaging underlying viscera, tenting is particularly important when making a laparotomy incision through the abdominal muscles (Figure 4).

When incising muscle, the fully rectified (unfiltered) waveform should always be used. If bleeding occurs, monopolar coagulation using a ball electrode or bipolar coagulation is recommended. When using a ball electrode, the ball should lightly touch the surface to be coagulated. Any blood should be sponged first, as coagulation does not occur in the presence of fluid. If an area is oozing, the ball electrode should be moved in a circular pattern over the area until the bleeding is controlled. If a discrete blood vessel is bleeding, the surgeon can coagulate the vessel by grasping it with a mosquito hemostat and touching the ball electrode to the hemostat or by the use of bipolar forceps. If the blood vessel is 2 mm or more in diameter, it should be ligated.

Planing, which is a rapid method of debulking tissue mass, is accomplished by passing a loop electrode back and forth over the area, making sure to take only a few millimeters of tissue at each stroke. The procedure can be performed by using either a filtered or unfiltered waveform; however, unfiltered current results in better hemostasis.

Taking a biopsy (particularly a liver biopsy) can be achieved by using a straight fine-wire electrode or a loop electrode. Filtered current must be used. If bleeding occurs after the sample has been harvested, a ball electrode can be used with partially rectified current to coagulate and stop the bleeding.

Radiosurgical units should be accessible to the surgeon at all times. I recommend keeping a unit on a cart or mounted on a wall bracket at the surgeon's fingertips. Radiosurgery should always be the technique of choice for every avian surgical procedure, regardless of the degree of difficulty involved.

About the Author

Dr. Altman has been involved with the practice of small animal, avian, and exotics specialties for almost 40 years. At present, he is Professor of Research at the Florida Atlantic University in Boca Raton, Florida. Dr. Altman is an honorary member of the American Board of Veterinary Practitioners and lectures and writes extensively on avian medicine and surgery.

REFERENCES

1. Sherman JA: *Oral Electrosurgery. An Illustrated Clinical Guide.* London, Martin Dunitz, 1992, pp 7–11.
2. White WF: Radiosurgery an advancement over the scalpel in many procedures. *Podiatry Products Rep*:16–17, 1986.
3. Coyne BE, Bednarski RM, Bilbrey SA: Thermoelectric burns from improper grounding of electrocautery units: Two case reports. *JAAHA* 29:7–9, 1993.
4. Fucci V, Elkins AD: Electrosurgery: Principles and guidelines in veterinary medicine. *Compend Contin Educ Pract Vet* 13(3): 407–414, 1991.
5. Kalkwarf KL, Krejci RF, Wentz FM: Healing of electrosurgical incisions in gingiva: Early histologic observations in adult men. *J Prosthet Dent* 46:662–669, 1981.
6. Maness WL, Roeber ES, Clark RE, et al: Histological evaluation of electrosurgery with varying frequency and waveform. *J Prosthet Dent* 40:304–312, 1978.
7. Harrison GJ: Surgical instrumentation and special techniques, in Harrison GJ, Harrison LR (eds): *Clinical Avian Medicine and Surgery.* Philadelphia, WB Saunders Co, 1986, pp 560–567.
8. Bennett RA: Surgical considerations in Ritchie B, Harrison GJ, Harrison LR (eds): *Avian Medicine: Principles and Applications.* Lake Worth, FL, Wingers Publishing, 1994, pp 1087–1090.
9. Altman RB: Principles and application of electrosurgery. *Assoc Avian Vet Annu Conf Practical Labs Proceed*:85–92, 1994.

Unique Features of the Avian Integumentary System

Karen Rosenthal, DVM, MS, ABVP

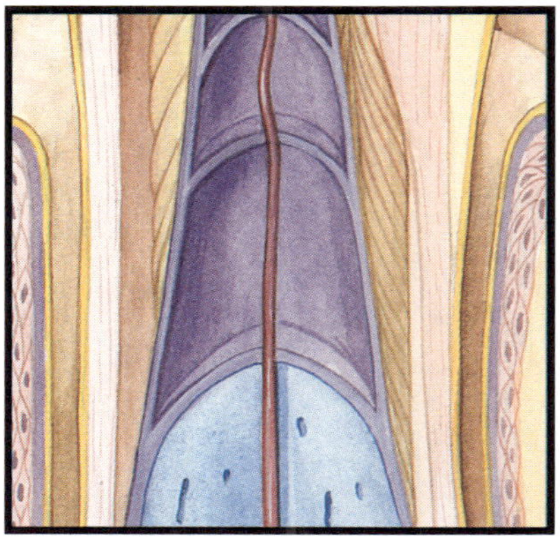

Illustration by Felecia J. Paras

Editor's note: Exotic animals are becoming increasingly popular as pets in the United States, with birds being among the most common. This article is meant to provide veterinarians with useful, hard to find, anatomical illustrations enhanced with explanatory text. These illustrations may be helpful for practitioners to use in demonstrations or in explaining a point to a client.

The integumentary system of birds is quite different from that of mammals and many of these differences are immediately obvious. For example, birds have feathers rather than hair as a body covering, a thin and delicate skin, and a specialized epidermal structure called the beak. All of these features contribute to the unique avian integumentary system and are adapted to the unique lifestyle of birds. Without feathers, birds could not fly, and their thin skin is an example of how the characteristics of birds limit their weight for flight. Feathers also serve an important aspect of courtship rituals and species recognition. They are essential in temperature regulation and, in the water birds, act as insulation. Finally, the great variety of beaks reflects the varied diets of avian species.

Originally published in May/June 1995 *Perspectives*

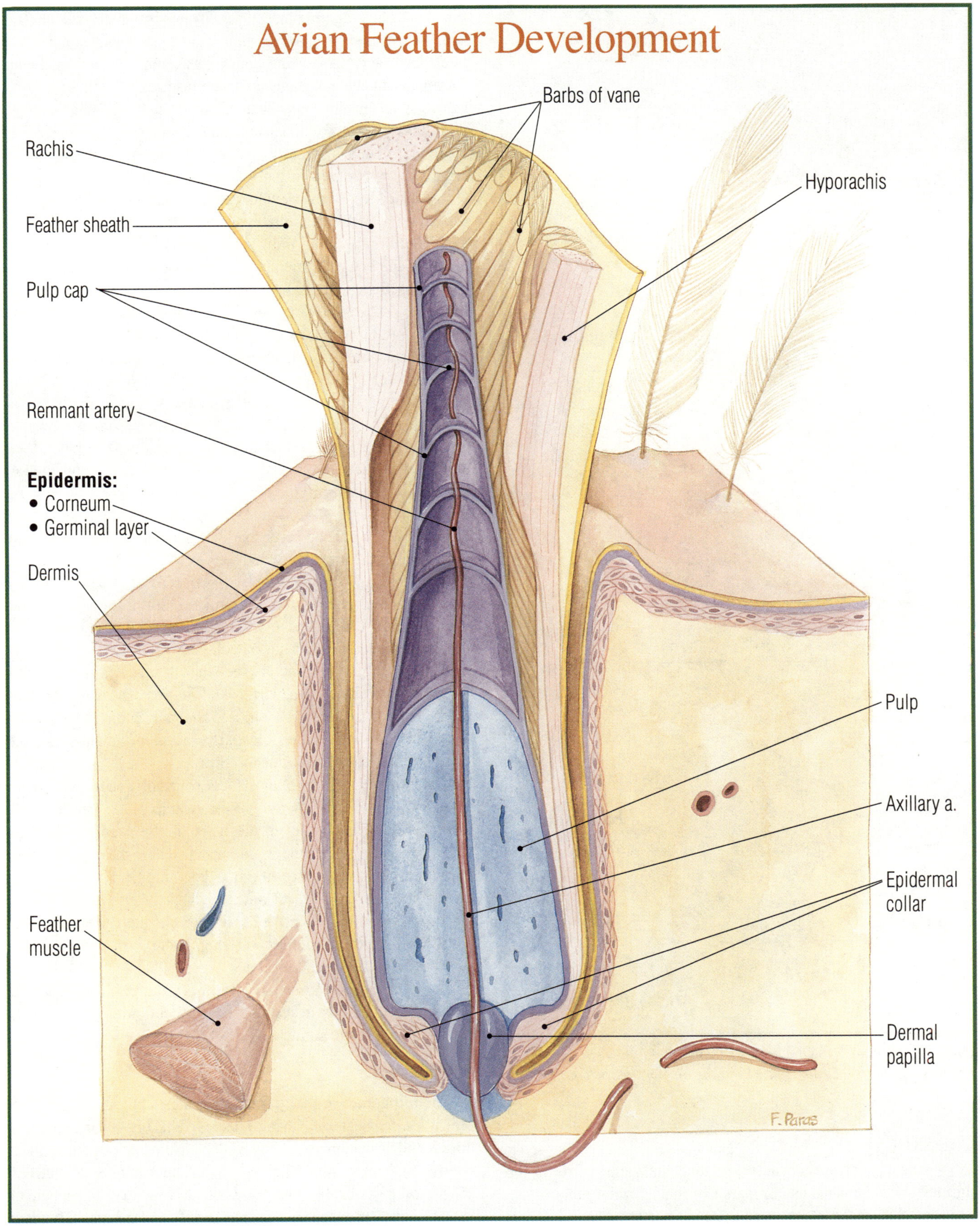

Illustration showing the layers of feather development.

Illustration by Felecia J. Paras

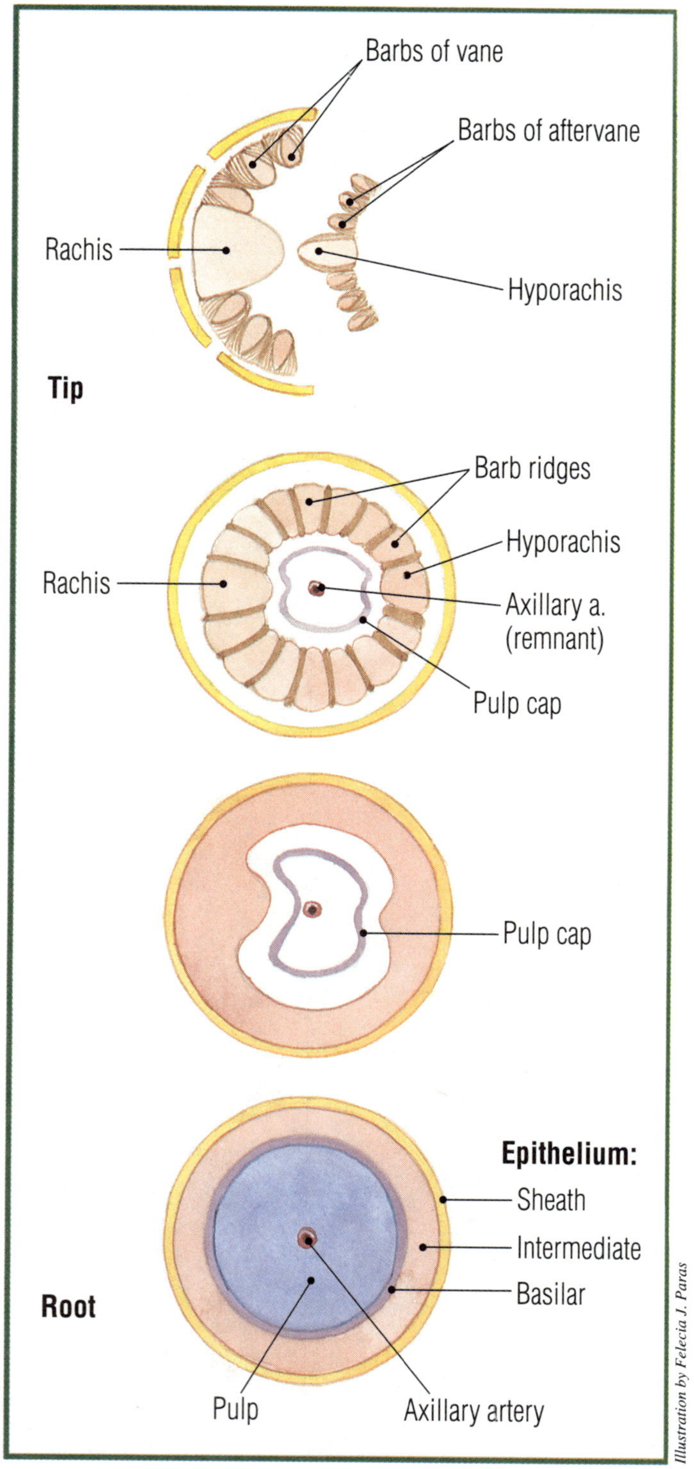

Cross sections of a growing contour feather, with the cross section progressing from the root (bottom) to the tip (top) of the feather.

THE SKIN

A striking difference between mammals and birds is the thinness of avian skin as compared to that of mammalian skin. Thinner skin means less weight; an important adaptation for flying animals. As is true in all animals, avian skin is the first line of defense against infections; it prevents mechanical damage, is involved in heat regulation, and prevents the escape of vital fluids and gasses. The delicate avian skin has extensive attachments to the skeleton but few muscular attachments. As a result of an absence of sweat glands, bird skin is essentially glandless except for the uropygial gland (preen gland). The uropygial gland is found just dorsal to the tail base and its secretions are involved in maintaining feather condition and waterproofing. It is most developed in waterfowl and its opening is marked by a tuft of feathers surrounding the gland.

In addition to being thin, avian skin is dry and inelastic over much of the body. Clinically, however, it seems no more prone to tearing than mammalian skin. Three skin layers are identified in birds, just as they are in mammals: the epidermis, the dermis, and the subcutaneous tissue. The epidermis consists of the stratum corneum (dead cells) and a germinal layer (living layer). In feathered areas, the epidermis may be only 10 cells thick. It is thicker in the unfeathered areas such as the beak and foot pads. The germinal layer of the epidermis has three strata: the basal, intermediate, and transitional zones. The basal layer lies next to the dermis and produces cells. The intermediate layer consists of polygonal cells. This layer merges with the transitional zone where cells become keratinized. The stratum corneum is a cornified layer made of dead cells that have a flattened shape and are vacuolated.

The dermis is comparatively thin in birds and consists of the superficial and deep layers. Within the dermis are the feather follicles and blood vessels. The superficial layer varies in thickness depending on the species and the area of the body while the deep layer contains the smooth muscles of the feathers and large blood vessels, fat, and nerves. The subcutaneous layer of the skin, formed by loose, connective tissue, is an area of fat storage. Striated muscles, also found in the subcutaneous layer, regulate the tension of the skin.

The thinness of the skin affects routine procedures. When giving subcutaneous injections, for example, the needle is directed somewhat parallel to the body. If the needle is injected at a more acute angle, the injection will enter the subcutaneous tissue. In birds, therefore, there is less margin for error when giving subcutaneous injections. The lack of tissue and the inelastic skin combine to afford few suitable sites: preferred sites are the right and left flanks, although others may use the dorsum between the shoulder blades.

Suturing avian skin also is sometimes challenging. The scarce subcutaneous tissue makes a subcuticular pattern difficult. A small gauge suture (e.g., 5-0) is preferred.

THE BEAK

The bill comes in many sizes and shapes but the basic structure is uniform among avian species. The beak consists of an upper and lower portion covered by a horny portion (rhamphotheca). This is a keratinized epidermal structure that covers the rostral parts of the upper and lower jaws. In some species it is horny and firm and in others it is soft and pliable. The beak is a reflection of what the particular species of bird consumes

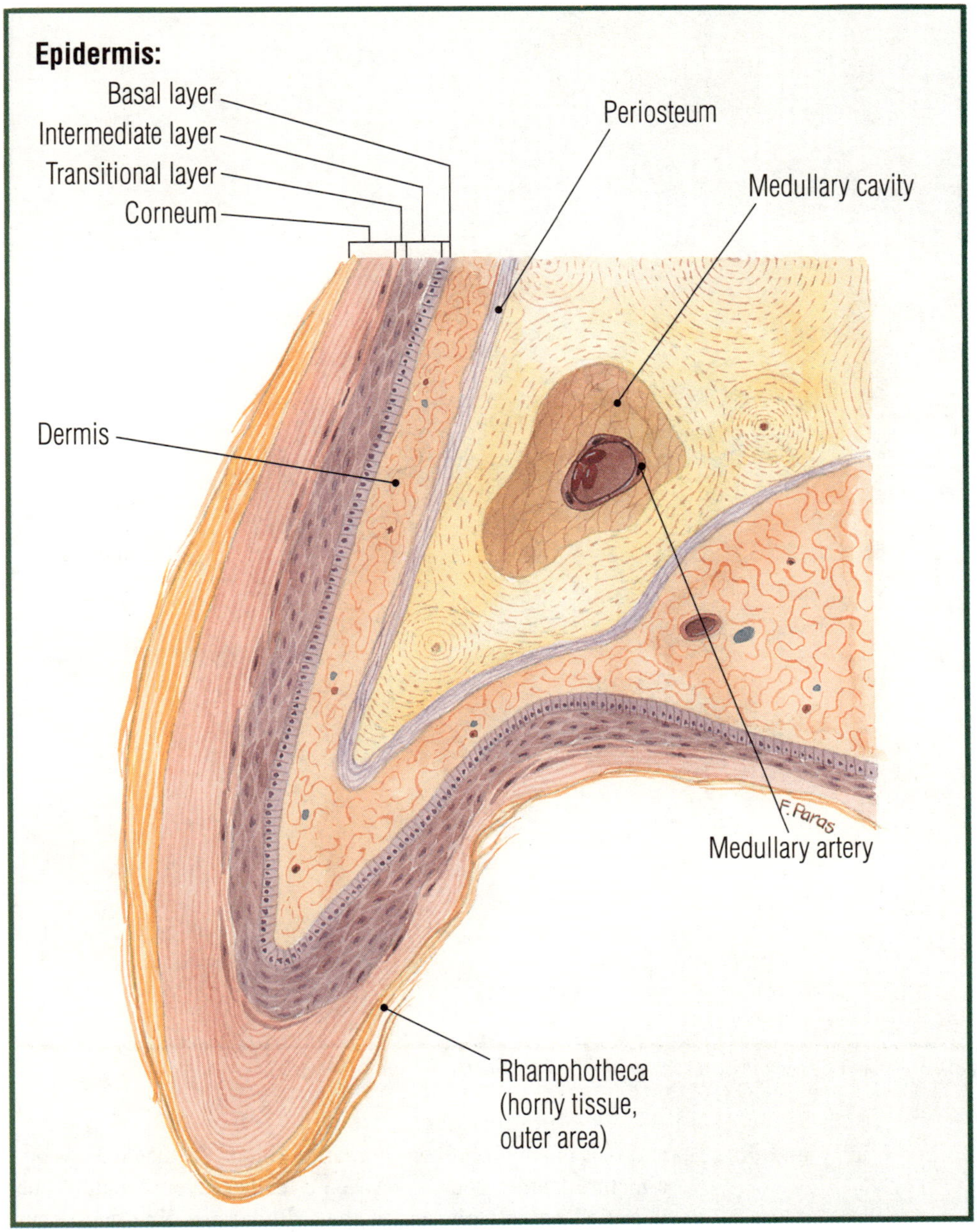

Illustration by Felecia J. Paras

Lateral view of the maxillary beak.

It is the epidermis that is greatly modified to form the beak. The stratum corneum, or rhamphotheca, is very thick and the addition of phosphate, hydroxyapatite, phospholipids, calcium, and abundant keratin to the epidermis gives the beak its characteristic hardness. In some birds, a "bill tip organ," a mechanoreceptor found at the distal end of the beak, aids in the sensory discrimination between food and other particles. The keratinized skin at the base of the beak, where the nares in psittacines are located, is called the cere.

Normally, the horny tissue of the bill is continually worn down by use and is constantly being replaced. In caged birds, the beak may have to be clipped because of a lack of suitable food items and surfaces on which to wear down the horny structure. Most newly hatched chicks have a projection at the rostral portion of the upper beak called the egg tooth. The hatchling uses the egg tooth to pip the shell and the tooth is sloughed within a few days after hatching.

in the wild: the parrot has a beak designed for cracking nuts, a woodpecker has a chisel-like bill for penetrating wood, the hummingbird has a long thin bill to suck out nectar and pollen, the anhinga has a dagger-like bill to spear fish. The bill contains both dermis and epidermis; therefore, histologically, it resembles skin. The dermis is closely attached to the periosteum of the jaws. Trauma or infection leading to necrosis of the dermis can lead to a loss of cells that form the normal beak and this in turn can lead to acquired beak deformities. Beak avulsions are a common traumatic injury and both the lower and upper beaks are vulnerable. This type of injury is usually caused by attacks by other animals or by such household dangers as slamming doors or closing hinges. In these injuries, part or all of the horny beak is torn from the skin.

THE NAILS

A nail is found at the distal end of the terminal phalanx of each digit. A hard, keratinized, dorsal plate forms the dorsal ridge and lateral walls of the nail and a softer ventral plate forms the sole of the nail. The dorsal plate grows faster than the ventral plate which produces a natural curve to the nails.

Owners usually have three concerns regarding nails: how often they should be cut, how short they should be, and what should be done if they bleed. Nail growth is individual and substrate is a factor in sharpness. The more a bird is handled, the more frequently the owner will want the nails clipped. Owners should be advised to try monthly grooming at home. If this is not possible, then visiting a veterinarian every 3 to 4 months normally suffices. Owners can be shown how to clip the nails by pointing out the quick and then demonstrating to the owner how they need to clip the nail distal to this area. Many birds have light colored nails so the blood vessel can be easily identified. Nail bleeding accidents are common, so owners should be advised to have a product in the house to aid

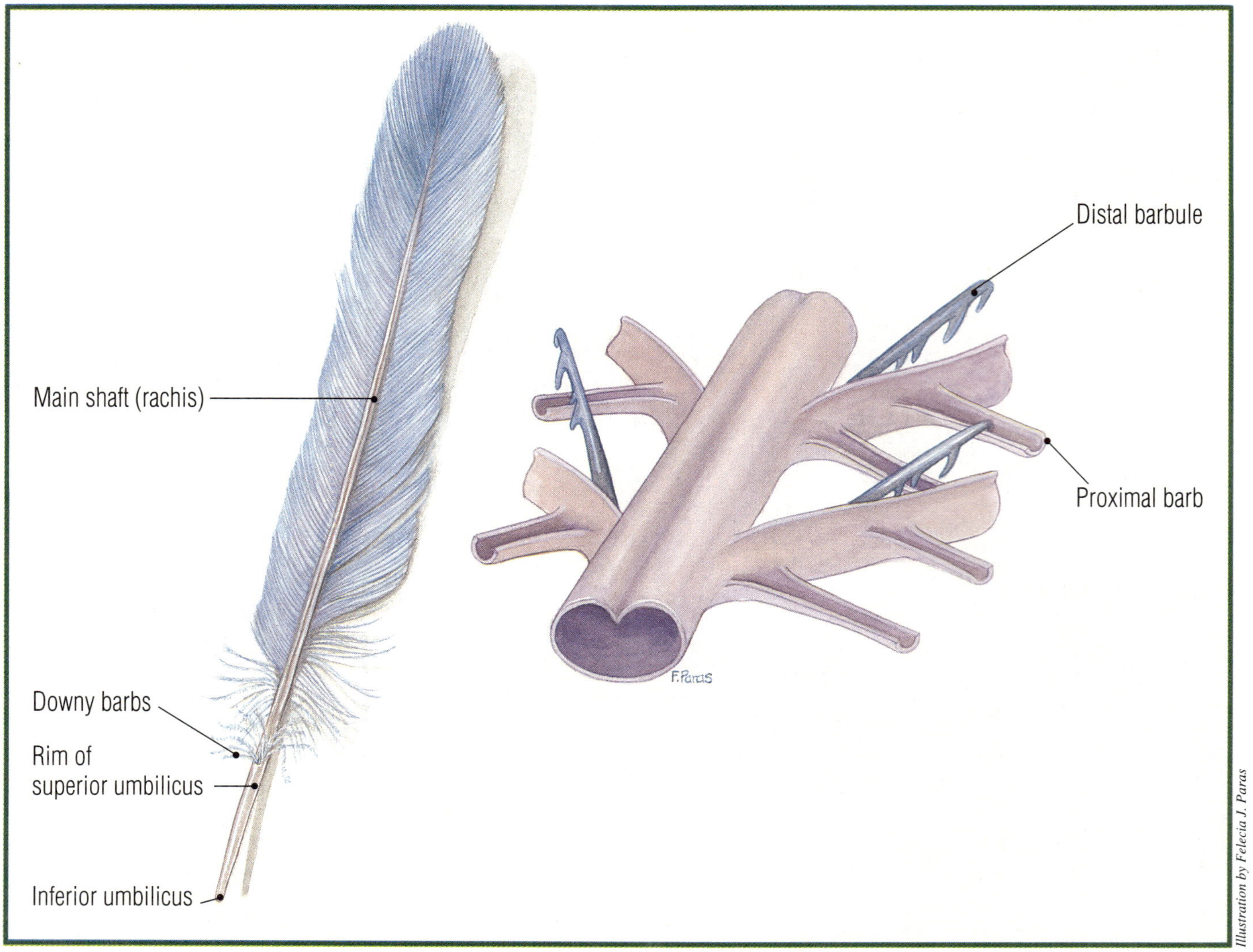

Illustration showing the parts of a flight feather (left) and how the barbules on the barb of the feather interlock (right).

in clotting. Powders are available commercially and corn starch can be used in an emergency.

THE FEATHERS

The size and number of feathers are physiologically and statistically related to the metabolic rate, temperature, body weight, and surface area of each species of birds. The color of feathers is determined by pigments, structural conditions, or a combination of both. The feathers themselves serve many functions: they provide flight, insulate the body, protect the skin, waterproof the bird, and function in courtship. There are seven main types of feathers which are distributed over the body in well defined tracts known as pterylae. The bare patches between these tracts are called apteria, and the number and distribution of the tracts varies among species.

The feather is embedded into the follicle and the section of the feather shaft embedded in the skin follicle, the calamus, is filled with, among other things, an artery and vein in the growing feather. These vessels degenerate when the feather matures and that is why a broken, immature (blood feather) bleeds and a mature feather does not. When a feather, even a mature one, is pulled completely out of the follicle, bleeding can occur. This happens because the vascular dermis is torn by the pulling motion.

Emerging from the calamus is the rachis, the central shaft of the feather. From the rachis, barbs branch out on each side and from each barb, barbules branch. Barbules have hooks (barbicles) that interlock with other barbules in a zipper-like fashion, giving the feather its characteristic smooth appearance.

The seven main types of feathers are as follows:

- **Contour** feathers are the largest and most prominent of all the feathers on a bird's body, making up the body and flight feathers. The typical contour feather contains the shaft (rachis and calamus), vanes, and after-feather.
- **Semiplumes** are feathers with a very long rachis and a vane that does not have a zipper effect.
- **Down** feathers have a small rachis, are fluffy, and are seen

in both hatchlings and adult birds.

- **Powder down** are specialized feathers, most notably found on cockatoos. They are responsible for the fine keratin debris resembling dust. This is a normal condition and its absence can be one of the first signs of Psittacine Beak and Feather Disease.
- **Hypopenna** are also called after-feathers. Bristles have a very stiff rachis and almost no barbules.
- **Filoplumes** resemble bristles, except that the shaft is very fine and there is a fine tuft of barbs at the tip.

The replacement of feathers is called a molt and can be complete or partial. Before the barbs of a new feather are released, they are encased in a feather sheath and the structure is called a pin feather. A new feather grows upward, out of the follicle.

All birds molt annually, some twice a year, and a few three times a year. Influential factors in molting are nutrition, reproduction, time of year, temperature, natural and artificial light cycles, and the species or sex of the bird. Young birds generally molt their juvenile feathers just before they mature.

Feather growth during molting periods puts an increased demand on body resources, so owners should be advised to pay extra attention to their bird's diet at this time.

About the Author

Dr. Rosenthal, who is board certified in avian practice, is a Staff Veterinarian for the avian and exotic pet service of The Animal Medical Center in New York City.

RESOURCES

Publications

Axelson DR, in Dermatology for the Small Animal Practitioner. Trenton, NJ, Veterinary Learning Systems, 1991.

King AS, McLelland J: *Birds: Their Structure and Function.* Philadelphia, Bailliere Tindall, 1984.

Lucas AM, Stettenheim PR: Anatomy: Integument. *Agriculture Handbook.* Washington, DC, US Government Printing Office, 1972.

Riche BW, Harridan GJ, Harridan IR, (eds): *Avian Medicine: Principles and Application.* Lake Worth, FL, Wingers, Inc, 1994.

Sturkie PD (ed): *Avian Physiology.* New York, Springer-Verlag, 1986.

Other

Association of Avian Veterinarians
P.O. Box 811720
Boca Raton, Florida 33481
Phone: (407) 393-8901

Avian Dermatology

Links Road Animal and Bird Clinic
North York, Ontario, Canada
R. Dean Axelson, DVM

STRUCTURE AND FUNCTION OF AVIAN SKIN

Diseases of the avian dermis involve many different disease processes and encompass not only skin but feathers, cere, uropygial gland, spurs, wattles, combs, claws, and beak.

Avian skin, which consists of dermis and epidermis, differs from that of mammals or reptiles in that the former is very thin and tears easily. Avian skin probably evolved to make birds lighter in weight to facilitate flight. The skin of the feet and legs is scaly and totally unlike the integument of the rest of the body. The only glands in avian skin are the uropygial gland, which is a holocrine gland at the base of the tail; holocrine glands in the external ear canal; mucous-producing glands around the vent; and meibomian glands in the eyelid. Claws, beak, cere, wattles, combs, and scales on feet and legs are all modifications of the skin. Some of these modified skin structures are very colorful and can vary between the sexes.

Adipose tissue is located mainly in the subcutis. Feather follicles are attached by smooth muscles to deeper tissues that control movement of the follicles when birds fluff out their feathers. Dermocutaneous muscles raise the feathered crests on the head. The wing web is called the *propatagium.* During nesting, the mid-ventral skin of the chest modifies with increased vascularity and thickness to form a brood patch that provides extra warmth during egg incubation; this happens in the female or in both sexes, depending on the species. Avian skin is lightly attached to underlying muscles but is strongly attached to underlying bone structures on the head, extremities, and dorsal midline.

Feathers are part of the avian integumentary system the same as hair is part of the mammalian system. The avian body is not totally covered with feathers; they grow in tracts or rows called *pterylae.* The bare skin areas between these tracts are called *apteria.* The avian body has two dorsal and two ventral pterylae that are placed roughly equidistant apart, with the mid-ventral and mid-dorsal areas bare. These pterylae extend up the neck of most birds. Some species, such as pigeons, have denser groupings of feather follicles all around the neck and no apteria. The wings are feathered differently in rows. There are 10 primary wing feathers that are the most distal, long flight feathers. Next to these are 10 secondary flight feathers. Flight feathers are also called *remiges.* Primary feathers are strongly attached to muscle, fascia, and bone of the wing by fibrous tissue and are not very movable; secondary feathers have more mobility. The rest of the wing feathers are called *coverts* (Figure 1). Right next to the

Originally published in *Dermatology for the Small Animal Practitioner*, Trenton, VLS Books, 1991 body, but still involved with the wing, are the humeral feathers.

Feathers are necessary insulators in maintaining body heat, which in the bird ranges from 39°C to 43°C (102°F to 109°F). Feather follicles are the areas from which the feathers grow and are tubular invaginations of the skin. Feathers also provide flight, flotation, and waterproofing and are used in sexual display rituals during the breeding season.

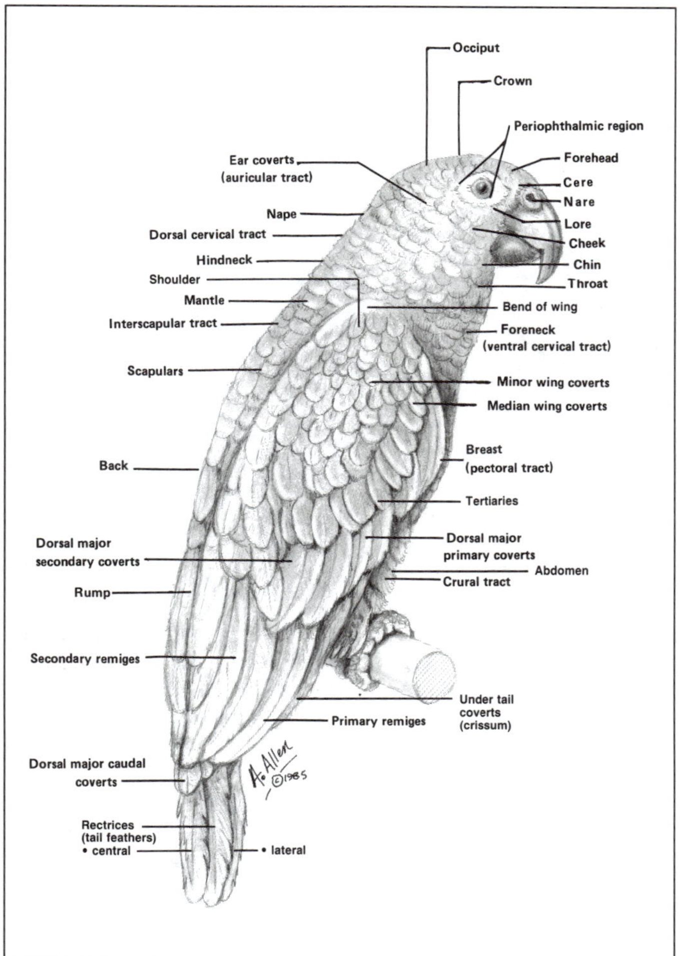

Figure 1—Topography of a bird showing normal plumage. (From Harrison GJ, Harrison LR [eds]: *Clinical Avian Medicine and Surgery*. Philadelphia, WB Saunders Co, 1986. Reprinted with permission.)

The three main types of feathers are the *contour feather* (*penna*), the *tufted bristle feather* (*filoplume*), and the *down feather* (*plume* or *plumule*) (Figure 2); three subtypes are the *powder down feather*, the *hypopenna*, and the *semiplume*. Bristle feathers that act as eyelashes and vibrissae around nasal openings are called *setae*. Contour feathers cover the contour of the body, tail, and wings. Each area of the body has a fairly fixed number of contour feathers. Semiplume feathers have a longer *rachis* (the distal part of the shaft) than *barbs* (side branches of the shaft) and lie along the edge of feather tracts acting as insulators. Down feathers have a shorter rachis than barbs, are the first feathers that grow on chicks, may grow in the apteria, and provide insulation in adult birds.

The long axis of a feather is divided into the *calamus* (the thick hollow part closest to the body) and the *rachis* (which contains the branches of the vane); together they make up the *scapus* (Figure 3). The *vexilla* is formed by barbs growing at 45° angles from each side of the rachis. Arising from each side of the barbs are barbules that interlock with adjacent barbules from neighboring barbs with a series of hooklets that latch onto a flange system from the next barb. One side of each barb has a row of barbules with hooklets, and the other side has a row of barbules with a flange system. The hooklets of one barbule attach to the flanges of the next barbule. This elaborate system keeps the feather parts together, thus allowing the bird to move air and not collapse.

Down feathers (plumes) are characterized by a rachis that is shorter than the longest barb. Slender and noninterlocking barbules give them their fluffy appearance. These feathers grow from the follicles of contour feathers and lie next to the body under these larger feathers. Certain species have modified plume feathers called *powder down feathers*. Powder is a keratin material originating from cells on the surface of barb-forming tissue in the feather germ. These feathers break open, lose their powder, and then take on the appearance of regular plume feathers. Powder down feathers are the only feathers that grow continuously. The function of powder is unknown.

The color of feathers is controlled by pigments, (such as melanins, carotenoids, and porphyrins) and by light diffraction on cells or layers of oil. The colors can be changed or modified by dirt, oils, hormones, bleaching agents, age, disease, diet, physical damage, and (temporarily) water. White is produced by the refraction and reflection of all light wavelengths. Green is produced by the combination of yellow pigments and structural scattering in the feathers. Carotene pigments produce reds, yellows, and oranges; are in fat globules in the feathers; and originate from plant material. Porphyrins are synthesized by the bird and produce reds and some greens. Melanin produces brown, reddish brown, and black.

Molting is the process of losing old feathers and growing new ones. All birds molt annually, some twice a year, and a few three times a year. Influential factors in molting are nutrition, reproduction, time of year, temperature, natural and artificial light cycles, and species or sex of the bird. Most birds molt after the end of the reproductive cycle. Some species, such as the Amazon parrot, molt continually during the year. Birds do not molt completely at one time, as they would be bald and incapable of flight. Certain areas lose feathers at different times than other areas so that enough feathers are in all areas to maintain body heat. Most birds also keep enough feathers on their wings to maintain flight; but a few species, such as some of the waterfowl, lose all their flight feathers within a short time and become flightless until they regrow. Young birds generally molt their juvenile feathers just before they mature, which in some species can be from 1½ to 2 years.

Molting usually starts with the inner primaries and follows a defined sequence in each bird. Cut feathers do not regrow until the feather shaft comes out during the next molt or is removed from the feather follicle. It takes about six weeks for feathers to regrow after they are lost or molted.

Molting is a stressful period for birds and can lower their resistance, making them more susceptible to disease at this time. Feather growth puts an increased demand on body resources. Attention should be given to a better diet during molting.

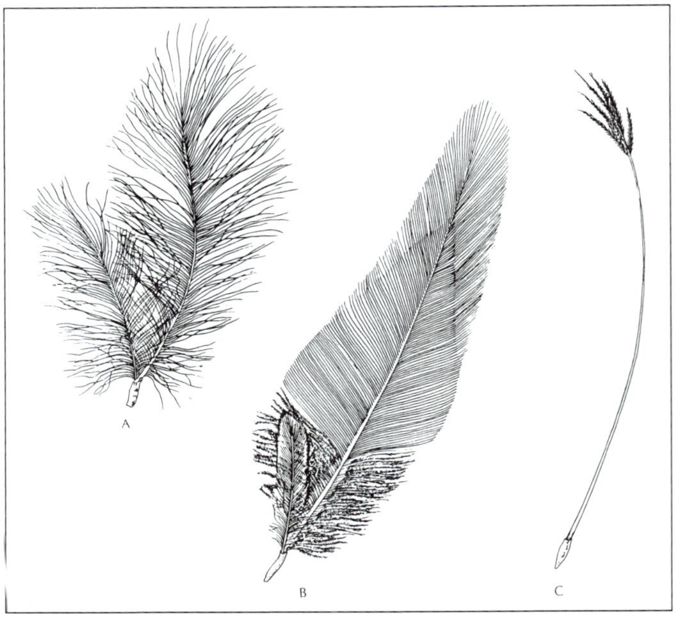

Figure 2—The three main types of feathers. *A,* Contour; *B,* down; *C,* filoplume. (From Macwhirter P [ed]: *Everybird, A Guide to Bird Health.* Melbourne/Sydney, Australia, Inkata Press, 1987. Reprinted with permission.)

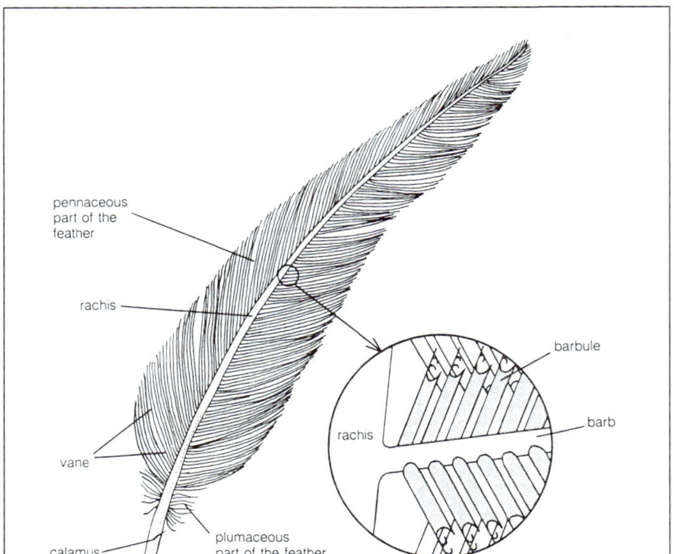

Figure 3—Anatomy of a feather showing the relationship of interlocking barbules. (From Petrak ML [ed]: *Diseases of Cage and Aviary Birds,* ed 2. Philadelphia, Lea & Febiger, 1982. Reprinted with permission.)

PARASITIC DISEASES

Cere Mites

Pathogenesis. Cere mites, usually members of the genus *Knemidokoptes* or *Procenemidokoptes* (Figure 4), are very small and are the most common mites parasitizing pet birds. Most budgerigars have this parasite on their bodies a majority of the time. Cere mites are usually transferred from parents to chicks. Most birds live asymptomatically with the mites, as the avian immune system apparently can control the mite population. Under certain conditions of stress, malnutrition, or other disease, the immune system can become impaired, allowing the mites to multiply; the infestation suddenly appears as a disease condition. Therefore, even with multiple birds in the same cage, not all are affected to the same degree.

Clinical Signs. Cere mites usually are first noticed around the bare areas of the face (Figure 5), spreading rapidly all over the face, including around the eyes, cere, and beak. The bird spreads them to the feet and legs and around the vent in the process of preening and cleaning itself. Crusty proliferation of the outer layers of the epithelium builds up; on close inspection, the tiny burrows of the mites appear as a tiny honeycomb. If not treated, this crusty layer can become so thick that the bird will have trouble opening its eyes. The beak itself can become honey-combed with mite burrows and start to grow in a deformed manner. The normal curvature to the beak lessens, and the beak begins to straighten out because of damage to the germinal cells at the base of the beak. Once this happens, the beak remains deformed and continuously overgrown; the beak has to be ground or trimmed back to normal length on a regular basis. In severe cases, birds can end up with beaks that look like canary beaks; with regular assistance, birds with this deformity can survive. The feet, legs, and vent areas also can become very heavily crusted if the disease is allowed to progress for a long time without treatment. The uropygial gland area has been observed to be involved occasionally as well.

Diagnosis. Clinical signs usually are enough for a diagnosis, but suspicions can be confirmed by using a scalpel blade with a little mineral oil on it to take a gentle scraping from one of the infected areas. Mites and eggs are plainly visible on the slide under low-power magnification.

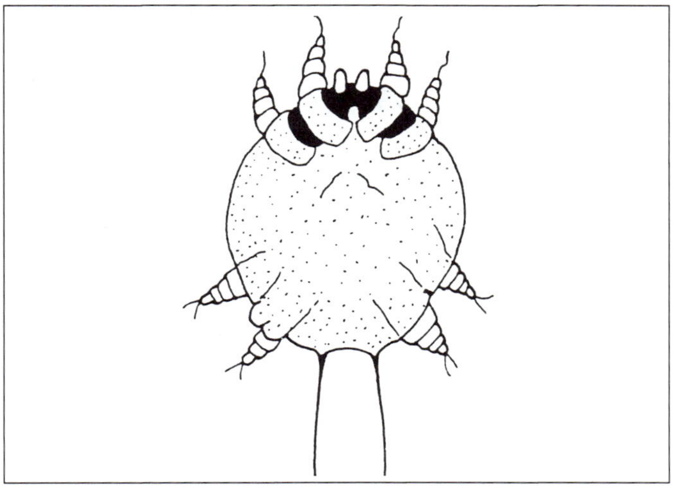

Figure 4—Knemidokoptic mite. (From Axelson RD: *Caring for Your Pet Bird.* Toronto, Canaviax Publications, 1981. Reprinted with permission.)

Treatment. A very effective method of eliminating cere mite infestation is to apply a mixture of 5% ivermectin in propylene glycol lightly to the affected areas. The entire face, around the eyes, below and around the beak, the feet and legs, and the vent area should always be treated even if there is no evidence of crusting. If all of these areas are not treated, the problem may recur. My program includes one treatment per week for three weeks and one more a month later. This product is never dispensed to the client. There may be some maintenance problems after recovery, but rarely are these insurmountable.

For birds with very severely infected cases, one drop of a 10% ivermectin and propylene glycol mixture can be applied to the bare area of skin on both sides of the neck. The mixture is absorbed through the skin and is an effective treatment. Bovine preparation can be diluted 1:4 with propylene glycol and given at 0.05 ml/lb (0.1 ml/kg), with a budgerigar dose of 0.01 ml (per bird) given either orally or intramuscularly. Some clinicians put one drop of pure bovine preparation on the neck of infected birds and have no problem with toxicity.

If an oil-based mixture is used to treat this disease, it must be applied *sparingly* so that the oil does not spread to the feathered areas. Too much oil (or glycerine) on feathers can cause them to stick together, which impairs the bird's ability to maintain its body heat. The bird may then get chilled, sicken, and die. The main reason that I do not dispense this product to clients is that they always apply too much, which can cause serious problems.

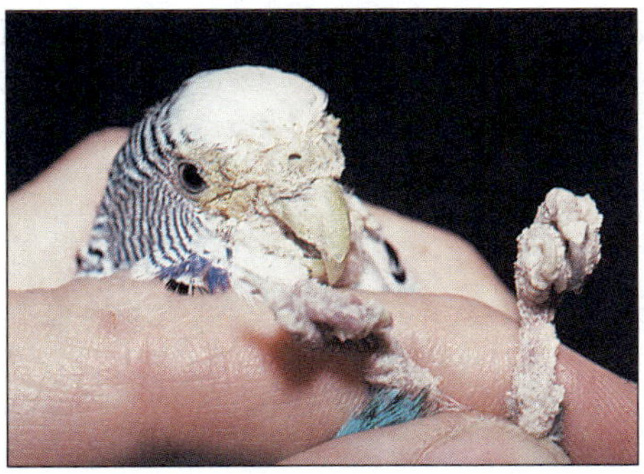

Figure 5—*Knemidokoptes* infestation on the face and feet of a budgerigar.

Red or Gray Mites

Pathogenesis. Red mites and gray mites (*Dermanyssus* spp.) are small but are visible to the naked eye. They generally do not live on the bird but inhabit the cage environment, hide in cracks and crevices or nesting material, and come out at night to feed on the blood of the bird. A mite may be seen on the bird only occasionally.

Clinical Signs. Infested birds are irritable, become itchy, have poor feather appearance, may preen excessively, or may become weak and anemic from excessive blood loss. A large number of mites can drain the blood of a nestling bird. Some skin irritation may be seen.

Diagnosis. These mites can be detected by covering the cage at night with a white cloth and later looking on the cloth's underside with a flashlight for dark gray or red "spots" that move fairly quickly. Cracks or crevices in the cage, nest box, or perches also should be checked.

Treatment. Strict cleanliness of the cage and environment is the best control method. Old nesting material should be removed. Dusting the bird and the cage with a mild insecticidal powder is effective in killing these mites. Products with a wide safety margin, such as pyrethrin and rotenone or pyrethrin combined with piperonyl butoxide, are effective and safe. Malathion and carbaryl in low concentrations also are fairly safe. In general, dusting powders that are safe for cats can be used on birds.

Depluming Mites

Clinical Signs. These mites (*Knemidokoptes laevis* and *Megninia* spp.) attack the feather shafts, causing broken, damaged feathers and feather loss. The damage starts in a small area and spreads to the head, neck, and legs (Figure 5). Psittacines are affected most often, and infestation occurs in the summer. A scaly alopecia around the face often is a sign of *Megninia* mite infestation.

Diagnosis. The mites are found by placing scrapings or acetate tape impressions of the affected area on a slide and observing through a microscope.

Treatment. Insecticidal powders should be applied; secondary bacterial skin infections can be controlled with antibiotic therapy.

Quill Mites

Pathogenesis. Several species of mites are involved, such as *Syrigophilus* spp., *Dermatoglyphus* spp., *Pterolichus* spp., and *Analges* spp.

Clinical Signs. These mites primarily attack new feathers and cause feather loss. The bottom part of the feather remains in the follicle and contains mites and debris.

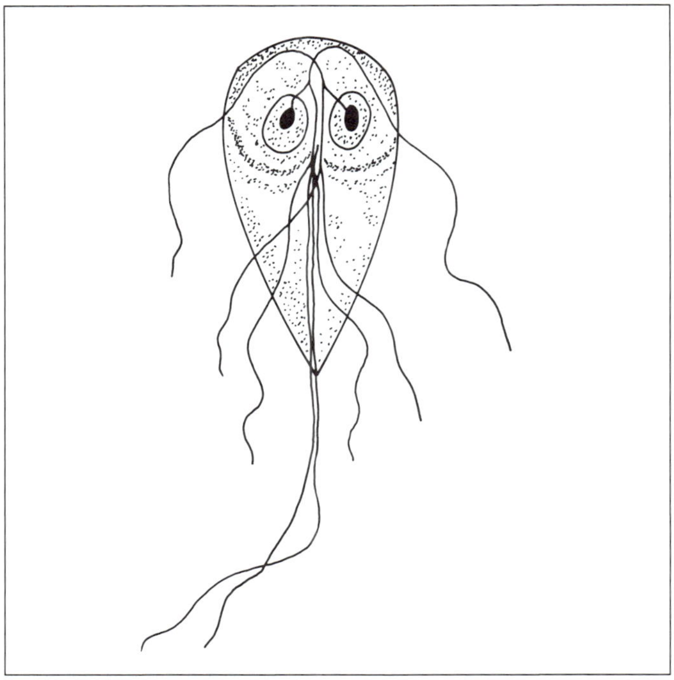

Figure 6—A *Giardia* organism.

Diagnosis. The presence of these mites can be confirmed by squeezing mites from the feather quill onto a slide with some mineral oil on it and examining microscopically.

Treatment. There is no totally effective treatment, but insecticidal dusts or sprays may help somewhat. Infested birds should be separated from healthy ones. An ivermectin spray may be helpful.

Fleas

Pathogenesis. Mammalian or avian fleas may infest birds on occasion if the population is high in a household or there is exposure to wild birds. Fleas are not commonly found on pet birds.

Clinical Signs. Affected birds may be irritable, scratch a lot, be unthrifty, and possibly be weak or anemic. Fleas might be seen running around on the body or embedded in the skin of the face, head, and neck.

Diagnosis. Finding fleas or flea feces is indicative of their presence. Nestlings are affected most often.

Treatment. The premises and environment should be cleaned using insecticidal powders and sprays. Other household pets should be treated as well. Residual sprays should be used in areas away from direct exposure to the birds. Direct access to wild birds should be prevented. Insecticidal powders should be applied to the flea-infested bird. Care should be taken when using sprays on birds. The treatment should be repeated weekly as necessary.

Lice

Pathogenesis. There are several genera and species of biting, sucking, and chewing lice; but they are not commonly found on house pets. Contact with wild birds is the usual source of these parasites. Lice usually are host-specific and do not survive very long off the bird.

Clinical Signs. Birds with lice may show feather damage, excessive preening, irritability, unthriftiness, and reduced productivity and vitality. Lice eggs or "nits" may be seen attached to the lower part of the feathers.

Diagnosis. Finding the lice or eggs confirms the diagnosis. They most commonly inhabit the neck, back, wings, and vent areas and are elongated, fairly fast moving, light brown, flattened creatures.

Treatment. Spraying or dusting with safe insecticides can eliminate lice. Repeating in two-week cycles for a few treatments totally eliminates the lice.

Giardia

Pathogenesis. Giardia lamblia is the species found in birds; because this species is the same that infects humans, there is some zoonotic potential. Giardiasis is seen most often in budgerigars and cockatiels and less often in toucans. It has been suggested that *Giardia* produces a malabsorption problem and allergic reaction that causes pruritus.

Clinical Signs. Affected birds may have soft green droppings, weight loss, and dry flaky skin; but the most significant dermatologic sign is that the pruritus leads to the bird scratching and chewing at itself until it actually chews lesions into the skin. These lesions can be very extensive and usually are found in the axillae, mid-dorsal back, or along the sides of the body under the resting wing. The lesions can become ulcerated if the bird does not leave them alone.

Diagnosis. It is not always possible to demonstrate the presence of these parasites (Figure 6). Clinicians can attempt to find *Giardia* on a wet-mount sample of very fresh droppings. More than one sample may be required. The basophil count in a complete blood count (CBC) may be quite high in *Giardia* infections. Eosinophilia is common. Visualization of the parasite in the wet-mount sample can be enhanced with the use of Gram's stain iodine or Lugol's iodine solution. False-negative results are common unless *very* fresh droppings are used (not more than 5 to 10 minutes old). The fecal trichrome stain may show a much higher sensitivity in finding positive samples; in this test, the sample must first be placed in polyvinyl alcohol, which is a preservative.

Treatment. At this time there is no known cure for this parasite, but some drugs can help reduce the population so that there is some improvement in clinical signs. Dimetridazole soluble powder (182 g/6.42 oz) mixed in the drinking water at 1 teaspoon/U.S. gallon (3.8 L) should be given as the only source of water for five days. Because this drug can be dangerous, the dose and interval should not be exceeded or toxic levels may be reached. It is advised that breeding birds not be treated because toxic levels can be reached in the female if the male is feeding her. Ipronidazole soluble powder (61 g/2.65 oz) mixed into drinking water at 500 mg/U.S. gallon and given for 7 to 21 days is another treatment. Metronidazole in the human injectable form, given at 25 to 35 mg/kg three times daily intramuscularly for 2 to 5 days, can be effective also. Clinical signs may recur after treatment.

The skin lesions also must be treated. It is necessary to break the self-trauma cycle long enough for healing to occur, which can take several weeks. An Elizabethan collar made of old x-ray film, custom fitted to the bird, can keep it from inflicting further injury to itself. The neck part of the collar should have a layer of adhesive tape along the edge to prevent the collar from cutting into the neck. If the skin damage is deep and extensive, the bird may require anesthesia so that an attempt can be made to debride and suture some of the worst areas. The skin edges should be freshened; some of the subcutaneous fascia may need to be dissected free to allow the skin to be moved to close the widest areas of damage. I use 4-0 Dexon® (Davis & Geck) with a CE-2 swedged-on needle; it is not necessary to remove these sutures, as they will dissolve. Systemic and topical antibiotic treatment can keep secondary infection under control during healing. The topical use of aloe vera gel on all skin lesions in birds decreases healing time, controls local infection, and reduces scarring. The gel has antimicrobial, antiinflammatory, and tissue-regenerative properties and is in a nongreasy base.

It is advisable to leave the collar on for at least a few days after the area appears to be totally healed, which may take several weeks.

Strict hygiene is a must in controlling this organism. Clinicians should be prepared for recurrences, as giardiasis is very difficult to eradicate. Chlorine as a disinfectant can effectively control *Giardia*. Water that has cycled through a water heater cannot contain live *Giardia*; temperatures of 60°C (140°F) can kill the organism.

Trichomonas

Pathogenesis. The flagellate *Trichomonas gallinae* causes disease in raptors, pigeons, canaries, finches, and budgerigars. Trichomoniasis in pigeons is commonly referred to as *canker.*

Clinical Signs. Caseous lesions are produced in the mouth as well as the esophagus and crop and also can involve the commissures of the beak and the sides of the face. These signs may be confused with other diseases. Anorexia and weight loss also are evident.

Diagnosis. The characteristic lesions associated with the host species are fairly diagnostic. Removing some of the caseous material and making a wet mount from a scraping of the raw tissue lesion under it confirms the diagnosis on microscopic examination. Motile, flagellated protozoa can be observed.

Treatment. All visible caseous material should be removed from the lesions. Local application of 5% Lugol's iodine daily, improved nutrition, and oral metronidazole at 10 mg/kg body weight daily for five days (up to 60 mg/kg) usually is successful. Antibiotics for secondary infection may be necessary. Vitamin-mineral supplementation should be part of the improved nutrition.

VIRAL DISEASES

Avian Pox

Pathogenesis. The various pox diseases of birds are caused by varieties of the genus *Avipoxvirus*, a member of the poxviridae. These viruses produce intracytoplasmic inclusion bodies in the epithelial layer of the skin. *Avipoxvirus* is very hardy and is resistant to drying, humidity, and light. It can remain viable in soil for up to 1½ years. Mosquitoes play an important part in transmission of the disease, as they penetrate the intact epithelium and allow entry of the virus. Susceptibility and transmission depend on the virulence of the strain of virus; but it generally spreads quickly, often with a high mortality in some species, such as canaries. Seventeen different types of poxvirus have been classified; most are host-specific, but some are not.

Clinical Signs. This infection manifests itself in different forms, the most common being the cutaneous form. Papular lesions appear mainly in the bare or unfeathered areas around the beak, nostrils, eyes, lower legs, and feet. It is unusual to find lesions in the feathered areas. The papules change color from yellow to dark brown and become crusty. If the bird survives, healing can occur after several weeks, often without scarring. Secondary bacterial or fungal infections can complicate the disease.

The wet or diphtheroid form of the disease starts out with papules similar to those of the cutaneous form, with the lesions appearing on the oral mucosa, larynx, and tongue. A fibrinous exudate is excreted and becomes caseous. Multiple small areas can enlarge to join and form large mucosal lesions that are difficult to remove without causing severe hemorrhage and tissue loss. These lesions make the bird very depressed, can interfere with swallowing, and can cause dyspnea and even death by blocking the larynx with exudate (Figure 7).

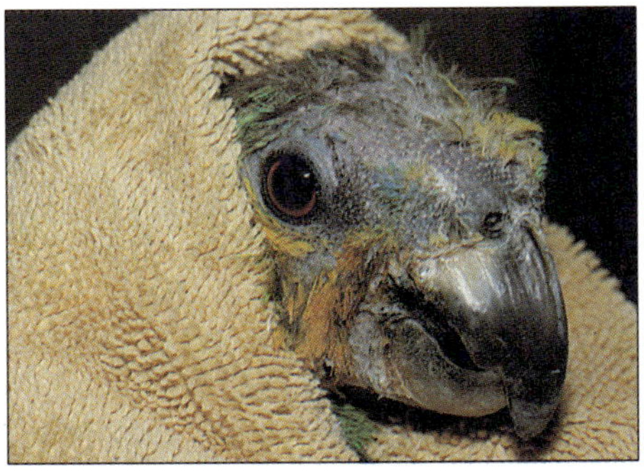

Figure 7—Amazon parrot recovering from parrot pox.

Both the cutaneous and diphtheroid forms of avian pox can appear in a given flock infection or even in one individual bird.

A septicemic form of the disease starts with fluffed plumage, listlessness, cyanosis, and inappetence. Affected birds usually die within a few hours to three days.

In psittacines, a diphtheroid enteritis and/or necrosis of the myocardium may be seen along with or without the other forms of the disease. Amazon parrots may show a serous nasal discharge (coryza), which later becomes mucoid or fibrinous. This usually is attributable to secondary bacterial or fungal infection. Occasionally, in severe cases, an acute conjunctivitis occurs.

Tumors of the skin, lungs, or respiratory tract may develop in survivors as a result of the oncogenic properties of the poxvirus.

Diagnosis. Confirmation of the diagnosis of pox infection in birds usually is done histologically. Clinical signs are a good indicator that the disease is present; but finding the typical Bollinger intracytoplasmic inclusion bodies in skin lesions, pharyngeal mucosa, and growing pin feathers is pathognomonic. The septicemic and coryzal forms usually are only diagnosed by culture on embryonated chicken eggs, where lesions appear on the chorioallantoic membrane that contains Bollinger bodies. Several passages may be necessary with some strains of virus.

Treatment. No specific treatment exists for avian pox, but risk can be minimized by controlling exposure to mosquitoes. Infected birds should be removed from the flock. Strict hygiene should be practiced and the premises kept clean and disinfected. Valuable birds can be given vitamin A at 2000 IU/kg body weight and vitamin C at 50 mg/kg body weight intramuscularly or per os. Antibiotics can be given for specific secondary bacterial infections. Clinicians should be careful with empirical use of antibiotics, as immunosuppression can be a side effect. Local use of chemical agents, such as mercurochrome or a mixture of tincture of iodine and glycerine, applied to the cutaneous or oral lesions may help. When using these products around the eye, care should be taken to keep them away from the eyeball. Antibiotic ointments can be used in the eye to help protect and lubricate it and keep the lids from adhering.

Vaccination with a pox vaccine in the face of an outbreak may have some beneficial effect in reducing the severity of the disease. A killed virus, psittacine poxvirus vaccine, is available in the United States and Canada. A canary poxvirus vaccine also is available. Preexposure use of these vaccines has great potential in controlling the disease.

Budgerigar Short Tail Disease

Pathogenesis. Believed to be of viral origin, this disease occurs in the lumbosacral and hip area, mainly in budgerigars. It is a gradually progressing disease and can involve other parts of the body. It appears initially in young immature birds and worsens as they mature.

Clinical Signs. The disease manifests itself as a folliculitis that causes the feathers to grow short, twisted, and deformed and several feathers to appear in one follicle that should only contain one feather. It usually is symmetric in pattern and varies from a few affected feathers to a large area of involvement. All birds in an infected aviary will not be affected, but the disease does seem to be infectious.

Peachface lovebirds have a disease that causes multiple feathers to grow in one follicle and is believed to be the same disease.

Diagnosis. Diagnosis can be suspected by the presence of typical signs and the failure to respond to all therapies.

Treatment. There is no known effective treatment. Control is by culling out all infected birds in a flock and practicing strict hygiene along with a disinfecting program.

Psittacine Beak and Feather Disease Syndrome

Pathogenesis. This disease is becoming a major economic factor in the pet bird industry in many parts of the world. One of the early names for this illness was *cockatoo beak and feather disease,* as it was first seen in cockatoos; but it has now been recognized in many other species, such as budgerigars, cockatiels, lorikeets, rosellas, hooded parrots, lovebirds, king parrots, Mallee ring-necks, and Port Lincoln parrots. It has been called by several other names as well, including *adrenal gland insufficiency.*

Australian researchers report that the disease frequently occurs in wild Australian psittacines. It has not been recognized in species other than psittacines; it may manifest differently in different species. Young birds of both sexes are more often affected, but all ages can be affected.

Clinical changes in the beak, nails, and feathers are caused by a combination of hyperplasia and dystrophy in the epidermis during the growing phase. Hyperkeratosis of the sheath of the feathers and outer layers of the beak and nails follows. Powder down feathers grow almost continually and thus are often the first feathers to be affected. The reduction or loss of this powder makes the beak appear black and glossy. These changes are the result of apparent epidermal cell necrosis.

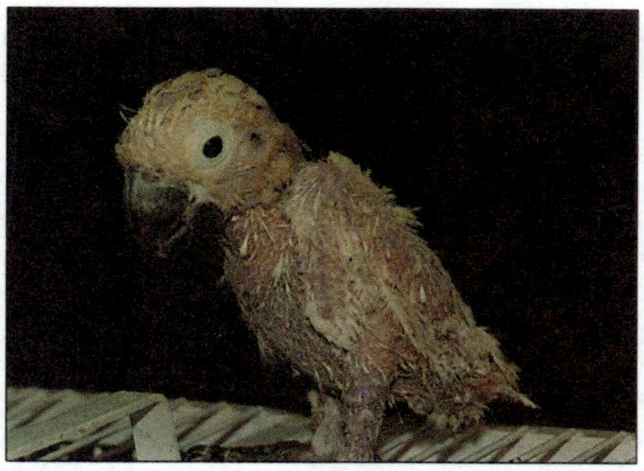

Figure 8—Cockatoo with beak deformed by psittacine beak and feather disease syndrome.

The virus has been isolated successfully and purified, and transmission to other birds has been perpetuated by oral and intracloacal routes. This virus is now classed as a *Diminuvirus*, which is a new species of microvirus, the smallest virus known to date. It is very infectious, causing clinical signs within seven days after injection into a susceptible host, and is shed by the fecal-oral route.

Clinical Signs. Beak involvement, feather changes only, or a combination of the two may be seen. Beak lesions can include progressive color changes from dull to glossy and growth pattern changes involving the appearance of fault lines, breakage, elongation, and other deformities. Large sections may break off. Secondary infections often invade the damaged beak and produce the so-called beak rot seen in some cases. Hemorrhage can occur in badly damaged beak areas. Necrosis of the palate and deformities of the toenails also can occur.

Feather changes are variable. The disease can occur as an overwhelming acute illness with symmetric loss of all growing feathers over a short period of time, followed by complete recovery, partial recovery, or death (Figure 8). It also can be a chronic progressive disease characterized by repeated loss and regrowth of feathers that are deformed and twisted, fail to mature, and are molted prematurely. Death can result from secondary infections. Green frothy diarrhea may be a clinical sign in some birds.

Initially, many of these cases are confused with feather picking (described under Miscellaneous Dermatoses). If the feathers of the head are involved in abnormal changes and/or the beak is affected, the psittacine beak and feather disease syndrome should be suspected.

Diagnosis. The proximal ends of affected feathers often show a characteristic nipple-like appearance when examined closely. A sampling of deformed growing feathers should be plucked, placed in formalin, and submitted to a laboratory for histopathologic examination. Skin biopsies are sometimes included. Some pathologists prefer to have at least one or more affected follicles along with the diseased feather. After preparing sections and staining with hematoxylin and eosin (H&E), intracytoplasmic inclusion bodies can be observed in macrophages and epidermal cells.

Treatment. No specific reliable treatment exists for this disease. Immunostimulants, such as autogenous bacterins, appear to help some birds while in others no change is noted. Antibiotic therapy and supportive care, such as vitamins, minerals, fluid therapy, improved nutrition, anabolic steroids, parasite control, improved hygiene and environment, and segregation of affected birds, should be carried out in an attempt at treating these cases. Many will die, some fairly quickly and some as long as two to four years later.

Contaminated cages and aviaries should be thoroughly scrubbed and disinfected. Nest boxes should be replaced regularly. Control measures include not breeding very young, very old, or pairs of birds that have produced affected young. A rest of one or two years in the breeding program also may help. Researchers are in the process of developing a vaccine that may help prevent this devastating disease.

Papovavirus

Pathogenesis. Papovavirus has been described as being responsible for various skin lesions in birds. It has been isolated in papillomas on the legs of European finches and in proliferative skin lesions on the head and eyelids of African grey parrots and has been identified as the causative agent for budgerigar fledgling disease, which is considered a generalized papovavirus infection. The virus may have oncogenic potential and may be a factor in the high incidence of tumors in budgerigars. Gerlach states that budgerigar fledgling disease seems to occur in other species as well, such as macaws, Amazon parrots, conures, pionus, African grey parrots, sulfur crested cockatoos, and eclectus parrots. Most of these species contract the disease as hand-fed babies, but some parent-raised birds do get it as well. The virus is highly infectious.

Clinical Signs. Adult budgerigars are known to be carriers. Incubation of the disease in baby birds from time of hatching is 10 to 21 days. Diseased baby birds show a lack of or malformation of down feathers, retarded growth of tail and body feathers, and a distended abdomen. Dehydration occurs from polyuria. The skin may be a reddish color. It is an acute disease, and secondary infections are common. Mortality can be quite high.

Diagnosis. On postmortem examination, hydropericardium, cardiomegaly, liver necrosis, and enlarged hyperemic kidneys are evident. Karyomegalic, clear or opaque inclusion bodies composed of virus particles are found in various tissues on histopathologic examination. Impression smears of the liver, spleen, and other organs can be examined for these inclusion bodies.

Treatment. There is no known specific treatment. Several control measures can be implemented, such as depopulation of infected flocks and restocking with disease-free birds, cessation of breeding for several months, and isolation of breeding flocks from cross-contamination. Strict hygiene, disinfection of the environment, and good nutrition are essential.

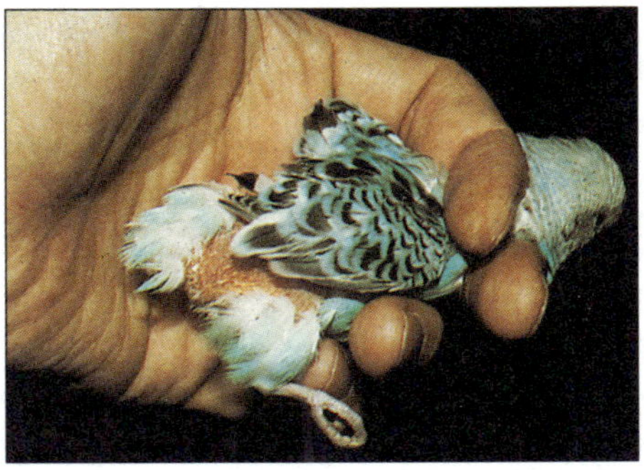

Figure 9—A young budgerigar with French molt.

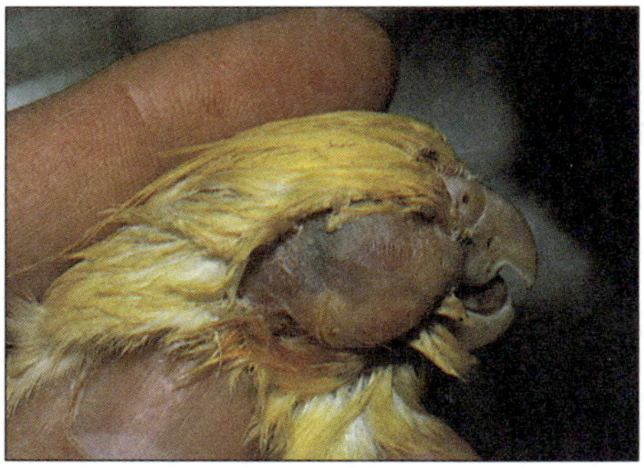

Figure 10—Cockatiel with a large abscess below the right eye.

French Molt

Pathogenesis. French molt is not conclusively documented to be viral in origin. Many other factors, such as parasites, nutrition, environment, and genetics, have been implicated. In Australia, French molt is believed to be caused by the psittacine beak and feather disease syndrome virus; and in North America and Japan, the papovavirus seems to be involved. The two viruses apparently produce a similar disease syndrome in the smaller species of psittacines.

Clinical Signs. In North America, French molt is a disease seen mainly in budgerigars, occasionally in lovebirds, and perhaps in some other small psittacines. It is a disease of baby birds and manifests itself primarily in the tail and long wing feathers (Figure 9). The feathers may break off at or beneath the skin surface or are molted prematurely. In the more severe form of the disease, the birds never do grow normal feathers but continue to molt their bent and twisted ones. In the milder form, the bird begins to grow normal-looking feathers after one or two molts. Birds with damaged wing feathers cannot fly and are often referred to as runners or creepers. The body feathers usually are not affected but can be in some birds.

Diagnosis. The condition can be suspected in young birds in which only the wing and tail feathers are affected.

Treatment. There is no effective treatment. Reproduction is not recommended for infected birds.

White Skin Wart Syndrome

Pathogenesis. The condition is also referred to as *herpesvirus warts* and is presumed to be caused by the herpes wart virus. This condition is seen primarily in cockatoos but also has been observed occasionally in Amazon parrots.

Clinical Signs. Usually one area of a single toe or sometimes two toes have a patch of whitish skin, generally near the distal end. This white area usually involves the ventral surface of the toe and may encircle it, involving 10% to 25% of the toe. The ventral skin layers often become overkeratinized to the point where it is necessary to grind them down.

Diagnosis. The condition can be suspected on the basis of the distinctive clinical signs.

Treatment. I suggest soaking this area with 5% Lugol's iodine solution daily as required. The warts appear to be self-limiting and eventually disappear, with no apparent aftereffects.

Warts can appear on the feet of other species of birds as well and rarely require removal by surgery.

MICROBIAL DISEASES

Abscesses

Pathogenesis. Abscesses can occur in various places on the body, but they are not a common problem in birds because of their high body temperature. Abscesses are accumulations of pus in pockets that are associated with infection or tissue irritation. Because birds lack lysozymes in their white blood cells (which liquefy mammalian pus), most avian pus is caseous in consistency and is impossible to aspirate with a needle.

Clinical Signs. Subcutaneous abscesses often are associated with feather loss over the involved area if in a feathered area of the body. They can be the result of blocked sebaceous glands, damaged feather follicles, feather cysts, foreign bodies, infected wounds, pressure, friction, and spread of infection from other areas. A common site for abscesses in canaries, budgerigars, cockatiels, and mynah birds is the periocular region (Figure 10). Lesions can be isolated above or below the eyelids, involve both lids, or be extensions of an acute sinus infection and involve a large area of the face below the eye. A frequent site of infection in large psittacines is the hard palate along the margins of the choana and the base of the tongue. The mucous glands in these areas are involved as a result of hypovitaminosis A.

Cockatiels sometimes get an accumulation of a hard mass of pus under the nictitating membrane in conjunction with a conjunctivitis as a result of local infection.

The uropygial gland is another frequent site for abscess formation in small birds. Canaries and finches sometimes get abscesses on the top of the head. The condition can develop in feather follicles as well.

Parrots, especially the African grey, and budgerigars are subject to abscess formation in the nares; the abscess often erodes the nasal opening and part of the cere to create a large pus-filled cavity (Figure 11). Abscesses may appear to be simply plugged, enlarged nares with some surrounding swelling. It is not until the huge mass of pus is removed that the full extent of the cavity is apparent. Response to treatment is good. A variety of organisms may be cultured from these lesions.

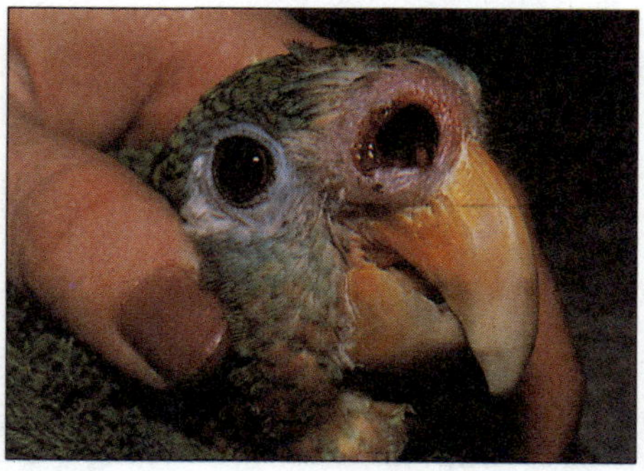

Figure 11—Yellow-billed Jamaican Amazon parrot with an erosive abscess of the right naris.

Chronic sinusitis with external abscessation may become very severe and involve both sides of the face with a joining passage inside the sinus cavity just above the cere in the frontal area. Serious curetting under general anesthesia may be required in such cases. Extensive chronic cases often require prolonged treatment to clear them up.

Diagnosis. The diagnosis of abscess is made clinically after finding a pocket or accumulation of pus.

Treatment. Treatment of abscesses should include nutritional and environmental improvement, elimination of contributory factors, lancing and curettage of the lesion, local application of 5% Lugol's iodine if possible, local application of antibacterial creams (e.g., chlorhexidine), and systemic antibiotics (Table I). Most abscesses respond rapidly to this sort of treatment. The use of bandages and possibly Elizabethan collars may be necessary.

Granulomatous Dermatitis

Pathogenesis. A nodular, granulomatous dermatitis that can be single or multiple is occasionally found on pet birds, mainly on the head. The pathogenesis of these lesions may involve avian tubercle bacilli (*Mycobacterium* spp.), fungi, or other granuloma-inducing agents.

Clinical Signs. The skin thickens as a result of the accumulation of large macrophages in the dermis and subcutis. Bacterial granulomas from overwhelming disease processes may appear as small scabs in the mouth of sick budgerigars. Bacterial granulomas on the cere, beak, or other skin areas may closely resemble malignant tumors.

Diagnosis. Histopathologic evaluation often is neces-

TABLE I
Drug Doses for Avian Patients

Generic Name	*Form*	*Route*	*Dosage*	*Comments*
Amikacin	Injectable (250 and 500 mg/ml)	IM	15–20 mg/kg bid–tid (0.015 mg/g)	Must be diluted (1:4) for birds; for gram-negative infections; less nephrotoxic than gentamicin
Chloramphenicol succinate	Injectable (100 mg/ml)	IM IV	80 mg/kg bid or tid 50 mg/kg tid or bid	Rapidly excreted
Chloramphenicol palmitate	Oral suspension (25, 30, 50 mg/ml)	PO	50 mg/kg qid (0.1 ml/g bid–qid)	Erratic absorption; palatable
Erythromycin	Oral suspension (40 mg/ml)	PO	45–90 mg/kg bid × 5–10 days	Good for sinusitis
Gentamicin	Injectable (50 mg/ml)	IM	10 mg/kg bid–tid	Dilute 1:4 with sterile water; can be nephrotoxic; do not use for more than 7 days; transient polyuria possible
Piperacillin	Injectable (50 mg/ml)	IM	100 mg/kg	Good general-purpose antibiotic
Tylosin	Injectable (50 mg/ml)	IM	10–40 mg/kg bid–tid	Nontoxic; good for respiratory disease

sary to confirm a diagnosis and to differentiate microbial granulomas from tumors. Acid-fast bacilli in large numbers can be found in macrophages in association with mycobacterial infections.

Treatment. Surgical excision of the lesions may be the best approach to therapy. The use of appropriate antibiotics may also be contemplated as an alternative to surgery (Table I).

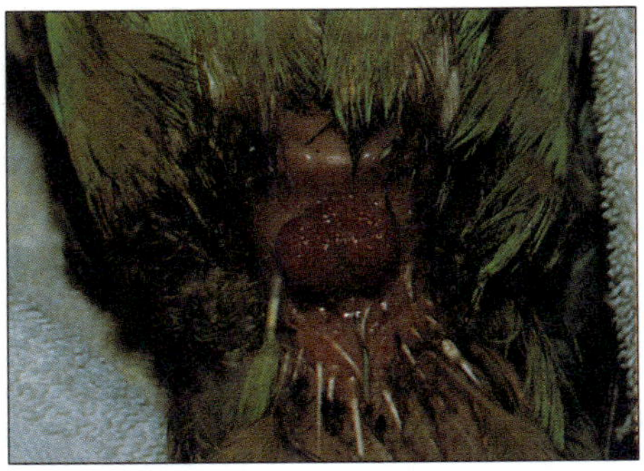

Figure 12—Cloacal papilloma.

Fungal Dermatitis

Pathogenesis. Fungal dermatitis is rare in pet birds and birds in general; yet more than 20 known species of dermatophyte fungi, including *Candida,* are capable of causing ringworm (also known as *favus, white comb, crete blanche*) by invading the keratinized layers of the skin and feathers. Birds with combs or wattles are more likely to be infected, especially in a wet, dirty environment.

Clinical Signs. Lesions are found mainly on the fleshy or thin-skinned areas of the head. Feather loss, scabs, and crusty areas appear. There may be extensive thickening of the epidermis producing crusty accumulations around the feather follicles. Neighboring feathered areas can become involved, resulting in extensive feather loss. The skin around the ears also may be involved. Fungal dermatitis may be secondary to other diseases in an immune-suppressed individual.

Diagnosis. A skin scraping using 10% to 20% potassium hydroxide solution may show the presence of septate hyphal fragments, which can confirm the diagnosis. Fungal cultures can identify the species involved.

Treatment. Cleaning up and improving the environment are important steps in the treatment and control of this disease. It is infectious to other birds and possibly to humans. Infected birds should be removed and separated from the others. Local antifungal products, such as chlorhexidine, iodine, formalin, tinactin, mycostatin, and carbolic acid, may help. Oral griseofulvin at 125 mg/kg body weight can also be given at the same time.

NEOPLASTIC DISEASES

Tumors of the Uropygial Gland

The uropygial gland (preen gland, oil gland) is situated dorsally at the base of the tail. It is not present in all species of birds and is not essential except in waterfowl, where it is needed to maintain feather condition and buoyancy. This gland is a common site for tumors, especially in the budgerigar and canary.

Enlargement of the gland and the appearance of a tissue mass in the area should draw attention to this problem. As the mass enlarges, the bird often chews at it, causing hemorrhage and secondary infection.

Close visualization can determine whether neoplasia is present, which must be differentiated from an abscess or blocked duct with simple enlargement. Histopathologic examination is necessary to identify the type of tumor tissue involved. The most common type of tumor found here is adenocarcinoma, followed by adenoma.

Surgical excision of the entire gland structure and tumor is essential to prevent recurrence. The use of an Elizabethan collar may be required as well during the healing period. Antibiotics and supportive care are usual accompaniments.

Papilloma

Papillomas, which are neoplasms originating from the nonglandular surface epithelium, occur most often on the skin of the feet, legs, neck, wing, eyelids, and uropygial area. The cause is unknown, although they may have a viral origin. Papillomas vary from finger-like projections to crusty, ulcerated masses and may bleed profusely when traumatized or excised. They can grow very large and usually are benign. Papillomas are subject to self-trauma and bleed easily.

The treatment of choice is complete surgical excision. Recurrence can be common. The use of an autogenous vaccine from some of the removed tissue has been suggested as an aid in preventing recurrence. The papovavirus group has been reported to cause papillomas in some parrot species.

Cloacal Papilloma

Cauliflower-like proliferation of tissue originating from the mucocutaneous junction of the vent, cloacal papillomas are most commonly observed in cockatoos, Amazon and hawk head parrots, and macaws but have been reported in many species. Because it protrudes from the vent, the cloacal papilloma is often misdiagnosed as a cloacal prolapse. Cloacal papillomas vary in size from a small piece of exposed tissue to large masses completely circumscribing the vent (Figure 12). They are benign, are believed to be of viral origin, and are very common in some geographic areas.

A high percentage of psittacines do not exhibit any clinical signs, but these cases may progress rapidly when the birds are subjected to various causes of stress. Subclinical cases can be diagnosed by close inspection of the vent by gently everting the cloaca with a cotton applicator.

Clinical cases may show straining to defecate, smelly droppings, pasting of the vent, decreased fertility, bloody feces, anemia, or persistent bacterial infections. Applying 5% acetic acid on the cloacal lining makes the papilloma lesions show up white. Preparation H® can help reduce the size of the cloacal lesion.

Improving the diet, reducing stress, and prescribing antibiotic therapy may help in some cases. Excision of involved tissue is the best therapy and can be done with cryosurgery or electrosurgery. Recurrence is common. Hemorrhage can be a problem unless care is taken. Some surgeons suture the defect closed. Care should be taken to prevent cloacal wall necrosis and strictures. Interrupted sutures are preferred rather than continuous sutures.

Controlling this disease by removing infected individuals in a breeding flock is important because of the infectivity of the disease and because breeding is impaired by it.

Inspection for cloacal papillomas should be a routine part of any complete physical examination of a potential breeding bird. The inside edge of the cloaca should be completely smooth all around, slightly moist, and pink.

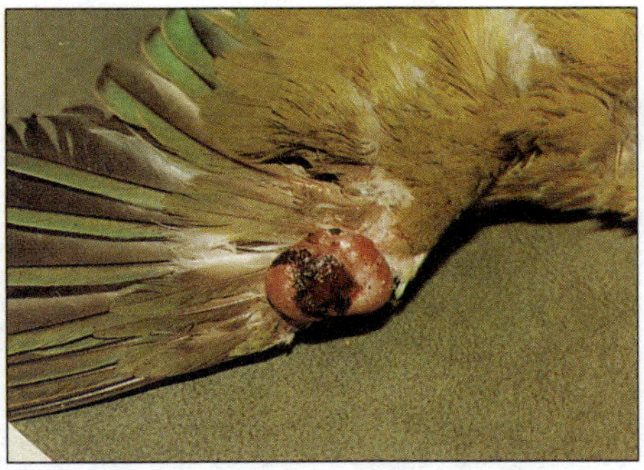

Figure 13—Fibrosarcoma on the wing of a lovebird.

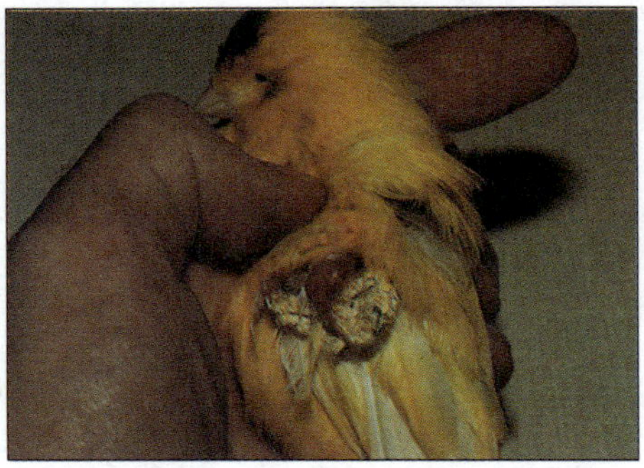

Figure 14—Large feather cysts on a canary's wing.

Fibroma and Fibrosarcoma

Fibrosarcoma is a malignant tumor of fibrous connective tissue, and fibroma is the benign form. Birds often get these tumors in the skin of the wings (Figure 13), legs, beak, and uropygial area. They usually are of firm consistency, are oval or round in shape, and may have a necrotic center. They tend to be locally invasive but rarely metastasize. A beak tumor also may invade the mouth. Budgerigars, males particularly, may get fibromas on the sternum. Surgical excision is the best therapy. Because some tumors involving areas of the beak and face make surgery impossible, euthanasia is recommended for these cases.

Lipoma and Liposarcoma

Lipomas and liposarcomas are neoplasms of adipose tissue; lipomas are benign tumors, and liposarcomas are the malignant form. Budgerigars of both sexes apparently are more prone to these tumors than other species; there may be a genetic predisposition. Lipomas are more common than liposarcomas, and both may be found anywhere there is subcutaneous fat tissue. The most common sites are the sternum, wings, abdomen, and rarely on the back, neck, and uropygial gland.

These tumors are more common on overweight birds; thus diet control and good nutrition are part of therapy. Lipomas typically are encapsulated and can be single or multiple, lobulated, subcutaneous masses. They should be differentiated from circumscribed lipogranulomas. Liposarcomas tend to be firm masses somewhat like fibrosarcomas and may be quite vascularized.

Surgical excision is the best therapeutic approach, and most of these tumors can be successfully removed.

Hemangioma and Hemangiosarcoma

Derived from vascular endothelium, these tumors are not commonly seen but are occasionally found as soft reddish to black subcutaneous swellings and often involve feather follicles. Hemangiosarcomas (the malignant form of the disease) can be locally invasive or metastatic. Treatment is by surgical excision.

Squamous Cell Carcinoma

Squamous cell carcinomas are found occasionally and occur mostly in the uropygial gland area and on the skin of the neck. Budgerigars appear to be the main host to these tumors.

Epidermal Cyst

An epidermal cyst occasionally may be found on a bird. These cysts are fluid-filled and collapse when punctured. I have seen epidermal cysts that contained a brownish fluid on the heads of canaries. An inclusion cyst in the area of the uropygial gland and a mucous cyst on the sternum, both in budgerigars, have been reported. Surgical removal is recommended.

Feather Cyst

Feather cysts are ingrown feathers that accumulate masses of necrotic feather material in the form of subcutaneous cysts that involve a feather follicle. They may occur as an isolated follicle that has been traumatized and healed before the new feather grew out or as generalized involvement of the feather tracts, as seen on canaries (Figure 14). The long wing feathers are common sites for these cysts to occur, where the follicles are easily damaged.

Certain strains of canaries appear to be genetically

susceptible to feather cyst formation. They may have an occasional cyst on the wings or the entire feather tracts of the body, dorsal and ventral, may be involved, producing extensive cyst formation.

Cysts show up as subcutaneous, whitish swellings over a feather follicle (often where a wing feather is missing). The swellings become progressively larger. The birds may pick at and even damage the cysts. Multiple cysts can occur in one small area. When a cyst is opened, it contains whitish, often caseous, necrotic debris; curled-up feather structures sometimes are observed inside. One cyst can involve several feather follicles.

If possible, with a wing feather, it is best to incise the end of the cyst, gently tease out the necrotic tissue, and leave the base of the feather attached so it can continue to grow from the incised end of the cyst to become a normal feather again. This may work in some cases; usually the whole mass, including the growing base, comes out in the mass of debris. If an opening is maintained in the end of the cyst, the new feather may grow from the opening. Risk of infection is high, and antibiotic ointment must be infused into the opening regularly. It may be necessary to remove the entire follicle surgically or destroy it with electrocautery in order to prevent frequent recurrence of the cyst.

In extensive feather tract involvement, it is pointless to try to remove all the cysts surgically. If the owners do not wish to keep a bird in this condition, euthanasia should be performed. If the owner is told that there is no cure and is willing to keep a heavily encysted bird, it may survive for a long time.

MISCELLANEOUS DERMATOSES

Disorders of the Feet and Legs

Leg Band Constriction

Leg band constriction is a common problem of small birds and occasionally is seen in large birds. Domestic-raised small birds usually have a closed band put on when they are a few days old. By the time these birds grow up, the bands may become a little snug. All birds exfoliate the outer layers of the skin on the legs, more so in some species than others. The skin layers build up under the band and gradually cause pressure between the band and the leg. This pressure triggers an inflammatory process that produces swelling. As the swollen tissue enlarges, more pressure develops under the band, circulation is impaired, infection develops, and all too frequently the leg dies from the band down. Dry gangrene results. The only treatment available at this point is amputation of the leg at the junction of healthy skin.

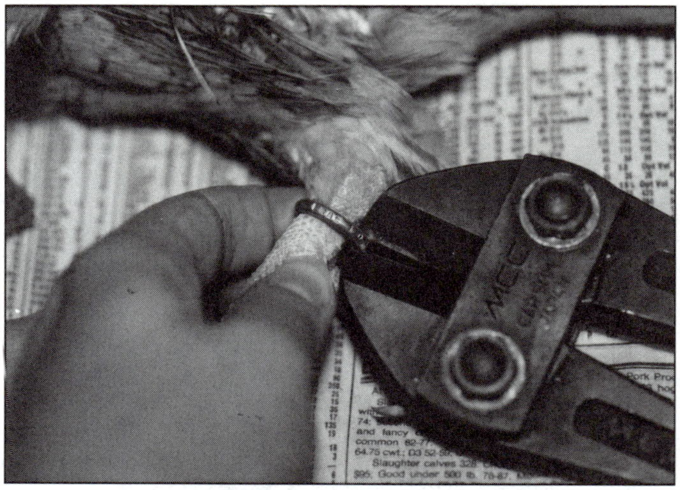

Figure 15—A safe way to remove heavy leg bands from large birds is with a bolt cutter.

If found early in the progression of the problem, careful removal of the leg band with local and systemic treatment of the leg lesion often restores the health of the leg. It is imperative that these leg bands be removed properly or the leg can be easily fractured at the site of the band. On small birds, it is best to cut the band with a side cutter that cuts close to the edge of the tool by placing it on the band so that it cuts out a piece of the band in one cut without further injuring the leg. The clinician should not try to get the tool under the band or the leg may get broken. Most small bird bands are made of aluminum or plastic and are easily cut. Large birds often have heavy stainless-steel bands that require the use of a heavy duty bolt cutter (Figure 15); these usually are split bands, so it is necessary to cut the band on the opposite side from the split.

Gout

Gout often is mistakenly diagnosed as abscesses of the foot. It is produced as a result of the body's failure to eliminate nitrogenous waste material from the blood via the kidneys. The result is the accumulation of urates, uric acid, and related substances in various parts of the body. This disease has been reported to be fairly common in southern Ontario, California, and Australia.

Birds suffer two different forms of the disease: visceral and articular gout. In cases of visceral gout, the urates are deposited in and around the major internal organs, particularly the kidneys. Articular gout takes a more obvious form. The urates are deposited in the joints of the limbs, particularly the feet and legs (Figure 16). The birds become painfully crippled. Lesions (tophi) show up as whitish nodular swellings along the bare area of the legs, ankles, and toes or more deeply involving the tissue around the joints. Affected birds exhibit acute lameness as the disease progresses. The joints become stiffened because of the mechanical encroachment of the deposits and tissue swelling. Polyuria may be evident.

If some of the whitish material is aseptically removed from a lesion and placed on a slide, the presence of uric acid crystals on microscopic examination can confirm the diagnosis. These crystals show up as thin, short, clusters of hair-like structures.

Attempts at surgically removing the deposits result in profuse hemorrhage, and no benefit is gained from this approach. Correcting the diet by reducing the protein level and increasing the vitamins, particularly vitamin A, and giving fruits and vegetables may help prolong the life of the patient. Antibiotics should be given to control secondary opportunistic infections.

Few birds respond to treatment because of permanent kidney damage, but some have been known to recover when their dietary deficiencies are corrected and treatment begins early in the disease. The use of allopurinol may have varying effects in arresting the progression of the disease. Crush one 100-mg tablet in 10 ml of water (10 mg/ml). Give one drop per os four times daily or 20 drops per ounce of drinking water. It will not cause resorption of the deposits but may assist in slowing the progression. The human drugs colchicine (an antigout drug) and probenecid (a drug used in venereal disease therapy) may provide additional options.

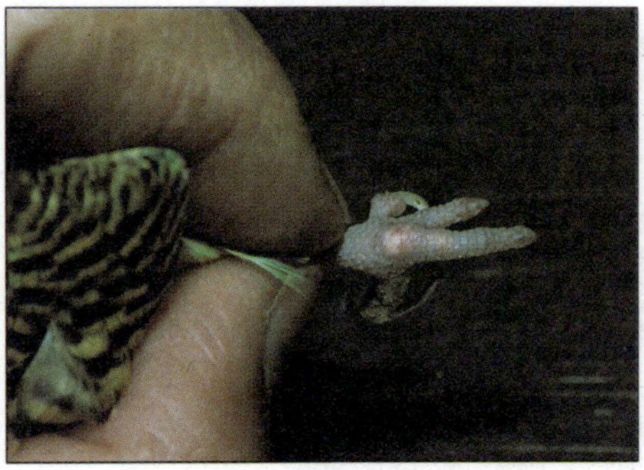

Figure 16—Uric acid deposits or tophi caused by gout on a budgerigar's foot.

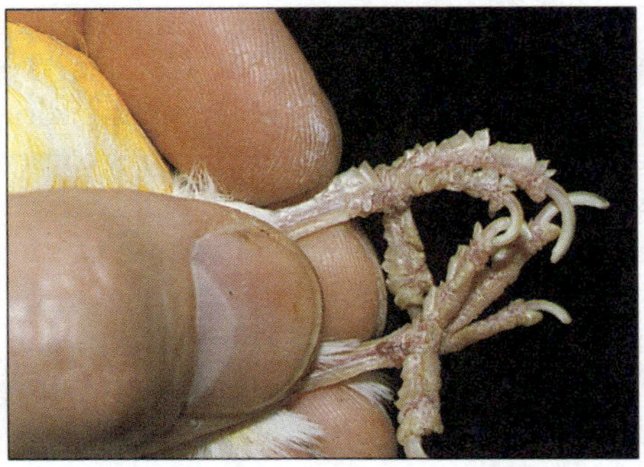

Figure 17—Hyperkeratosis of the feet on a canary.

Self-Mutilation

Birds of many species have been known to start chewing on their feet and legs for no apparent reason. They may constantly work at them until they peel off large areas of epithelium, resulting in open sores that do not heal. The toes are a favorite site for self-mutilation. The lesions may start from small wounds caused by trauma from something in the cage or may be the result of an overzealous neurotic feather picker. Stress of various sorts also can contribute to the problem.

Treatment involves correcting nutritional and environmental factors and breaking the chewing habit by applying an Elizabethan collar. The skin lesions can be treated with local chlorhexidine or antibiotic cream, protective bandages, and if necessary, systemic antibiotics. Once healing is complete, the collar can be removed. Medroxyprogesterone at 30 mg/kg given subcutaneously may help control these cases.

Nesting Fiber Constriction

A common finding in finches particularly as well as canaries and some other small birds is the presentation with one or often several swollen and sore toes. The end of the toe may even be gangrenous and dry. Under magnification, fine strands of plastic fiber can be seen in a circumscribed indentation in the skin of the toe, ankle, or foot. These strands originate from the synthetic fibers sold commercially as nesting material. Natural fibers used as nesting material are less likely to cause this problem than the synthetic fibers, although human hair is sometimes implicated. By carefully inserting a pointed scalpel blade under the fibers, they can be cut and removed. Once the fibers are removed, the damaged tissues heal quickly with topical treatment. The necrotic areas should be amputated and the foot bandaged for protection during healing. Systemic and local antibiotics usually are necessary.

Hyperkeratinization

This is a condition most commonly affecting canaries, finches, and mynah birds. It also has been observed in a few species of captive wild birds, such as starlings, crows, grackles, and evening grosbeaks. The condition results from excessive exfoliation of keratin on the skin surface and can result in scaling, swelling, irritation, cracking, and splitting (Figure 17). If a leg band is present, serious constriction of the band on the leg develops. In some species, the abnormal keratinization is noted on the ventral aspects of the toes.

It is recommended that this material be removed manually on a regular basis before it develops to an advanced state. The layers of dead skin (keratin) can be carefully removed by using a narrow, blunt-pointed instrument, such as the pointed end of a small pair of suture removal scissors. The daily application of chlorhexidine cream or moisturizing cream can help soften this material and control infection. It should be rubbed into the feet and legs well until it disappears and not left on in excessive amounts. Vitamin A has long been known for its normalizing effect on keratinization and may be indicated in some cases.

Trauma

Trauma can take many different forms, such as bites, fractures, burns, scalds, and frostbite; the feet and legs are commonly traumatized. These problems are treated according to the degree of injury, with some requiring only cleansing and the application of antiseptics and others requiring more intensive treatment.

Burns from heat sources should have cold water put on them immediately. The treatment of burns should include initial shock therapy if needed, parenteral fluids (1 ml/100 g body weight) if lesions are severe, topical vitamin A and E creams, aloe vera gel, antibiotics, and bandaging of areas that need protection and can be bandaged. Grease- or oil-based products should not be used. Treatment may be prolonged, as severe burns take considerable time to heal. Some patients may require tube feeding or force feeding; an Elizabethan collar may be required as well.

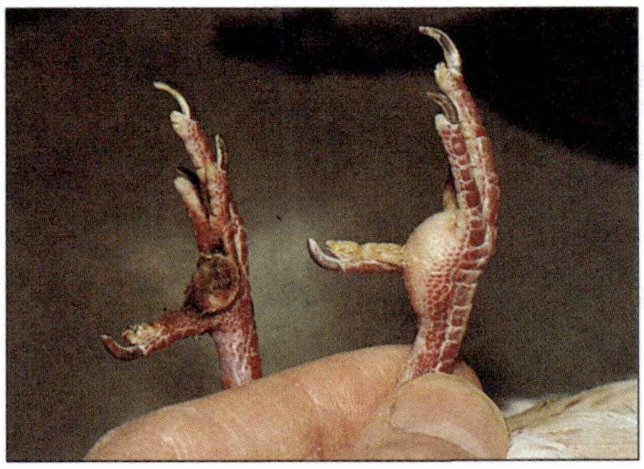

Figure 18—Pododermatitis in a ring-necked dove.

Chemical burns are treated similarly, except that acids must be neutralized with sodium bicarbonate solution and caustics with diluted white vinegar solution. Antihistamine and corticosteroid incorporated into a topical antibiotic cream initially may help reduce the shock and pain of the trauma. A moderately warm, humid environment is better than a hot dry environment.

Pododermatitis (Bumblefoot)

Pododermatitis is quite common in budgerigars, canaries, and cockatiels and is occasionally seen in other species. The problem occurs on the ventral surface of the foot and may progress from there to involve other areas (Figure 18). It starts as a thinning of the epithelial layer; inflammation and swelling develop and then scabs and ulcers appear, along with a severe lameness. Progression of the lesion to involve the tendons and joints, as occurs in raptors at times, is rarely seen in psittacines or passerines. Contributory factors are hypovitaminosis (particularly vitamin A), dirty cages and perches, sandpaper perch covers, rough corrugated perches or sometimes perches that are too smooth, stress, hypothyroidism, and obesity. A variety of shapes and thickness of perches are better for birds than perches that are all the same size. A variety of perches that are round, oval, flat, and square in cross section are healthier for the feet than all round ones of the same size. The use of natural tree branches also can be of benefit.

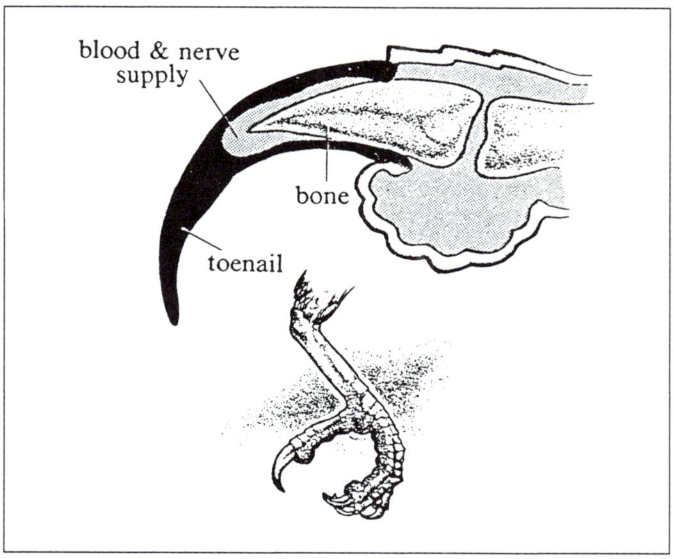

Figure 19—Cross section of a toenail. (From Axelson RD: *Caring for Your Pet Bird.* Toronto, Canaviax Publications, 1981. Reprinted with permission.)

It is necessary to debride these lesions and remove the necrotic tissue. Topical 5% Lugol's iodine and chlorhexidine cream followed by a protective bandage can assist in the healing of these areas. Bandages should be changed regularly during the healing period. The use of Vetrap® bandaging tape (3M Company) and systemic antibiotics administered parenterally initially, followed by oral dosing, usually results in recovery (Table I). Certain individuals appear to be highly susceptible to recurrences.

Padding of the perches with such materials as Moleskin tape (Dr. Scholl's Foot Products), which is available in any pharmacy foot products department, is quite helpful in protecting the bottom of the feet of affected birds.

Improvements in nutrition and environment are essential. Injections of B-complex and A, D_3, and E vitamins should be followed by continued use of oral supplementation of multivitamin–mineral–amino acid preparations.

Various organisms may be involved in these infections, such as *Staphylococcus* spp., *Streptococcus* spp., *Escherichia coli*, *Mycobacterium* spp., *Klebsiella* spp., *Pseudomonas* spp., *Proteus* spp., and *Candida albicans*. *Staphylococcus* spp. are the most common.

Nail Overgrowth

Nails that are allowed to overgrow (Figure 19) may curl into a spiral shape and get caught in cages and toys and can result in broken nails, toes, or legs. Injured and misshapen toes often produce long nails that grow out straight or at abnormal angles.

The use of sandpaper perch covers or sandpaper on the bottom of bird cages is not recommended. It does not help to wear the nails down; and it can cause abrasion and wear to the skin on the bottom of the feet, resulting in pressure sores and bumblefoot with secondary infection. A bird walking on sandpaper is comparable with a human walking on a gravel road in bare feet. It is better to put white, absorbent paper on the bottom of the cage, as the paper can show the state of the droppings better and absorb moisture, which keeps the feet cleaner.

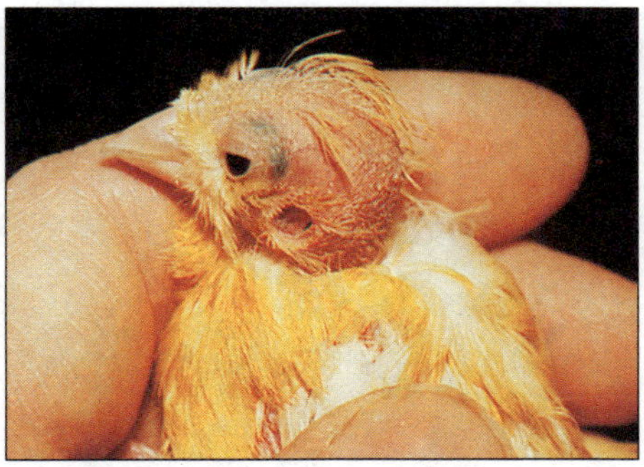

Figure 20—A bald canary.

Placing gravel or grit on the bottom of the cage also does nothing to wear the nails down. The only purpose for gravel is for the bird to eat. It acts as teeth and helps to grind the food in the gizzard. A few grains a week are normally eaten, mainly by the smaller species. It is doubtful that larger psittacines require grit, but they could be offered it at least quarterly.

One way to help larger birds wear their nails and sometimes their beaks down normally is to place a brick or coarse rock on or in the cage. In the process of walking on the brick, the nails are worn down. They often rub their beaks on it as well, which helps wear them down.

Feather Disorders

Cockatiel Feather Syndrome

This disease can be very frustrating to the avian veterinarian, the owner, and particularly the bird. It is peculiar to cockatiels and is commonly associated with giardiasis. A viral cause also has been proposed. The bird is presented as a chronic feather picker, often starting in the carpal-metacarpal area, the flank, and legs. The bird often picks intensely and cries as if the area hurts. On examination, the bird may have atrophy of the pectoral muscles, dry flaky skin, feather loss in different areas of the body, chewed feathers, and watery droppings that may be diarrheic. As the condition progresses, the bird begins to chew the skin and produce large, nonhealing ulcers, especially in the axillae and on the back. Some birds work on the wing tips. The lesions often bleed, and the sight of blood may alert the owner that there is a serious problem. Broken pin or blood feathers can be involved. Some of these birds may have secondary infections and may show anorexia and depression.

Diagnosis involves fecal assessment of fresh samples for *Giardia*, a complete blood count (CBC), fecal Gram's stain, and perhaps a fecal culture. Eosinophilia may be a fairly consistent finding. Serum lactate dehydrogenase (LDH) and serum aspartate aminotransferase (ASAT) levels often are elevated.

Treatment for *Giardia*, regardless of whether it was recovered, is usually the first therapeutic option. Nutrition should be evaluated closely. Supportive treatment (vitamins A, D_3, E, and B-complex and selenium) should be started with injections and maintained orally. Antihistamines may provide temporary relief. The use of corticosteroids should be discouraged, as many of these birds are already immunocompromised. Antibiotics should be given systemically or orally, as some birds do respond to this therapy.

A shifting leg lameness present in some birds seems to respond rapidly to injections of the above vitamins and selenium.

Skin lesions must be treated with topical nongreasy antibacterial agents, such as chlorhexidine cream. An Elizabethan collar usually is required to keep the bird from continuing to chew at the open lesions. Recurrence is common.

Baldness

Balding disease is prevalent in canaries and is sometimes seen in finches. The feather loss starts on the back of the neck and spreads up onto the head, sometimes involving the entire head (Figure 20). The skin may become thickened or scaly and wrinkled. If this condition spreads to the eyelids, it may pose a physical problem for the bird. In general, the health of the bird is not affected by the baldness, as it is a localized problem. Maintaining body temperature might be a factor, but the feather loss usually is not severe enough for this. Owners tend to become alarmed when feather loss occurs.

The cause may be fungal or bacterial infections of the skin; thyroid deficiencies; or in male canaries, hormonal imbalances. It has not been proven that thyroid deficiencies are a contributory factor, but it is suspected and some birds do respond to treatment with thyroid replacement. It is believed that hereditary factors could be involved in some cases. In some birds, baldness is the result of an arrested molt. Birds that are "stuck-in-molt" lose the feathers on the head and neck but do not grow replacements. The usual cause of this phenomenon is stress. Perhaps the hen has been forced into egg-laying through too rich a diet, or babies have been stressed from training before they finished their primary molt. Sudden weather changes may be enough stress to interrupt a bird's molt cycle. Poor nutrition and irregular photoperiods may predispose to this problem.

Some species, such as lutino cockatiels and cockatoos, have a genetic baldness on the top of the head under the crest. Another cause of baldness is over-aggressive birds that pick the feathers off the heads of their mates.

Birds that are "stuck-in-molt" often regrow their lost

feathers during the next normal molt cycle if their stress is reduced and nutrition improved. Treatment for the baldness in canaries and finches should include improved nutrition, vitamin-mineral supplements, hormone replacements (such as testosterone), thyroid replacement, and reduced stress.

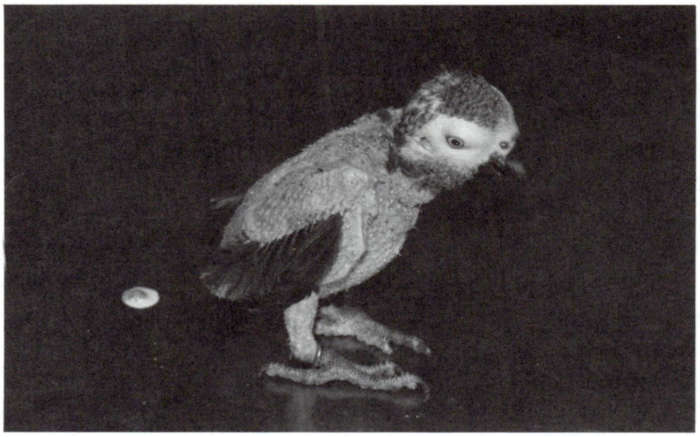

Figure 21—A badly feather-picked bird.

Many cases do not respond to any treatment. These birds remain bald permanently; their feather follicles apparently cannot generate new feathers.

Feather Hemorrhage

Newly growing feathers have a thick, dark-colored base filled with blood and nerve supply. Those growing in on the tail and wings may be very large. These feathers are called *pin feathers* or *blood feathers.* At this stage in their development, they are very susceptible to injury. As these feathers grow out, they are covered by a protective sheath that is preened off by the bird before the feather fans out into its normal shape. Occasionally a bird may overzealously preen the sheath off too close to the distal growth area and cause some hemorrhage. These bleeders can be controlled with local clotting powders, such as styptic powder.

Pin feathers often get traumatized down in the thick vascular area and bleed profusely. This hemorrhage is more difficult to control, and it is better to pluck these feathers out by pulling the feather straight out in the line of growth. The feathers should not be bent or twisted. Moderate pressure and the use of clotting powder in the follicle area soon stop the bleeding. It is better to grasp the feather near the skin when removing it to prevent it from breaking. Pliers may be needed for extra large feathers. Regrowth usually starts immediately after removal and takes about six weeks to complete.

Stress Lines on Feathers

Stress marks can appear on feathers that are in the growth stage in a bird that undergoes severe stress, usually from some disease. They appear as lines or bands of incomplete feather development across the feather from side to side. These lines appear in the same places on all the feathers that were growing in at the same time and remain until those feathers are molted. Stress marks may weaken the feather somewhat and may be the site of feather breakage but usually cause no problems. Variation in the nutritional supply to the feathers caused by the stress of the disease is a contributory factor.

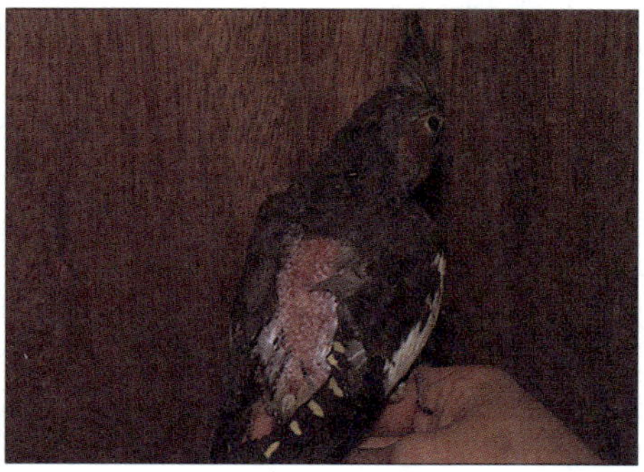

Figure 22—A self-mutilated cockatiel.

Feather Picking

Feather chewing or plucking is a common problem in pet birds (Figure 21), especially the psittacines, and can be very frustrating for both the owner and the attending avian veterinarian. It also has been observed in captive native North American wild birds.

Feather picking is most commonly seen in African grey parrots, cockatoos, and cockatiels; but it has been seen in most psittacines and occasionally in other species as well (Figure 22). There are many contributory factors involved, many of which are environmental and behavioral irregularities. Some of the most common factors include nutritional inadequacies, boredom, emotional frustration, stress, insecurity, parasitism, infections (viral, bacterial, or fungal), and low humidity.

When wild birds are upset or frightened, they fly away to escape. Caged birds cannot do this. Some are more nervous than others and like to have a place to hide. A privacy box, which is built like a nest box except it has a perch inside plus an open bottom, or an open paperbag in the cage can give the bird a place to hide and get away from some of its stresses. Covering the cage at night gives darkness if the owner has a light on while the bird is trying to sleep and does provide some privacy.

Birds should be kept in a cage big enough to provide ample room for exercise. The bird that only eats and sleeps in its cage and is out all day can get along with a smaller cage than one that is kept caged all the time. Rectangular cages that are longer than they are high or wide are far superior to the tall, narrow, or round cages because most birds are not able to fly straight up and down like a helicopter.

Birds require 9 to 12 hours of sleep each night, preferably in darkness. Insufficient sleep can make a bird irritable, stresses it, and can cause it to start picking. Birds should be put in a dark room or have the cage covered at a reasonable hour at night. They awaken at dawn. Bird bedtime habits should be routine.

Abnormal increases or decreases in the various hormones can cause feather loss or trigger feather picking. This is most often seen as canary balding disease and hypothyroidism. Canary baldness can be caused by other factors as well.

Sexual frustration or a desire to breed and nest may induce a bird to feather pick. These birds should be sexed (surgically or otherwise) and paired with an appropriate mate in a breeding cage with nest box. Seasonal or intermittent picking can sometimes be controlled with injections of medroxyprogesterone or testosterone. Some birds that are paired already may only feather pick during their breeding cycle and may use their feathers to line their nest.

Self-mutilation can be a progression of feather picking. Self-mutilation also can result from bacterial or fungal dermatitis, folliculitis, lacerations, ingrown feathers, *Giardia* infection, irregular photoperiods, allergic reactions, malnutrition, insect bites or stings, internal abscesses, tumors, arthritis, stress, puncturing foreign bodies, external parasites, thyroid problems, or such foreign objects as fibers wrapped around parts of the body.

Discomfort in an internal organ from infection, neoplasia, or other causes may induce a bird to chew the skin and/or feathers over that area; but this is an uncommon situation.

Treatment must include a method to break the self-chewing cycle, and an Elizabethan collar usually solves this problem. Local and systemic therapy must be combined with an attempt to find the original cause and correct it as well. Suturing may be required. The administration of medroxyprogesterone at 30 mg/kg subcutaneously may help control this problem in some birds; one of the side effects of this product, however, is obesity.

Preening Complications

Part of a bird's personal grooming procedure is to remove the feather sheaths that grow out around each feather. They also rearrange the feathers, lining up the hooklets and flanges on the barbules to assist the feathers in keeping their normal shape and appearance and to help keep them clean. This grooming procedure is called *preening* and usually is done with the beak.

Anatomic or physical disabilities, such as spinal injuries, fractures, malformation of the beak, long-term use of Elizabethan collars, or disinterest from illness, may interfere in a bird's ability to preen the feather sheaths off growing feathers or to accomplish other preening procedures. Birds often have difficulty in reaching their head and neck and prefer to rely on a cage mate or owner to preen these areas. The bird may end up looking like a porcupine, with quills sticking out of various parts of its body and tattered and unkempt feathers. The owner needs to remove these coverings by rubbing them between the fingers or allowing another bird to do it. Young birds learn how to preen from their parents.

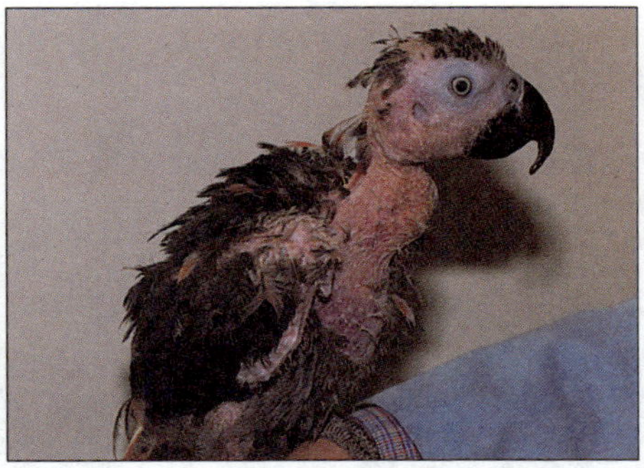

Figure 23—An African grey parrot that had a low thyroxine (T_4) level and responded to thyroid therapy.

Canary Dysplastic Feather Syndrome

Canary dysplastic feather syndrome is also referred to as *straw feather disease,* as the feathers somewhat resemble the appearance of straw. The disease affects all or most of the feathers of baby birds symmetrically in their first molt. The feathers often retain their sheaths and are very narrow as a result of improper development of the barbs and barbules. Dorsally the feathers appear glossy, and ventrally they appear dull. These birds cannot fly and may not survive long because they have trouble maintaining body heat. Genetic factors are suspected as the cause, and no treatment is known.

Hypothyroidism

History and Clinical Signs. One of the clinical signs of suspected thyroxine deficiency in some birds (mainly budgerigars and occasionally cockatiels) is an elongation of the down feathers. This phenomenon generally starts bilaterally on the lateral body under the wing (Figure 23); as it progresses, other parts of the body become involved. The down feathers grow longer than the regular feathers; and in an advanced case, the bird may have fluffy down feathers sticking out all over its body (Figure 24). Other clinical signs may develop later, such as nonpruritic feather loss, cardiac problems, and predisposition to bacterial and fungal diseases. Lethargy, depression, and sensitivity to cold may develop. Many of these birds become obese, which can occur before any feather changes. Hypothyroidism can occur in conjunction with thyroid hypertrophy (goiter) caused by iodine deficiency and insufficient thyroxine production.

Diagnosis. It is recommended that the confirmation of thyroxine deficiency be verified by using the thyroid-stimulating hormone (TSH) stimulation test rather than the measurement of a low thyroxine (T_4) level. The suggested protocol involves collection of baseline T_4 values followed by giving ¼ to 1 IU of TSH intramuscularly (depending on the size of the bird) and collecting a second sample six hours later to measure the T_4 level again. Samples should be submitted to reliable avian laboratories. Serum cholesterol levels may be high.

Treatment. Empirical doses of thyroid replacement often produce dramatic improvement. L-thyroxine added to the water is quite effective. (I use a stock mixture of one 50-mg tablet in ½ ounce of water and give eight to ten drops per ounce of fresh drinking water daily.)

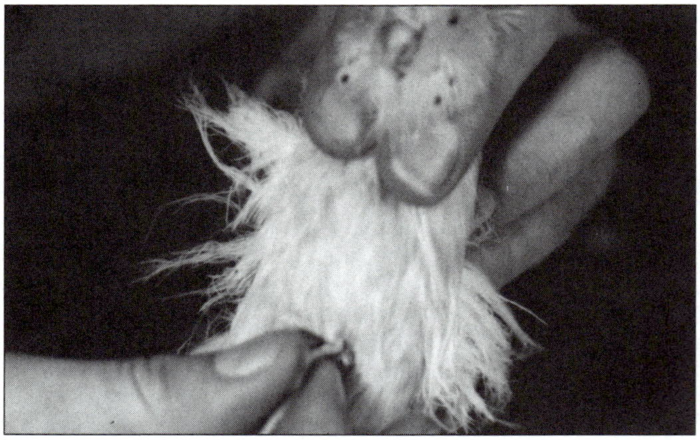

Figure 24—Budgerigar showing the long down feather syndrome that responds to thyroid supplementation.

The long down feathers should be plucked at the beginning of therapy, as these can be a guide to monitoring the dose of L-thyroxine supplementation. If they start to grow in long again, this indicates that the dose needs to be increased. Thyroxine replacement should continue for the duration of the bird's life. Iodine in the form of one drop of 5% Lugol's iodine should be put in the drinking water daily or every other day as well.

If the bird is obese, the diet should be improved and the volume of food reduced. A vitamin–mineral–amino acid supplement is added to fresh water daily or sprinkled on moist fruit and greens. It is necessary to weigh the bird initially and at least monthly until the desired weight is reached. The volume of seed can then be adjusted so that this weight level is maintained. It usually is necessary to keep the bird on this controlled diet and thyroid replacement continuously with regular rechecks every four to five months.

As long as the overgrowth of the long down feathers and any other disease-related clinical signs are controlled, the dose of thyroid supplementation is maintained. Clinical signs of thyroid overdose range from hyperactivity and nervousness to diarrhea and vomiting. Untreated birds often progress to death over a fairly long period of time.

Trauma

Breast or ventral chest sores are skin lesions found on the ventral chest over the sternal bone. They are actually decubital ulcers or pressure sores caused by a bird lying on its chest too much. After prolonged sternal recumbency the skin gets pressed between the sternum and the surface of whatever the bird is lying on. The constant pressure causes tissue necrosis, and an ulcer develops. These sores are seen in birds that are chronically ill and weak and in birds recovering from fractures or leg problems that cannot stand properly. Breast sores also can occur from a bad fall or flying into a wall, and the concussion from the fall or trauma splits the skin open in this area.

If not discovered early, the bird may self-traumatize the lesion with its beak and make it worse or prevent it from healing. Treatment involves a general anesthetic, debridement of the lesion, freshening the wound edges, disinfecting the area, and suturing the skin closed. It may be necessary to put an Elizabethan collar on until the skin heals. Antibiotic therapy can help control secondary infection.

Birds can fall prey to other household pets, such as dogs, cats, ferrets, and other birds, and receive skin lacerations varying in severity from minor scratches to extensive skin tears and punctures, even involving fractures.

Air movement fans that have no protective screen, especially ceiling fans, can do a great deal of damage to birds. They also can fly into walls, windows, and furniture and receive injuries. Birds that fly freely may swoop too high and scalp themselves on a rough textured ceiling. I have even seen birds that flew out a building door and were hit by a car as they crossed the street.

The traumatized area should be cleansed and the lesions sutured if needed. Local application of an antibacterial powder containing chlorhexidine or an antibiotic can help keep the area dry and control infection. Oral or systemic antibiotics along with multivitamin supplementation should help the injury to heal. General anesthesia may or may not be required.

Lipogranuloma

Budgerigars very commonly get lipogranulomas, which often are associated with obesity. In obese birds, the fat is deposited primarily over the pectoral and abdominal areas. Fatty degeneration sometimes occurs in these fat pads, precipitating the formation of a small nodular granuloma that rapidly enlarges. Fat necrosis also can occur in the center of the mass. These granulomas are often confused with lipomas. It is best to remove them surgically and to control food consumption of the bird strictly. Improved nutrition with proper control of volume consumed can bring the bird's weight down. Xanthomas may occasionally develop over a large distended obese chest or abdomen of a bird.

Xanthoma and Xanthomatosis

Pathogenesis. Xanthomas are relatively common in cockatiels, are seen less frequently in budgerigars, and may be seen occasionally in other species. The usual site of involvement in cockatiels is the tips of the wings. In humans and other animals, xanthomas represent alterations in lipid metabolism; and although they are sometimes categorized as tumors, they should be considered metabolic disorders.

Clinical Signs. In the cockatiel, a thickening of the skin develops in the form of a lobular mass on the distal end of one or both wings. It gradually progresses down the wing toward the body (Figure 25). The lesion is yellowish-tan and gets thicker as it grows. It may surround the wing in its progression. As wing joints become involved and the mass gets heavier, the wing may droop and flight may be impaired. These masses can occur on other parts of the body as well. The bird may traumatize the mass as it enlarges, and bleeding does occur. Xanthomas may occur as discrete tumor masses or as diffuse thickening of the skin as described. Xanthomas often occur over protruding parts of the body, such as abdominal hernias, tumor masses, or obese fat pads.

Diagnosis. Xanthomas and xanthomatosis have a typical unmistakable appearance and can be confirmed by histopathologic examination.

Treatment. It is impossible to remove xanthomatosis and leave the wing intact. Usually by the time the owner notices it, the condition has progressed to the point that amputation of at least part of the wing is necessary. If the entire tumor is removed in the amputation, recovery is usually complete unless it starts in the opposite wing as well. Many birds have continued as useful pets with one or both wing tips removed.

If amputation is not done, the mass encroaches on the entire wing and severely inhibits the use of it. If the condition occurs as a discrete mass and not as the diffuse type, excision of the mass alone with some of the immediate surrounding tissue is possible.

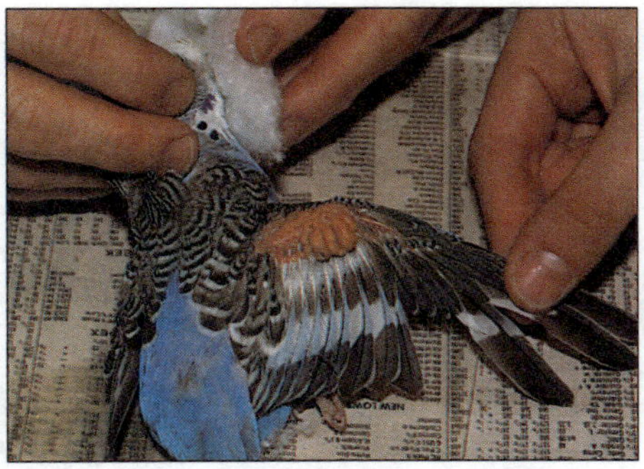

Figure 25—Xanthomatosis on a budgerigar's wing.

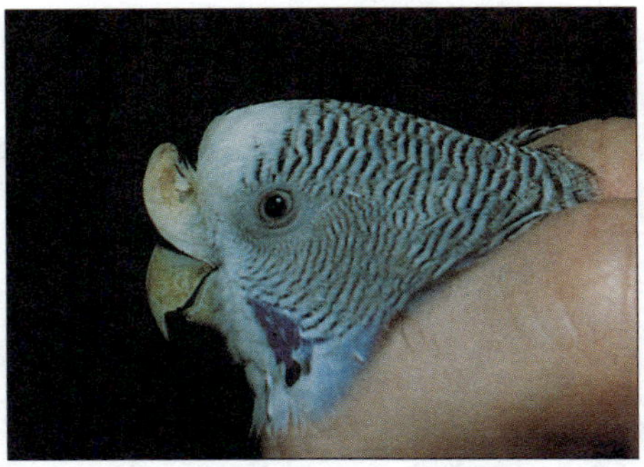

Figure 26—Brown hypertrophy of the cere.

Blocked Uropygial Gland

Occasionally the uropygial gland (commonly called the oil gland), which is located on the dorsal base of the tail, becomes blocked and distended from the buildup of glandular secretion. This is most commonly seen in canaries, finches, and budgerigars. The gland may become quite large and cause discomfort to the bird, which may pick at the area, sometimes traumatizing the gland or the surrounding skin. The bird frequently plucks feathers from around the gland area and the base of the tail.

Very often the problem can be corrected by placing gentle pressure with the fingernails on the gland, forcing the contents out through the gland opening, which is a little protruding papilla. If the gland cannot be emptied in this manner, it may require lancing or even surgical removal. All species of birds do not have uropygial glands; they are absent in Amazon parrots and hyacinth macaws.

Local treatment of irritated skin should be done by applying soothing nongreasy antiseptic creams.

Disorders of the Beak and Cere

Brown Hypertrophy of the Cere

The cere is the soft raised skin area surrounding some birds' nostrils. It is quite prominent in certain species, such as budgerigars, hawks, and falcons, and absent in other species, such as canaries and finches.

Brown hypertrophy or hyperplasia of the cere is seen mostly in budgerigars, most frequently in females, and is more common as they get older. The color of the cere may turn a medium or dark brown, or it may build up excessive layers of keratin that can proliferate into a horn-like protuberance over the cere (Figure 26). Sometimes the nostrils are blocked. Except for the blockage of the nares and the appearance of the buildup, there is little discomfort to the bird.

The buildup of dead skin layers can be gently removed by scraping or peeling it off the cere. Occasionally, overly aggressive removal may produce some hemorrhage that can be quickly controlled with clotting powder. Local application of chlorhexidine or moisturizing cream can soften the tissue and make removal easier if it adheres tightly. The buildup of cere tissue can recur. Regular removal of these layers is part of the maintenance program done on birds in my practice. The exact cause is unknown, but it may be associated with hormonal changes.

Demineralization of the Beak

Certain species, such as doves and pigeons, normally have a fairly soft beak. Demineralization of the beak to the point of being very soft, pliable, and rubbery can be the aftermath of pronounced malnutrition causing a severe nutritional secondary hyperparathyroidism, which produces this syndrome in the beak. Insufficient calcium, vitamin D_3, and methionine contribute to beak demineralization. In addition, birds in this state often have a rubbery, twisted sternum and the ribs may be deformed, which is seen most frequently in cockatiels, doves, and pigeons.

Correcting the diet and supplementing calcium, vitamins, and other minerals may save some of these birds. A badly twisted upper beak can be difficult to correct and may require some form of supportive splint to hold it straight while the beak firms up with remineralization. The ribs and sternum of some of these birds have so much deformity because of lack of rigidity that respiration is severely impaired and death may follow.

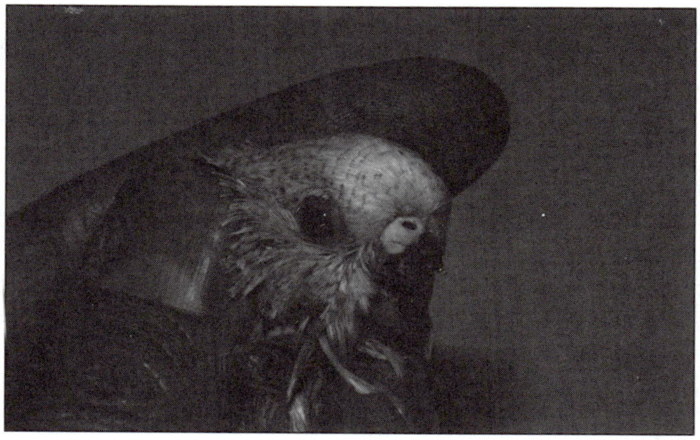

Figure 27—Budgerigar with upper beak chewed off to the cere by an Amazon parrot.

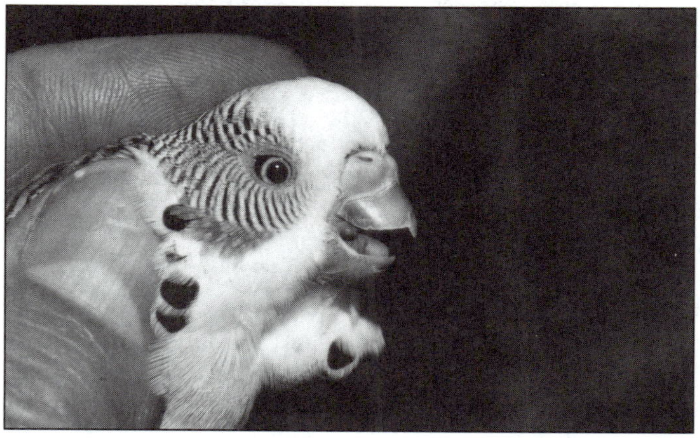

Figure 28—Same budgerigar as in Figure 27 with beak almost completely grown back.

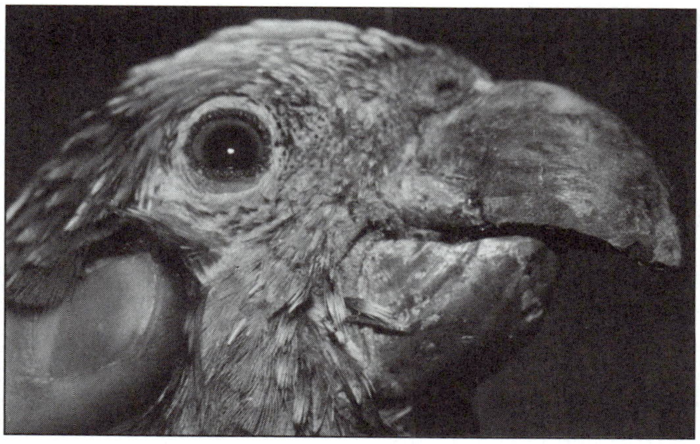

Figure 29—Acrylic prosthesis on an Amazon parrot with a severely damaged beak.

Beak Trauma

Beaks can be traumatized in a variety of ways. Birds can get their beaks caught in metal clips, rings, and wires in a cage; be bitten by animals or other birds; or get caught in doors or other objects, as well as a multitude of other accidents that can happen.

Large birds can chew the beak of a smaller bird right off. Beakless birds cannot eat very well and usually have to be tube-fed until new beak tissue grows back, if in fact it does. I treated two budgerigars with this trauma, and their beaks did regrow (Figures 27 and 28). The beaks were chewed off, upper bill only, right back to the nostrils. The birds were tube-fed for many weeks. Gradually, the upper beak regenerated to be about three quarters of the original length; but the birds eventually were able to eat on their own.

Treatment of beak trauma can be relatively simple or quite complex. It may only require a little trimming or grinding plus some clotting powder, or a beak prosthesis may have to be made. Some beak defects can be repaired with five-minute epoxy. Split beaks can be drilled and wired together with stainless-steel wire, which holds the pieces together as the beak grows out. Most glues and epoxies do not adhere to beak tissue very long because the outer layers continually exfoliate and detach the adhesive.

Beak prostheses can be made from dental acrylics. A strengthening powder is mixed with the acrylic liquid; and while it is pliable, it can be molded into the desired shape or molded to fit contours of the damaged beak. As the acrylic hardens, heat is produced and once it has hardened, it can be ground and polished. Coloring agents can be added in the early stage of preparation to match the tissue being repaired. The prosthesis can be attached to the beak stump with stainless-steel wire, Steinmann pins, K-wires, and epoxies or skin glue. As the damaged beak grows out, the prosthesis often comes off and has to be redone to fit again. The material can be molded around preset anchor pins or wires and then hardened quickly with a coating of quick-setting solution.

Acrylic resins that were originally developed for dentists can be very useful as adhesives and prosthesis material in birds (Figure 29). Ethyl acrylic becomes very hard and is suitable for beak repair. Dental methacrylate can be used with exothermic catalytic polymerization. Super Glue is a methylacrylic resin but contains ingredients that are toxic to tissue.

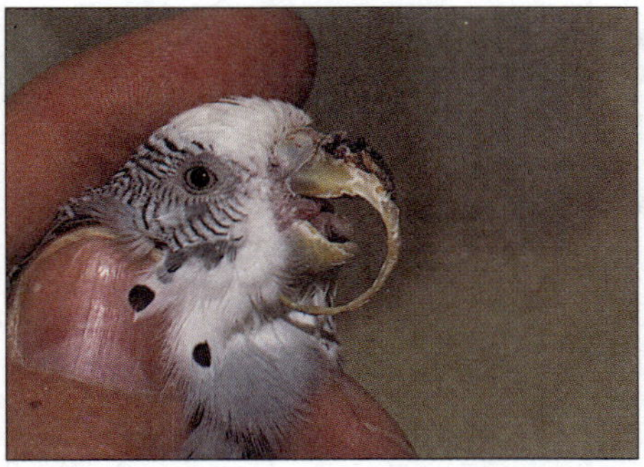

Figure 30—An overgrown beak resulting from a tumor on the dorsal surface near the cere of a budgerigar.

Damage to the growth area at the base of the beak usually results in a permanently deformed beak. A fracture of the lower jaw that splits the lower beak may never heal so that the beak is a solid unit. The split may always remain in the beak even though the bone of the jaw heals.

Even if the damaged beak cannot be repaired completely, many birds learn to eat and adapt to a severe beak deformity.

Beak Overgrowth

Beaks often overgrow as a result of injury to the growth area or other trauma (Figure 30). Prolonged irritation from the *Knemidokoptes* mite can produce some bizarre beak shapes that need continual regular trimming or grinding (Figure 31). Even normal undamaged beaks and nails need regular maintenance care if they are not being worn down naturally. Overgrown upper beaks can grow long enough to impair eating and on occasion grow into the neck in a long curve if neglected.

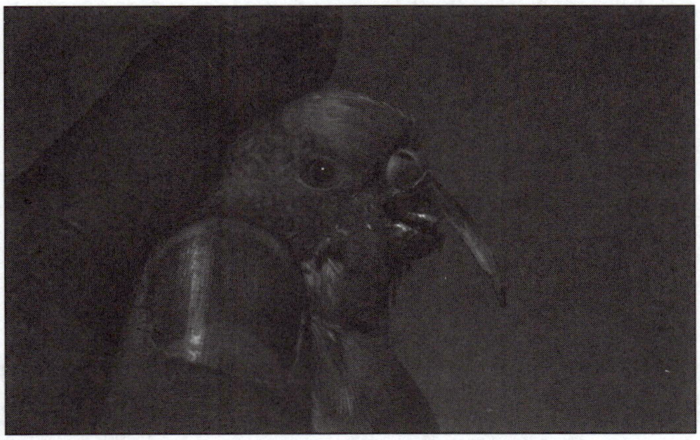

Figure 31—Budgerigar with beak deformed by *Knemidokoptes* mites.

Beak tissues grow continuously; and when they are trimmed, care must be taken not to cut them back too close or the inner quick area, which is the area containing the blood and nerve supply, will be exposed. When cut too short, these areas bleed profusely and are painful.

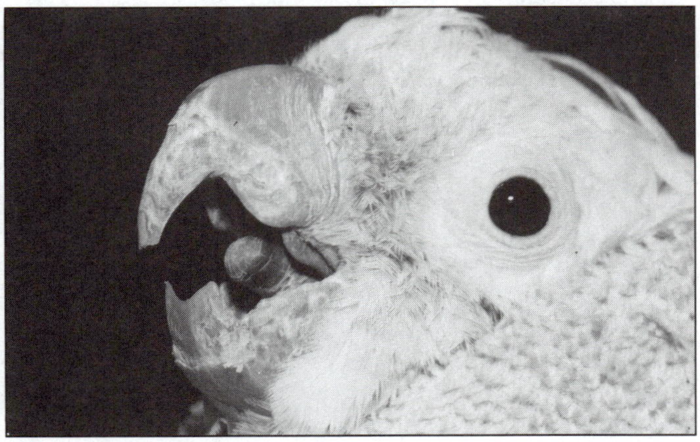

Figure 32—A Goffin cockatoo with excessive beak flakiness resulting from malnutrition.

It is better to grind the beak and nails with a portable hand grinder using a small rotary grinding wheel about ½ inch in diameter. Flexible shaft grinders are available from jewelry supply outlets and hand-held grinders from hobby shops or hardware stores. The beak can be shaped easily and quickly with these tools. If an area starts to bleed, it can be easily stopped by holding the grinder lightly on the bleeding spot for a few seconds, creating enough heat to cauterize the bleeder quickly.

Most psittacine birds produce flaking or crumbly buildup of beak tissue in the normal growth of the beak; in some birds this can leave unsightly platforms or steps of beak layers. This buildup should be ground off the beaks of larger birds and scraped off the beaks of smaller ones as a part of their regular maintenance program, which helps to maintain a healthier beak and better cosmetic appearance of the bird. Some birds require this more frequently than others, but it should be done two to four times a year. A bird with a beak that is too soft and excessively flaky needs mineral and vitamin supplements (especially calcium) plus dietary improvement (Figure 32).

A condition seen mostly in budgerigars and cockatiels causes the central part of the upper beak, including the point, to become longitudinally porous and crumbly. It may start as dark areas on the beak tissue and usually results in a change in the angle of growth from the normal curve to a larger curve and sometimes a gradual straightening of the beak. Because the lower beak can no longer help to wear it down, the upper part continues to grow and becomes very long unless a regular clipping or grinding program is maintained. Liver disease, vitamin deficiency, internal neoplasia, psittacine beak and feather disease syndrome, and even clotting abnormalities have been proposed; but the true cause is unknown. Once this problem starts, there is no way to reverse it and return to normal tissue. The clinician should improve the general health of the bird with nutrition, test for liver disease, and continue to groom the beak regularly.

About the Author

Dr. Axelson has been in private practice since 1960; he currently practices at the Links Road Animal and Bird Clinic in North York, Ontario, Canada. He is past president of the Association of Avian Veterinarians and lectures extensively on various avian topics throughout North America.

BIBLIOGRAPHY

Altman RB: Conditions involving the integumentary system, in Petrak ML (ed): *Diseases of Cage and Aviary Birds*, ed 2. Philadelphia, Lea & Febiger, 1982, pp 368–381.

Arnall L: Conditions of the beak and claw in the budgerigar. *J Small Anim Pract* 6:135–144, 1965.

Arnall L, Keymer IF: *Bird Diseases.* London, Bailliere Tindall, 1975.

Axelson RD: *Caring for Your Pet Bird*, rev ed. New York, Sterling, 1989, p 160.

Axelson RD: Possible chlorhexidine toxicity in finches. *Assoc Avian Vet Today* 1(5):208, 1987.

Campbell TW: Neoplasia, in Harrison GJ, Harrison LR (eds): *Clinical Avian Medicine and Surgery.* Philadelphia, WB Saunders Co, 1987, pp 500–505.

Choudary C: Neoplasms, cysts, and obstructive diseases, in Burr EW (ed): *Companion Bird Medicine.* Ames, IA, Iowa State University Press, 1987, pp 231–233.

Clubb SL: Therapeutics in avian medicine—Flock vs. individual bird treatment regimens. *Vet Clin North Am Small Anim Pract* 14:345–361, 1984.

Clubb SL: Therapeutics, in Harrison GJ, Harrison LR (eds): *Clinical Avian Medicine and Surgery.* Philadelphia, WB Saunders Co, 1988, p 340.

Fudge A, McEntee L: A feather syndrome in cockatiels associated with giardiasis. Unpublished data, Sacramento, CA (private practice), 1986.

Fudge AM: Avian giardiasis: Syndromes, diagnosis, and therapy, in *Proceedings of the Association of Avian Veterinarians' Conference, 1986.* E. Northport, NY, Association of Avian Veterinarians, 1986, pp 155–164.

Epple A, Stetson MH (eds): *Avian Endocrinology.* New York, Academic Press, 1980.

Gerlach H: Viral diseases, in Harrison GJ, Harrison LR (eds): *Clinical Avian Medicine and Surgery.* Philadelphia, WB Saunders Co, 1986, pp 172–173.

Gough JF: Outbreaks of budgerigar fledgling disease in three aviaries in Ontario. *Can Vet J* 30:672–674, 1989.

Gould J: Liver disease in psittacines, in *Proceedings of the Association of Avian Veterinarians' Conference, 1989.* E. Northport, NY, Association of Avian Veterinarians, 1989, pp 125–128.

Harrison GJ: Disorders of the integument, in Harrison GJ, Harrison LR (eds): *Clinical Avian Medicine and Surgery.* Philadelphia, WB Saunders Co, 1987, pp 509–524.

Hillyer EV: Basic avian dermatology, in *Proceedings of the Association of Avian Veterinarians' Conference, 1989.* E. Northport, NY, Association of Avian Veterinarians, 1989, pp 101–121.

Martin SL: Skin and feather diseases of pet birds, in Nesbitt GH (ed): *Contemporary Issues in Small Animal Practice. Dermatology*, vol 8. New York, Churchill Livingstone, 1987, pp 295–321.

McCluggage DM: Parasitology in caged birds, in *Proceedings of the Association of Avian Veterinarians' Conference, 1989.* E. Northport, NY, Association of Avian Veterinarians, 1989, pp 97–100.

McDonald SE: Clinical experiences with cloacal papillomas, in *Proceedings of the Association of Avian Veterinarians' Conference, 1988.* E. Northport, NY, Association of Avian Veterinarians, 1989, pp 27–30.

Paster MB, Isaacs M: Repair of damaged beaks in cherry-headed conures using cyanoveneer acrylic. *Bird World Magazine.* March 1983, pp 52–53, 55.

Perry R: Avian dermatology, in Burr EW (ed): *Companion Bird Medicine.* Ames, IA, Iowa State University Press, 1987 pp 40–50.

Perry R: Skin, beak, claw and feather disorders, in Macwhirter P (ed): *Everybird, A Guide to Bird Health.* Melbourne/Sydney, Australia, Inkata Press, 1987, pp 98–121.

Rosskopf WJ, et al: Normal thyroid values for common pet birds. *VM SAC* 77:409–412, 1982.

Rosskopf WJ, et al: Treatment of feather folliculitis in a lovebird. *Mod Vet Pract* 64:923–924, 1983.

Stunkard JA: *Diagnosis, Treatment and Husbandry of Pet Birds*, ed 2. Edgewater, MD, Stunkard Publishing Co, 1984.

Taylor TG: French molt, in Petrak ML (ed): *Diseases of Cage and Aviary Birds*, ed 2. Philadelphia, Lea & Febiger, 1982, pp 361–367.

VanDerHeyden N: Psittacine papillomas, in *Proceedings of the Association of Avian Veterinarians' Conference, 1988.* E. Northport, NY, Association of Avian Veterinarians, 1988, pp 23–25.

Avian Mites

Babson College
Babson Park, Massachusetts
James R. Philips, PhD

KEY FACTS

- **Avian mites can infest feathers, quills, skin, subcutaneous tissue, and the respiratory tract.**
- **Avian mites feed on blood, tissue fluid, skin and feather lipids and debris, keratin, fungi, algae, and other mites.**
- **Most mite infestations are not pathologic; however, mange, hyperplasia, secondary infections, anemia, respiratory distress, and death can occur.**
- **Treatment involves internal or external use of acaricides; treatment of the cage is also often necessary.**

Birds are hosts to a diverse microcommunity of mites. Most adult mites are 0.3 to 1.5 millimeters in length. Mite eggs develop into larvae with three pairs of legs, undergo two or three nymphal stages, and then develop into adults with four pairs of legs. Under optimum conditions, this life cycle can be completed in as few as five days. Habitats of avian mites include the feathers, quills, skin and subcutaneous tissue, and respiratory tract. Available food sources include blood, tissue fluid, skin and feather lipids and debris, keratin, fungi, algae, and other mites.[1] Krantz has written the most comprehensive general overview of mite biology and taxonomy; the work includes keys to families.[2] The classification scheme used in the book is used for most of this article; however, the Hypoderidae family mentioned by Krantz is now known as Hypoderatidae and the Ascouracaridae family is a newer taxon—it was a subfamily of Syringobiidae at the time of Krantz's writing. Most of the figures contained in this article are of parasitic mites of raptors, on which my research has concentrated, but the discussion focuses on mites of cage birds and poultry. The taxa and treatments discussed are summarized in Table I.

FEATHER MITES

Feather mites (Figure 1A) live between the barbs on the ventral surface of contour, wing, and tail feathers (Figures 1B). Feather mites feed on feather fragments and lipids, scaly skin debris, fungal spores, and algae. Nymphs often move to the plumulaceous barbs near the calamus to molt, and shed skins may accumulate there (Figure 1C). Masses of mites on a feather can look like many grains of sand. When wing and tail feathers are fanned out against background light, mites may appear as tiny dark spots.

Large populations are sometimes deleterious to the health of the bird, and populations can explode if birds are too sick to beat their wings.[3] Budgerigars can be infested with two species of feather mites: *Protolichus lunula*, which is found on wing and tail feathers, and *Dubininia melopsittaci*, which is found on smaller body feathers.[4] When overcrowded, mites move from feathers to the skin (Figure 1D). The irritation causes feather pulling, and skin lesions result. Mites of the genus *Proctophyllodes* congregate harmlessly under the primaries and secondaries of passerines; this genus of mite includes *P. pinnatus*, which is found on the canary.[5]

In chickens, masses of *Pterolichus obtusus* turn flight and tail feathers gray and cause reduced vigor of the bird. The genus *Megninia* is also found on chickens, turkeys, and other galliform birds. In addition to being present on feathers and skin, *Megninia* has been found in quills, under the skin, and in

Originally published in Volume 15, Number 5, May 1993

TABLE I
Mite–Host Relationships and Treatment

Habitat	*Mite*	*Host*	*Treatment*
Feathers	*Proctophyllodes pinnatus*	*Serinus canaria*	Acaricidal dusts and sprays
	Megninia species	*Gallus gallus, Meleagris gallopavo*	
	Pterolichus obtusus	*Gallus gallus*	
	Protolichus lunula	*Melopsittacus undulatus*	
	Dubininia melopsittaci	*Melopsittacus undulatus*	
	Chiasmalges species	*Aratinga* species	
	Diplaegidia columbae	*Columba livia*	
	Falculifer rostratus	*Columba livia*	
Quills	*Dermoglyphus elongatus*	*Serinus canaria, Gallus gallus*	None known
	Syringophilus bipectinatus	*Gallus gallus*	
	Peristerophila columba	*Gallus gallus*	
	Ascogastra species	Psittacidae	
	Cytoidosoma species	Psittacidae	
	Petersonsascus species	Psittacidae	
	Fainocoptinae	Columbiformes, Galliformes, Psittaciformes	
Skin	*Knemidocoptes jamaicensis*	*Serinus canaria*	Ivermectin and levamisole
	Microlichus avus	*Serinus* species	
	Passeroptes species	*Serinus canaria,* Columbidae	
	Harpypalpus serini	*Serinus mozambicus*	
	Bakericheyla chanayi	Fringillidae	
	Epidermoptes bilobatus	*Gallus gallus*	
	Knemidocoptes mutans	*Gallus gallus*	
	Neocnemidocoptes gallinae	*Gallus gallus*	
	Rivoltasia species	Phasianidae	
	Harpyrhynchus species	Psittacidae	
	Knemidocoptes pilae	*Melopsittacus undulatus,* other Psittacidae	
	Neocheyletiella species	Psittacidae, *Leiothrix lutea*	
	Ornithocheyletia species	Psittacidae, *Columba livia, Leiothrix lutea*	
	Procnemidocoptes species	Psittacidae	
	Psittophagoides species	Psittacidae	
	Promyialges species	Passeriformes	
	Harpyrhynchus columbae	*Columba livia*	
	Picicnemidocoptes laevis	*Columba livia*	
	Trombiculidae	Many orders	Acaricidal spray plus antibiotics, antihistamines, and corticosteroids
	Dermanyssus gallinae	Many orders	Carbaryl, deltamethrin, bendiocarb, tetrachlorvinphos, or permethrin
	Ornithonyssus sylviarum	Many orders	Bendiocarb, monocrotophos, cythioate, or famphur
	Ornithonyssus bursa	Many orders	
Subcutaneous areas	Hypoderatidae	Columbiformes, Psittaciformes	Ivermectin
	Laminosioptes cysticola	Columbiformes, Passeriformes, Psittaciformes	
Respiratory tract	*Sternostoma tracheacolum*	*Serinus canaria, Erythrura gouldiae, Melopsittacus undulatus,* and many others	Dimethyl carbinol, dichlorvos, malathion, ivermectin, trichlorfon, carbaryl, or sulfaquinoxaline
	Cytodites species	Columbiformes, Galliformes, Psittaciformes	
	Ereynetidae	Many orders	
	Turbinoptidae	Many orders	

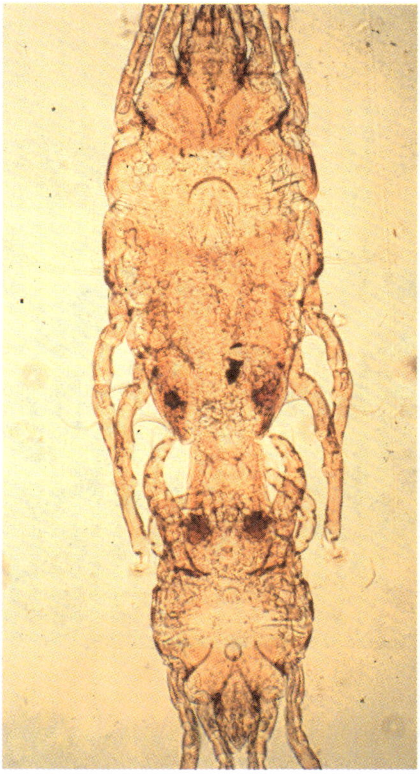

Figure 1A

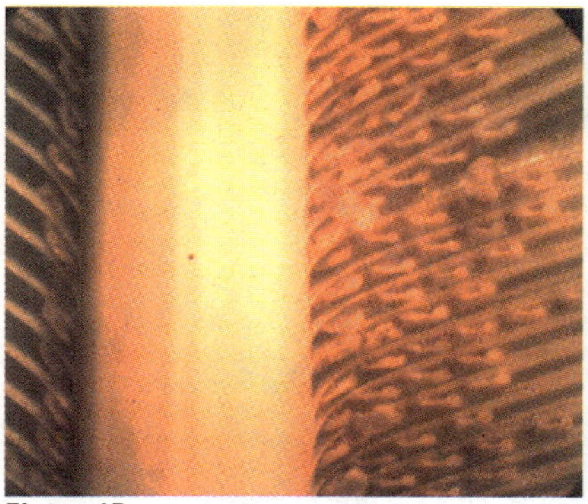

Figure 1B

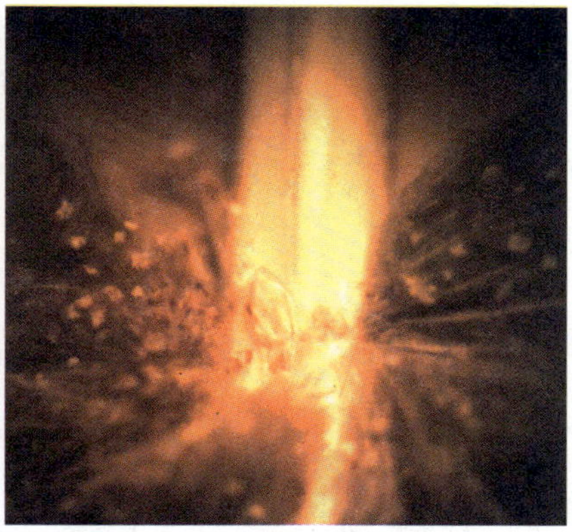

Figure 1C

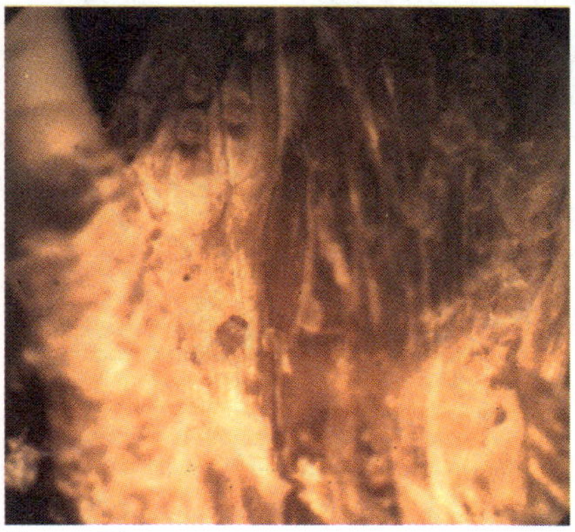

Figure 1D

Figure 1—Feather mites. (**A**) *Pseudalloptinus aquilinus* (Pterolichidae family) from a bald eagle. (**B**) Many *Kramerella* species (Kramerellidae family) occupying the spaces between the barbs near the rachis on an alula feather of a great horned owl. (**C**) Nymphs and molted skins on the plumulaceous barbs on an alula feather of a great horned owl. (**D**) Adult *Kramerella* species on the skin at the base of an upper primary covert of a great horned owl (×160).

the respiratory tract. Infestation with this genus of mite causes severe scratching, a 10% decrease in egg laying in chickens,[6] and some feather loss in turkeys.

Chiasmalges lives on the exposed quill surface of rectrices and the tail coverts of Mexican conures. Nymphs damage feathers by cutting into the dorsal rachis and tunneling through the medulla to the quill.[7] Conures host more than 15 species of feather and quill mites, and at least seven genera of such mites are found on African parrots.[8]

Domesticated pigeons can support many *Diplaegidia columbae* and *Pterophagus strictus* on body feathers without ill effects. *Falculifer rostratus*, a wing feather mite of domesticated pigeons and doves, can damage the feathers.[9,10]

In total, there are more than 25 families, 400 genera, and 1400 described species of feather mites. Acaricidal dusts and sprays are effective against feather mites.

QUILL MITES

Quill mites live and reproduce inside quills. Most of these mites probably feed on available secretions and quill materials; however, mites of the Syringophilidae family have long, needlelike chelicerae with which the quill wall is pierced and tissue fluid is obtained from the feather follicle. Infested quills can be detected by the yellowish accumulation of mites; empty mite exuviae from molts; and mite excreta, which fill the quill and change its appearance from transparent to opaque (Figure 2A). Adult female syringophilid mites (Figure 2B) leave mature feathers during the molting process by means of the superior umbilicus or through nearby channels that they have created and enter developing quills through the superior umbilicus.[11]

Dermoglyphidae[12] (Figures 2C and 2D), Syringophilidae,[13] and Ascouracaridae[14] are the most important quill mite families. *Dermoglyphus elongatus* lives in the quills of canaries and chickens. In canaries infested with these mites, feather loss results from excessive digging with the beak to alleviate irritation. When a large number of syringophilid mites is present, feathers may epilate easily and secondary bacterial infections occur. *Syringophilus bipectinatus* has been associated with feather loss and breakage in chickens, and *Peristerophila columba* causes similar problems in pigeons. Three genera of the Ascouracaridae family, *Ascogastra*, *Cytoidosoma*, and *Petersonascus*, are found on parrots; *Cytoidosoma* damages feathers by destroying the medulla from the quill to the rachis.[7]

Quill wall mites (Laminosioptidae and Fainocoptinae) parasitize developing feathers (usually primaries) of columbiform, galliform, psittaciform, and other birds. These mites feed on the outer, unkeratinized

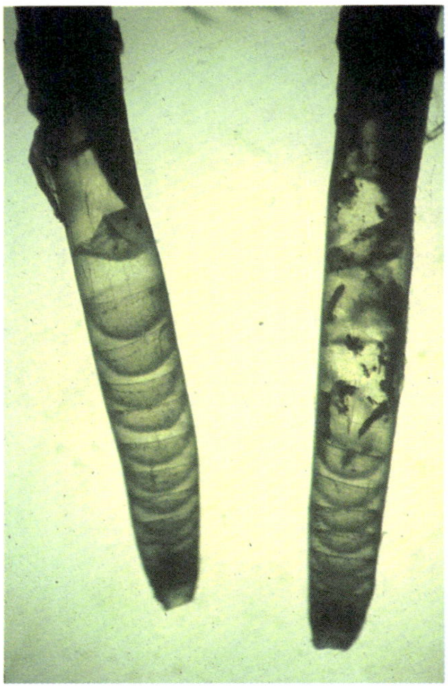

Figure 2A

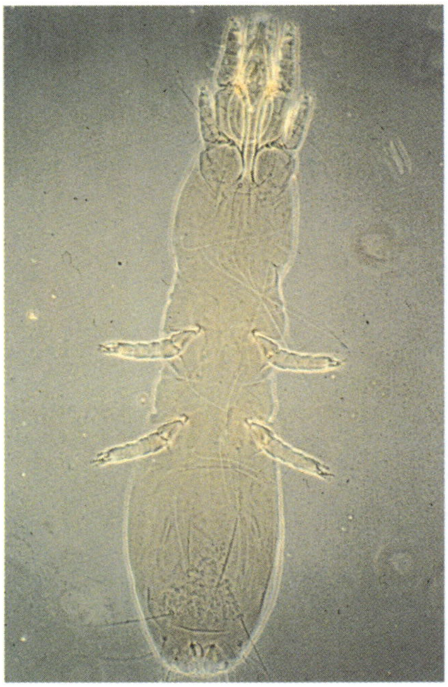

Figure 2B

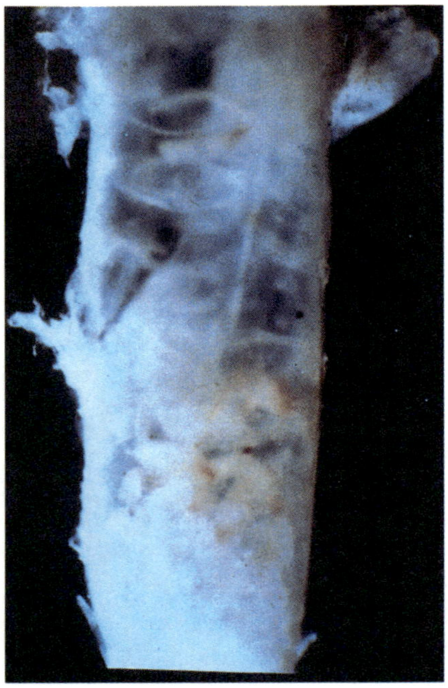

Figure 2C

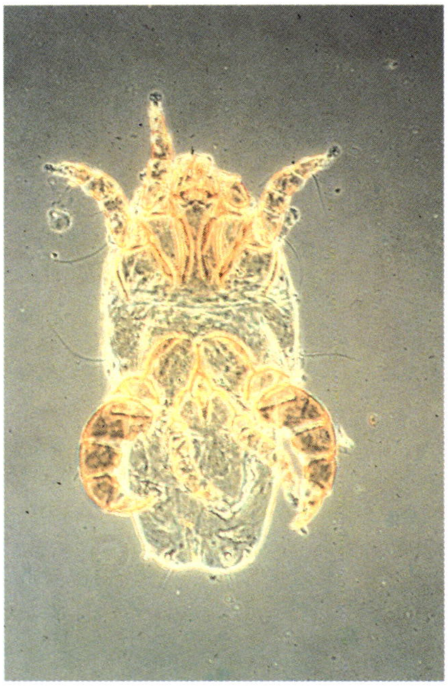

Figure 2D

Figure 2—Quill mites. (**A**) Uninfested (*left*) and syringophilid-colonized (*right*) quills of a great horned owl. Several elongate mites and mite excreta can be seen. The quill will become opaque when the mites fill it completely. (**B**) Female of an undescribed genus of syringophilid mites from bald eagles (×160). (**C**) *Paralges* (Dermoglyphidae family, undescribed species) in an upper lesser covert quill of a great horned owl. (**D**) Male *Paralges* (undescribed species) from a boreal owl (×160).

layers of the feather germ, thereby triggering hyperkeratosis of the feather sheath. Attachment of the feather sheath to the quill wall traps and kills some mites, but others remain inactive in the epidermis to wait for the next feather molt or to seek developing feathers.[15] Although no satisfactory treatment for quill mites has been described, ivermectin has yet to be tested.

SKIN MITES

Sources of food for skin mites include surface skin debris, keratin, tissue fluid, blood (which is obtained by piercing the skin), or other mites. Burrowing mites include the Epidermoptidae, Knemidocoptidae, Harpyrhynchidae, Cheyletiellidae, and Trombiculidae (chiggers) families. Surface-feeders include the Trombiculidae, Dermanyssidae, and Macronyssidae families as well as some genera of the Epidermoptidae family.

Epidermoptid mites, such as *Psittophagoides* from parrots, *Passeroptes* from pigeons and canaries, and *Rivoltasia* from fowl, lack the clawlike process on the anterior legs that enables other taxa, such as *Microlichus avus* from canaries, *Epidermoptes bilobatus* from chickens, and *Promyialges* from passerines, to burrow into the corneous layers of skin; this burrowing causes long, winding galleries.[16] These epidermoptids can, however, cause severe itching, craterlike lesions, scurf, pityriasis, and mange. *Microlichus* lives mainly in feather bulbs; these mites produce congestion and swelling. Like *Promyialges*, adult female *Microlichus* mites use louseflies to transport their eggs to new host birds (Figure 3A). Microscopic examination of skin scrapings is necessary for diagnosis.

Knemidocoptid mites invade feather follicles and

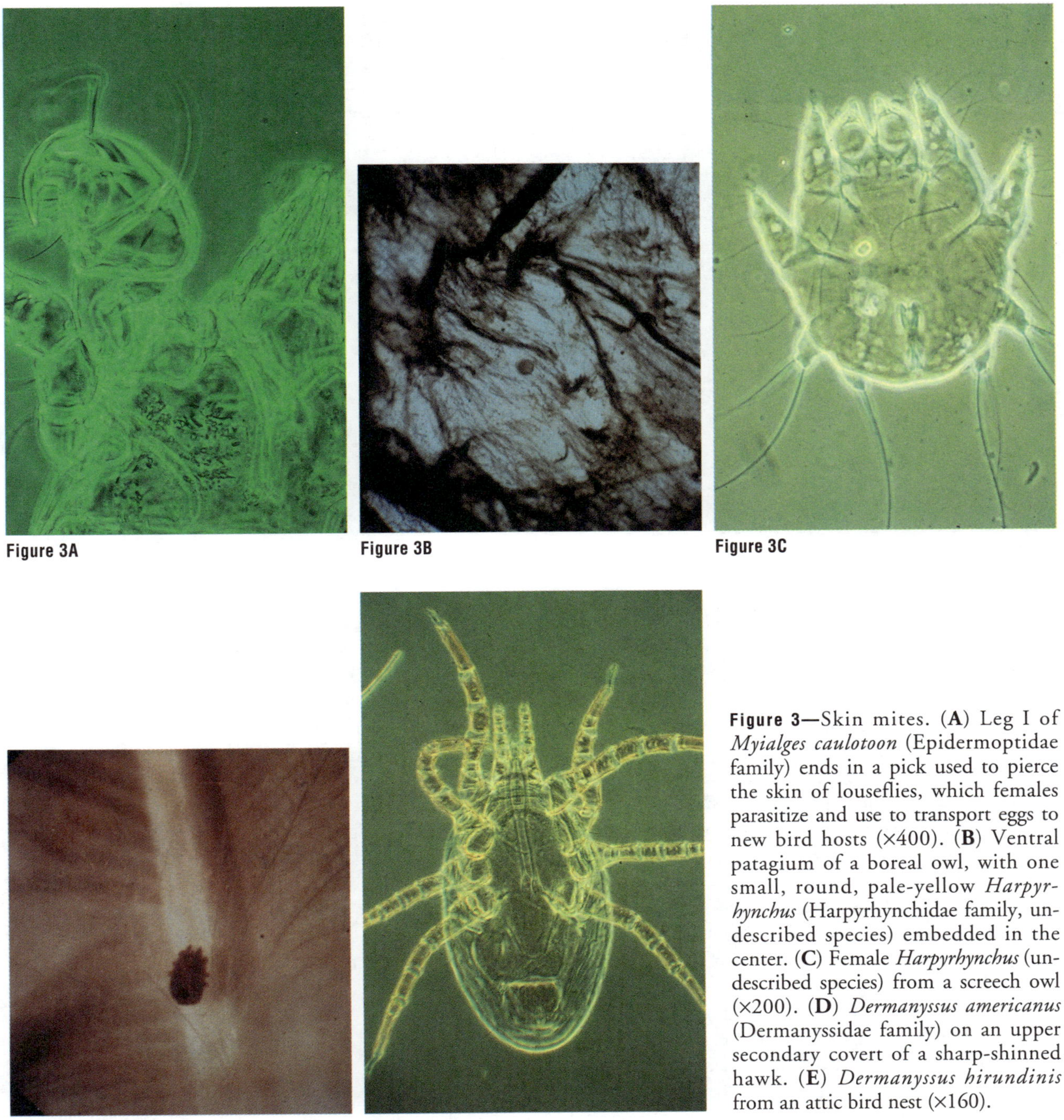

Figure 3A

Figure 3B

Figure 3C

Figure 3D

Figure 3E

Figure 3—Skin mites. (**A**) Leg I of *Myialges caulotoon* (Epidermoptidae family) ends in a pick used to pierce the skin of louseflies, which females parasitize and use to transport eggs to new bird hosts (×400). (**B**) Ventral patagium of a boreal owl, with one small, round, pale-yellow *Harpyrhynchus* (Harpyrhynchidae family, undescribed species) embedded in the center. (**C**) Female *Harpyrhynchus* (undescribed species) from a screech owl (×200). (**D**) *Dermanyssus americanus* (Dermanyssidae family) on an upper secondary covert of a sharp-shinned hawk. (**E**) *Dermanyssus hirundinis* from an attic bird nest (×160).

the stratum corneum of the face, feet, and cere; these mites feed on keratin and produce honeycomb cavity networks.[17] The result is scaly leg or scaly face disease, which is characterized by scaling and hyperkeratosis as well as intense irritation, pruritus, and feather loss. *Knemidocoptes pilae* parasitizes psittaciform birds, and many photographs of the cere and foot lesions caused by these mites have been published.[18–21] *Procnemidocoptes* also parasitizes parrots. *Knemidocoptes jamaicensis* infests the feet of many passerine birds, including canaries. The scaly leg mite, *Knemidocoptes mutans*, and the depluming mite, *Neocnemidocoptes gallinae*, infest chickens; these mites cause crippling, weight loss, and lowered egg production. *Picicnemidocoptes laevis* causes mange in pigeons.

Although various topical acaricidal treatments can be used,[20–22] Ryan[20] concluded that one or two intramuscular or oral doses of ivermectin (200 µg/kg) was the optimum regimen. Ryan emphasized that knemidocoptid infestation is typically a secondary problem

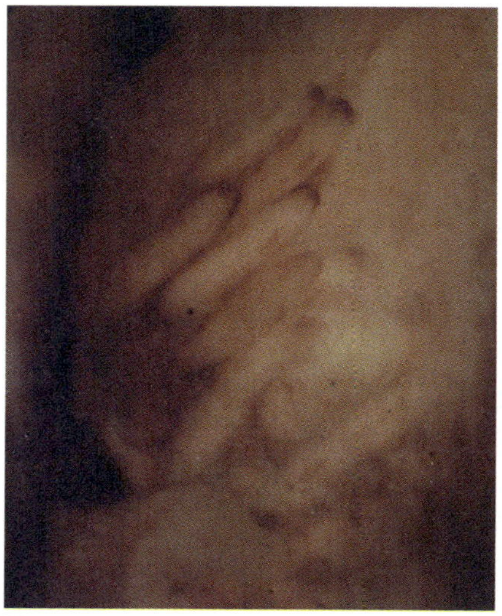

Figure 4A

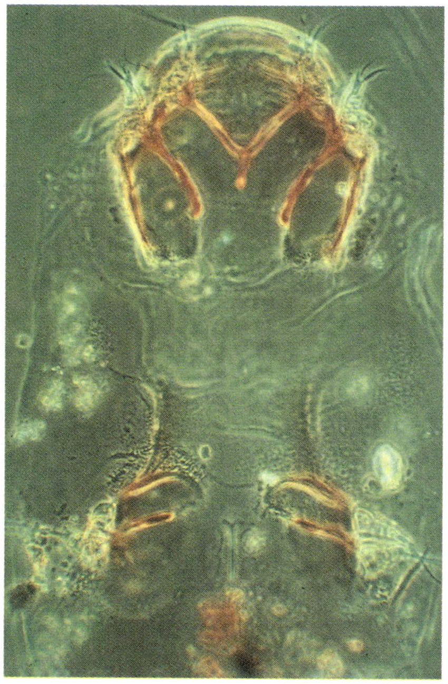

Figure 4B

Figure 4—Subcutaneous mites (Hypoderatidae family). (**A**) *Hypodectes nycticoracis* deutonymphs in the subcutaneous fascia of a black-crowned night heron. (**B**) *Tytodectes cerchneis* from an American kestrel nest (×400). The legs are extremely reduced, and the anterior end is smooth with no mouthparts.

associated with stress or dietary deficiency, and adjunct therapy should address the primary susceptibility factor. Another adjunct therapy involves levamisole hydrochloride in water at 2.5 mg/lb for 30 days; the agent acts as an immunostimulant to help eliminate mite infestation.

A few species of harpyrhynchid mites attach to skin at the base of a feather calamus, and females and their eggs become covered by a semifibrous sheath on the calamus.[23] The most pathogenic species of this family inhabit hyperkeratotic epidermal cysts that appear as pea-sized white lumps or yellowish-orange nodules.[24,25] Several species of *Harpyrhynchus* (Figures 3B and 3C) occur on parrots, whereas *H. columbae* parasitizes the pigeon and *Harpypalpus serini* was discovered on the yellow-fronted canary. Schulz[26] treated an eagle with loss of feathers on the head and neck caused by harpyrhynchid-induced scratching with 200 µg/kg of intramuscular ivermectin.

Cheyletiellid mites cause skin lesions and mange, as illustrated in photographs in a work by Guilhon and Euzeby[27] of a red-billed leiothrix (*Leiothrix lutea*, also known as the domesticated Japanese nightingale) with *Neocheyletiella*; cheyletiellid mites also parasitize several species of canaries. The leiothrix hosts *Ornithocheyletia*, a genus found on parrots and other birds, which does extensive damage. The burrows of these mites in the stratum corneum of a pigeon cause hyperkeratosis and are colonized by mold (*Micromonospora*); fungal breakdown products of the keratinous tissue are probably part of the mite's food.[28] *Bakericheyla chanayi* feeds on blood and spins webbing microshelters on the skin of its fringillid hosts.[29]

Chiggers are larval mites of the Trombiculidae family; they are 0.1 to 0.3 millimeters in length. Nymphal and adult stages of this family are predators in soil and litter. The mites attach to skin and inject tissue-dissolving saliva, which causes intense itching. After about three days, they become engorged and drop off the host. The most common attachment sites on birds are the thighs, under the wings, and around the anus. Host ranges are broad, and some species infest mammals as readily as birds. Severe skin reactions can be treated with antibiotics and antihistamines, and corticosteroids help decrease extreme irritation and swelling[30]; the ground should also be treated with an ascaricide.

Dermanyssid[31] and macronyssid[32] mites are much larger (0.7 to 1.1 millimeters in length) and more mobile. These mites appear white when unfed; depending on how recently a bloodmeal was consumed, their color may change to red, black, or gray (Figures 3D and 3E). Both families have low host specificity and cause irritation, crusting, weight loss, listlessness, and anemia. Severe infestation of these mites causes severe anemia and subsequent death of the host. If the mite population reaches 50,000 per chicken on poultry farms, daily blood loss is approximately 6% per bird.

Although *Dermanyssus gallinae* is known as the chicken red mite, it has been reported in 30 species of birds. It hides near the bird during the day, feeds at night, and lays as many as 20 eggs in the nest material. These mites can be difficult to detect unless the

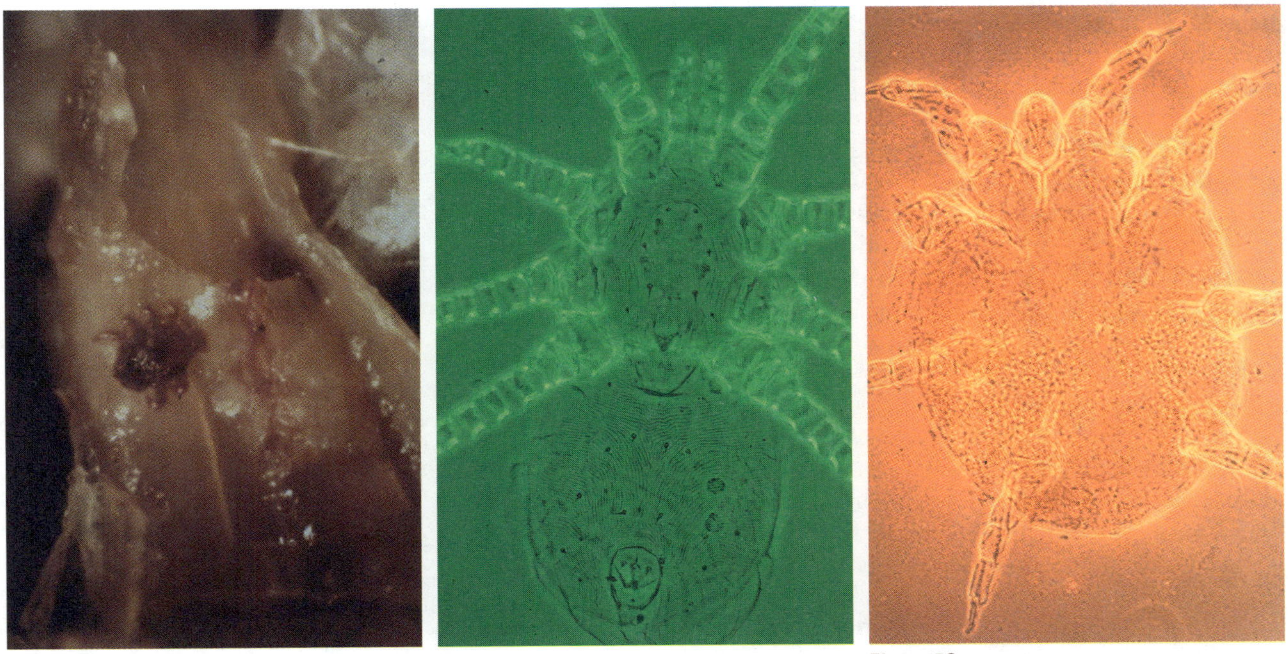

Figure 5A **Figure 5B** **Figure 5C**

Figure 5—Respiratory mites. (**A**) *Rhinoecius aegolii* (Rhinonyssidae family) in the nasal passages of a boreal owl. The dark red color indicates that a bloodmeal was recently consumed. (**B**) *Ptilonyssus melissae* from a purple finch (×200). (**C**) *Cytodites nudus* (Cytoditidae family), the air sac mite of chickens and turkeys (×160).

cage is examined at night. They can survive as long as five months without food, overwintering in the nest. Some other species of this genus spend most of their lives on the host and lay eggs on feathers. Acaricides that are most effective against *D. gallinae* are carbaryl, deltamethrin, bendiocarb, tetrachlorvinphos, and permethrin.[33,34]

The macronyssid genus *Ornithonyssus* can complete its life cycle on the bird; eggs may be laid on the feathers or off the bird. *Ornithonyssus sylviarum*, the northern fowl mite, and *O. bursa*, the tropical fowl mite, have many host species and are among the most important pests in the poultry industry. They feed day and night, preferring the vent region. The literature on the northern fowl mite is particularly extensive.[35] The most effective acaricides against *O. sylviarum* are bendiocarb and three organophosphorus compounds: monocrotophos, cythioate, and famphur.[34,36] External application is required; adding famphur, ivermectin, or many anticoccidials to feed has no effect on these mites.

SUBCUTANEOUS MITES

Subcutaneous mites of the families *Laminosioptidae*[37] and *Hypoderatidae*[38] (Figures 4A and 4B) form nodules in the subcutaneous tissue of the breast and other areas, sometimes burrowing in muscles and internal organs. *Laminosioptes cysticola*, the fowl cyst mite, and related species from passerine, columbiform, and psittaciform birds are more pathogenic than are hypoderatid mites and can be fatal. Only the deutonymph of hypoderatid mites parasitizes birds; other stages are free-living in nests. Among the hosts are pigeons, doves, macaws, and parrots. Infesting mites become surrounded by macrophages and, in some cases, fibrous encapsulation. Ivermectin may be an effective treatment.[39]

RESPIRATORY TRACT MITES

Mites from the families Turbinoptidae, Ereynetidae, Rhinonyssidae, and Cytoditidae[40] occupy different parts of the respiratory tract and use different food sources. Turbinoptid mites live in the nares of birds, such as fowl, and feed on the corneous skin there. Ereynetid mites feed on mucus mainly in the deeper part of the nasal cavity of columbiform, galliform, psittaciform, and other birds. Both types of mites are relatively harmless to the host.

Rhinonyssid mites (Figures 5A and 5B) feed on blood and inhabit the anterior part of the nasal cavity in small numbers; *Sternostoma tracheacolum*, the canary lung mite, is an exception—these mites reside in the trachea and air sacs of canaries, Gouldian finches, budgerigars, and other birds. *Sternostoma tracheacolum* can cause death resulting from bronchopneumonia and air sacculitis.[41] Signs resemble those caused by *Syngamus trachea*, *Aspergillus fumigatus*, and pharyngeal pox infections; such signs include respiratory distress and a characteristic clicking-smacking sneeze or cough. Dimethyl carbinol fumigation, dichlorvos vapors, malathion powder inhalation, intramuscular ivermectin, trichlorfon in drinking water, and carbaryl or sulfaquinoxaline in feed are among the recommended treatments[22,42] for rhinonyssid and cytoditid mite infestations. *Cytodites nudus*, the air sac mite (Figure 5C), feeds on serous secretions in the air sacs of chickens and turkeys. Signs of infestation, which can be fatal, include coughing, mucus accumulation, and loss of equilibrium. Four related species of these mites are found on psittaciform birds, and one related species is found on columbiform birds.[43]

SUMMARY

Birds host a diverse microcommunity of feather, quill, skin, subcutaneous, and respiratory tract mites. Avian mites feed on blood, tissue fluid, skin and feather lipids and debris, keratin, fungi, algae, and other mites. Feather mites are normally commensals, but a large population can be irritating and result in feather loss and skin lesions from scratching and secondary infections. Quill and burrowing skin mites can cause mange and hyperkeratosis; anemia can result from other skin mites. Nasal mites can cause respiratory distress and bronchopneumonia. New species of avian mites are continually being discovered, and it is unlikely that we are aware of all parasitic avian mites, even those that affect common cage birds.

About the Author

Dr. Philips is affiliated with the Mathematics and Science Division, Babson College, Babson Park, Massachusetts.

REFERENCES

1. Philips JR: What's bugging your birds? Avian arthropod parasites, in Ludwig DR (ed): *Wildlife Rehabilitation*, vol 8. Edina, MN, Burgess Publishing Co, 1990, pp 155–203.
2. Krantz GW: *A Manual of Acarology*. Corvallis, OR, Oregon State University Bookstores, 1978, pp 1–509.
3. Atyeo WT, Gaud J: Feather mites and their hosts, in Rodriguez GE (ed): *Recent Advances in Acarology*, vol II. New York, Academic Press, 1979, pp 355–361.
4. Atyeo WT, Gaud J: Feather mites (Acarina) of the parakeet, *Melopsittacus undulatus* (Shaw) (Aves:Psittacidae). *J Parasitol* 73:203–206, 1987.
5. Atyeo WT, Braasch NL: The feather mite genus *Proctophyllodes* (Sarcoptiformes:Proctophyllodidae). *Bull Univ Nebraska State Mus* 5:1–354, 1966.
6. Rosen S, Hadani A, Perlstein Z: The occurrence of *Megninia hologastra* (Analgidae Gaud, 1974) on poultry in Israel. *Avian Pathol* 17:921–923, 1988.
7. Pérez TM, Atyeo WT: Site selection of the feather and quill mites of Mexican parrots, in Griffiths DA, Bowman CE (eds): *Acarology VI*, vol I. Chichester, Ellis Horwood Ltd, 1984, pp 563–570.
8. Gaud J: Acariens Sarcoptiformes plumicoles parasites sur les oiseaux Psittaciformes, Strigiformes et Caprimulgiformes en Afrique. *Ann Mus r Afr cent, Série in-8°, Zool* 230:1–106, 1980.
9. Gaud J: Acariens Sarcoptiformes plumicoles parasites sur les oiseaux Lariformes et Columbiformes d'Afrique. *Ann Mus r Afr cent, Série in-8°, Zool* 214:1–101, 1976.
10. Rosen S, Hadani A, Shoham D: Parasitic mites (Arachnida, Arachnoidea) in wild birds trapped in poultry farms in Israel. 1. Species of mites and their hosts. *Acarologia* 26:79–85, 1985.
11. Casto SD: Entry and exit of syringophilid mites (Acarina:Syringophilidae) from the lumen of the quill. *Wilson Bull* 86:272–278, 1974.
12. Gaud J: Quelques espèces nouvelles de Sarcoptiformes plumicoles (Analgidae & Dermoglyphidae) parasites d'oiseaux d'Europe. *Acarologia* 15:727–758, 1973.
13. Kethley J: A revision of the family Syringophilidae. *Contrib Am Entomol Inst* 5:1–76, 1970.
14. Gaud J, Atyeo W: Ascouracarinae, n. sub-fam. des Syringobiidae, Sarcoptiformes plumicoles. *Acarologia* 18:143–162, 1976.
15. Lukoschus FS, Lombert HAPM: Five new species of quill wall mites from European birds (Astigmata:Laminosioptidae:Fainocoptinae). *Int J Acarol* 6:63–78, 1980.
16. Fain A: A review of the family Epidermoptidae Trouessart parasitic on the skin of birds (Acarina:Sarcoptiformes). Part I. *Verhand. Koninklijke Vlaamse Acad Wetenschappen, Letteren Schone Kunsten Belgie* 27:1–176, 1965.
17. Fain A, Elsen P: Les acariens de la famille Knemidocoptidae producteurs de gale chez les oiseaux. *Acta Zool Pathol Antverp* 45:1–142, 1967.
18. Perry RA, Gill J, Cross GM: Disorders of the avian integument. *Vet Clin North Am Small Anim Pract* 21:1307–1327, 1991.
19. Pass DA: The pathology of the avian integument: A review. *Avian Pathol* 18:1–72, 1989.
20. Ryan T: Cnemidocoptic mite infestation in cage birds. *Mod Vet Pract* 67:525–526, 1986.
21. Keymer IF: Parasitic diseases, in Petrak ML (ed): *Diseases of Cage and Aviary Birds*. Philadelphia, Lea & Febiger, 1982, pp 535–598.
22. Stauber E, Schussman S: Parasites of pet and aviary birds—Part 2. *Mod Vet Pract* 66:539–543, 1985.
23. Moss WW, Oliver JH Jr, Nelson BC: Karyotypes and developmental stages of *Harpyrhynchus novoplumaris* sp. n. (Acari:Cheyletoidea:Harpyrhynchidae), a parasite of North American birds. *J Parasitol* 54:377–392, 1968.
24. Morley LC, Shillinger JE: Parasitic tumors in wild birds. *JAVMA* 91:94–97, 1937.
25. Filippich LJ, Domrow R: Harpyrhynchid mites in a scalybreasted lorikeet, *Trichoglossus chlorolepidotus* (Kühl). *J Wildl Dis* 21:457–458, 1985.
26. Schulz TA: New and unusual ectoparasites of raptors, in Ludwig DR (ed): *Wildlife Rehabilitation*, vol 8. Edina, MN, Burgess Publishing Co, 1990, pp 205–213.
27. Guilhon J, Euzeby J: Une nouvelle espèce de Cheylétidé parasite des oiseauz de volière. *Bull Acad Vét France* 57:495–500, 1984.
28. Haarlov N, Morch J: Interaction between *Ornytocheyletia hallae* Smiley 1970 (Acarina, Cheyletiellidae) and *Micromonospora chalcea* (Foulerton 1905) Orskov 1923 (Streptomycetaceae, Actinomycetales) in the skin pigeon. *Acarologia* 17:284–299, 1975.
29. Furman DP, Sousa OE: Morphology and biology of a nestproducing mite, *Bakericheyla chanayi* (Acarina: Cheyletidae). *Ann Entomol Soc Am* 62:858–863, 1969.
30. Arnall A, Keymer IF: *Bird Diseases*. Neptune City, NJ, TFH

Publishing, 1975, pp 1–528.
31. Moss WW: An illustrated key to the species of the acarine genus Dermanyssus (Mesostigmata:Laelapoidea:Dermanyssidae). *J Med Entomol* 5:67–84, 1968.
32. Micherdzinski W: Eine taxonomische analyse der familie Macronyssidae Oudemans, 1936. I. Subfamilie Ornithonyssinae Lange, 1958 (Acarina, Mesostigmata). *Polska Akad Nauk Zak Zool Syst Doswiad*:1–263, 1980.
33. Zeman P, Zelezny J: The susceptibility of the poultry red mite, *Dermanyssus gallinae* (DeGeer, 1778), to some acaricides under laboratory conditions. *Exp Appl Acarol* 1:17–22, 1985.
34. Fletcher MG, Axtell RC: Susceptibilities of northern fowl mite, *Ornithonyssus sylviarum* (Acarina:Macronyssidae) and chicken mite, *Dermanyssus gallinae* (Acarina:Dermanyssidae), to selected acaricides. *Exp Appl Acarol* 13:137–142, 1991.
35. Hogsette JA, Butler JF, Miller WV, Hall RD: Annotated bibliography of the northern fowl mite, *Ornithonyssus sylviarum* (Canestrini & Fanzago) (Acari:Macronyssidae). *Misc Publ Entomol Soc Am* 76:1–62, 1991.
36. Crystal MM, Demilo AB: Susceptibility of laboratory-reared northern fowl mites, *Ornithonyssus sylviarum* (Acari:Macronyssidae), to selected acaricides. *Exp Appl Acarol* 4:353–358, 1988.
37. Fain A: Notes on the genus *Laminosioptes* Megnin, 1880 (Acari, Astigmata) with description of three new species. *Syst Parasitol* 2:123–132, 1981.
38. Fain A: Les hypopes parasites des tissus cellulaires des oiseaux (Hypodectidae:Sarcoptiformes). *Bull Inst r Sci nat Belg* 43:1–139.
39. Hendrix CM, Kwapien RP, Porch JR: Visceral and subcutaneous acariasis caused by hypopi of *Hypodectes propus bubulci* in the cattle egret. *J Wildl Dis* 23:693–697, 1987.
40. Pence D: Keys, species and host list, and bibliography for nasal mites of North American birds (Acarina:Rhinonyssinae, Turbinpotinae, Speleognathinae and Cytoditidae). *Spec Publ Mus Texas Tech Univ* 8:1–148, 1975.
41. Tidemann SC, McOrist S, Woinarski JCZ, Freeland WJ: Parasitism of wild Gouldian finches (*Erythrura gouldiae*) by the air-sac mite *Sternostoma tracheacolum*. *J Wildl Dis* 28:80–84, 1992.
42. Losson B, Coignoul F, Vindevogel H: L'acariose respiratoire du canari. *Ann Méd Vét* 123:327–331, 1979.
43. Fain A, Bafort J: Les acariens de la famille Cytoditidae (Sarcoptiformes). Description de sept espèces nouvelles. *Acarologia* 6:504–528, 1964.

KEY FACTS

- Trauma is the most common underlying cause of ocular lesions in birds of prey.
- Because of the large size of the globe and relative lack of orbital protection, any form of cranial trauma frequently involves the eye and its accessory structures.
- The sequelae of lid defects are minimal if the membrana nictitans is functioning normally.

Raptor Ophthalmology*

Christopher J. Murphy, DVM, PhD
Section of Ophthalmology
Veterinary Medical Teaching Hospital
University of California
Davis, California

A bird is a wing guided by an eye. . . .
Rochon-Duvigneaud: ***Les Yeux et La Vision Des Vertebres***

Raptors are birds of prey that belong to the orders Falconiformes and Strigiformes. Hawks, eagles, harriers, kites, falcons, ospreys, and vultures belong to the Falconiformes, while owls compose the Strigiformes. Both orders display remarkable variation in morphology, geographic distribution, and ecologic habits. Major advances in raptor medicine have been made in recent years, with an ever-increasing number of veterinarians participating in the delivery of medical care to this group of birds. The majority of raptors requiring medical attention are free-living birds that have sustained some form of injury; but an individual raptor may belong to a falconer, a zoo, or a captive propagation project.

Ocular lesions are a common finding during physical examination of birds of prey.[1-4] A retrospective study[3] found that 14.5% of all raptors admitted to the Avian Clinic at the New York State College of Veterinary Medicine, Cornell University, and the Owl Rehabilitation Research Foundation in Ontario, Canada, had some form of ocular lesion. Of the lesions, 90% resulted from physical injury. Collisions accounted for 33% of ocular lesions and gunshot wounds for 11%. Unilateral lesions were more common than bilateral lesions, with the anterior segment being most frequently involved. Hyphema was the most common clinical finding. A prospective study was later conducted, and 28% of raptors admitted to the Avian Clinic (Cornell) were found to have some form of ocular lesion. The higher incidence in the latter study was attributed to a lower number of juveniles (which frequently have no medical problems) being admitted and to an increased detection of subtle lesions. Clearly, with such a high prevalence of ocular lesions, a complete ophthalmoscopic examination should be performed on every bird of prey admitted for medical attention.

Assessment of Visual Function

Evaluation from a Distance

The ideal situation would be to observe a bird while it is flying, hunting, perching, and interacting with conspecifics. For this reason, visual deficits

*This article is based on a presentation at the Annual Meeting of the Association of Avian Veterinarians, Toronto, Ontario, Canada, 1984.

Originally published in Volume 9, Number 3, March 1987

are often detected earliest in falconers' birds. Valuable information can be gained from direct observation or thorough questioning of the bird's caretaker as regards the following points.

Food Intake

Oftentimes a bird that has recently become blind fails to find food left in its cage but will eat readily when hand-fed. Some birds adjust to the situation and learn to feed themselves if food is left in a consistent location. A blind bird can be encouraged to feed itself by placing food in its talons.

Reluctance to Fly

Generally, in cases of severely impaired vision, the affected birds are reluctant to fly, although we[a] have recently observed a peregrine falcon that would take short flights in a familiar flight chamber despite dense bilateral senile cataracts.

Abnormal Head Posture

Head posture may vary from a subtle tilt favoring one side to opisthotonos. If a bird is unilaterally blind, it will try to keep its sighted eye positioned toward activity in its environment. A bird with a head tilt but *without* any other neurologic deficit is likely to have a severe unilateral ocular lesion, such as a detached retina (Figure 1). A case has been reported[5] in which a barred owl showed opisthotonos similar to the neurologic deficit seen with raptor thiamine deficiency.[6] It was presumed the bird assumed the position in order to make use of the clear peripheral zones surrounding dense central corneal opacities.

Accentuated Startle Reaction

Birds with severely impaired vision become very apprehensive about activity in their environment. An affected bird may demonstrate exaggerated defensive reactions to benign conspecific activity.

Evaluation of Restrained Birds

Familiarity with the "personalities" of the various species can be important in assessing visual function under restraint. Buteos (soaring hawks, e.g., red-tailed hawk, rough-legged hawk, broad-winged hawk) are generally fairly calm when restrained. They are less likely to respond to a menacing gesture than the accipiters or falcons. Accipiters (goshawk, Cooper's hawk, sharp-shinned hawk) are high-strung creatures that are very susceptible to the stresses imposed by excessive handling. They demonstrate very brisk pupillary reflexes initially, but after excessive handling even a normal bird will develop dilated pupils with a diminished pupillary light reflex. Indeed, excessive handling may cause a clinically normal bird to die.

Falcons (peregrine, kestrel) lie somewhere between these two extremes. The owls are the most sedate of raptorial species when adequately restrained. When both the feet and head are restrained, owls become focused for distant vision. When so restrained, it is very difficult to elicit any response from them with a menacing gesture. The susceptibility of the various species to the stresses of handling must also be taken into account when deciding on a therapeutic regimen.

The procedure for a complete ophthalmic examination is covered adequately elsewhere.[7] It should be stressed, however, that adequate restraint is essential both for the completeness of the examination and for the clinician's safety. A prolonged procedure is best performed with the bird tranquilized or under general anesthesia.

Orbit and Associated Structures

The bony orbit is made up of a number of individual elements with contributions from the frontal, prefrontal, sphenoid, ethmoid, palatine, and quadrate bones as well as the bony components of the jugal arch. The two globes are separated from each other by the exceedingly thin interorbital septum. The osseous septum is complete in owls; while in diurnal birds of prey, an aperture is present that is covered by a tough fibrous membrane in life (Figure 2). The bony component of the posterior orbital wall is less than 1 mm thick in some locations. Many of the larger bony elements are pneumatized, which increases their susceptibility to surgical trauma. The posterior aspect of the eye fits snugly within the orbit, but the majority of the globe's temporal and dorsal aspects remains completely outside of its protection.

The avian eye has four rectus and two oblique extraocular muscles associated with it (Figure 3). There is no retractor bulbi complex, which is replaced by the pyramidalis and quadratus muscles that move the membrana nictitans and are innervated by cranial nerve VI. At least a portion of cranial nerves I through VI has an intraorbital course. A number of vessels are associated with the orbit. The most significant of these is the ophthalmic plexus, which assumes a ventrolateral position. Severence of this complex is the primary source of orbital hemorrhage during enucleation procedures.

The harderian gland or gland of the membrana nictitans (third eyelid) is the major source of tears in birds and is attached to the posterior aspect of the globe in raptors, ventral to the medial rectus muscle. A lacrimal gland is reported to be present and associated with the ventromedial orbital rim in most raptors but absent in the eagle owl.[2] The orbit of the great horned owl lacks an orbital lacrimal gland and contains the slender body of a nasal salt gland in its dorsonasal aspect.[8]

Lids

The upper and lower lids of birds are sparsely feathered, with the palpebral margin of most species having delicate

[a]*Author's Note:* In this text, *we* refers to such notables as Drs. Thomas Kern, Howard Evans, Alexander deLahunta, Ronald Riis, and David Graham, Cornell University; Dr. Doug MacCoy, University of Illinois; Dr. Dennis Brooks, University of Tennessee; Kay and Larry McKeever at the Owl Rehabilitation Research Foundation in Ontario, Canada; and Drs. Joanne Paul-Murphy, Nedim Buyukmihci, Roy Bellhorn, and Dennis Hacker, University of California, Davis.

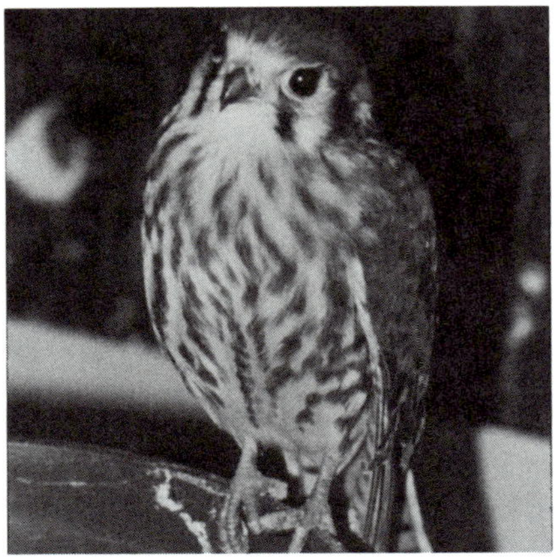

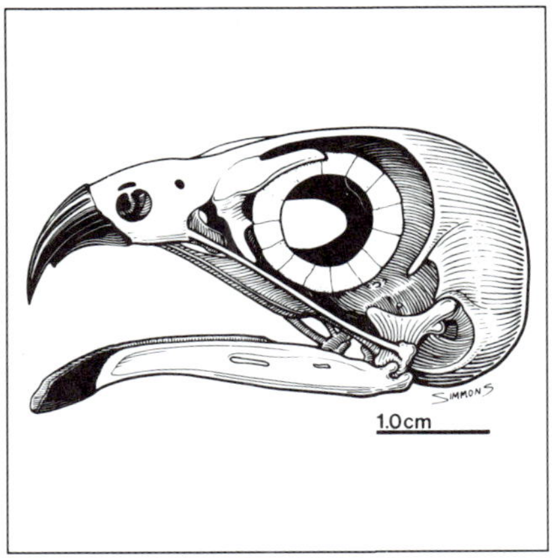

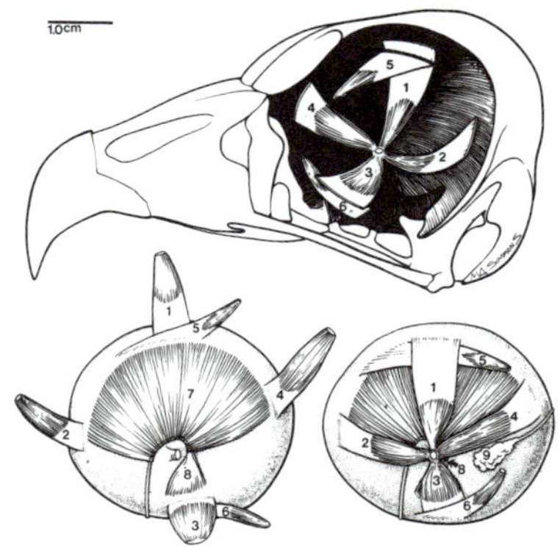

Figure 1 (left)—A mature female kestrel (*Falco sparverius*) shows a persistent left head tilt because of a detached retina in its right eye.

Figure 2 (center)—Skull and scleral ossicles of the kestrel (*Falco sparverius*). Note the aperture present in the osseous interorbital septum. This aperture is covered by a fibrous membrane in life. The interorbital septum is completely bony in owls.

Figure 3 (right)—Extraocular muscles and gland of the membrana nictitans of the great horned owl (*Bubo virginianus*). *Top*, muscles in situ with globe removed; quadratus and pyramidalis muscles not included. *Bottom left*, posterior view of left eye with muscles reflected to demonstrate the pyramidalis and quadratus muscles. *Bottom right*, posterior view of left eye with muscles in situ. Note the position of the gland of the nictitans at the medial aspect. *1* = dorsal rectus muscle; *2* = lateral rectus muscle; *3* = ventral rectus muscle; *4* = medial rectus muscle; *5* = dorsal oblique muscle; *6* = ventral oblique muscle; *7* = quadratus muscle; *8* = pyramidalis muscle; *9* = gland of the nictitans.

filoplumes associated with it. The palpebral margin is usually pigmented, and there are no modified sebaceous glands (meibomian glands). Both upper and lower lids are mobile, with the lower lid covering the majority of the cornea when the lids are closed. Nocturnal species blink less frequently than diurnal species.[9] In all species, the necessity of blinking is diminished because of the ability of the third eyelid to spread the precorneal tear film adequately across the cornea. The lower lid of most raptors contains a fibrous plate that is roughly semicircular in outline with the flat edge facing the palpebral margin. The palpebral reflex can be elicited, although, especially in excited birds, the lids may only partially close while the membrana nictitans is observed to make a complete excursion. It may be more appropriate to refer to a membrana nictitans–palpebral reflex in birds. Running near the lid margin and sending off fine ramifications are small-caliber palpebral arteries that are commonly severed when lacerations occur. These are branches of the supraorbital artery, which is often transected when performing a lateral canthotomy. The inner lid surface is lined by the palpebral conjunctiva. The nasolacrimal puncta of raptors are well developed and extremely so in owls (Figure 4). The nasolacrimal duct empties into the nasal cavity dorsal to the choanal cleft.

Bilateral agenesis of the temporal aspects of the upper lids has been reported in a peregrine falcon.[57] The most common lesions associated with lids are lacerations of varying extent. It is common to observe lid defects resulting from improperly healed lacerations. Usually, topical anesthesia (0.5% proparacaine hydrochloride) and adequate restraint are all that is necessary to repair an acute laceration surgically. Lacerations are debrided and repaired using 6-0 absorbable suture material. The thinness of the lid precludes a double-layer closure, but care should be taken that split-thickness sutures are placed to prevent corneal abrasions. The sequelae of lid defects in birds are minimal *if* the membrana nictitans in the affected eye is functioning normally.

Temporary tarsorrhaphy is commonly performed. This procedure provides a good biologic bandage for a severely compromised cornea. It may also be performed bilaterally in extremely excitable birds, such as accipiters, when a prolonged hospital stay is unavoidable. In such species, tarsorrhaphy has the same effect as "hooding" a bird of prey in that it calms the bird, thus decreasing the amount of self-inflicted trauma. Falconers have used this technique for centuries and refer to the procedure as *sealing*. Good restraint and topical anesthesia are used. In larger species, topical anesthesia is supplied by holding the lid between two to four cotton-tipped swabs that have been soaked in 0.5% proparacaine hydrochloride. The lids are then apposed using one to three simple interrupted or horizontal mattress split-thickness sutures of 6-0 silk (Figure 5).

Vitamin A deficiency has been reported to cause swell-

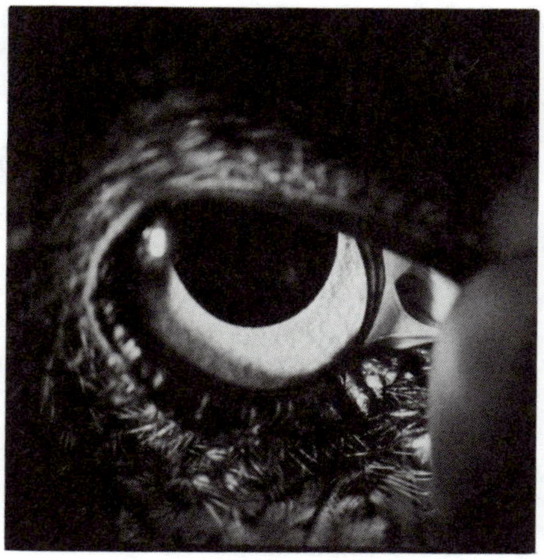

Figure 4—Dorsal puncta of the right orbit in an adult screech owl (*Otus asio*).

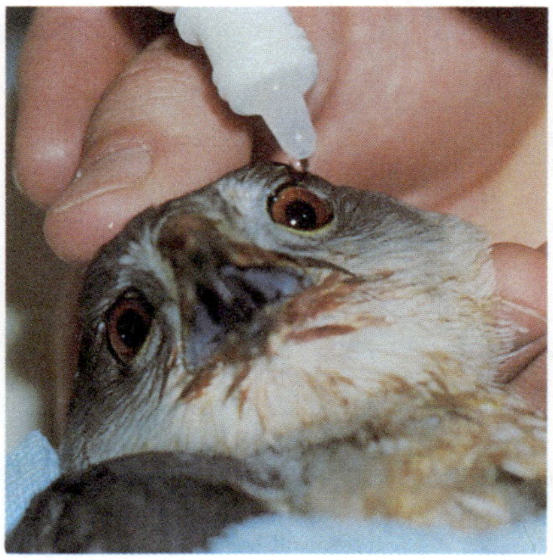

Figure 5A

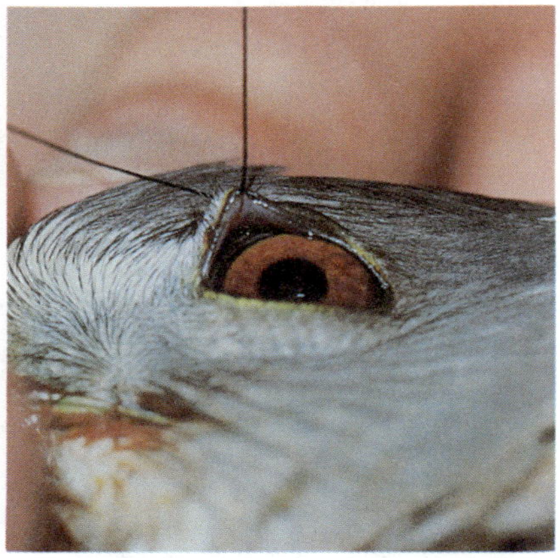

Figure 5B

Figure 5 (**A** and **B**)—Placement of a temporary tarsorrhaphy in an adult sharp-shinned hawk (*Accipiter striatus*). (**A**) Several drops of topical anesthetic (0.5% ophthalmic proparacaine hydrochloride) are placed in the conjunctival sac. (**B**) Split-thickness sutures of 6-0 silk are placed so that they exit through the pigmented palpebral margin. Care should be taken to avoid dragging suture material over the corneal surface.

ing of the lids as a result of conjunctival hyperkeratosis.[6] Pox lesions have been observed affecting the skin around the orbital region in birds of prey.[10] A large pox lesion located anterior to the orbit could interfere with normal visual function. We observed a screech owl after it had been attacked by a swarm of bees. More than 15 stingers were removed from the bird. Its lids became severely swollen, with one dorsal lid margin undergoing ischemic necrosis over the next two weeks despite systemic steroid therapy.

Membrana Nictitans (Third Eyelid)

The membrana nictitans (third eyelid) is developed to the extreme in avian species. A membrana nictitans excursion is usually elicited simultaneously with the palpebral reflex (Figure 6). In the normal bird, the membrana nictitans component should be brisk and complete. It is one of the last reflexes to cease during general anesthesia. The leading edge of the membrana nictitans is pigmented and is characterized by the presence of a marginal plait (plica marginales). The direction of movement is from dorsonasal to ventrotemporal. It assumes a more dorsoventral direction in owls. The temporal edge of the membrana nictitans is tightly secured to the associated conjunctiva and underlying sclera (Figure 7). The nasal edge is where the tendon of the pyramidalis muscle inserts.

Muscles that effect movement of the membrana nictitans are the pyramidalis and quadratus, which originate in the posterior aspect of the globe. They are covered by the overlying extraocular muscles (see Figure 3). Both muscles are innervated by the sixth cranial nerve. The insertion of the quadratus muscle forms a sleeve dorsal to the optic nerve through which the tendon of the pyramidalis muscle passes. This unique arrangement allows the quadratus muscle to act as a pulley of variable diameter, amplifying the action of the pyramidalis muscle. The tendon of the pyramidalis muscle passes first dorsally, then temporally, then ventrally around the optic nerve. The pyramidalis tendon then passes anteriorly and nasally en route to its final insertion on the membrana nictitans. Owls have a peculiar bony trochlea associated with a ventral scleral ossicle around which the tendon passes.

The pigmented flange that characterizes its leading edge allows the membrana nictitans to act as a "squeegee," pushing tears and debris in front of it as it passes ventrotemporally. It then collects tears that fill the trough of the marginal plait and carries these dorsally, thus remoisturizing the cornea. There are specialized "featherlike" epithelia, which assist in sweeping debris from the corneal surface, associated with the bulbar surface of the membrana nictitans near its leading edge.[11] The degree of their development is species variable. These have been erroneously referred to as modified feathers in a previous publication.[2]

Foreign bodies can be found in the membrana nictitans, and lacerations can occur. Occasionally, depigmented areas indicative of previous trauma are found associated with the marginal plait. We have observed several kestrels that had benign subconjunctival calcific deposits on the palpebral surface of the membrana nictitans. Care must be taken to preserve the tendon of the pyramidalis muscle when performing conjunctival surgery.

The Eye as a Whole

Raptors depend heavily on vision in order to compete successfully for survival. The avian eye is a relatively and absolutely large structure that makes up a major portion of the entire cranial mass (Figure 8). Indeed, the impression given is that the head and neck of a raptor evolved merely to suspend a large pair of forwardly directed eyes.

The shape of the raptor eye is species variable and is determined by the shape and extent of the scleral ossicles. The eye is relatively flat in some of the small diurnal raptors, such as the kestrel; globose in large diurnal raptors, such as the red-tailed hawk; and tubular in all owls. In all birds, the temporal aspect of the globe is more elongate

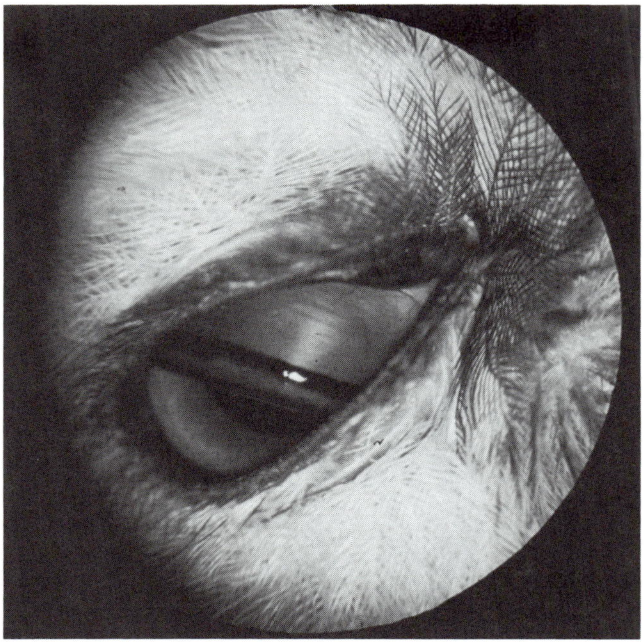

Figure 6—Membrana nictitans excursion in a saw-whet owl (*Aegolius acadicus*). Note the pigmented marginal plait and orientation of the leading edge.

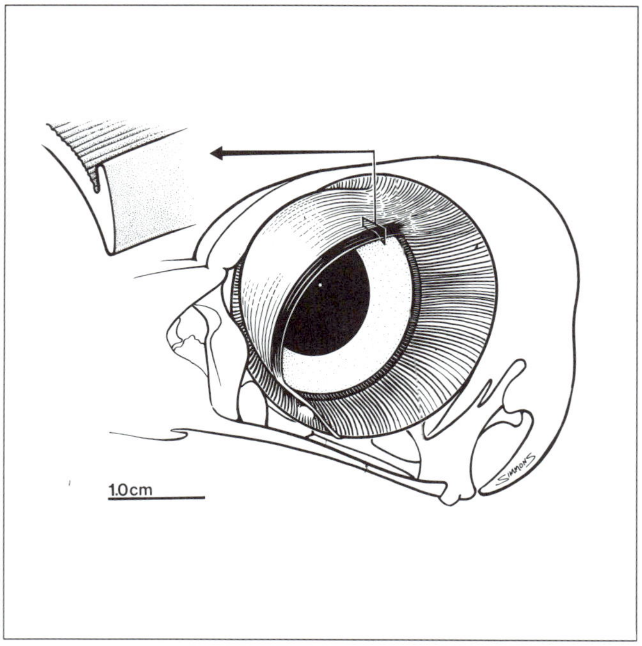

Figure 7—Membrana nictitans of the great horned owl. The membrana nictitans is firmly anchored at its dorsotemporal margin. The leading edge of the membrana nictitans is characterized by the pigmented marginal plait (*insert*), which forms a trough. Ventrally, the tendon of the pyramidalis muscle is seen passing around a bony tubercle en route to its insertion on the medial aspect of the membrana nictitans.

than the nasal aspect. This intrinsic asymmetry optically acts to converge the visual fields, thereby assisting in the construction of a large binocular field.

The eyes of predatory birds are directed forward in the skull creating a large field of binocular vision. This is most marked in owls. Such a primatelike feature is one explanation for human fascination with owls through the millennium. Ocular mobility is more limited in birds than in domestic mammals. Diurnal raptors are capable of ocular convergence, and vestibular nystagmus can be elicited. For years it was stated that owls were incapable of ocular movement. Studies have demonstrated that the great

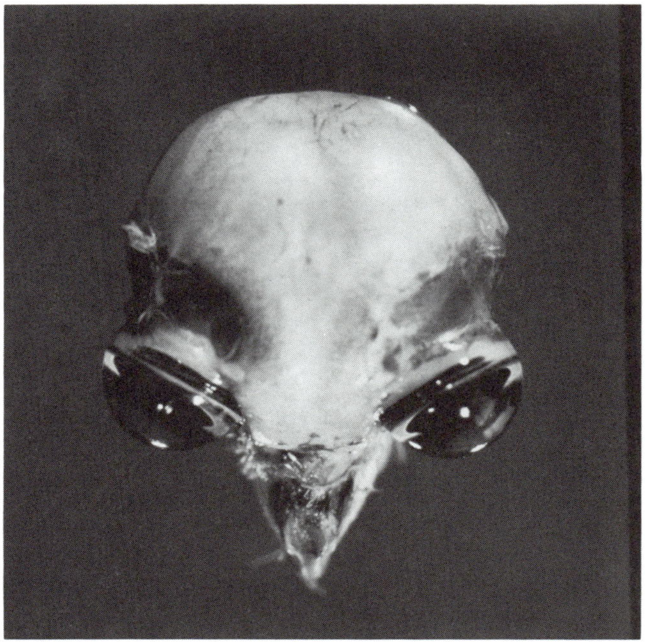

Figure 8—Dorsal view of the skull and globes of the screech owl. Note the large size of the globes and their tubular shape, which are characteristic of owls.

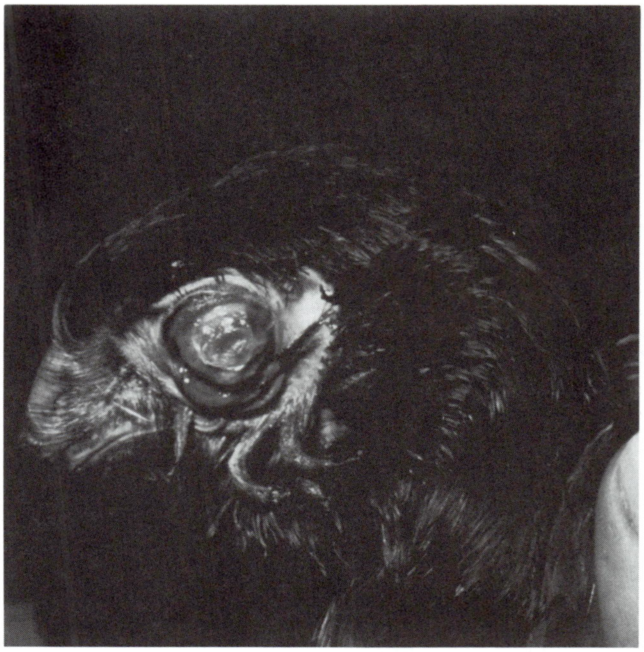

Figure 9—Panophthalmitis resulting from trauma in a marsh hawk (*Circus cyanus*).

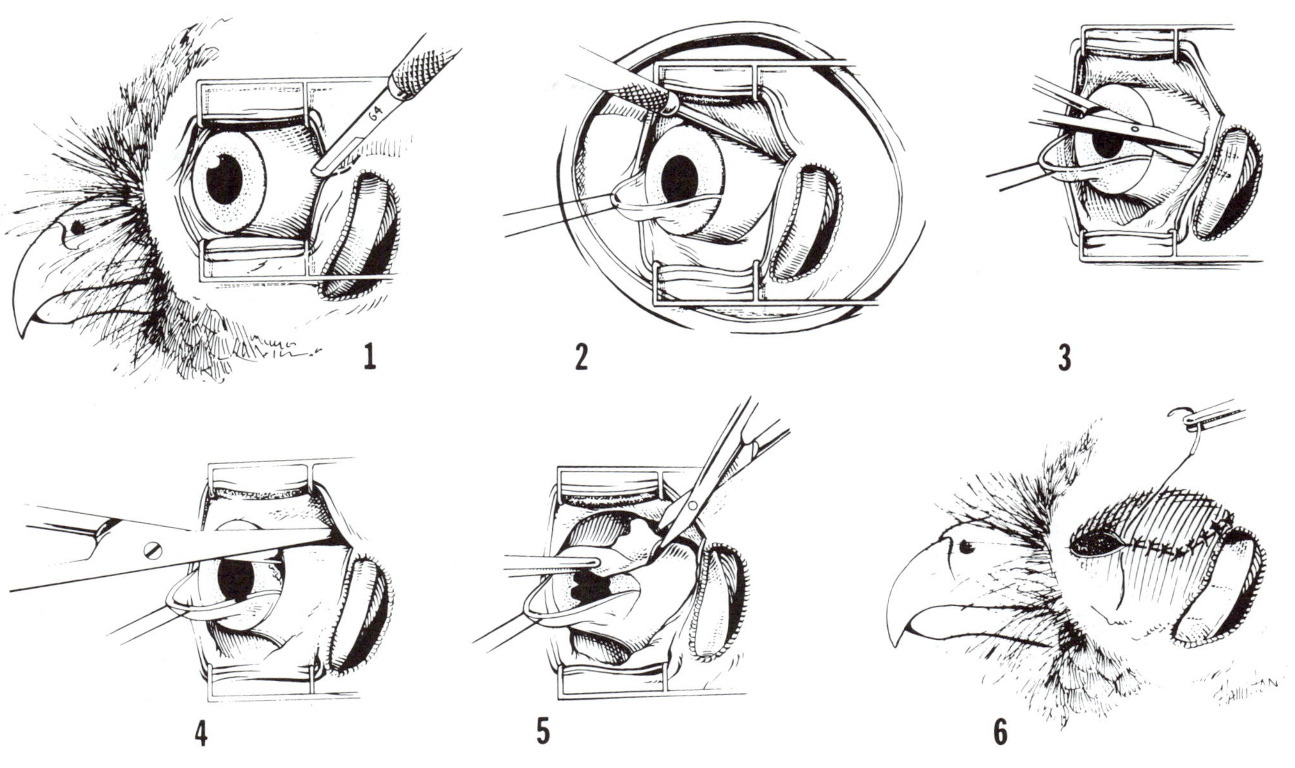

Figure 10—Globe-collapsing procedure for enucleation. (*1*) The bird is anesthetized and placed in lateral recumbency. The orbital region is plucked and prepared for aseptic surgery. A fine-wire lid speculum is placed under the membrana nictitans and lower lid. A lateral canthotomy extends dorsal to the anterior auricular margin. (*2*) A 180° dorsal limbal incision is made, and a stay suture is placed in the incised cornea. A 360° subconjunctival dissection undermines the conjunctiva, membrana nictitans, and periorbital fascia. (*3*) The region deep to the auricular skin is gently undermined. (*4*) Mayo scissors are placed carefully between the uveal tract and sclera so that only the sclera and its associated ossicles are severed. (*5*) A forceps is used to collapse the cut margins of the sclera inward, allowing access to the posterior aspect of the orbit. Excessive traction should be avoided to prevent damage to the optic chiasm. The extraocular attachments to the globe and the optic nerve are severed, and the eye is removed. (*6*) The conjunctiva and membrana nictitans are removed and a 2-mm strip of lid margin is resected. Closure is accomplished by the use of a fine (5-0 to 7-0) absorbable suture in a simple interrupted pattern. (From Murphy CJ, Brooks DE, Kern TJ, et al: Enucleation in birds of prey. *JAVMA* 183:1236, 1983. Reprinted with permission.)

horned owl is capable of very small-amplitude movements in all planes (less than 3° torsional, less than 1.5° in horizontal and vertical planes).[12,13] Because of the close fit of the globe within the orbit and the absence of retractor bulbi muscles, birds are unable to withdraw the globe into the orbit. In owls, the posterior aspect of the globe is visible through the delicate skin associated with the external aspect of the aural canal. This allows a transaural approach for enucleation in most species of owl.

A case of severe bilateral microphthalmia has been observed in a screech owl. This wild-hatched, captive-raised bird had no externally visible ocular structures and the palpebral fissure was notably reduced. The orbits were hypoplastic, and 3×7-mm ocular remnants were found tightly adherent to the orbital wall. Unilateral microphthalmia has been seen in a red-tailed hawk. The affected eye had a normally formed anterior segment except for a diminished diameter. The retina was detached and had pigment clumps associated with it. Insufficient evidence was available to determine whether this represented a congenital lesion or resulted from neonatal trauma. The former is suggested by the completely normal appearance of the anterior segment despite its diminished diameter. Extensive colobomas have been reported in hawks.[14]

As a result of its large size and relative lack of orbital protection, any form of cranial trauma frequently involves the eye and its associated structures. Enucleation is recommended for birds on which extensive ocular damage has occurred or if secondary infection has resulted in panophthalmitis (Figure 9). Two procedures have been described for enucleation in raptors.[15] The globe-collapsing procedure involves severing the scleral ossicles and collapsing the globe on itself to gain surgical access to the retrobulbar elements (Figure 10). This procedure may be employed in any avian species but precludes a complete histologic examination of the globe. The transaural approach for enucleation is feasible only in owl species that have extensive external ear openings (Figure 11). This procedure results in removal of an intact globe, which allows for complete histologic examination. Use of topical epinephrine for hemo-

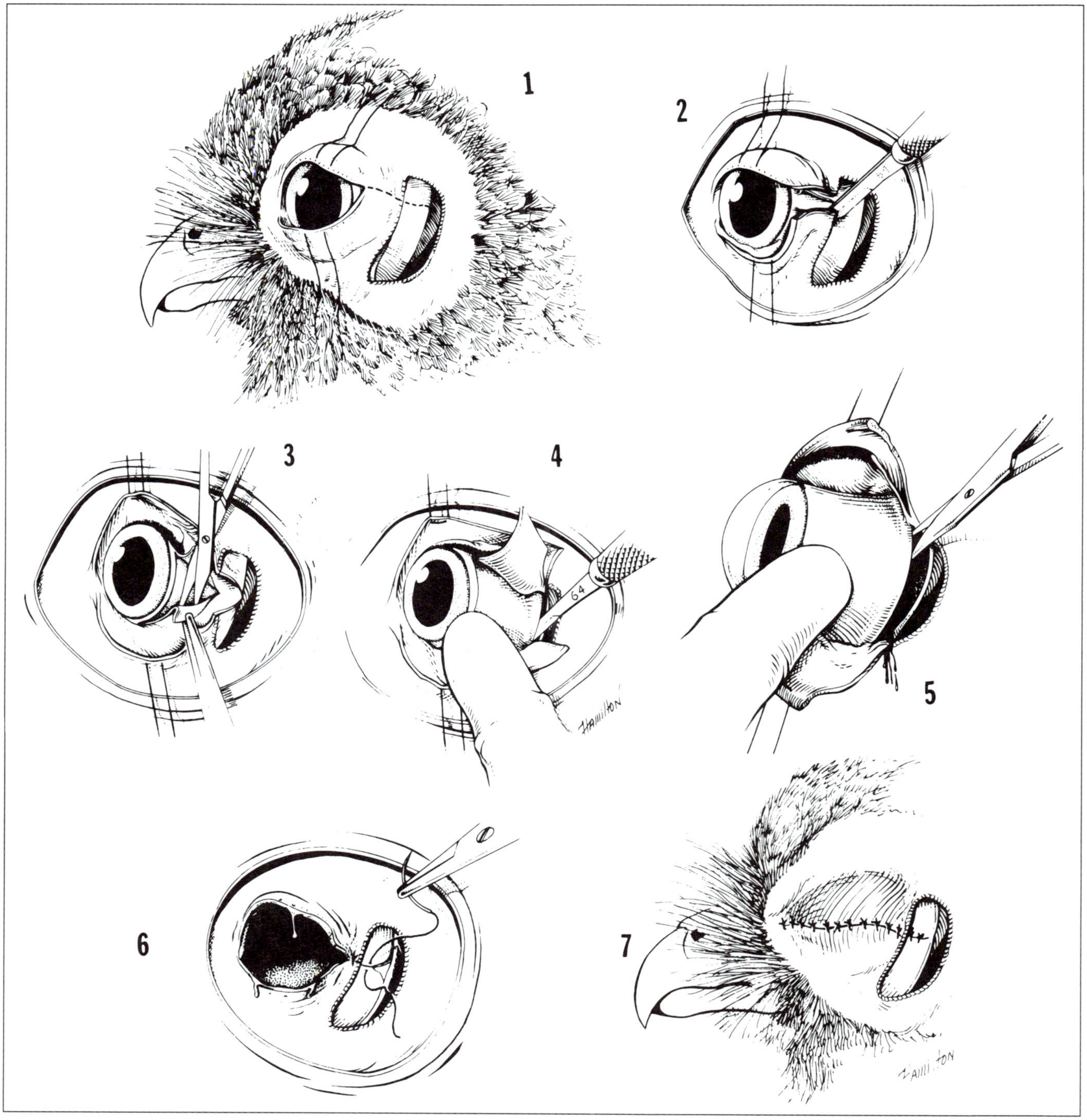

Figure 11—Transaural approach for enucleation. (*1*) The bird is anesthetized and placed in lateral recumbency. The feathers over the orbital and auricular regions are plucked, and the area is prepared for aseptic surgery. Two stay sutures of 4-0 silk are placed in the lid margins. The anterior auricular margin is extended rostrally to expose the posterior aspect of the globe. The incision line is indicated by the broken line. (*2*) A small scalpel blade is used to perform a lateral canthotomy that extends through the anterior auricular margin to the junction of the tubular globe within the postorbital process. A small vessel is encountered at the anterior auricular margin. Hemorrhage from this vessel can be controlled by electrocautery. The incision passes through conjunctiva and an extension of periorbital fascia. (*3*) The skin is gently dissected free, exposing the posterior limit of the tubular globe. A 360° subconjunctival dissection is extended posteriorly under the extension of periorbital fascia. An additional incision of this fascia at the 12-o'clock position may be necessary to mobilize the globe. (*4*) A finger is placed at the limbus, and pressure is applied medially while a small scalpel blade is used to create a gap between the globe and the bony orbital elements. (*5*) After a gap is created, tenotomy scissors are used to dissect the globe free from its extraocular elements and to sever the optic nerve. The globe is then delivered through the lateral aperture. Some bleeding occurs as the vessels are severed, but blood loss will be minimized if the surgeon rapidly proceeds with removal of the globe. Blood loss then can be controlled by packing the orbit with gauze pads. The gauze is removed before closure. (*6*) After hemostasis is obtained, the membrana nictitans and conjunctiva are removed, and a 2-mm strip of lid margin is resected. Closure is accomplished by use of fine absorbable suture material (5-0 to 7-0) in a simple interrupted pattern. The first suture is used to recreate the anterior auricular margin. The aural closure is then completed, followed by apposition of the lid margins. (*7*) Appearance after closure. (From Murphy CJ, Brooks DE, Kern TJ, et al: Enucleation in birds of prey. *JAVMA* 183:1235, 1983. Reprinted with permission.)

stasis in this procedure should be done with caution as systemic hypertension can result, exacerbating the situation.

Cornea

The circumference of the cornea approximates a circle, with the horizontal diameter being slightly larger than the vertical. The corneal diameter in diurnal birds of prey is much smaller than in owls of similar size. This gives the illusion that the diurnal raptor eye is smaller than it actually is. Viewed from the side, the cornea has a smaller radius of curvature (i.e., it is more highly curved) than the posteriorly situated sclera. Compared with diurnal raptors, owls possess a cornea of wide diameter that is relatively flat. Contrary to a previous report,[2] the raptor cornea is not exceptionally thick.[8] The role of corneal participation in avian visual accommodation is currently being debated.[8,12]

From external to internal, the five distinct components of the raptor cornea are:

- *Anterior corneal epithelium*—composed of a stratified squamous nonkeratinized epithelium that is two to four cells thick. The most superficial cells have numerous microplicae, which may assist in adherence of the precorneal tear film (Figure 12).
- *Anterior limiting lamina (Bowman's layer)*—represents an acellular layer composed of collagen fibrils organized into fibers that are arranged in an irregular fashion. This layer may play a role in epithelial adherence to the corneal stroma.
- *Substantia propria (stroma)*—composes the bulk of the cornea. It is made up of collagen fibrils of uniform size that are arranged in lamellae. These lamellae have varying orientation relative to each other, but all run parallel to the corneal surface.

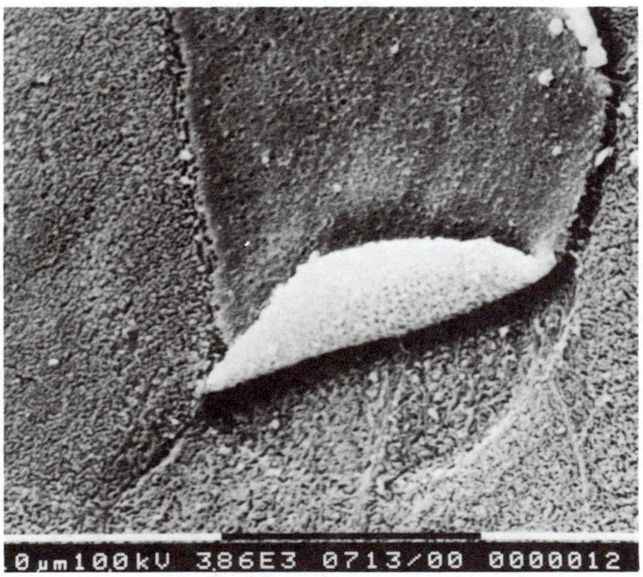

Figure 12—Scanning electron micrograph of the external surface of the cornea of a screech owl. Note the numerous microplicae associated with the individual epithelial cells. One cell is in the process of sloughing into the precorneal tear film. (Bar = 10 μ.)

- *Posterior limiting lamina (Descemet's membrane)*—the exaggerated basement membrane of the posterior epithelium.
- *Posterior epithelium (endothelium)*—simple cuboidal epithelium that is hexagonal in outline (Figure 13).

Corneal opacities are commonly found associated with ulceration and scarring. Corneal ulcers are readily demonstrated with water-soluble fluorescein dye. Ulcers are treated with topical broad-spectrum antibiotics (e.g., chloramphenicol) three times daily for three to five days. The cornea should be restained with fluorescein periodically to monitor healing. Most corneal ulcers heal readily, thus paralleling the clinical course of uncomplicated ulcers in domestic mammals. Corneal vascularization occurs rarely in birds. Several cases have been observed, however, in which chronic ulceration resulted in superficial corneal vascularization with pigmentation (Figure 14). Focal corneal opacities may occur as sequelae to keratic precipitates pursuant to uveitis. Diffuse corneal

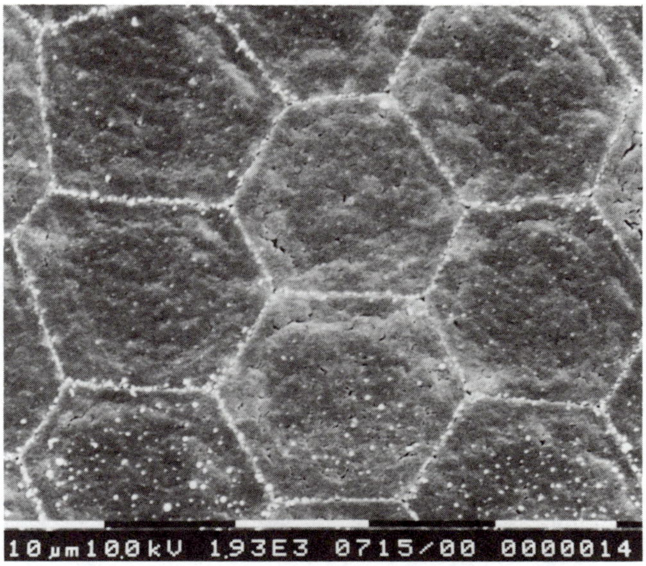

Figure 13—Scanning electron micrograph of the posterior epithelium of the screech owl cornea. Note the regular polygonal outline characteristic of these cells. (Bar = 10 μ.)

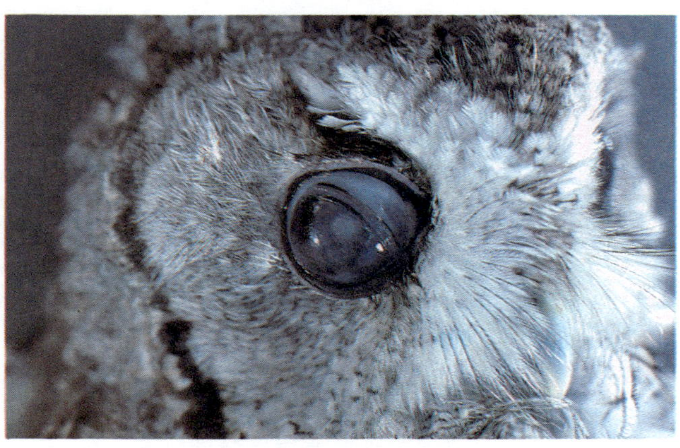

Figure 14—Perilimbal pigmentation with vascularization caused by chronic ulceration in an adult screech owl.

edema resulting from an anterior luxated lens in a juvenile screech owl has been recently observed. Other reported corneal disorders associated with opacification in raptors include a bilateral keratopathy with microcornea of unknown cause in a barred owl[5] and corneal dystrophy.[2] The optical significance of a corneal opacity is dependent on its density, size, and location.

Keratoconjunctivitis or conjunctivitis of variable extent is frequently present in birds that have fallen into chimney hearths. To date, only screech owls and kestrels have been admitted with this history. Any burns incurred are complicated by soot foreign bodies in the conjunctival sac. Several birds that fell into inactive hearths have been admitted to the clinic, with soot-associated inflammation being the only sequela. Affected eyes are gently irrigated with sterile saline and stained with fluorescein. A topical antibiotic-steroid combination is applied three times daily for three to five days to treat the conjunctivitis *if* the cornea is *not ulcerated*. A temporary tarsorrhaphy may be helpful for severely irritated eyes.

Sclera

A hallmark of the avian eye is its anteriorly located bony scleral ring and its posteriorly located cartilage cup, both of which are embedded in the sclera. The scleral ring is composed of 10 to 18 (15 in most raptors) small interdigitating bones.[16] These ossicles determine the shape of the eye, provide protection for the internal ocular structures and serve as the site of origin for the striated ciliary muscles (Figure 15). Their shape and extent must be taken into account when performing enucleation using the globe-collapsing procedure. An additional scleral bone, the os nervi optici, is present in many diurnal species but is lacking in owls.[17] It has also been referred to as the *os opticus* and *Gemminger's ossicle*.[18] It is embedded within the cartilage cup and partially or totally surrounds the exit of the optic nerve. The presence of the scleral ossicles necessitates decalcification before histologic processing.

The scleral rings are a constant feature in skull radiography. We have seen two cases of ocular trauma that resulted in fracture of the scleral ring. Attempts to demonstrate the fracture radiographically with the eye in situ were unsuccessful. In both cases, the defect in the scleral ring could be digitally palpated. The fracture of the scleral ring was radiographically demonstrable in the enucleated globe (Figure 16).

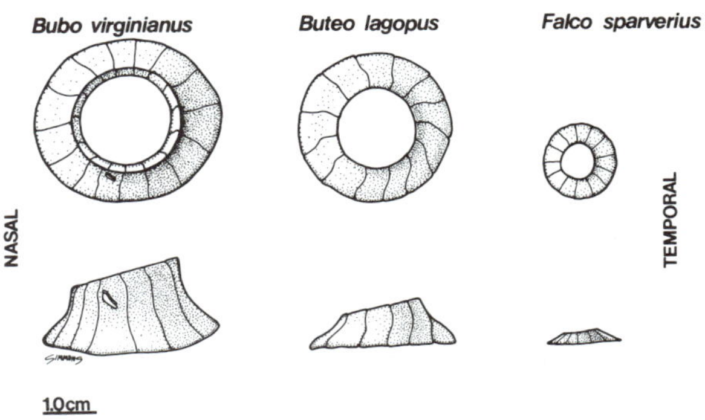

Figure 15—Anterior and ventral views of the scleral ossicles of the left eye of the great horned owl compared with two diurnal birds of prey. *Left*, great horned owl. Note tubular shape, asymmetric outline and tubercle associated with the ventral aspect of the ossicle. The tendon of the pyramidalis muscle passes around the tubercle en route to its insertion on the membrana nictitans. *Middle*, Rough-legged hawk. Note the asymmetry and conical outline that imparts a globose shape characteristic of the larger diurnal birds of prey. *Right*, American kestrel. Note the relatively flattened shape of the ossicles.

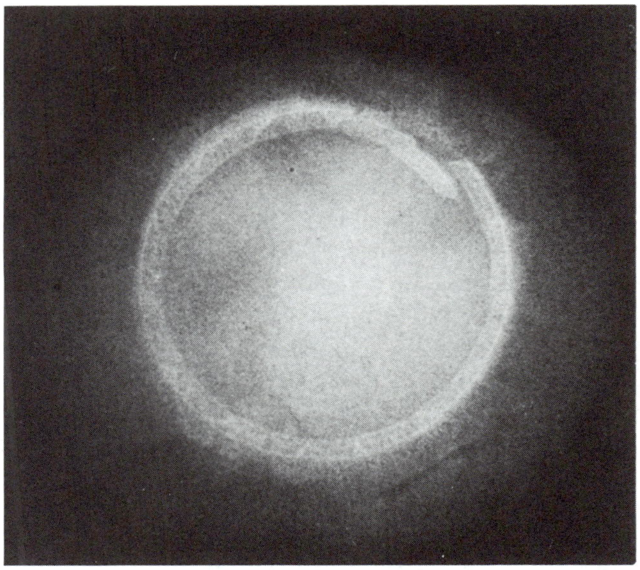

Figure 16—Anterior to posterior radiograph of the enucleated globe of an adult screech owl, which had sustained a fracture of its scleral ring. The fracture was not demonstrable with the eye in situ.

Iris

Iris coloration is species variable; brown, yellow, and red are predominant. In raptors, iris coloration may provide information as to the relative age of an individual in certain species. The juvenile red-tailed hawk has a yellow-gray iris, which becomes more darkly pigmented with increasing age until it achieves a deep chocolate-brown appearance by four years of age. The iris of accipiters (goshawk, Cooper's hawk, sharp-shinned hawk) is gray in nestlings, yellow in juveniles and young adults, orange in middle-aged adults, and ruby red in older adults (five years)[19] (Figure 17).

The iris contains chromatophores of variable type, blood vessels, connective tissue, nerves, and muscle. A recent study of the iris in great horned owls demonstrated a complex iridic musculature consisting of smooth muscle, striated muscle, and myoepithelium.[20] Clinically, a circumferential striated muscle appears to be the primary pupillary sphincter in all species examined, which necessitates the use of curariform drugs to achieve mydriasis.[21]

I have found topically applied curariform drugs to be in-

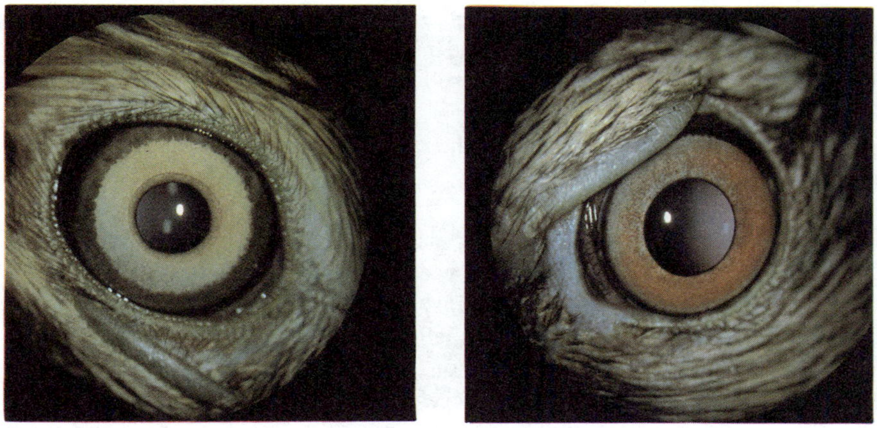

Figure 17A **Figure 17B**

Figure 17—The iris coloration typical of a juvenile (**A**) and a mature (**B**) goshawk (*Accipiter gentilis*).

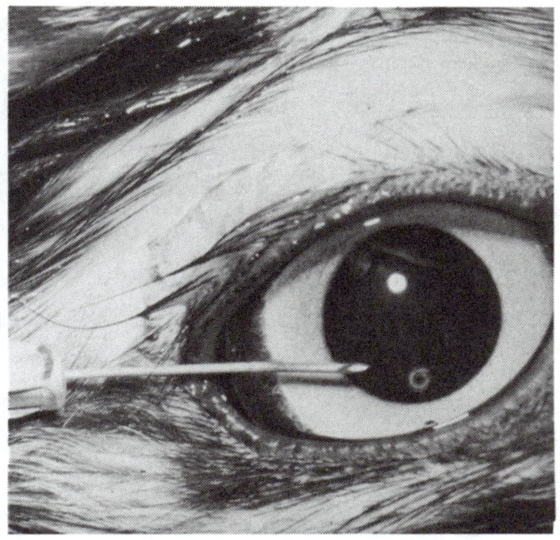

Figure 18—Placement of a fine-gauge needle for intracameral injection of *d*-tubocurarine in a red-tailed hawk (*Buteo jamaicensis*).

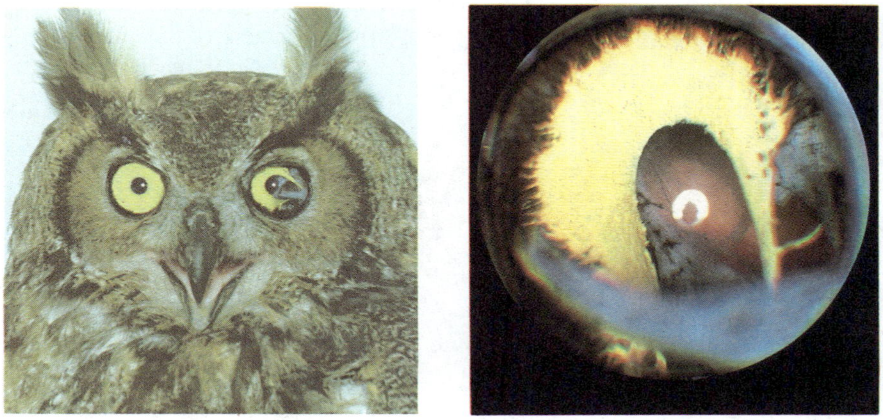

Figure 19A **Figure 19B**

Figure 19—(**A**) Sequelae of a perforating injury in the left eye of a mature great horned owl. (**B**) Closer view of the damaged left eye. Note the corneal scar, iridic tear with anterior synechia, and cataractous changes.

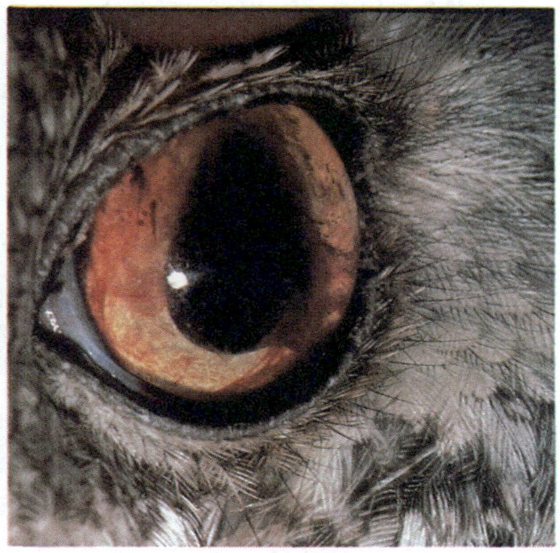

Figure 20—Hyphema in an adult screech owl. Ocular lesions are very common in this species.

effective in most species of raptors. To dilate a raptor's pupil before cataract extraction, I have used the following technique on numerous owls (as small as screech owls), rough-legged hawks, red-tailed hawks, and peregrine falcons. Adequate restraint is essential. The eye is topically anesthetized and a 27-gauge needle on a tuberculin syringe is introduced under the bulbar conjunctiva just posterior to the temporal limbus. Picking up a tag of conjunctiva before entering the anterior chamber may not be possible in all species (e.g., peregrine falcon) because of its tight adherence to underlying stroma. The needle is then passed through the limbus into the anterior chamber and 0.01 to 0.03 ml of aqueous *d*-tubocurarine chloride (Tubocurarine Chloride Injection USP—E.R. Squibb & Sons; 3 mg/ml) is injected (Figure 18). Dilation may occur immediately or may take up to 15 minutes and lasts for 4 to 12 hours. Some salivation may occur, but no other clinical signs have been noticed. It has been observed that a sharp-shinned hawk stopped breathing after insertion of this amount of *d*-tubocurarine.[b] Because of the fragile nature of this species, it cannot be ascertained whether this resulted from stress or was directly related to the instillation of curare. We are currently trying to determine the minimum effective and lethal doses for *d*-tubocurarine delivered by this route. It should be emphasized that *an intracameral injection should not be performed for routine examination.* Most raptors have large enough pupillary apertures to allow a fairly complete examination of the fundus in a darkened room. Examination of the fundus is also facilitated by minimizing the intensity of the examination light.

In contradiction to the report of Greenwood and Barnett,[2] pupillary light reflexes are very brisk and contraction occurs faster than dilation.[20,22] A slow reflex is usually indicative of profound cranial trauma. There is 100% decussation of the optic nerve at the optic chiasm,[23] and a *true* consensual pupillary light reflex has not been

[b]Buyukmihci N: Personal communication, University of California, Davis, 1984.

documented. In addition, a small degree of anisocoria can be normal. Clinically, a slight, aberrant consensual response may be noted when light passes directly into the contralateral globe across the exceedingly thin interorbital septum.[24] One investigation has demonstrated remarkable similarities of the neural substrate mediating the pupillary light reflex in birds and mammals.[25] A degree of pupillary contraction occurs when a raptor accommodates for near vision.[26]

Iridic tears occur commonly with penetrating foreign bodies. Anterior and posterior synechiae are common findings secondary to severe uveitis and hyphema (Figure 19). We have observed a cyst in the iris of a screech owl as an incidental finding, and an iridic melanoma in a great horned owl has been reported.[27]

Anterior Chamber

Hyphema is the most common abnormal finding on ocular examination of birds of prey[3] (Figure 20). The blood generally organizes into a clot within a day or two and, depending on its size, resolves over a period of days to weeks. If uncomplicated by infection, resorption occurs regardless of medication.

Iridocorneal Angle

The *iridocorneal angle* is a regional term that includes the most posterior internal aspect of the cornea, the most anterior internal aspect of the sclera, the most anterior external aspect of the ciliary body, and the root of the iris. Trabeculae that constitute the pectinate ligament cross the angle as they pass from the cornea to the root of the iris. This region is well developed in raptors and is most extensive in owls (Figure 21). Fine trabecular veins are a constant feature, and pigment is usually associated with the trabeculae. Ciliary body detachment or dialysis associated with rupture of the pectinate ligament has been observed after trauma to the raptor eye.

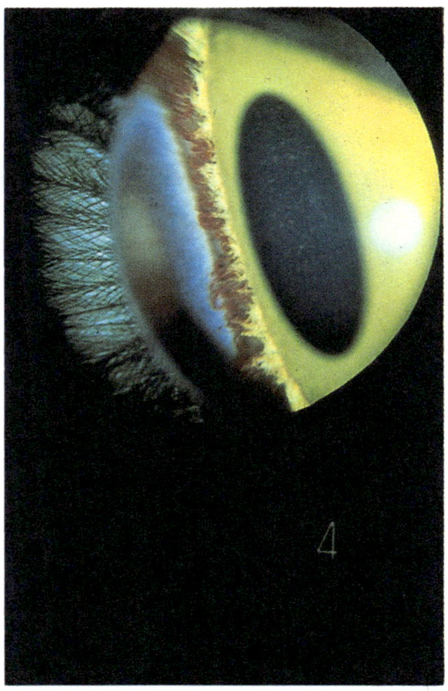

Figure 21—Iridocorneal angle of the great horned owl. Note the depth of the anterior chamber, the extensive development of the pectinate ligament, and the ciliary processes fusing to the lens capsule (visualized behind the plane of the pupil).

Ciliary Body

As in other vertebrates, the avian ciliary body consists of blood vessels, connective tissue, muscle, and two layers of epithelium lining its internal aspect. The ciliary muscles in birds are striated, allowing a very swift mechanism for visual accommodation.[26]

The ciliary processes fuse to the lens capsule in the region of the equator (Figure 22), thus minimizing the role of the zonular fibers in supporting the lens. The ciliary processes can be visualized on ophthalmoscopic examination in the region of the lens equator (see Figure 21). Hemorrhage in this region may be associated with ocular trauma. Intracapsular cataract removal has not been attempted in raptors because of the firm attachment of the ciliary processes to the lens capsule. A successful intracapsular proce-

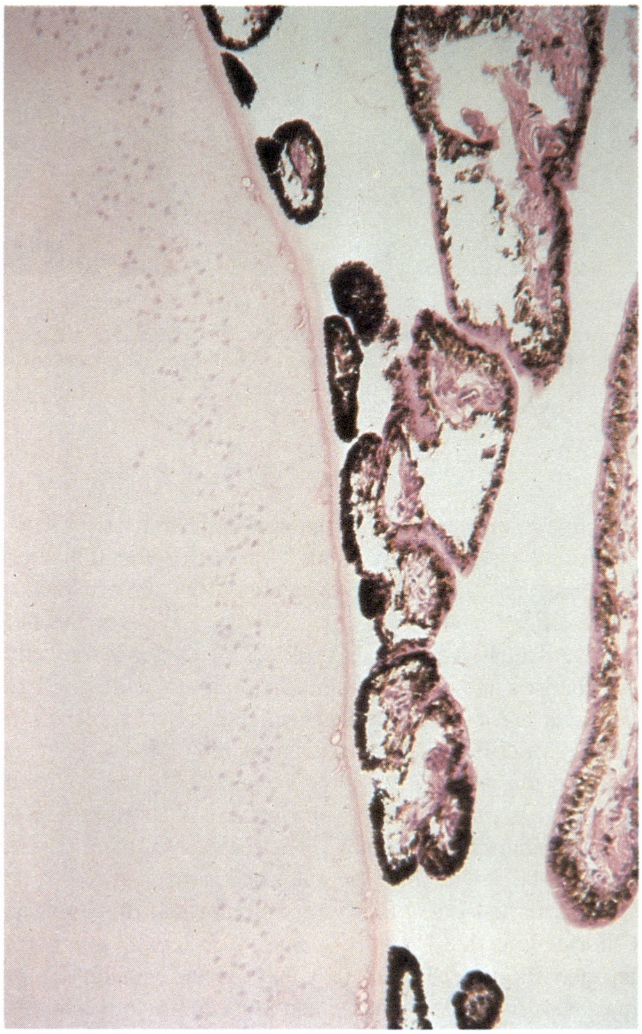

Figure 22—Photomicrograph of the equatorial region of the lens of the great horned owl demonstrating fusion of the ciliary processes to the lens capsule (original magnification ×100).

dure has been performed, however, in a penguin.[c] The applicability of this procedure in raptor ophthalmology remains to be determined.

Choroid and Pecten

The choroid is well developed in avian species. A choroidal tapetum has not been described for any avian species. A retinal pigmented epithelial tapetum has been described in caprimulgiforms (e.g., poorwill), which are closely related to owls.[28]

During ophthalmoscopic examination, the choroidal vasculature is clearly visible in most owls, which have a paucity of pigment in the retinal pigmented epithelium. At the dorsal limit of the fundus, a point may be visualized in owls (and many other birds) where a dorsal vascular cascade emanates (Figure 23). The choroidal vessels are most prominant in young animals and become more obscure peripherally with increasing age because of increased pigment deposition. The choroidal vessels are harder to appreciate in most diurnal raptors and in many cases are totally obscured by the overlying retinal pigmented epithelium. Choroidal lesions are a very common finding on ophthalmoscopic examination of raptors and will be described along with the retina.

The pecten is a pigmented, pleated vascular structure that is typically located temporal and ventral within the raptor eye (Figure 24). It protrudes into the vitreous from a base situated on the optic disk, which it largely obscures. The pecten was first described in 1687 and has had approximately 30 different functions ascribed to it. Despite intensive investigation, its function is still under debate. Currently, the most supported theories are that it is involved in meeting the nutritional needs of the internal layers of the avascular retina,[29] that it is involved in aqueous formation,[30] or that it is involved in maintenance of intraocular acid–base balance[31] or all three. The avian pecten has been demonstrated to be permeable to sodium fluorescein.[30,32,33]

During ophthalmoscopic examination, the pecten serves as a valuable landmark. At the base of the pecten, a thin white line may be seen surrounding its perimeter. This represents the periphery of the myelinated optic disk. The pecten is more extensively developed in diurnal raptors than in owls.

Because of its vascular nature, the pecten may be the source of extensive hemorrhage in the posterior segment of the eye when there is intraocular trauma[34] (Figure 25). A red-tailed hawk with disseminated tuberculosis was described histologically as having a tuberculous lesion in its pecten, yet the lesion was inapparent ophthalmoscopically.[35] The pecten may be obscured from view in cases of detached retina.

Retina

The retina in birds of prey is similar to retinas in other vertebrates in that it consists of a three-neuron chain and an externally situated retinal pigmented epithelium. Within the retina, 10 discrete layers can be recognized histologically. Owls possess a single temporal fovea (depression) within the retina that is used in binocular vision (Figure 26). It is typically located dorsal and temporal to the pecten. Many diurnal raptors have the remarkable specialization (along with hummingbirds, kingfishers, and others) of having two foveae in each eye (Figure 27). In these birds, it is hypothesized that the temporal fovea is used in binocular vision, while the more medially located deep central fovea is used in monocular vision. This provides the basis for the construction of a visual trident in which an animal could simultaneously have three separate objects located in areas of high visual acuity. Curiously, the physiologic optics of this system have never been investigated. Ophthalmoscopically, the foveae of many diurnal raptors appear to have translucent concentric rings surrounding them as a result of reflections from the internal limiting membrane.

Diurnal raptors have been reported to have visual acuity between 2 and 2.6 times better than humans.[36,37] One possible explanation for the increased acuity observed in these birds is that the base of the deep central fovea may act as a negative lens projecting a magnified image onto the externally located photoreceptor layer.[38] Despite their nocturnal habits, the owl retina comprises both rods and cones and color vision has been verified.[39,40] The ability to perceive infrared wavelengths has historically been attributed to owls,[41] but experimental evidence demonstrates that they are incapable of using wavelengths in this portion of the electromagnetic spectrum.[42,43]

There is 100% decussation of the optic nerves at the optic chiasm. Previously, it was felt that this precluded the possibility for true stereoscopic vision (depth perception); but recent studies[44,45] have demonstrated that there is partial decussation between the thalamus and the visual cortex (visual wulst). Indeed, stereopsis has been verified in the American kestrel (*Falco sparverius*) using psychodynamic techniques.[46]

The ophthalmoscopic appearance of various avian species may be found in Wood's book *The Fundus Oculi of Birds Especially as Viewed by the Ophthalmoscope*,[1] which is also the first reference that points out the high frequency of chorioretinal lesions found in birds of prey. This has been supported by more recent works.[2–4] The majority of these lesions in raptors probably represents chorioretinal scars resulting from trauma[3,34]; toxoplasmosis and nutritional deficiencies have been proposed as additional causes[2] (Figure 28).

Focal to complete retinal detachments have been observed in numerous species with and without associated choroidal hemorrhage (Figure 29). As previously noted, an extensive retinal detachment may obscure the pecten during ophthalmoscopic examination. In birds of prey as in domestic mammals, pigmented retinal lesions are indicative of chronicity.

Retinal dysplasia has been reported in a prairie falcon[47] and in a peregrine–kestrel hybrid falcon.[58] We have observed a number of owls with small, punctate, well-circumscribed bilateral retinal lesions located in the ventral

[c]Bellhorn RW: Personal communication, University of California, Davis, 1985.

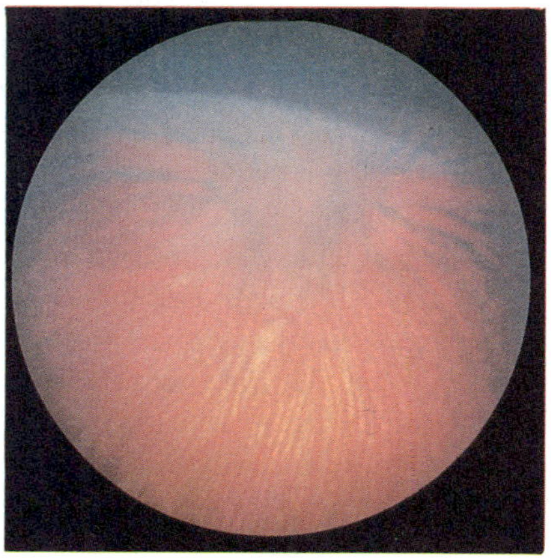

Figure 23—Dorsal choroidal cascade in a great horned owl.

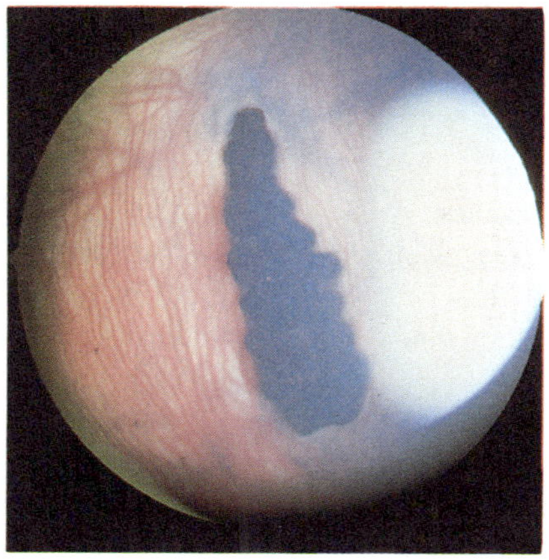

Figure 24A

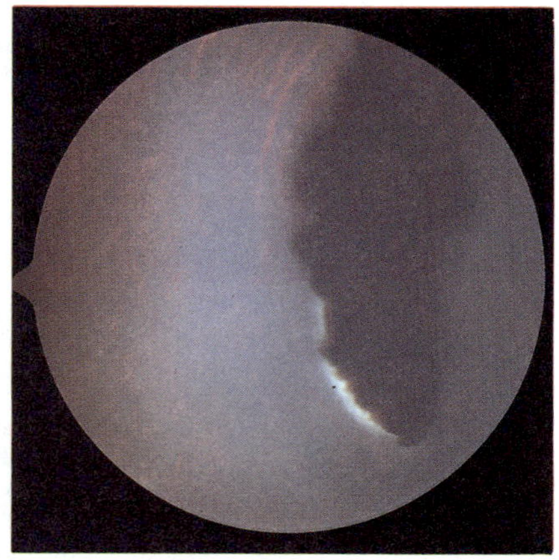

Figure 24B

Figure 24—Ophthalmoscopic appearance of the pecten in a great horned owl (**A**) and in a barn owl (**B**). The pecten is much more extensive in the diurnal birds of prey. Note the choroidal vessels visible through the avascular retina. (Figure 24B courtesy of Dr. R. Bellhorn, University of California, Davis)

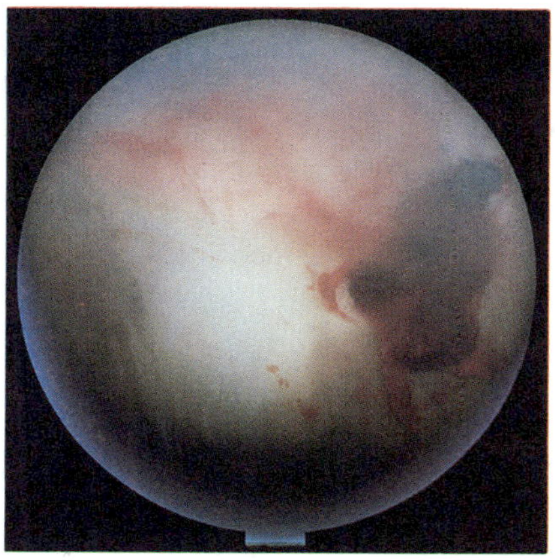

Figure 25—Extensive pecten hemorrhage in the eye of a screech owl that was hit by a car.

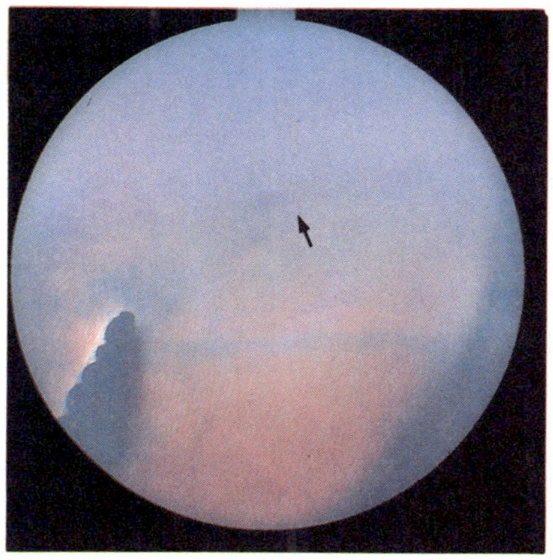

Figure 26—The fovea of the left eye of the great horned owl. The fovea appears as a small dark spot located dorsal and temporal to the pecten.

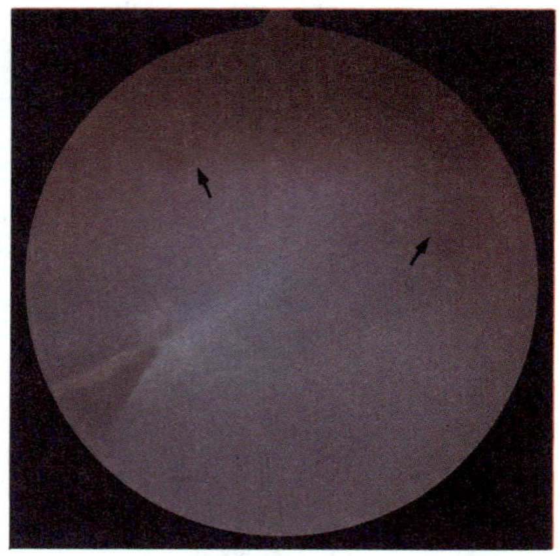

Figure 27—Fundus photograph of the left eye of an adult black-shouldered kite (*Elanus leucurus*). Note the two foveae present dorsomedial and dorsolateral to the pecten.

aspect of the fundus (Figure 30). These have been observed in owls with and without other ocular lesions. Histologic evaluation of the retinas of two great horned owls with lesions revealed only focal degeneration of the photoreceptors (Figure 31). While other species have not been evaluated histologically, the similarity in funduscopic appearance suggests they may share a common morphologic defect. The cause of these lesions is unknown at this time; but the histologic appearance, location and size of the lesions suggest this focal degeneration might result from the imaging of the sun on the retina as the bird views distant objects.

Central visual deficits occur after severe cranial trauma. The visual wulst of birds is the equivalent of the occipital cortex of mammals and is located rostrally in the telencephalon. A case has been reported in which a red-tailed hawk was bilaterally blind because of a combination of ocular and central visual lesions.[34]

Lens

The lens is generally softer in birds than in mammals.[48] This characteristic accounts for the extremely fast visual accommodative mechanism birds possess. Surrounding the cortex in the equatorial zone is the annular pad, or ringwulst, that is composed of hexagonal fibers oriented in a radial fashion. It lies directly under the lens capsule in the region of attachment of the ciliary processes. Functions ascribed to the annular pad include participation in visual accommodation[48,49] and the provision of nutritive substances to the remainder of the lens.[50] In diurnal birds of prey, the annular pad is much more extensive than it is in owls. The cortical fibers of the lens interdigitate by means of their hexagonal shape and by ball-and-socket junctions between adjacent fibers.[8] The soft nature of the avian lens makes phacoemulsification an ideal method for lens removal[51] (Figure 32). Extracapsular cataract extraction has been reported in an Andean condor.[59]

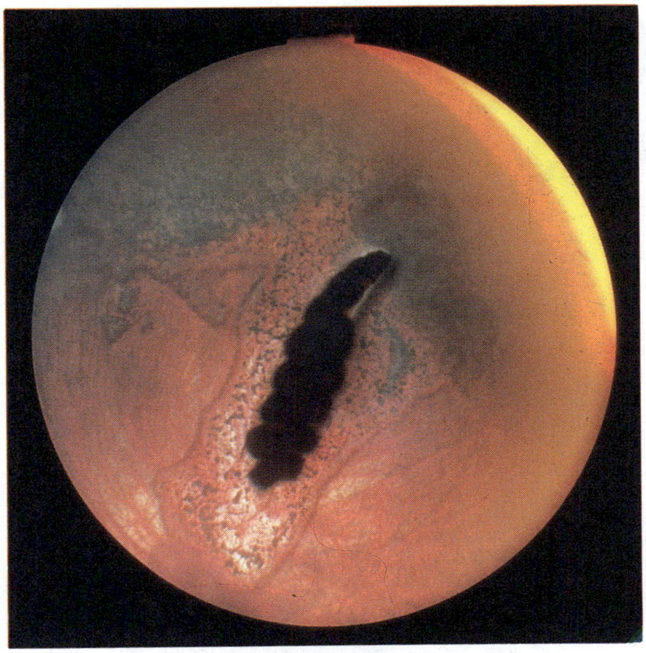

Figure 28—Extensive chorioretinal scarring surrounding the pecten in the left eye of a mature screech owl one year after it sustained severe cranial trauma.

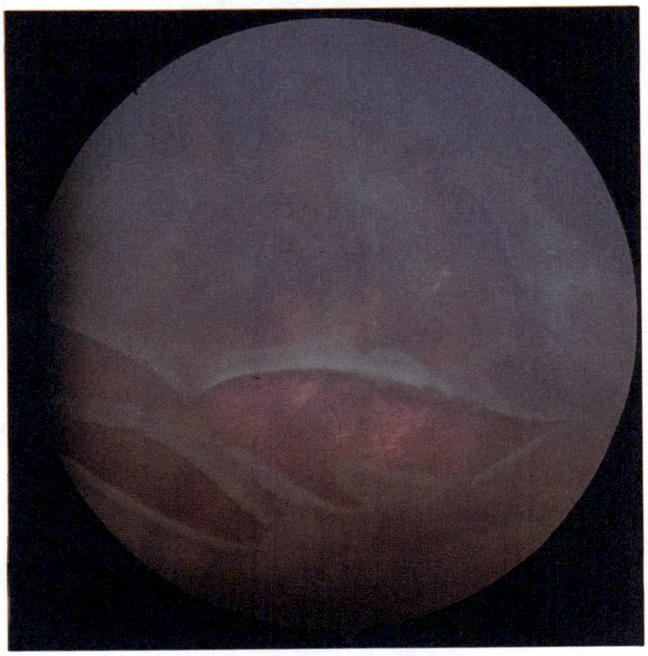

Figure 29—Focal peripheral nasal retinal detachment in the eye of a mature great horned owl (*Bubo virginianus*).

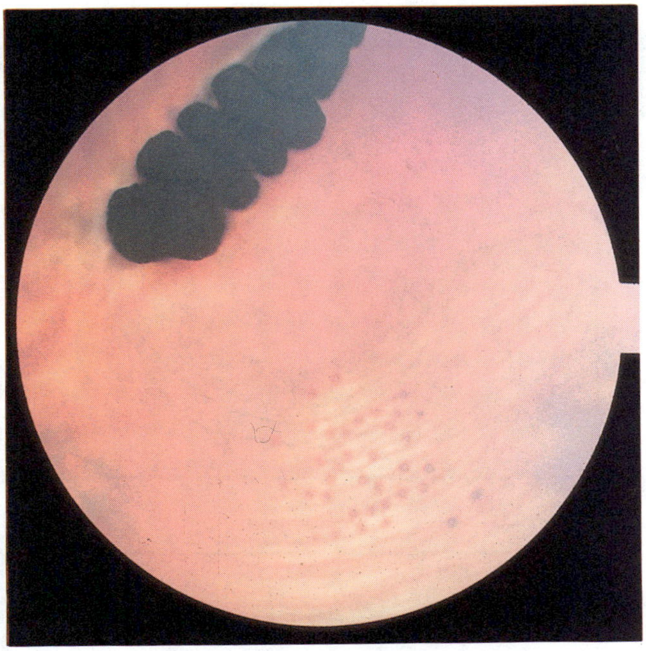

Figure 30—Punctate retinal lesions as a result of focal photoreceptor degeneration ventrotemporal to the pecten in the left eye of a mature great horned owl.

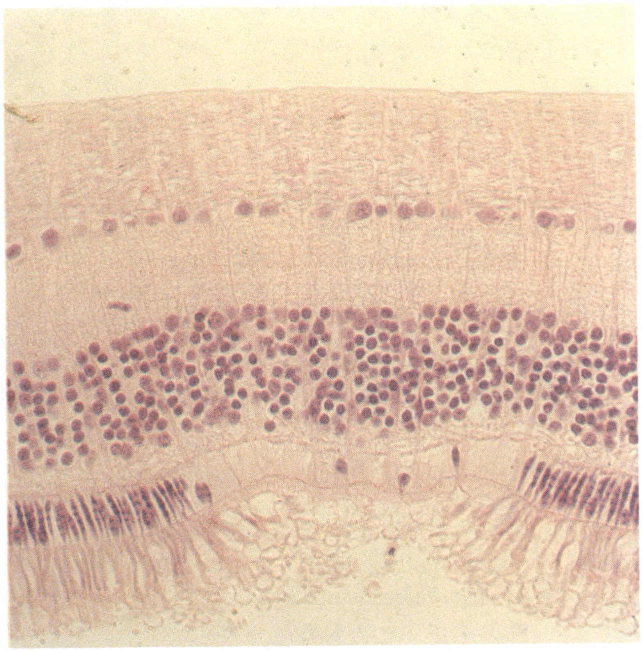

Figure 31—Photomicrograph of the histologic lesion depicted funduscopically in Figure 30. Note the focal loss of the external nuclear layer and associated photoreceptors.

Cataracts are seen in birds of prey and may be divided into juvenile, senile, and traumatic types. In captive birds, the majority have been reported in diurnal raptors and appear to be senile in type.[51,52] An 18-year-old male peregrine falcon with bilateral mature cataracts has been reported.[51] The bird was blind but had intact direct pupillary light reflexes. The lenses were removed bilaterally by phacoemulsification, and the bird responded to visual stimuli on recovery from anesthesia. In free-living birds, the majority of cataracts have been considered traumatic in origin; these have occurred primarily in owls[2,3,53] (Figure 33). Idiopathic juvenile cataracts have been reported in the tawny owl.[2] We have observed bilateral juvenile-onset cataracts in two screech owls. In one bird, the cataracts pro-

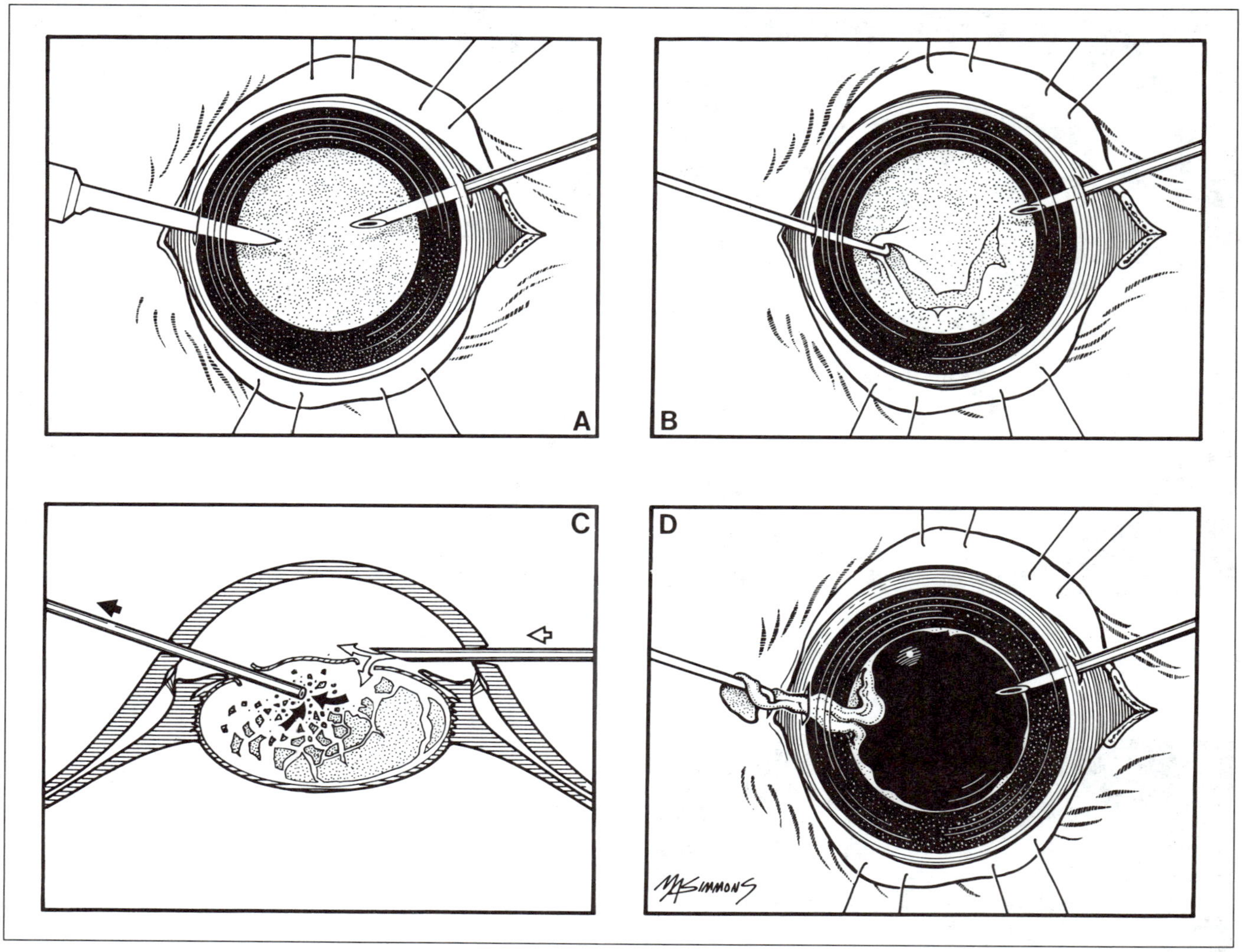

Figure 32—The procedure of phacoemulsification for lens removal in raptors. (*A*) Infusion tip in place through limbal incision. Corneal incision being made with von Graefe knife for access by cystotome and ultrasonic probe tip. (*B*) Annular peripheral anterior capsulotomy made by 27-gauge needle with bent tip or cystotome. (*C*) Continuous lactated Ringer's solution infusion through infusor tip maintains the depth of the anterior chamber while the ultrasonic probe tip fragments, then aspirates, lens material under cover provided by the anterior capsule. (*D*) After phacoemulsification and aspiration, the anterior capsule is hooked with a cystotome or 27-gauge needle tip and is removed through the corneal incision. (From Kern TJ, Murphy CJ, Riis RC: Lens extraction by phacoemulsification in two raptors. *JAVMA* 185:1403, 1984. Reprinted with permission.)

gressed until they impaired vision and were removed bilaterally by phacoemulsification.[51] In the other bird, they began as punctate subcapsular opacities, progessed to involve a small portion of the posterior cortex, then remained static. Their visual significance diminished as the bird continued to grow.

Cranial trauma may result in lens luxation.[3,53] The luxated lens may have a pigmented ring demarcating the equatorial region. This ring represents the avulsed tips of ciliary processes, which normally fuse to the lens capsule. A completely luxated lens should be surgically removed to decrease the likelihood of secondary complications. We have observed uveitis, corneal opacification, and peripheral anterior synechiae associated with anterior lens luxation (Figure 34). An inflammatory condition resulting from leakage of lens proteins (phacoanaphylactic uveitis) has been described in a screech owl.[54]

Vitreous

The vitreous body is the largest single structure in the eye and fills the vitreous chamber. It contains fibrocytes (hyalocytes) and collagen and is at least 98% water. It has firm attachments to the apical bridge of the pecten (Figure 35).

Vitreous hemorrhage is a common finding associated with pecten and/or choroidal hemorrhage. As in domestic mammals, vitreous hemorrhage often persists for long periods. In addition, foreign bodies are occasionally found within the vitreous (Figure 36).

Assessment Before Release

Although there is currently insufficient data to predict accurately the impact of specific ocular lesions on survival potential after release back to the wild, assessment of visual function must certainly be taken into account when de-

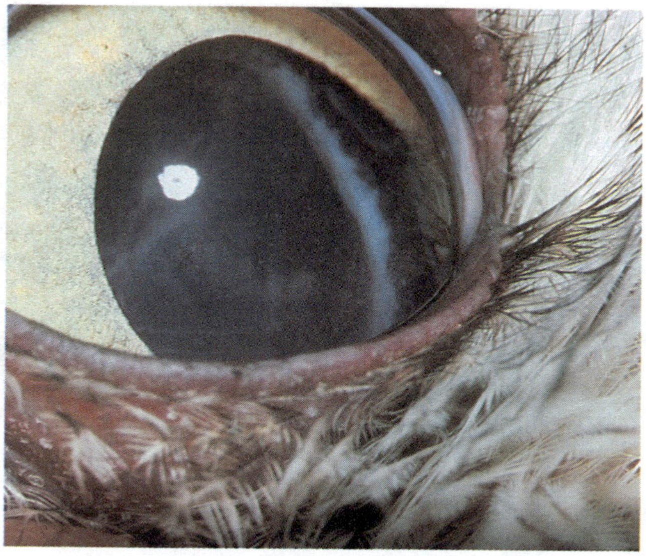

Figure 33—Equatorial traumatic cataract in an adult screech owl 18 months after it was hit by a car (same eye as in Figure 20).

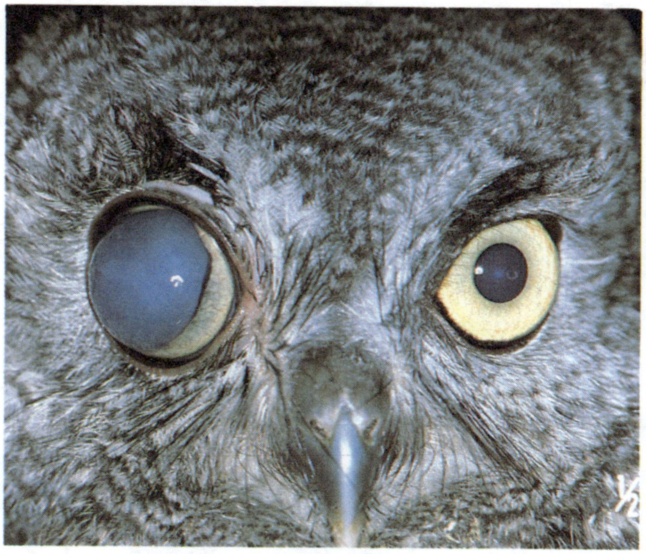

Figure 34—Peripheral anterior synechia and corneal opacification associated with an anterior luxated lens in the right eye of a juvenile screech owl.

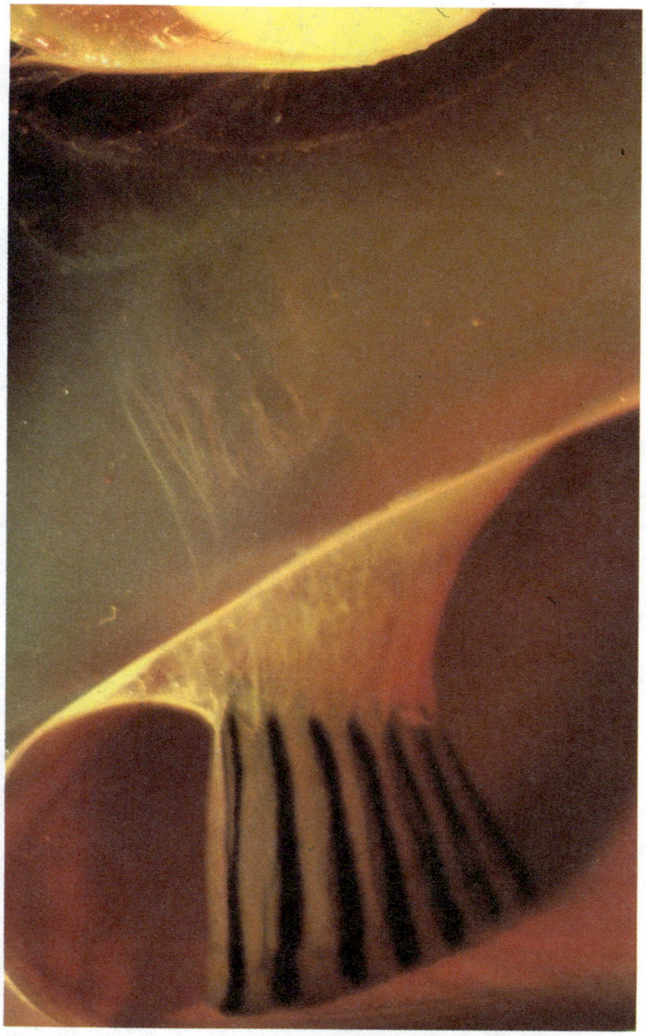

Figure 35—Pecten and vitreous in a great horned owl. The vitreous has contracted in this specimen as a result of fixation. Note the firm attachments of the hyaloid membrane to the apical bridge of the pecten.

termining a bird's suitability for release. The following are prerelease parameters that I take into account.

Lesion chronicity: A lesion that has obviously been present for months should not be weighted as heavily as a recent injury. Numerous birds have been admitted for treatment with evidence of previous ocular disease that resulted in scarring. These birds had clearly been able to compete successfully in the wild despite moderate to marked visual impairment. It should be noted that the majority of birds with extensive ocular damage had sustained unilateral lesions.

Lesion location: Axial lesions of the optical media and foveal lesions of the retina are the most severe. Peripheral lesions may have little effect on visual function.

Lesion extent: Small focal lesions are less significant than extensive lesions or lesions involving multiple ocular structures.

Lesion symmetry: Bilateral lesions should be weighted more heavily than unilateral lesions, especially if they involve the axial optical media and/or foveae.

Lesions of other body systems: The impact of an ocular lesion may enhance the debilitating effects of lesions incurred in other body systems. For example, while a bird may be able to compete successfully with mild, unilateral impairment of wing function, it might starve to death if it had also sustained loss of an eye.

Age of bird: Raptors normally have a very high attrition rate during their first year of life.[55] For this reason, I weight lesions more heavily in young, inexperienced birds than in mature birds that have honed their hunting skills.

Species involved: Generally, ocular lesions are weighted more heavily in diurnal birds of prey than in owls because the latter possess a highly developed acoustic sense, which

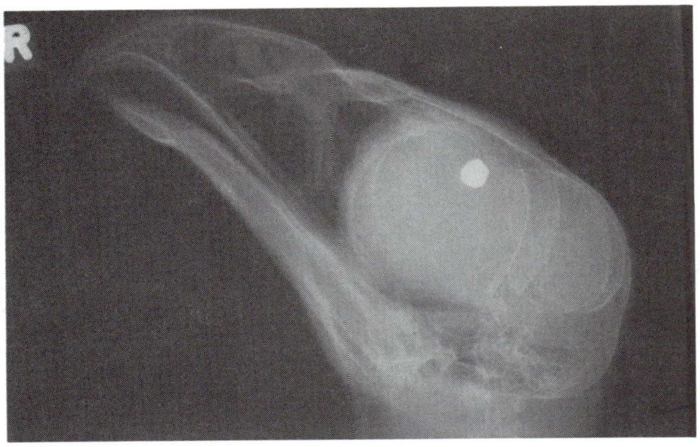

Figure 36A

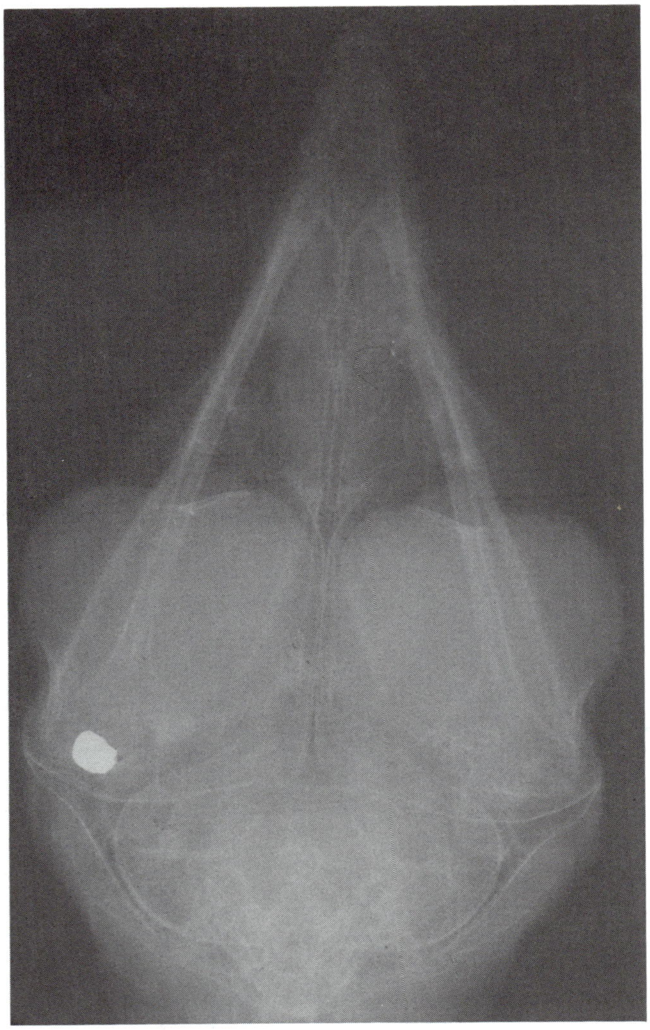

Figure 36B

is used extensively during predation. The barn owl (*Tyto alba*) is capable of capturing mice in absolute darkness using only auditory cues.[56]

Should a one-eyed raptor be released? This is a question commonly posed by rehabilitators. In answering it, several facts should be considered. A number of well-fleshed birds

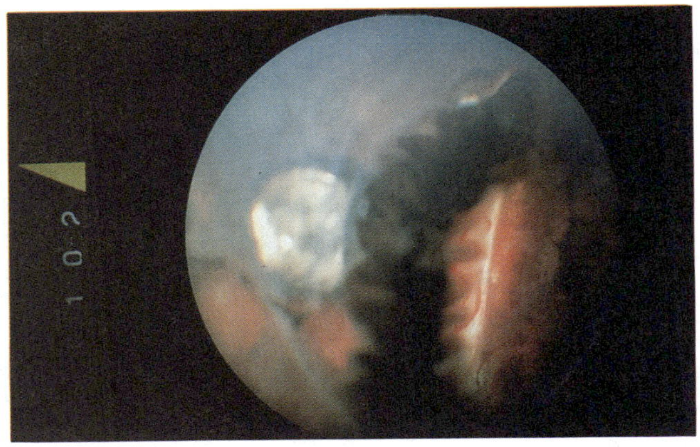

Figure 36C

Figure 36—Lead pellet in the left eye of a mature red-tailed hawk. Initially, this pellet was freely movable within a liquified vitreous. Fourteen weeks later the pellet had become fibrosed adjacent to the pecten. (**A** and **B**) Radiographs demonstrating the intraocular location of the lead pellet. (**C**) Ophthalmoscopic appearance of the pellet after it became fibrosed adjacent to the pecten. The periphery of the optic nerve is visible as a thin white line surrounding the base of the pecten.

that had been unilaterally blind for prolonged periods before admission (evidenced by the chronicity of lesions present) have been seen. Bird banders have also reported observing at banding stations migrating raptors that had extensive unilateral ocular lesions but were in good flesh.

The bottom line in assessment for release is whether the raptor can capture live prey species. For this reason, I strongly advocate the use of release-training enclosures that allow an accurate determination.

Acknowledgments

Special thanks to Drs. Nedim Buyukmihci, Roy Bellhorn, and Dennis Hacker, University of California, Davis, as well as Dr. Thomas Kern, Cornell University, and an anonymous reviewer for constructive criticism of the manuscript. The anatomic plates were prepared by Michael Simmons and William Hamilton, Department of Veterinary Anatomy, New York State College of Veterinary Medicine, Cornell University.

REFERENCES

1. Wood CA: *The Fundus Oculi of Birds Especially as Viewed by the Ophthalmoscope*. Chicago, Lakeside Press, 1917.
2. Greenwood AG, Barnett KC: The investigation of visual defects in raptors, in: *Recent Advances in the Study of Raptor Diseases*. West Yorkshire, England, Chiron Publications Ltd, 1981, pp 131–135.
3. Murphy CJ, Kern TJ, McKeever K, et al: Ocular lesions in free-living raptors. *JAVMA* 181:1302–1304, 1982.
4. Buyukmihci N: Lesions in the ocular posterior segment of raptors. *JAVMA* 187:1121–1124, 1985.
5. Murphy CJ, Kern TJ: Bilateral keratopathy in a barred owl. *JAVMA* 179:1271–1273, 1981.
6. Graham DL, Halliwell WH: Malnutrition in birds of prey, in Fowler M (ed): *Zoo and Wild Animal Medicine*. Philadelphia, WB Saunders Co, 1978, pp 236–242.
7. Slatter DH: *Fundamentals of Veterinary Ophthalmology*, Philadelphia, WB Saunders Co, 1981.

8. Murphy CJ: "Physiological Optics and Comparative Ocular Anatomy of the Strigiformes with Notes on Clinical Features of the Eyes of Birds of Prey." PhD thesis, Cornell University, 1984.
9. Kirsten SJ, Kirsten EB: Spontaneous blink rates of birds. *Condor* 85:92–93, 1983.
10. Graham DL, Halliwell WH: Viral diseases of birds of prey, in Fowler M (ed): *Zoo and Wild Animal Medicine*. Philadelphia, WB Saunders Co, 1981, pp 260–265.
11. Leeson CR: The fine structure of the "feather epithelium" in the dove, *Columba domestica*. *Anat Rec* 140:359–366, 1961.
12. Steinbach MJ, Money KE: Eye movements of the owl. *Vision Res* 13:889–891, 1973.
13. Steinbach MJ, Angus RG, Money KE: Torsional eye movement of the owl. *Vision Res* 14:745–746, 1974.
14. Lord RD: An anomolous condition in the eyes of some hawks. *Auk* 73:457, 1956.
15. Murphy CJ, Brooks DE, Kern TJ, et al: Enucleation in birds of prey. *JAVMA* 183:1234–1237, 1983.
16. Curtis EL, Miller RC: The sclerotic ring of North American birds. *Auk* 55:225–254, 1938.
17. Tiemeier OW: The os opticus of birds. *J Morphol* 86:25–46, 1950.
18. Evans HE: Organa sensoria, in Baumel J, et al (eds): *Nomina Anatomica Avium*. New York, Academic Press, 1979, pp 505-532.
19. Snyder NF, Snyder HA: Function of eye coloration in North American accipiters. *Condor* 76:219–222, 1974.
20. Oliphant LW, Johnson MR, Murphy C, Howland H: The musculature and pupillary response of the great horned owl iris. *Exp Eye Res* 37:583–595, 1983.
21. Campbell HS, Smith JL: The pharmacology of the pigeon pupil. *Arch Ophthalmol* 67:501–504, 1962.
22. Bishop LG, Stark L: Pupillary response of the screech owl, *Otus asio*. *Science*. 148:1750–1752, 1965.
23. Bravo H, Pettigrew JD: The distribution of neurons projecting from the retina and visual cortex to the thalamus and tectum opticum of the barn owl, *Tyto alba*, and the burrowing owl, *Speotyto cunicularia*. *J Comp Neurol* 199:419–441, 1981.
24. Levine J: Consensual pupillary response in birds. *Science* 122:690, 1955.
25. Gamlin PPR, Reiner A, Erichsen JT, et al: The neural substrate for the pupillary light reflex in the pigeon (*Columba livia*). *J Comp Neurol* 226:523–543, 1984.
26. Murphy CJ, Howland HC: Owl eyes: Accommodation, corneal curvature, and refractive state. *J Comp Physiol* 151:277–284, 1983.
27. Fournier GA, Albert DM, Bachrach AB, Lampiz KA: Symbol of Boston's Museum of Science has eye tumor. *N Engl J Med* 38:782–783, 1983.
28. Nicol JAC, Arnott HJ: Tapeta lucida in the eyes of goatsuckers (Caprimulgidae). *Proc R Soc Lond B* 187:349–352, 1974.
29. Wingstrand KG, Munk O: The pecten oculi of the pigeon with particular regard to its function. *Biol Skr Danske Viden Selsk* 14:1–64, 1965.
30. Bellhorn RW, Bellhorn MS: The avian pecten I. Fluorescein permeability. *Ophthalmic Res* 7:1–7, 1975.
31. Brach V: The effect of intraocular ablation of the pecten oculi of the chicken. *Invest Ophthalmol* 14:166–168, 1975.
32. Bellhorn MB, Bellhorn RW, Poll PS: Permeability of fluorescein-labbelled dextrans in fundus fluorescein angiography of rats and birds. *Exp Eye Res* 24:595-605, 1977.
33. Abelsdorf G, Wesseley K: Vergleichend Physiologische Untersuchungen uber den Flussigkeitswechsel des Auges in der Wirbeltierreihe. I. Vogel. *Arch Augenheik* 64:65–124, 1909.
34. Murphy CJ, Kern TJ, Riis RC: Intraocular trauma in a red-tailed hawk. *JAVMA* 181:1390–1391, 1982.
35. Sykes GP: Tuberculosis in a red tailed hawk (*Buteo jamaicensis*). *J Wildl Dis* 18:495–499, 1982.
36. Fox R, Lehmkuhle SW, Westendorf DH: Falcon visual acuity. *Science* 192:263–265, 1976.
37. Shlaer R: An eagle's eye: Quality of the retinal image. *Science* 176:920–922, 1972.
38. Snyder AW, Miller WH: Telephoto lens system of falconiform eyes. *Nature* 275:127–129, 1978.
39. Fite KV: Anatomical and behavioral correlates of visual acuity in the great horned owl. *Vis Res* 13:219–230, 1973.
40. Martin GR, Gordon IE, Cadle DR: Electroretinographically determined spectral sensitivity in the tawny owl (*Strix aluco*). *J Comp Physiol Psychol* 89:72–78, 1975.
41. Vanderplank FL: The effect of infra-red waves on tawny owls (*Strix aluco*). *Proc Zool Soc Lond* II:505–507, 1934.
42. Matthews LH, Matthews BHC: Owls and infra-red radiation. *Nature* 143:983, 1939.
43. Hocking B, Mitchell BL: Owl vision. *Ibis* 103:284–288, 1961.
44. Pettigrew JD, Konishi M: Neurons selective for orientation and binocular disparity in the visual wulst of the barn owl (*Tyto alba*). *Science* 193:675–678, 1976.
45. Karten HJ, Hodos W, Nauta WJ, Revzin AM: Neural connections of the "visual wulst" of the avian telencephalon. Experimental studies in the pigeon (*Columba livia*) and owl (*Speotyto cunicularia*). *J Comp Neurol* 150:253–278, 1973.
46. Fox R, Lehmkuhle SW, Bush RC: Stereopsis in the falcon. *Science* 197:79–81, 1977.
47. Dukes TW, Fox GA: Blindness associated with retinal dysplasia in a prairie falcon, *Falco mexicanus*. *J Wildl Dis* 19:66–69, 1983.
48. Duke-Elder S: *The Eye in Evolution*. London, Henry Kimpton, 1958.
49. Walls GL: *The Vertebrate Eye and Its Adaptive Radiation*. Bloomfield Hills, MI, Cranbrook Institute of Science, 1942.
50. Slonaker JR: A physiologic study of the anatomy of the eye and its accessory parts in the English sparrow (*Passer domesticus*). *J Morphol* 31:351–459, 1918.
51. Kern TJ, Murphy CJ, Riis RC: Lens extraction by phacoemulsification in two raptors. *JAVMA* 185:1403–1406, 1984.
52. Keymer IF: Cataracts in birds. *Avian Pathol* 6:335–341, 1977.
53. Brooks DE, Murphy CJ, Quesenberry KE, Walsh MT: Surgical correction of a luxated cataractous lens in a barred owl. *JAVMA* 183:1298–1299, 1983.
54. Anderson GA, Buyukmihci N: Phacoanaphylactic endophthalmitis in an owl. *Vet Pathol* 20:776–778, 1983.
55. Brown L, Amadon D: *Eagles, Hawks and Falcons of the World*. New York, McGraw-Hill Book Co, 1968, pp 136–137.
56. Payne RS: Acoustic location of prey by barn owls. *J Exp Biol* 54:535–573, 1971.
57. Kern TJ, Murphy CJ, Heck WR: Partial upper eyelid agenesis in a peregrine falcon. *JAVMA* 187:1207, 1985.
58. Murphy CJ, Buyukmihci NC, Bellhorn RW, et al: Retinal dysplasia in a hybrid falcon. *JAVMA* 187:1208–1209, 1985.
59. Moore CP, Pickett JP, Beehler B: Extracapsular extraction of a senile cataract in an Andean condor. *JAVMA* 187:1211–1213, 1985.

INDEX

A

B

C

D

E

F

G

H